CRITICAL CARE

SECRETS

T0195355

CRITICAL CARE

SECRETS

SIXTH EDITION

POLLY E. PARSONS, MD
E. L. Amidon Professor and Chair of
    Medicine
Robert Larner College of Medicine at
    the University of Vermont
Burlington, VT

JEANINE P. WIENER-KRONISH, MD
Henry Isaiah Dorr, Professor of
    Research and Teaching in
    Anesthetics and Anesthesia
Department of Anesthesia, Critical
    Care and Pain Medicine
Harvard Medical School;
Anesthetist-in-Chief
Massachusetts General Hospital
Boston, MA

RENEE D. STAPLETON, MD, PHD
Associate Professor of Medicine
University of Vermont, Larner College
    of Medicine
Burlington, VT

LORENZO BERRA, MD
Anesthesiologist and Critical Care
    Physician
Department of Anesthesia, Critical
    Care and Pain Medicine,
Medical Director of Respiratory Care
Massachusetts General Hospital;
Assistant Professor
Harvard Medical School
Boston, MA

ELSEVIER

ELSEVIER

1600 John F. Kennedy Blvd.
Ste 1800
Philadelphia, PA 19103-2899

CRITICAL CARE SECRETS, SIXTH EDITION   ISBN: 978-0-32351064-6
Copyright © 2019 by Elsevier, Inc.

All rights reserved. No part of this publication may be reproduced or transmitted in any form or by any means, electronic or mechanical, including photocopying, recording, or any information storage and retrieval system, without permission in writing from the publisher. Details on how to seek permission, further information about the Publisher's permissions policies and our arrangements with organizations such as the Copyright Clearance Center and the Copyright Licensing Agency, can be found at our website: www.elsevier.com/permissions.

This book and the individual contributions contained in it are protected under copyright by the Publisher (other than as may be noted herein).

Notices

Practitioners and researchers must always rely on their own experience and knowledge in evaluating and using any information, methods, compounds or experiments described herein. Because of rapid advances in the medical sciences, in particular, independent verification of diagnoses and drug dosages should be made. To the fullest extent of the law, no responsibility is assumed by Elsevier, authors, editors or contributors for any injury and/or damage to persons or property as a matter of products liability, negligence or otherwise, or from any use or operation of any methods, products, instructions, or ideas contained in the material herein.

Previous editions copyrighted 2013, 2007, 2003, 1998 and 1992.

Library of Congress Cataloging-in-Publication Data
Names: Parsons, Polly E., 1954-editor. | Wiener-Kronish, Jeanine P., 1951-editor. | Stapleton, Renee Doney, editor. | Berra, Lorenzo, editor.
Title: Critical care secrets / [edited by] Polly E. Parsons, Jeanine P. Wiener-Kronish, Renee D. Stapleton, Lorenzo Berra.
Other titles: Secrets series.
Description: Sixth edition. | Philadelphia, PA : Elsevier, [2019] | Series: Secrets series | Includes bibliographical references and index.
Identifiers: LCCN 2017061385 | ISBN 9780323510646 (pbk.) | ISBN 9780323527897 (ebook)
Subjects: | MESH: Critical Care | Examination Questions
Classification: LCC RC86.9 | NLM WX 18.2 | DDC 616.02/8—dc23 LC record available at https://lccn.loc.gov/2017061385

Content Strategist: James Merritt
Content Development Specialist: Meghan B. Andress
Publishing Services Manager: Deepthi Unni
Project Manager: Beula Christopher
Design Direction: Bridget Hoette

Working together
to grow libraries in
developing countries

www.elsevier.com • www.bookaid.org

Printed in India
Last digit is the print number: 9 8 7 6

To our spouses Jim, Daniel, and Jonathan, and to all our colleagues in the ICU, as well as our patients, students, residents, and fellows. This book is dedicated to the patients that we have had the privilege to care for, to the ICU nurses who have been so important in the care of the patients, and to the medical students, residents, and fellows who have helped in caring for all the patients. Thank you all for allowing us to work and be with you.

Polly E. Parsons, MD

Jeanine P. Wiener-Kronish, MD

Renee D. Stapleton, MD, PhD

Lorenzo Berra, MD

CONTRIBUTORS

Varun Agrawal, MD, FACP, FASN
Assistant Professor of Medicine
Division of Nephrology and Hypertension
University of Vermont
Burlington, VT

Paul H. Alfille, MD
Executive Vice Chairman
Department of Anesthesia, Critical Care and Pain
  Management
Massachusetts General Hospital
Boston, MA

Gilman B. Allen, MD
Pulmonary Critical Care Department
University of Vermont
Burlington, VT

Michael N. Andrawes, MD
Instructor
Harvard Medical School;
Adult Cardiothoracic Anesthesiology Fellowship
  Program Director
Department of Anesthesia, Critical Care and Pain
  Medicine
Massachusetts General Hospital
Boston, MA

Amir Azarbal, MD
Fellow
Cardiology Unit, Department of Medicine
University of Vermont-Larner College of Medicine
Burlington, VT

Aranya Bagchi, MBBS
Assistant in Anesthesia
Massachusetts General Hospital;
Instructor in Anesthesia
Harvard Medical School
Boston, MA

Keith Baker, MD, PhD
Associate Professor of Anesthesia
Harvard Medical School;
Vice Chair for Education
Department of Anesthesia, Critical Care and
  Pain Medicine
Massachusetts General Hospital
Boston, MA

Rita N. Bakhru, MD, MS
Assistant Professor
Wake Forest University School of Medicine
Department of Internal Medicine
Pulmonary, Critical Care Medicine, Allergy and
  Immunology
Medical Center Blvd
Winston-Salem, NC

Arna Banerjee, MD, FCCM
Associate Professor of Anesthesiology/Critical Care
Associate Professor of Surgery, Medical Education
  and Administration
Assistant Dean for Simulation in Medical Education
Director, Center for Experiential Learning and
  Assessment
Nashville, TN

Caitlin Baran, MD
University of Vermont
Burlington, VT

Pavan K. Bendapudi, MD
Instructor in Medicine
Harvard Medical School;
Division of Hematology
Massachusetts General Hospital
Boston, MA

William J. Benedetto, MD
Department of Anesthesia, Critical Care and Pain
  Medicine
Massachusetts General Hospital
Boston, MA

Sheri Berg, MD
Department of Anesthesia, Critical Care and Pain
  Medicine
Massachusetts General Hospital
Boston, MA

Lorenzo Berra, MD
Anesthesiologist and Critical Care Physician
Department of Anesthesia, Critical Care and Pain
  Medicine
Medical Director of Respiratory Care
Massachusetts General Hospital;
Assistant Professor
Harvard Medical School
Boston, MA

Edward A. Bittner, MD, PhD, MSEd
Department of Anesthesia, Critical Care and Pain
  Medicine
Massachusetts General Hospital
Boston, MA

M. Dustin Boone, MD
Department of Anesthesia, Critical Care and Pain
  Medicine
Beth Israel Deaconess Medical Center
Harvard Medical School
Boston, MA

William E. Charash, MD, PhD
Associate Professor
Division of Acute Care Surgery,
Director
Trauma Critical Care
University of Vermont Larner College of Medicine
Burlington, VT

Sreedivya Chava, MD, FACC
Interventional Cardiology
Tricity Cardiology consultants
Mesa, AZ

Katharine L. Cheung, MD, MSc, FRCPC
Assistant Professor of Medicine
Division of Nephrology
Larner College of Medicine at The University of
  Vermont
Burlington, VT

Hovig V. Chitilian, MD
Department of Anesthesia, Critical Care and Pain
  Medicine
Massachusetts General Hospital
Boston, MA

Jaina Clough, MD
Assistant Professor of Medicine
University of Vermont College of Medicine
University of Vermont Medical Center
Burlington, VT

Ryan Clouser, DO
Assistant Professor of Medicine, Critical Care/
  Neurocritical Care
University of Vermont Medical Center
Burlington, VT

Lane Crawford, MD
Instructor
Harvard Medical School;
Department of Anesthesia, Critical Care and Pain
  Medicine
Massachusetts General Hospital
Boston, MA

Jerome Crowley, MD, MPH
Staff Intensivist and Anesthesiologist
Clinical Instructor
Harvard Medical School;
Department of Anesthesia, Critical Care and Pain
  Medicine
Massachusetts General Hospital
Boston, MA

Adam A. Dalia, MD, MBA
Clinical Instructor in Anesthesia
Division of Cardiac Anesthesiology
Department of Anesthesia, Critical Care and Pain
  Medicine
The Massachusetts General Hospital-Harvard Medical
  School
Boston, MA

Harold L. Dauerman, MD
Professor of Medicine
University of Vermont Larner College of Medicine;
Network Director
UVM Health Network Interventional Cardiology
McClure 1 Cardiology
Burlington, VT

Hill A. Enuh, MD
Department of Pulmonary Critical Care
University of Vermont
Burlington, VT

Peter J. Fagenholz, MD, FACS
Assistant Professor of Surgery
Harvard Medical School;
Attending Surgeon
Department of Surgery
Division of Trauma, Emergency Surgery and Surgical
  Critical Care
Massachusetts General Hospital
Boston, MA

Joshua D. Farkas, MD, MS
Department of Pulmonary and Critical Care
  Medicine
University of Vermont
Burlington, VT

Corey R. Fehnel, MD, MPH
Department of Neurology
Beth Israel Deaconess Medical Center
Harvard Medical School
Boston, MA

Amanda Fernandes, MD
Clinical Instructor
Larner College of Medicine at The University of
  Vermont
Burlington, VT

Daniel F. Fisher, MS, RRT
Department of Respiratory Care
Boston Medical Center
Boston, MA

Michael G. Fitzsimons, MD
Assistant Professor
Harvard Medical School;
Director
Division of Cardiac Anesthesia
Department of Anesthesia, Critical Care and Pain
  Medicine
Massachusetts General Hospital
Boston, MA

Joseph D. Frasca, MD
Clinical Instructor
University of Vermont College of Medicine
Burlington, VT

Zechariah S. Gardner, MD
Assistant Professor of Medicine
Division of Hospital Medicine
University of Vermont College of Medicine
University of Vermont Medical Center
Burlington, VT

Garth W. Garrison, MD
Assistant Professor of Medicine
Division of Pulmonary and Critical Care Medicine
University of Vermont Medical Center
Burlington, VT

Matthew P. Gilbert, DO, MPH
Associate Professor of Medicine
Larner College of Medicine at The University of
  Vermont
Burlington, VT

Christopher Grace, MD, FIDSA
Professor of Medicine, Emeritus
University of Vermont College of Medicine;
Infectious Diseases Unit
University of Vermont Medical Center
Burlington, VT

Cornelia Griggs, MD
Chief Resident
Department of Surgery
Massachusetts General Hospital
Boston, MA

Dusan Hanidziar, MD, PhD
Attending Anesthesiologist and Intensivist
Department of Anesthesia, Critical Care and Pain
  Medicine
Massachusetts General Hospital;
Instructor in Anesthesia
Harvard Medical School
Boston, MA

Michael E. Hanley, MD
Professor of Medicine
University of Colorado Denver School of Medicine;
Staff Physician
Pulmonary and Critical Care Medicine
Denver Health Medical Center
Denver, CO

T.J. Henry, MD
Resident
Department of Surgery
University of Iowa
Iowa City, IA

Dean Hess, PhD
Respiratory Care
Massachusetts General Hospital,
Teaching Associate in Anesthesia
Harvard Medical School
Boston, MA

David C. Hooper, MD
Department of Medicine
Division of Infectious Diseases
Massachusetts General Hospital
Boston, MA

Catherine L. Hough, MD, MSc
Professor of Medicine
Division of Pulmonary, Critical Care and Sleep
  Medicine
University of Washington
Seattle, WA

James L. Jacobson, MD
Professor
Department of Psychiatry
Larner College of Medicine at The University of
  Vermont and University of Vermont Medical Center
Burlington, VT

Paul S. Jansson, MD, MS
Department of Emergency Medicine
Massachusetts General Hospital
Brigham and Women's Hospital
Harvard Medical School
Boston, MA

Daniel W. Johnson, MD
Assistant Professor
Department of Anesthesiology
University of Nebraska Medical Center
Omaha, NE

Robert M. Kacmarek, PhD, RRT
Department of Respiratory Care
Department of Anesthesia, Critical Care, and Pain
  Medicine
Massachusetts General Hospital
Boston, MA

Rebecca Kalman, MD
Department of Anesthesia, Critical Care and Pain
  Medicine
Massachusetts General Hospital
Boston, MA

Brinda B. Kamdar, MD
Program Director
Regional Anesthesia and Pain Medicine Fellowship,
Instructor
Harvard Medical School;
Department of Anesthesia, Critical Care and Pain
Medicine
Massachusetts General Hospital
Boston, MA

David A. Kaminsky, MD
Pulmonary Critical Care Department
University of Vermont
Burlington, VT

Mark T. Kearns, MD
Assistant Professor of Medicine
University of Colorado Denver School of Medicine;
Staff Physician
Pulmonary and Critical Care Medicine
Denver Health Medical Center
Denver, CO

C. Matthew Kinsey, MD, MPH
Director, Interventional Pulmonary
University of Vermont Medical Center;
Assistant Professor
Larner College of Medicine at the University of
Vermont
Division of Pulmonary and Critical Care
Burlington, VT

Themistoklis Kourkoumpetis, MD
Gastroenterology and Hepatology Fellow
Department of Medicine, Section of Gastroenterology
Baylor College of Medicine
Houston, TX

Erin K. Kross, MD
Associate Professor of Medicine
Division of Pulmonary, Critical Care and Sleep
Medicine
University of Washington
Seattle, WA

Leandra Krowsoski, MD
Division of Trauma, Emergency Surgery and
Surgical Critical Care
Department of Surgery
Massachusetts General Hospital
Boston, MA

Abhishek Kumar, MD
Assistant Professor of Medicine/Transplant Medicine
Division of Nephrology and Hypertension
University of Vermont
Burlington, VT

Alexander S. Kuo, MS, MD
Assistant in Anesthesia
Department of Anesthesia, Critical Care, and Pain
Medicine
Massachusetts General Hospital;
Instructor
Harvard Medical School
Boston, MA

David Kuter, MD, DPhil
Professor of Medicine
Harvard Medical School;
Chief, Division of Hematology
Massachusetts General Hospital
Boston, MA

Jean Kwo, MD
Assistant Professor
Department of Anesthesia, Critical Care and Pain
Medicine
Harvard Medical School
Massachusetts General Hospital
Boston, MA

Daniela J. Lamas, MD
Brigham and Women's Hospital
Division of Pulmonary and Critical Care Medicine,
Instructor in Medicine
Harvard Medical School;
Associate Faculty
Ariadne Labs
Boston MA

Stephen E. Lapinsky, MBBCh, MSc, FRCPC
Director
Intensive Care Unit
Mount Sinai Hosptal;
Professor of Medicine
University of Toronto
Toronto, Canada

John L. Leahy, MD
Professor of Medicine
Larner College of Medicine
The University of Vermont
Burlington, VT

Timothy Leclair, MD
Department of Medicine, Division of Pulmonary
and Critical Care Medicine
University of Vermont Medical Center
Burlington, VT

Jarone Lee, MD, MPH
Medical Director Blake 12 ICU
Massachusetts General Hospital/Harvard Medical
School
Boston, MA

Robert Y. Lee, MD
Senior Fellow
Division of Pulmonary, Critical Care and Sleep Medicine
University of Washington
Seattle, WA

Martin M. LeWinter, MD
Professor of Medicine and Molecular Physiology
    and Biophysics
Cardiology Unit, Department of Medicine
University of Vermont-Larner College of Medicine
Burlington, VT

Eva Litvak, MD
Fellow in Adult Cardiothoracic Anesthesia
Division of Cardiac Anesthesia
Department of Anesthesia, Critical Care and Pain
    Medicine
Massachusetts General Hospital
Boston, MA

Kathleen D. Liu, MD, PhD, MAS
Professor
Divisions of Nephrology and Critical Care Medicine
Departments of Medicine and Anesthesia
University of California, San Francisco
San Francisco, CA

Yuk Ming Liu, MD, MPH
Clinical Assistant Professor
Department of Surgery, Division of Acute Care Surgery
University of Iowa
Iowa City, IA

Lowell J. Lo, MD
Associate Professor
Division of Nephrology
Department of Medicine
University of California, San Francisco
San Francisco, CA

Johnathan P. Mack, MD, MSc, FRCPC
Assistant Director of Blood Transfusion Service
Department of Pathology
Massachusetts General Hospital
Boston, MA

Annis Marney, MD, MSCI
Diabetes and Endocrinology
The Frist Clinic
Nashville, TN

Annachiara Marra, MD, PhD
University of Naples Federico II
Naples, Italy;
Visiting Research Fellow
Division of Allergy, Pulmonary and Critical Care
    Medicine
Vanderbilt University Medical Center
Nashville, TN

Anthony Massaro, MD
Department of Medicine
Pulmonary and Critical Care
Brigham and Women's Hospital
Boston, MA

Alexis McCabe, MD
Resident
Department of Emergency Medicine
Massachusetts General Hospital/Harvard Medical
    School
Boston, MA

Prema R. Menon, MD, PhD
Assistant Professor of Medicine
University of Vermont
Burlington, VT

Katherine Menson, DO
Fellow
Division of Pulmonary and Critical Care Medicine
University of Vermont Medical Center
Burlington, VT

Matthew J. Meyer, MD
Department of Anesthesia, Critical Care and Pain
    Medicine
Massachusetts General Hospital
Boston, MA

Lydia Miller, MD
Department of Anesthesia, Critical Care and Pain
    Medicine
Massachusetts General Hospital
Boston, MA

Jimmy L. Moss, MD
Fellow, Anesthesia Critical Care Program
Massachusetts General Hospital;
Clinical Fellow in Anesthesia
Harvard Medical School
Boston, MA

Marc Moss, MD
Professor
University of Colorado School of Medicine
Division of Pulmonary Sciences and Critical Care
    Medicine
Aurora, CO

Maged Muhammed, MD
Research Fellow
Harvard Medical School;
Division of Infectious Diseases and Division of
    Gastroenterology
Boston Children's Hospital;
Department of Adult Inpatient Medicine, Department
    of Medicine
Newton Wellesley Hospital
Newton, MA

Eleftherios Mylonakis, MD, PhD, FIDSA
Charles C.J. Carpenter Professor of Infectious Disease
Chief, Infectious Diseases Division
Alpert Medical School of Brown University;
Division of Infectious Diseases
Rhode Island Hospital
Providence, RI

Jennifer Nelli, MD
Department of Anesthesia
Hamilton General Hospital
McMaster University
Hamilton, ON

Cindy Noyes, MD
Assistant Professor of Medicine, Infectious Disease
University of Vermont Medical Center/University of
    Vermont College of Medicine
Burlington, VT

Ala Nozari, MD, PhD
Associate Professor
Harvard Medical School;
Department of Anesthesia, Critical Care and Pain
    Medicine
Massachusetts General Hospital
Boston, MA

Haitham Nsour, MD
Assistant Professor of Medicine
Larner College of Medicine
University of Vermont
Burlington, VT

Jacqueline C. O'Toole, DO
Pulmonary and Critical Care Fellow
Johns Hopkins University
Division Pulmonary and Critical Care Medicine
Baltimore, MD

Pratik Pandharipande, MD, MSCI, FCCM
Professor of Anesthesiology and Surgery
Chief, Division of Anesthesiology Critical Care
    Medicine
Vanderbilt University Medical Center
Nashville, TN

Alan C. Pao, MD
Assistant Professor
Departments of Medicine and Urology
Stanford University School of Medicine
Veterans Affairs Palo Alto Health Care System
Palo Alto, CA

Kapil Patel, MD
Assistant Professor of Medicine
Director, Center for Advanced Lung Disease
Division of Pulmonary and Critical Care Medicine
Morsani College of Medicine, University of South
    Florida
Tampa, FL

Alita Perez-Tamayo, MD
University of Vermont Medical Center
Burlington, VT

Kristen K. Pierce, MD
Associate Professor of Medicine
Division of Infectious Diseases
University of Vermont College of Medicine
Burlington, VT

Louis B. Polish, MD
Associate Professor of Medicine
Division of Infectious Diseases
Director, Internal Medicine Clerkship
University of Vermont College of Medicine
Burlington, VT

Nitin Puri MD, FCCP
Program Director Critical Care Medicine Fellowship
Cooper University Hospital;
Associate Professor Medicine
Cooper Medical School of Rowan University
Camden, NJ

Molly L. Rovin, MD
Psychiatry Resident
Department of Psychiatry
Larner College of Medicine at The University of
    Vermont and University of Vermont Medical
    Center
Burlington, VT

Sten Rubertsson, MD, PhD, EDIC, FCCM, FERC
Professor
Anaesthesiology and Intensive Care Medicine
Department of Surgical Sciences/Anaesthesiology
    and Intensive Care Medicine
Uppsala University
Uppsala, Sweden

Noelle N. Saillant, MD
Division of Trauma, Emergency Surgery and
    Surgical Critical Care
Massachusetts General Hospital
Harvard Medical School
Boston, MA

Jason L. Sanders, MD, PhD
Department of Medicine
Massachusetts General Hospital
Boston, MA

Joel J. Schnure, MD FACE, FACP
Director
Division of Endocrinology and Diabetes
University of Vermont Medical Center;
Professor of Medicine
Larner College of Medicine
The University of Vermont
Burlington, VT

Kenneth Shelton, MD
Department of Anesthesia, Critical Care and Pain
 Medicine
Massachusetts General Hospital
Boston, MA

Tao Shen, MBBS
Department of Anesthesia, Critical Care and Pain
 Medicine
Massachusetts General Hospital
Boston, MA

Erica S. Shenoy, MD, PhD
Department of Medicine
Division of Infectious Diseases
Massachusetts General Hospital
Boston, MA

Stephanie Shieh, MD
Assistant Professor
Division of Nephrology, Department of Medicine
Veterans Affairs St. Louis Health Care System;
Division of Nephrology, Department of Medicine
St. Louis University
St. Louis, MO

Bryan Simmons, MD
Critical Care Fellow
Massachusetts General Hospital
Boston, MA

Alexis C. Smith, DO
Fellow
Wake Forest University School of Medicine
Department of Internal Medicine
Pulmonary, Critical Care, Allergy and Immunology
 Medical Center Blvd
Winston-Salem, NC

Lindsay M. Smith, MD
Assistant Professor of Medicine
Division of Infectious Diseases
Director, Antimicrobial Stewardship
University of Vermont College of Medicine
Burlington, VT

Peter D. Sottile, MD
Assistant Professor
University of Colorado School of Medicine
Division of Pulmonary Sciences and Critical Care
 Medicine
Aurora, CO

Peter S. Spector, MD
Professor of Medicine
Director of Cardiac Electrophysiology
The University of Vermont Medical Center
Burlington, VT

Antoinette Spevetz, MD, FCCM, FACP
Professor of Medicine
Cooper Medical School of Rowan University;
Designated Institution Official
Graduate Medical Education,
 Director
Intermediate Care Unit
Section of Critical Care Medicine
Cooper University Hospital
Camden, NJ

Krystine Spiess, DO
Assistant Professor of Medicine
University of Vermont College of Medicine;
Infectious Diseases Unit
University of Vermont Medical Center
Burlington, VT

Renee D. Stapleton, MD, PhD
Associate Professor of Medicine
University of Vermont, Larner College of Medicine
Burlington, VT

Scott C. Streckenbach, MD
Department of Anesthesia, Critical Care and Pain
 Medicine
Massachusetts General Hospital
Boston, MA

Benjamin T. Suratt, MD
Professor of Medicine and Cell and Molecular Biology
Vice Chair of Medicine for Academic Affairs
Associate Chief, Pulmonary and Critical Care Medicine
University of Vermont College of Medicine
Burlington, VT

Charlotte C. Teneback, MD
Associate Professor of Medicine
University of Vermont, College of Medicine
Burlington, VT

Susan A. Vassallo, MD
Department of Anesthesia, Critical Care and Pain
 Medicine
Massachusetts General Hospital
Boston, MA

Mario J. Velez, MD
Assistant Professor
University of Vermont College of Medicine
Burlington, VT

Rodger White, MD
Department of Anesthesia, Critical Care and Pain
 Medicine
Massachusetts General Hospital
Boston, MA

Elizabeth Cox Williams, MD
Instructor in Anesthesia
Massachusetts General Hospital
Boston, MA

Elliott L. Woodward MB, Bch, BAO, MSc
Cardiothoracic Anesthesia Fellow
Massachusetts General Hospital
Boston, MA

D. Dante Yeh, MD
Ryder Trauma Center
University of Miami Miller School of Medicine
DeWitt Daughtry Family Department of Surgery/
    Division of Trauma
Miami, FL

Jing Zhao, MD, PhD
Anesthesiologist
Department of Anesthesia
Xijing Hospital
Xi'an, China

Hui Zhang, MD, PhD
Anesthesiologist
Department of Anesthesia
Xijing Hospital
Xi'an, China

Pierre Znojkiewicz, MD
Assistant Professor, Cardiac Electrophysiology
The University of Vermont Medical Center
Burlington, VT

PREFACE

Since publishing the first edition of *Critical Care Secrets* in 1992, critical care medicine has continued to become increasingly complex. Medical knowledge, clinical skills, and understanding of technology required to care for critically ill patients continue to transcend subspecialties, so in this edition we have again included chapters from a wide range of specialists, including intensivists, pulmonologists, surgeons, anesthesiologists, psychiatrists, pharmacists, and infectious disease and palliative care experts. The chapters in this edition contain key questions in critical care followed by succinct answers so practitioners can identify effective solutions to their patients' medical and ethical problems.

A broad understanding of anatomy, physiology, immunology, and inflammation is fundamentally important to effectively care for critically ill patients. For example, it is hard to imagine understanding the principles of mechanical ventilation without being aware of the principles of gas and fluid flow, pulmonary mechanics, and electronic circuitry. Accordingly, the authors have again incorporated these key elements into this edition. In addition, critical care medicine requires knowledge of protocols and guidelines that are continuously evolving and that increasingly dictate best practices.

In this sixth edition of *Critical Care Secrets*, we continue to be fortunate that many clinical and thought leaders in critical care have contributed chapters in their areas of expertise. In addition to substantially revising and updating chapters from the previous edition, we have included new chapters on timely topics such as neurologic monitoring, obesity in the intensive care unit (ICU), new ultrasound practices, ICU survivorship, and the latest cardiac technology such as ventricular assist and percutaneous support devices.

We immensely appreciate all the authors who contributed their time and expertise to this edition. We believe they have captured the essence of critical care medicine and have presented it in a format that will be useful to everyone, from students to experienced clinicians.

Polly E. Parsons, MD

Jeanine P. Wiener-Kronish, MD

Renee D. Stapleton, MD, PhD

Lorenzo Berra, MD

CONTENTS

III PROCEDURES

IV PULMONARY

V CARDIOLOGY

VI INFECTIOUS DISEASE

VII RENAL DISEASE

XII SURGERY AND TRAUMA

XIII EMERGENCY MEDICINE

XIV TOXICOLOGY

XV UNIQUE PATIENT POPULATIONS

TOP SECRETS

1. Hyperglycemia is common in critically ill patients and has been independently associated with increased ICU mortality.

2. Oral medications and noninsulin injectable therapies should not be used to treat hyperglycemia in critically ill patients.

3. An intravenous insulin infusion is the safest and most effective way to treat hyperglycemia in critically ill patients.

4. ICU-acquired weakness is a syndrome characterized by the development of generalized diffuse muscle weakness after onset of critical illness and is defined by standard functional muscle tests.

5. Early mobilization of critically ill patients is safe, feasible, and can improve short-term outcomes including functional status.

6. Delirium monitoring and management is critically important since it is a strong risk factor for increased time on mechanical ventilation, length of ICU and hospital stay, cost of hospitalization, long-term cognitive impairment, and mortality.

7. Psychoactive medications, and in particular benzodiazepines, may contribute to delirium.

8. In delirious patients pharmacologic treatment should be used only after giving adequate attention to correction of modifiable contributing factors. The ABCDEF bundle (**A**ttention to analgesia, **B**oth awakening and breathing trials, **C**hoosing right sedative, **D**elirium monitoring and management, **E**arly exercise and **F**amily involvement) is recommended and associated with improved outcomes including reduction in delirium.

9. Inadequate analgesia is common in the ICU and has detrimental effects on patients.

10. Critically ill patients are often especially vulnerable to adverse side effects and toxicity from both opioid and nonopioid analgesic drugs.

11. Early, high-quality, and interdisciplinary communication improves shared decision making around end-of-life care in the ICU.

12. When difficult cases are causing moral distress and/or conflict among family members or team members, consider an ethics consultation to alleviate these issues.

13. Lung protection ventilation is less guided by volume than lung pressures. Minimizing both volumes and pressures is essential for a lung protective ventilation strategy.

14. Managing patient-ventilator interactions is crucial to outcome. The more control granted to a patient during assisted ventilation, the greater the patient-ventilator synchrony.

15. Definition of high-flow nasal cannula (HFNC). HFNC oxygen therapy uses an air/oxygen blender, active humidifier, heated tubing, and a nasal cannula capable of high flows (Fig. 9.1). The HFNC delivers adequately heated and humidified gas at flows up to 60 L/min. The traditional oxygen cannula is limited to a flow of 6 L/min because higher flows are not tolerated. Due to the conditioning of the gas and the design of the prongs, the HFNC is comfortable at high flows.

16. Patient population that benefits most for use of NIV. The strongest evidence for use of NIV is for patients with exacerbation of chronic obstructive pulmonary disease (COPD). For such patients, the use of NIV has a mortality benefit, with a relative risk of 0.56

(95% CI 0.38–0.82), which translates to a number needed to treat (NNT) of 16. The use of NIV for acute cardiogenic pulmonary edema is associated with a relative risk of 0.64 (95% CI 0.45–0.90), with a NNT of 16. Available evidence also supports a mortality benefit for NIV in patients with postoperative acute respiratory failure (NNT 11) and prevention of postextubation acute respiratory failure (NNT 12).

17. High-flow nasal cannula use immediately following extubation may decrease risk for reintubation in patients who remain in the ICU and at risk for recurrent respiratory failure.

18. The primary goal of hemodynamic monitoring is to assess the ability of the cardiovascular system in delivering oxygen to organs and peripheral tissues to meet metabolic demands.

19. *Fluid responsiveness* refers to an increase in stroke volume in response to a fluid challenge. Methods used to predict fluid responsiveness include the passive leg raise test as well as systolic pressure, pulse pressure, and stroke volume variation.

20. Neuroprognostication after cardiac arrest depends on a combination of history of arrest, clinical exam, electroencephalography features, evoked potentials, and magnetic resonance imaging findings. The depth of temperature management also can have a major impact on how these tools can be used to make a prognosis.

21. Point-of-care ultrasound by intensivists is a vital tool in the rapid assessment of critically ill patients presenting with shock, respiratory failure, or cardiac arrest.

22. PVADs improve cardiac function by unloading a failing ventricle, thereby reducing ventricular wall stress and oxygen consumption, and augmenting systemic perfusion pressure to maintain end-organ perfusion.

23. Left-sided PVADs require a well-functioning right ventricle (otherwise biventricular support is indicated), no evidence of respiratory compromise, and structural anatomy that is amenable to insertion.

24. IABP improves coronary blood flow by increasing perfusion pressure during diastole.

25. The major benefit of the IABP may be the reduction in myocardial oxygen consumption via a reduction in the isovolumic contraction phase of systole.

26. There is little evidence that an IABP improves outcomes in myocardial infarction complicated by cardiogenic shock. There is some indication that management of mechanical complications of myocardial infarction such as papillary muscle rupture associated or ventricular septal rupture may be an indication for an IABP.

27. ECMO is a method for providing temporary oxygenation, ventilation and circulatory support for patients with lung or heart diseases.

28. ECMO is not identical to cardiopulmonary bypass in that ECMO does not have a reservoir for additional fluid, there are no pumps for the administration of cardioplegia and the heart chambers are not vented while on peripherally cannulated ECMO.

29. VA ECMO primarily supports cardiopulmonary failure while VV ECMO only supports the failing lungs.

30. Never push a rigidly styletted ETT against resistance if the ETT tip is not in view.

31. Most ETTs have an identifiable mark 1 to 2 cm from the cuff. Maintaining the video view of the glottic opening during ETT insertion and placing this mark at the vocal cords will guard against main stem intubation (and virtually guarantee against esophageal intubation).

32. Upper airway obstruction can be addressed with humidified air followed by racemic epinephrine, heliox, and, ultimately, surgical airway placement if airway patency cannot be secured via the laryngeal route.

33. Bleeding from a tracheostomy site 48 hours after procedure should always prompt investigation for tracheoarterial fistula formation.

34. Bronchoalveolar lavage should be considered when there is a suspected atypical pneumonia or nonresolving infiltrate.

35. Bronchoscopy has limited value in the diagnosis of idiopathic interstitial pneumonias.

36. Exercise therapy has significant benefits in both the acute and chronic setting for patients with COPD. It can be started in the ICU and continued on an outpatient basis in a formal pulmonary rehabilitation program.

37. Many patients with COPD and acute respiratory failure can be supported with noninvasive ventilatory support; however, intubation when needed is relatively well tolerated.

38. The five causes of hypoxemia are:
    - V/Q (ventilation/perfusion) mismatch
    - Alveolar hypoventilation
    - Shunt: physiologic (alveolar level) and anatomic (proximal to lung)
    - Diffusion limitation
    - Low inspired oxygen fraction

39. Two therapies proven to reduce mortality in patients with ARDS are:
    - Low tidal volume ventilation (6mL/kg predited body weight)
    - Prone positioning

40. Death from massive hemoptysis is more commonly due to asphyxiation than exsanguination.

41. Bronchial embolization is the initial treatment of choice for most patients with massive hemoptysis.

42. Clinical findings, including laboratory and EKG results, are neither sensitive nor specific for the diagnosis of PE. CT chest angiography or V/Q scan is necessary to confirm the diagnosis.

43. Duration of therapy in an unprovoked PE in a low-risk bleeding patient is at least 3 months, with a recommendation for life-long anticoagulation and annual reassessment of the risk versus benefit of long-term anticoagulation.

44. Clinical assessment of volume status and perfusion is critical in treatment of acute decompensated heart failure.

45. Valve replacement is the only treatment for symptomatic severe aortic stenosis. No medical options have been shown to be effective.

46. It is important to distinguish hemodynamically unstable arrhythmias that need immediate cardioversion/defibrillation from more stable rhythms.

47. In patients with out-of-hospital cardiac arrest who have recovered a perfusing rhythm but have neurologic deficits, therapeutic hypothermia has been shown to dramatically improve outcomes.

48. Aortic dissection carries high morbidity and mortality if untreated and should be suspected in a patient presenting with acute onset severe chest, back, or abdominal pain.

49. All patients presenting with aortic dissection should be immediately evaluated by a surgeon. Type A dissections require emergent open repair. Type B dissections complicated by end-organ ischemia, rupture, rapidly expanding dissection or aneurysm, or intractable pain or hypertension require surgery; endovascular repair is preferable if possible.

50. Pericardial tamponade is a medical emergency, diagnosed based upon clinical physiology, and treated by emergent pericardiocentesis or drainage.

51. Pericarditis can result in diffuse ST and T wave changes on ECG, and mild troponin elevation, without coronary artery disease.

52. Early diagnosis and initiation of treatment for sepsis is associated with improved outcomes.

53. Obtain 2 to 3 sets of blood cultures before giving antibiotics in cases of suspected endocarditis.

54. Streptococcus pneumoniae remains the most common cause of community acquired bacterial meningitis and treatment directed to this should be included in initial empiric antibiotic regimens.

55. Most patients do not require CT scan prior to lumbar puncture; however, signs and symptoms that suggest elevated intracranial pressure should prompt imaging. They include: new onset neurologic deficits, new onset seizure and papilledema. Severe cognitive impairment and immune compromise are also conditions that warrant consideration for imaging.

56. Refractory fever among critically ill patients despite proper antibiotics may warrant antifungal introduction for possible fungal infection.

57. Reducing multidrug-resistant bacteria can only be accomplished by reduced use of antibiotics, not by increased use.

58. During influenza season, all persons admitted to the ICU with respiratory illness should be presumed to have influenza and be tested and treated.

59. Patients with influenza may develop secondary bacterial infections and should be treated with ceftriaxone and vancomycin pending cultures.

60. In a patient presenting with hypertensive crisis (SBP ≥200 or DBP ≥120 mm Hg), the presence of acute end organ injury (cerebral, renal, or cardiac) constitutes "hypertensive emergency" and should be immediately treated in the intensive care unit.

61. Short-acting titratable intravenous antihypertensive agents such as nicardipine, clevidipine, labetalol, esmolol, or phentolamine are administered in hypertensive emergency to prevent further end organ injury.

62. Chronic renal failure is more likely than acute kidney injury to be associated with anemia, hypocalcemia, normal urine output, and small shrunken kidneys on ultrasound examination.

63. While contrast dye can be removed with hemodialysis, there is no evidence that this is beneficial, perhaps because the volume of contrast administered is minimal and delivery of contrast to the kidney is almost immediate.

64. Hypokalemia can be caused by low potassium intake, intracellular potassium shift, gastrointestinal potassium loss (diarrhea), and renal potassium loss. Hyperkalemia can be caused by high potassium intake, extracellular potassium shift, and low renal potassium excretion.

65. Drugs that can cause hyperkalemia include those that release potassium from cells (succinylcholine or, rarely, β-blockers), those that block the renin-angiotensin-aldosterone system (spironolactone, angiotensin-converting enzyme inhibitors, heparin, or nonsteroidal anti-inflammatory drugs), and those that impair sodium and potassium exchange in cells (digitalis) or specifically in the distal nephron (calcineurin inhibitors, amiloride, or trimethoprim).

66. Upper endoscopy is the first diagnostic tool used in patients with suspected upper gastrointestinal bleeding and can also be used therapeutically.

67. For localized lower gastrointestinal bleeding refractory to endoscopic or angiographic intervention, segmental resection of the intestine involved in the bleeding is the usual treatment.

68. Steroids should be considered for the treatment of severe alcoholic hepatitis.

69. Management of variceal bleeding should include antibiotics to prevent spontaneous bacterial peritonitis.

70. The most common cause of thrombocytopenia in the intensive care unit is idiopathic.

71. Platelets should only be transfused in the setting of active bleeding, indications for a procedure, or an absolute value less than 10,000/mm^3.

72. Although disseminated intravascular coagulation (DIC) typically presents with bleeding or laboratory abnormalities suggesting deficient hemostasis, *hyper*coagulability and accelerated thrombin generation actually underlie the process.

73. The use of blood products in the treatment of DIC should be reserved for patients with active bleeding, those requiring invasive procedures, or those otherwise at high risk for bleeding. Heparin, via its ability to reduce thrombin generation, may be useful in some patients with DIC and bleeding that has not responded to the administration of blood products.

74. The immediate approach to the comatose patient includes measures to protect the brain by providing adequate cerebral blood flow and oxygenation, reversing metabolic derangements, and treating potential infections and anatomic or endocrine abnormalities.

75. The differential diagnosis for coma is broad and includes structural injury, metabolic and endocrine derangements, and physiologic brain dysfunction.

76. Brain death is the irreversible loss of both brain and brainstem function from a known cause.

77. Brain death is a clinical diagnosis.

78. Status epilepticus is defined as a seizure lasting 5 minutes or more or recurrent seizure activity between which there is incomplete recovery of consciousness or function.

79. Benzodiazepine therapy is the first-line treatment for seizure termination.

80. Blood pressure should *not* be treated in acute ischemic stroke unless it is greater than 220/110 mm Hg or SBP greater than 185/110 mm Hg if intravenous tissue plasminogen activator is to be administered.

81. If a patient diagnosed with delirium tremens becomes sedated following low-dose benzodiazepine, reconsider the diagnosis.

82. If intravenous lorazepam is re-dosed before the previous dose took full effect, this may eventually lead to oversedation ("dose-stacking").

83. Only second- and third-degree injuries count for calculation of total body surface area and Parkland resuscitation.

84. Burn patients require aggressive fluid resuscitation with lactated Ringer solution.

85. The patient's own palmar surface is the equivalent of 1% body surface area and can be used to quickly assess scattered areas of burns.

86. Effective responses to large-scale disasters, both natural and man-made, depend upon extensive communication and collaboration between local, state, and federal agencies.

87. Biologic and epidemiologic factors make influenza the single greatest infectious threat to global health.

88. The standard hallmarks of death do not apply in a hypothermic patient—no one is dead until WARM (>35°C) and dead.

89. Therapeutic hypothermia for a comatose patient following cardiac arrest and return of spontaneous circulation is no longer recommended—temperature should be targeted to avoid hyperthermia.

90. In an individual from a hot environment or undergoing strenuous exercise who presents with an altered mental status, think of heat stroke.

91. Heat stroke is a true medical emergency requiring immediate action: delay in cooling increases mortality.

92. A standardized approach focusing on airway, breathing, circulation, disability, exposure, and expert consultation should be used for all critically ill poisoned patients.

93. Poisonings with antidotes must be recognized and treatment initiated promptly. Focusing on toxidromes can expedite this process.

94. Sedation and intubation in a salicylate-intoxicated patient can be a precursor to rapid clinical decompensation and increased mortality.

95. Administering an additional NAC bolus or extending the 6.25 mg/kg per hour infusion beyond 21 hours may be indicated in a persistent acetaminophen-toxic patient.

96. The toxic alcohols are methanol, ethylene glycol, isopropyl alcohol, and propylene glycol; like ethanol, they are metabolized in the liver by the enzyme alcohol dehydrogenase (ADH).

97. The mainstay of toxic alcohol ingestion involves limiting the amount of toxic metabolites produced, either by competitive inhibition of ADH by fomepizole or ethanol, or by dialysis in severe cases.

98. Cardiovascular medications should be chosen based on their characteristics, evidence of effectiveness in specific conditions, and the pathophysiology of the individual patient.

99. Use of cardiovascular medications necessitates adequate monitoring, including continuous cardiac telemetry, invasive blood pressure monitoring, and continuous pulse oximetry.

100. Although radiologic investigations and drug treatment may carry some risk of harm to the fetus, necessary tests and treatment should never be avoided in the pregnant woman.

101. Intubation in the critically ill pregnant woman may be very difficult due to airway edema and friability, as well as rapid oxygen desaturation despite optimal preoxygenation.

102. Fever may be the only sign of serious infection in oncologic patients with neutropenia. Patients with low absolute neutrophil counts lack the ability to mount appropriate inflammatory response. For example, patients with intra-abdominal catastrophe may not have peritonitis clinically. Erythema, swelling, or tenderness may be absent in patients with soft tissue infection. Chest radiograph may be without infiltrates in patients with pneumonia.

103. Patients with cancer have a four-fold increase in venous thromboembolism; their risk is further increased when they have indwelling vascular catheters, they receive chemotherapy, they undergo recent surgeries or when they are immobile.

104. It is important for clinicians treating patients in the intensive care unit and after critical illness to recognize that life does not return to normal for most survivors of critical illness.

105. Impairments in physical, cognitive, and mental health domains may burden patients and families for months or even years after critical illness.

106. The diagnosis of sepsis includes a widely heterogeneous patient population that has hitherto been treated with a "one size fits all" approach, with a notable lack of success. Leveraging the tools of modern technology and "big data" should allow a more biologically sound classification of the different subgroups of patients with sepsis, paving the way for rational therapies.

I

GENERAL INTENSIVE CARE UNIT CARE

GLYCEMIC CONTROL IN THE INTENSIVE CARE UNIT

Matthew P. Gilbert and Amanda Fernandes

1. Who is at risk for development of hyperglycemia?

   Hyperglycemia can occur in patients with known or undiagnosed diabetes mellitus. Hyperglycemia during acute illness can also occur in patients with previously normal glucose tolerance, a condition called *stress hyperglycemia*.

2. How common is hyperglycemia in critically ill patients?

   Acute hyperglycemia is common in critically ill patients. It is estimated that 90% of all patients develop blood glucose concentrations greater than 110 mg/dL during critical illness. Stress-induced hyperglycemia has been associated with adverse clinical outcomes in patients with trauma, acute myocardial infarction, and subarachnoid hemorrhage.

3. What causes hyperglycemia in critically ill patients?

   In healthy individuals, blood glucose concentrations are tightly regulated within a narrow range. The cause of hyperglycemia in critically ill patients is multifactorial. Glucose toxicity and activation of inflammatory cytokines, and counterregulatory hormones such as cortisol and epinephrine cause an increase in peripheral insulin resistance and hepatic glucose production. The use of glucocorticoids and parenteral and enteral nutrition is an important contributor to hyperglycemia.

4. What is the relationship between hyperglycemia and acute illness?

   The relationship between hyperglycemia and acute illness is complex. Severe hyperglycemia (>250 mg/dL) has been shown to have a negative impact on the vascular, hemodynamic, and immune systems. Hyperglycemia can also lead to electrolyte imbalance, mitochondrial injury, and both neutrophil and endothelial dysfunction. Acute illness increases the risk for hyperglycemia through the release of counterregulatory hormones, increased insulin resistance, and immobility. Fig. 1.1 illustrates the relationship between acute illness and hyperglycemia.

5. Should oral medications used to treat diabetes be continued in the intensive care unit?

   Given the high incidence of renal and hepatic impairment, oral medication to treat diabetes should not be continued in the intensive care unit (ICU). Medications such as metformin are contraindicated in patients with renal and/or hepatic dysfunction and congestive heart failure. Long-acting formulations of sulfonylureas have been associated with episodes of prolonged severe hypoglycemia in hospitalized patients. Oral medications are not easily titrated to meet glycemic targets and may take weeks to effectively lower blood glucose levels.

6. Should noninsulin, injectable medications be used in the intensive care unit?

   Noninsulin, injectable medications such as glucagon-like peptide-1 receptor agonists (GLP-1 RAs) stimulate insulin release in a glucose dependent manner. These medications have been shown to cause nausea and emesis and slow gastric emptying. GLP-1 RAs have similar limitations as oral agents with regards to titration and should not be used in the ICU setting.

7. What is the most effective way to treat hyperglycemia in the intensive care unit?

   An intravenous insulin infusion using regular insulin is the safest and most effective way to treat hyperglycemia in critically ill patients. Because of the short half-life of circulating insulin (minutes), an insulin infusion can be frequently adjusted to match the often-variable insulin requirements of critically ill patients. Intravenous insulin therapy should be administered by validated written or computerized protocols that outline predefined adjustments in the insulin dose based on frequent blood glucose measurements.

8. When should treatment with an intravenous insulin infusion be initiated?

   Intravenous insulin therapy should be initiated for the treatment of persistent hyperglycemia starting at a blood glucose concentration of no greater than 180 mg/dL.

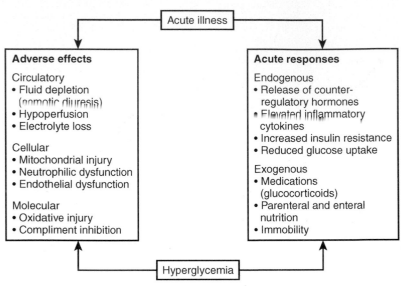

Figure 1-1. Hyperglycemia and acute illness.

9. **What is the appropriate glycemic target for critically ill patients?**
   Recognizing the importance of glycemic control in critically ill patients, a number of professional societies have developed treatment guidelines and/or consensus statements that provide evidence-based glycemic targets. Although the glycemic targets are not identical, all of the groups advocate for good glycemic control while avoiding hypoglycemia (Table 1.1).

10. **What is the evidence supporting the current glycemic targets?**
    The first randomized controlled trial (RCT) comparing tight glycemic control (target blood glucose concentration of 80–110 mg/dL) with conventional insulin therapy (target blood glucose concentration of 180–200 mg/dL) was conducted by Van den Berghe and colleagues (2001). This single-center trial enrolled more than 1500 surgical ICU patients and showed a 34% reduction in mortality associated with tight glycemic control. However, subsequent studies in both medical and surgical ICU populations have not shown consistent reductions in mortality with tight glycemic control. A meta-analysis of RCTs that included 8432 critically ill adult patients did not show a significant difference in mortality between tight glycemic control and control groups.

11. **What was the normoglycemia in intensive care evaluation–survival using glucose algorithm regulation study?**
    The Normoglycemia in Intensive Care Evaluation–Survival Using Glucose Algorithm Regulation (NICE-SUGAR) was a multicenter, multinational RCT that evaluated the effect of tight glycemic control (target glucose level of 81–108 mg/dL) to conventional glucose control (<180 mg/dL) on a number of clinical outcomes in 6104 critically ill adults, greater than 95% of whom required mechanical ventilation. The 90-day mortality was significantly higher in the tight glycemic control group (78 more deaths;

Table 1-1. Summary of Glycemic Targets from the Medical Literature

Professional society/consensus statement	Glycemic target for critically ill patients
American Diabetes Association	140–180 mg/dL
American Association of Clinical Endocrinologists	140–180 mg/dL
Surviving Sepsis Campaign	150–180 mg/dL
American College of Physicians	140–200 mg/dL
American Thoracic Society	<180 mg/dL (in patients undergoing cardiac surgery)

27.5% vs. 24.9%; $P = .02$). Cardiovascular mortality and severe hypoglycemic events were also more common in the tight glycemic control group. The results of the NICE-SUGAR trial have resulted in a shift from tight glycemic control to good control in critically ill patients, and standard of care is now to target glucose level between 140 and 180 mg/dL.

12. **How should patients be transitioned from an intravenous insulin infusion to subcutaneous insulin therapy?**
Patients should be transitioned from an insulin infusion to a subcutaneous insulin program when clinically stable. In patients who are eating, once- or twice-daily administration of basal insulin in combination with scheduled mealtime rapid-acting insulin and a supplemental (correction) component has been shown to maintain adequate glycemic control without clinically significant hypoglycemia. Subcutaneous insulin therapy should be initiated at least 2 hours before the discontinuation of the insulin infusion to reduce the risk of hyperglycemia. The use of a sliding-scale insulin regimen as the sole means of treatment of hyperglycemia is ineffective and should be avoided.

13. **How is hypoglycemia defined?**
Hypoglycemia is defined as any blood glucose level less than 70 mg/dL. This level correlates with the initial release of counterregulatory hormones. Cognitive impairment begins at a blood glucose concentration of approximately 50 mg/dL, and severe hypoglycemia occurs when blood glucose concentrations are less than 40 mg/dL.

14. **What is the clinical impact of hypoglycemia?**
Hypoglycemia has been associated with mortality, although whether it serves as a marker of illness or a causal agent remains to be established. Patients with diabetes who experience hypoglycemia during hospitalization have longer lengths of stay, higher costs, and greater odds of being discharged to a skilled nursing facility than their counterparts without hypoglycemia. Insulin-induced hypoglycemia and subsequent endothelial injury, abnormal coagulation, and increases in counterregulatory hormones are all associated with increased risk for cardiovascular events and sudden death. The true incidence of inpatient hypoglycemia is underestimated because of a lack of standardized definitions and varying models of data collection and reporting among hospitals. Despite this, iatrogenic hypoglycemia remains a top source of inpatient adverse drug events.

15. **How do we prevent severe hypoglycemic events in the intensive care unit?**
Critically ill patients are likely not able to report symptoms of hypoglycemia; thus it is important that patients be closely monitored. Early recognition and treatment of mild hypoglycemia can prevent the adverse outcomes associated with severe hypoglycemia. The establishment of a system for documenting the frequency and severity of hypoglycemic events and the implementation of policies that standardize the treatment of hypoglycemia are essential components of an effective glycemic management program.

16. **Is intensive treatment of hyperglycemia cost-effective?**
Intensive treatment of hyperglycemia not only reduces morbidity and mortality but is also cost-effective. The cost savings have been attributed to reductions in laboratory and radiology costs, decreased ventilator days, and reductions in ICU and hospital length of stay.

ACKNOWLEDGMENT

The authors wish to acknowledge Dr. Alison Schneider, MD, for the valuable contributions to the previous edition of this chapter.

KEY POINTS: GLYCEMIC CONTROL IN THE INTENSIVE CARE UNIT

Management of Hyperglycemia in Critically Ill Patients
1. Hyperglycemia is common in critically ill patients and has been independently associated with increased ICU mortality.
2. Oral medications and noninsulin injectable therapies should not be used to treat hyperglycemia in critically ill patients.
3. An intravenous insulin infusion is the safest and most effective way to treat hyperglycemia in critically ill patients.
4. A glycemic target of 140 to 180 mg/dL is recommended for critically ill patients.
5. Early recognition and treatment of mild hypoglycemia can prevent the adverse outcomes associated with severe hypoglycemia.

BIBLIOGRAPHY

1. Chow E, Bernjak A, Williams S, et al. Risk of cardiac arrhythmias during hypoglycemia in patients with type 2 diabetes and cardiovascular risk. *Diabetes*. 2014;63:1738.
2. Clement S, Braithwaite S, Magee M, et al. Management of diabetes and hyperglycemia in hospitals. *Diab Care*. 2004;27:856.
3. Cryer P, Davis S, Shamoon H. Hypoglycemia in diabetes. *Diab Care*. 2003;26:1902.
4. Curkendall SM, Natoli JL, Alexander CM, Nathanson BH, Haidar T, Dubois RW. Economic and clinical impact of inpatient diabetic hypoglycemia. *Endocr Pract*. 2009;15:302.
5. Dellinger R, Levy M, Carlet J, et al. Surviving Sepsis Campaign: international guidelines for management of severe sepsis and septic shock. *Crit Care Med*. 2008;36:1394.
6. Egi M, Bellomo R, Stachowski E, et al. Hypoglycemia and outcomes in critically ill patients. *Mayo Clin Proc*. 2010; 85:217.
7. Egi M, Finfer S, Bellomo R. Glycemic control in the ICU. *Chest*. 2011;140:212.
8. Farrokhi F, Smiley D, Umpierrez GE. Glycemic control in non-diabetic critically ill patients. *Best Pract Res Clin Endocrinol Metab*. 2011;25:813.
9. Goto A, Arah OA, Goto M, Terauchi Y, Noda M. Severe hypoglycemia and cardiovascular disease: systemic review and meta-analysis with bias analysis. *BMJ*. 2013;347:f4533.
10. Inzucchi SE. Management of hyperglycemia in the hospital setting. *N Engl J Med*. 2006;355:1903.
11. Lazar H, McDonnnell M, Chipkin S, et al. The Society of Thoracic Surgeons practice guideline series: blood glucose management during adult cardiac surgery. *Ann Thorac Surg*. 2009;87:663.
12. Levetan C, Salas J, Wilets I, Zumoff B. Impact of endocrine and diabetes team consultation on hospital length of stay for patients with diabetes. *Am J Med*. 1995;99:22.
13. McCowen K, Malhotra A, Bistrian B. Stress-induced hyperglycemia. *Crit Care Clin*. 2001;17:107.
14. Moghissi E, Korytkowski M, DiNardo M, et al. AACE/ADA consensus statement on inpatient glycemic control. *Endocr Pract*. 2009;15:1.
15. NICE-SUGAR Study Investigators; Finfer S, Chittock D, Su S, et al. Intensive versus conventional glucose control in critically ill patients. *N Engl J Med*. 2009;360:1283.
16. Qaseem A, Humphrey LL, Chou R, Snow V, Shekelle P; Clinical Guidelines Committee of the American College of Physicians. Use of intensive insulin therapy for the management of glycemic control in hospitalized patients: a clinical practice guideline from the American College of Physicians. *Ann Intern Med*. 2011;154:260.
17. Umpierrez G, Smiley M, Zisman A, et al. Randomized study of basal-bolus insulin therapy in the inpatient management of patients with type 2 diabetes (RABBIT 2 Trial). *Diabetes Care*. 2007;30:2181.
18. Van den Berghe G, Wouters P, Weekers F, et al. Intensive insulin therapy in the critically ill patients. *N Engl J Med*. 2001;345:1359.
19. Wiener R, Wiener D, Larson R. Benefits and risk of tight glucose control in critically ill adults: a meta-analysis. *JAMA*. 2008;300:933.

CHAPTER 2

EARLY MOBILITY

Alexis C. Smith and Rita N. Bakhru

1. **What is intensive care unit–acquired weakness?**
   Intensive care unit–acquired weakness (ICU-AW) is a syndrome encompassing generalized diffuse muscle weakness that develops after the onset of critical illness and is not attributable to a primary neurologic cause. It is defined by standard muscle strength testing with the Medical Research Council (MRC) strength testing scale.

2. **How is intensive care unit–acquired weakness diagnosed?**
   MRC testing is performed (Table 2.1) by assessing upper and lower extremity strength at three points per limb on a 0 (no visible contraction) to 5 (active movement against full resistance) scale. A total sum score of less than 48 (of a total of 60) is suggestive of ICU-AW. In patients with ICU-AW, muscle strength testing will reveal a symmetric proximal weakness. However, of note, is that muscle strength testing with the MRC scale is not possible in the sedated or unconscious patient. In these patients, facial grimace may be helpful because the facial muscles are spared in ICU-AW and thus will respond to pain. In the sedated or unresponsive patient, ICU-AW should be a diagnosis of exclusion and additional differential diagnoses include but are not limited to stroke, infectious diseases, hypoglycemia, spinal cord injuries, demyelinating diseases, myasthenia gravis, and Guillain-Barré. If necessary, nerve conduction studies and electromyography (EMG) or muscle biopsy can be performed, although neither of these modalities provides a definitive diagnosis.

3. **Who is at risk for intensive care unit–acquired weakness?**
   Most data regarding ICU-AW center around mechanically ventilated patients. However, there are other known risk factors, both intrinsic and iatrogenic. Possible intrinsic risk factors include systemic inflammatory response syndrome (and the entire sepsis spectrum), multisystem organ failure, acute respiratory distress syndrome (ARDS), increasing age, and a low functional status at baseline. Possible iatrogenic risk factors include high-dose corticosteroids and neuromuscular blockade, particularly when the two medications are administered concomitantly. Persistently elevated blood glucose levels, delirium, deep sedation, and prolonged bed rest are also iatrogenic risk factors for ICU-AW. Other risk factors may be associated with ICU-AW in some studies, but these relationships have not been fully elucidated.

Table 2-1. MRC Scale for Muscle Examination*

Functions assessed
    Upper extremity: wrist flexion, forearm flexion, shoulder abduction
    Lower extremity: ankle dorsiflexion, knee extension, hip flexion
Score for each movement
    0–No visible contraction
    1–Visible muscle contraction but no limb movement
    2–Active movement but not against gravity
    3–Active movement against gravity
    4–Active movement against gravity and resistance
    5–Active movement against full resistance
    Maximum score: 60 (four limbs, maximum of 15 points per limb) [normal]
    Minimum score: 0 (quadriplegia)

MRC, Medical Research Counsel.

Medical Research Council scale for evaluation of intensive care unit–acquired weakness (ICU-AW). Three muscle groups in each limb are tested and score on a 0- to 5-scale. A total score of 60 is possible; a score of <48 is suggestive of ICU-AW. Taken from Schweickert WD, Hall J. ICU-acquired weakness. *Chest.* 2007;131:1541-1549.

*Modified with permission from Kleyweg et al.

4. How common is intensive care unit–acquired weakness?

ICU-AW is very common, with incidence rates reported in up to 25% to 100% of patients, depending on the population studied (e.g., mechanical ventilation for >7 days, sepsis, multiorgan failure).

5. What are short- and long-term complications that are associated with intensive care unit–acquired weakness?

Studies have demonstrated that ICU-AW is a predictor of prolonged mechanical ventilation, increased ICU and hospital lengths of stay, and increased mortality. In addition, muscle wasting and long-term physical impairments are very common in patients with ICU-AW.

6. Can we prevent or mitigate intensive care unit–acquired weakness?

Minimization of risk factors for ICU-AW is a central tenet of prevention of ICU-AW.

Glycemic control, intermittent and targeted sedation, and minimization of steroid use are all important to prevent or mitigate ICU-AW. Efforts to minimize the duration of mechanical ventilation (including sedative minimization and daily breathing trials) may decrease the incidence of ICU-AW. In addition, early mobilization of ICU patients is emerging as a potential mechanism to lessen the long-term debility associated with ICU-AW. Given the complex nature of this evolving field, it is important to note that there are some conflicting studies. However, the overall evidence to date demonstrates improvement in functional outcomes. Optimal timing, duration, intensity, and composition of an early rehabilitation program has not been established.

7. What is an early mobilization program?

Many studies of early mobilization have used a mobilization protocol. Use of a mobility protocol rather than simply having a culture of early mobilization has been associated with patients achieving higher levels of mobilization. Some of these protocols have been published, but there is currently no single protocolized approach to mobility that is accepted. Fig. 2.1 demonstrates an example of how a patient may progress through a mobility protocol. Efforts focus initially on passive, or nurse-driven, range-of-motion exercises and then advance to active exercises, often physical therapist driven, when the patient is alert and able to follow commands. Patients will then progress through the following exercises: sitting in the chair position in bed, sitting on the side of the bed, standing, marching in place, and ultimately walking. Progression through activities, duration and timing of therapies, and other types of exercise are just some of the many details that vary between different mobility protocols and practices. Additional modes of muscle exercise, beyond physical therapy–driven protocols, include in-bed cycle ergometry and neuromuscular electrical stimulation (NMES). No specific modality has been shown to be superior.

8. How "early" is early mobilization?

At this time, there is no consensus to clearly define a timeline for initiation of early mobility. Some studies have reported mobilizing ICU patients as soon as 1 to 2 days after intubation, whereas others mobilized patients on the fifth or even the eighth day of ICU stay. There are no national or societal guidelines that define "early" as it pertains to mobility, but most experts agree that patients should be mobilized as soon as safely possible.

9. Is it safe to mobilize mechanically ventilated patients?

Yes. More than a dozen studies to date have examined the safety of early mobility of mechanically ventilated patients. In fact, most studies of early mobilization focus on mechanically ventilated patients given the risk of ICU-AW in these patients. Collectively, adverse events are reported infrequently during the thousands of therapy sessions in these studies. Arrhythmia, hypertension or hypotension, inadvertent removal of catheters, falls, and oxygen desaturations happen rarely (<1% of sessions). No cardiac arrests or patient deaths have been reported in the setting of mobilization. In general, these studies have used standard criteria to safely initiate and continue mobilization exercises.

10. What are contraindications to initiation or continuation of early mobility exercises?

Contraindications are commonly grouped into cardiac, respiratory, and other contraindications. There are also other patient-specific contraindications.

Cardiac Contraindications:
- Evidence of active myocardial ischemia
- Mean arterial pressure (MAP) <55 millimeters mercury (mm Hg) on minimal to moderate vasopressors; new or escalating vasopressor requirement
- Hypertensive emergency on an antihypertensive infusion
- New, uncontrolled arrhythmia

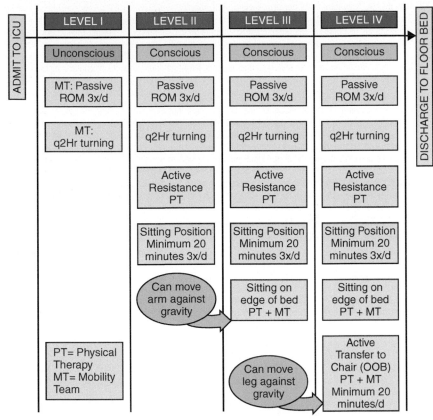

Figure 2-1. A mobility protocol example. Mobility protocols vary but are designed to safely advance patients to different levels of therapeutic exercise as their condition tolerates. Here, level 1 begins passive range of motion (PROM), level II initiates a sitting position, level III mobilizes a patient to sitting on the edge of the bed, level IV initiates transfers out of bed (OOB), or ambulating. *(From Morris PE, Goad A, Thompson C, et al. Early intensive care unit mobility therapy in the treatment of acute respiratory failure. Crit Care Med. 2008;36:2238–2243.)*

Respiratory/Ventilator Contraindications:
- Pulse oximetry <88% for greater than 3 minutes during mobility
- Requiring high levels of oxygen or positive end expiratory pressure (PEEP) (e.g., fraction of inspiratory oxygen (FIO_2) >80% or PEEP >15)

Other Patient-Specific Contraindications
- Active gastrointestinal bleeding
- Sustained intracranial hypertension requiring treatment
- Uncontrolled seizures
- Spinal Precautions

11. **Who performs early mobilization with patients?**
    In a few intensive care units, ICU nurses have been reported to be the primary discipline mobilizing patients. However, given high bedside demand, ICU nurses are not routinely the sole providers for early mobilization. Programs that use physical and occupational therapists have had some of the best success with early mobility. In addition, other programs have had success using a dedicated mobility team, consisting of nursing assistants, nurses, and physical therapists. In many instances, respiratory therapists will be involved as well to assist with ventilators and other oxygen delivery devices.

12. Why do intensive care units perform early mobilization?

Early mobilization is performed in ICU patients, in particular mechanically ventilated patients. In many studies, early mobilization has been found to improve functional outcomes (earlier time to get out of bed, increased independence at hospital discharge, increased rates of discharge to home), increase strength and endurance (including walk distance and quadriceps strength), improve neurocognitive outcomes, reduce hospital dependence, and improve long-term outcomes such as readmissions and deaths.

13. What are the global barriers to an ICU mobility program?

There are a variety of barriers to an ICU mobility program that may be separated into the following categories: institutional barriers, patient-level barriers, and provider-level barriers. Institutional barriers may include lack of institutional protocols or guidelines for mobilization, insufficient equipment or financial support, and insufficient staffing. Patient-level barriers to mobility include medical instability, excessive sedation, and lines/tubes. Finally, provider-level barriers often include lack of knowledge about early mobility, safety concerns, and delays in recognition of patients who are appropriate for early mobility. It is important for ICUs and institutions as a whole to recognize their site-specific barriers, so that these can be addressed in such a way as to make an early mobility program successful.

KEY POINTS: EARLY MOBILITY

1. ICU-AW is a syndrome characterized by the development of generalized diffuse muscle weakness after onset of critical illness and is defined by standard muscle strength testing.
2. ICU-AW is common, and debility often persists long after discharge from the hospital.
3. Early mobilization of mechanically ventilated patients is safe and feasible.
4. Short-term outcomes including decreased delirium, shorter ICU and hospital lengths of stay, and better functional performance at hospital discharge can be improved with early mobilization of critically ill patients soon after onset of critical illness.

BIBLIOGRAPHY

1. Hashem MD, Parker AM, Needham DM. Early Mobilization and rehabilitation of patients who are critically ill. *Chest.* 2016;150(3):722-731.
2. Hermans G, Van Mechelen H, Clerckx B, et al. Acute outcomes and 1-year mortality of intensive care unit-acquired weakness. A cohort study and propensity-matched analysis. *Am J Respir Crit Care Med.* 2014;190(4):410-420.
3. Herridge MS, Tansey CM, Matte A, et al. Functional disability 5 years after acute respiratory distress syndrome. *N Engl J Med.* 2011;364:1293-1304.
4. Iwashyna TJ. Survivorship will be the defining challenge of critical care in the 21st century. *Ann Intern Med.* 2010; 153(3):204-205.
5. Kress JP, Hall JB. ICU-acquired weakness and recovery from critical illness. *N Engl J Med.* 2014;371(3):287-288.
6. Latronico N, Bolton CF. Critical illness polyneuropathy and myopathy: a major cause of muscle weakness and paralysis. *Lancet Neurol.* 2011;10:931-941.
7. Morris PE, Goad A, Thompson C, et al. Early intensive care unit mobility therapy in the treatment of acute respiratory failure. *Crit Care Med.* 2008;36:2238-2243.
8. Needham DM, Korupolu R, Zanni JM, et al. Early physical medicine and rehabilitation for patients with acute respiratory failure: a quality improvement project. *Arch Phys Med Rehabil.* 2010;91:536-542.
9. Schweickert WD, Pohlman MC, Pohlman AS, et al. Early physical and occupational therapy in mechanically ventilated, critically ill patients: a randomised controlled trial. *Lancet.* 2009;373:1874-1882.
10. Schweickert WD, Hall J. ICU-acquired weakness. *Chest.* 2007;131:1541-1549.

CHAPTER 3

SEDATION, ANALGESIA, DELIRIUM

Annachiara Marra, Pratik Pandharipande, and Arna Banerjee

1. **What is delirium?**
   Delirium is defined by the Diagnostic and Statistical Manual of Mental Disorders (DSM-4) as:
   A. Disturbance in attention (i.e., reduced ability to direct, focus, sustain, and shift attention) and awareness (reduced orientation to the environment).
   B. The disturbance develops over a short period of (usually hours to a few days), represents an acute change from baseline attention and awareness, and tends to fluctuate in severity during the course of a day.
   C. An additional disturbance in cognition (e.g.memory deficit, disorientation, language, visuospatial ability, or perception).
   D. The disturbances in Criteria A and C are not better explained by a pre-existing, established or evolving neurocognitive disorder and do not occur in the context of a severely reduced level of arousal such as coma.
   E. There is evidence from the history, physical examination or laboratory findings, that the disturbance is a direct physiological consequence of another medical condition, substance intoxication or withdrawal (i.e. due to a drug of abuse or to a medication), or exposure to a toxin, or is due to multiple etiologies.

2. **What is the prevalence of delirium?**
   The true prevalence and magnitude of delirium has been poorly documented because a myriad of terms, such as acute confusional state, intensive care unit (ICU) psychosis, acute brain dysfunction, and encephalopathy have been used historically to describe this condition. Although the overall prevalence of delirium in the community is only 1% to 2%, the prevalence increases with age, rising to 14% among those more than 85 years old. Delirium rates range from 14% to 24% with incidence up to 60% among general hospital populations, especially in older patients and those in nursing homes and post–acute care settings. In critically ill patients (medical, surgical, trauma, and burn ICU patients) the reported prevalence of delirium is 20% to 80%, with the higher rates seen in mechanically ventilated patients. Up to 30% to 40% of adults, regardless of age, may be delirious during ICU stay.

   In spite of this, delirium is often unrecognized by clinicians or the symptoms are incorrectly attributed to dementia or depression or considered as an expected, inconsequential complication of critical illness. Numerous national and international surveys have shown a disconnection between the perceived importance of delirium, the accuracy of diagnosis, and the implementation of management and treatment techniques.

   Given that delirium is one of the most problematic and life-threatening neuropsychological complications of ICU patients, it is important to diagnose and manage the disease by implementation of validated screening protocols.

3. **What morbidity is associated with delirium?**
   Delirium itself is a strong predictor of increased length of mechanical ventilation, longer ICU stays, increased cost, long-term cognitive impairment, and mortality. Delirium is also a significant risk factor for death while in the ICU, after discharge from the ICU while still hospitalized, and after discharge from the hospital, with each additional day with delirium increasing the risk for dying by 10% in some studies.

   Recently, in the study of Klein Klouwenberg et al., delirium was not associated with mortality after adjustment for time-varying confounders in a marginal structural model. According to the authors, increased mortality could be mediated through a prolonged ICU length of stay rather than by a direct effect on the daily risk of death, though longer duration of delirium (>2 days) still had some attributable mortality risk.

   Patients with longer periods of delirium have more cognitive decline, when evaluated after 1 year, attesting to the importance of detecting and managing delirium early in the course of illness.

The post-ICU long-term cognitive impairment involves memory, attention, and executive function problems and leads to inability to return to work, impaired activities of daily living, increased risk of hospitalization, and decreased quality of life. While post-traumatic stress disorder (PTSD) after critical illness is common, delirium has not been shown to be a strong risk factor.

4. Describe the clinical features of delirium.
Delirium manifests as a reduced clarity of awareness of the environment and ability to focus, sustain, or shift attention. This may be accompanied by memory impairment, disorientation, or language disturbance. Speech or language disturbances may be evident as dysarthria, dysnomia, dysgraphia, or even aphasia. In some cases, speech is rambling and irrelevant, in others pressured and incoherent with unpredictable switching from subject to subject. Perceptual disturbances may include misinterpretations, illusions, or hallucinations. Delusion is often associated with a disturbance in the sleep-wake cycle. Patients may also exhibit anxiety, fear, depression, irritability, anger, euphoria, and apathy.
In the new DSM-5 criteria, the core feature of delirium is disturbance in attention and awareness that develops over a short period of time and tends to fluctuate in severity during the course of a day. This shift towards attention was driven by a recognition that the consciousness was difficult to assess objectively.
According to the European Delirium Association and American Delirium Society inclusive interpretation of the DSM-5 criteria, patients who are not comatose but have impaired arousal, resulting in an inability to engage in cognitive testing or interview (e.g., drowsiness, obtundation, stupor, or agitation), must be understood as effectively having inattention. Including such patients under the umbrella of delirium will result in increased patient safety through broader delirium prevention and identification.

5. What are the sub-types of delirium?
Delirium can be classified by psychomotor behavior into the following:
A. **Hypoactive** delirium, which is very common and often more deleterious in the long term, is characterized by decreased responsiveness, apathy, decreased physical and mental activity, and inattention.
B. **Hyperactive** delirium is characterized by agitation, restlessness, and emotional lability. Manifestations may include groping or picking at the bedclothes or attempting to get out of bed when it is unsafe or untimely. This puts both patients and caregivers at risk for serious injuries. Fortunately, this form of delirium occurs in the minority of critically ill patients.
C. Patients with both features have **mixed** delirium.
D. **Sub-syndromal** delirium. Patients who have some features of delirium but do not meet all the criteria are considered to have sub-syndromal delirium.

6. What is the pathophysiology of delirium?
The pathophysiology of delirium is poorly understood, although a number of hypotheses exist.
Neurotransmitter hypothesis. The most commonly described neurotransmitter changes associated with delirium are reduced availability of acetylcholine (Ach); excess release of dopamine (DA), norepinephrine (NE), and/or glutamate (GLU); and alterations (e.g., both a decreased and increased activity depending on circumstances and etiologic factors) in serotonin (5HT), histamine (H1 and H2), and/or γ-aminobutyric acid (GABA).
Neuroinflammatory hypothesis. An acute peripheral inflammatory stimulation (from infectious, surgical, or traumatic etiologies) could induce the activation of brain parenchymal cells and expression of pro-inflammatory cytokines and inflammatory mediators in the central nervous system (CNS), inducing a neuronal and synaptic dysfunction, ischemia, and neuronal apoptosis resulting in acute brain dysfunction and delirium.
Neuroaging hypothesis. Numerous studies in ICU and non-ICU patient populations have identified age as an independent risk factor for delirium. Aging is associated with age-related cerebral changes in stress-regulating neurotransmitters, brain–blood-flow decline, decreased vascular density, neuron loss, and intracellular signal transduction systems that may render it more susceptible to exogenous insults such as acute inflammatory states in the body. In addition, the aging brain may mount a more exuberant CNS inflammatory response when stimulated by peripheral inflammatory states.
Oxidative stress hypothesis. Many stimuli can increase oxygen consumption in and/or decrease oxygen delivery to the CNS, causing increased CNS energy expenditure and reduced cerebral oxidative metabolism resulting in CNS dysfunction. Delirium may be a result of cerebral

insufficiency caused by a global failure of oxidative metabolism. Oxidative stress is one of the mechanisms by which neurotransmitter derangement imbalance could occur.

Neuroendocrine hypothesis. Delirium represents a reaction to acute stress mediated by abnormally high glucocorticoid levels which induce a general vulnerability in brain neurons by impairing the ability of neurons to survive after various metabolic insults. Chronically, high levels of physiologic stress are also associated with increased levels of inflammation in the body, connecting the neuroinflammatory and neuroendocrine theories of delirium.

Diurnal dysregulation hypothesis. This hypothesis suggests that disruptions to the 24-hour circadian cycle and the usual stages of sleep may lead to the development of delirium. Derangements in melatonin levels may cause delirium, due to its central role in the regulation of circadian rhythm and sleep-wake cycles. Sleep deprivation has been associated with increased levels of inflammatory substances, connecting this hypothesis to the neuroinflammatory theory of delirium.

Network disconnectivity hypothesis. The brain is a highly organized and interconnected structure functioning to allow complex integration of sensory information and motor responses. According to this hypothesis, delirium could represent a variable failure in the integration and appropriate processing of sensory information and motor responses. The clinical forms of delirium, hypoactive versus hyperactive, may be determined by which neural networks break down in response to stressors such as aging, sleep deprivation, infection/inflammation, or medication exposure. How they will break down in the face of a particular stressor is thought to be related to the degree of baseline network connectivity and the level of inhibitory tone, mediated by GABA levels in that particular neural network.

Large neutral amino acids. Changes in large neutral amino acids (LNAAs), which are precursors of several neurotransmitters that are involved in arousal, attention, and cognition, may play a role in the development of delirium. All LNAAs (isoleucine, leucine, methionine, phenylalanine, tryptophan, tyrosine, and valine) enter the brain by using the same saturable carrier in competition with each other. Increased cerebral uptake of tryptophan and tyrosine (amino acid precursors) can lead to elevated levels of serotonin, DA, and NE in the CNS, leading to an increased risk for development of delirium.

None of these theories by themselves explains the full phenomenon of delirium but rather that two or more of these, if not all, act together to lead to the biochemical derangement we know as delirium.

7. What are the risk factors for delirium?
The average medical ICU patient has 11 or more risk factors for developing delirium. These risk factors can be divided into predisposing baseline (as underlying characteristics and comorbidities) and hospital-related (precipitating) factors (as acute illness, its treatment and ICU management) (Table 3.1). Many of these factors are modifiable. Several mnemonics can aid clinicians in recalling the list as IWATCHDEATH and DELIRIUM (Table 3.2).

8. Which drugs are most likely to be associated with delirium?
Many drugs are considered to be risk factors for the development of delirium. Benzodiazepines showed a trend toward stronger association with delirium. The class of benzodiazepines does not seem to change the risk profile, with both lorazepam and midazolam being significant risk factors for delirium. The Society of Critical Care Medicine's ICU Pain Agitation Delirium (PAD) guidelines recommend that non-benzodiazepine sedative options may be preferred over benzodiazepine-based sedative regimens.

Although targeted pain control has been shown to be associated with improved rates of delirium, overzealous administration of opiates has been associated with worse delirium outcomes as well. Marcantonio found that delirium was significantly associated with postoperative exposure to meperidine and benzodiazepines, although not to other commonly prescribed opiates. Pandharipande et al. found that every unit dose of lorazepam was associated with a higher risk for daily transition to delirium. Similarly, Seymour et al. confirmed that benzodiazepines are an independent risk factor for development of delirium during critical illness even when given more than 8 hours before a delirium assessment.

Opioids and benzodiazepines are risk factors for delirium in medical and surgical ICU patients, though trauma and burn patients, who have pain, appear to be protected from development of delirium with intravenous opiates.

Table 3-1. Risk Factors for Delirium

	UNMODIFIABLE/UNPREVENTABLE RISK FACTORS	POTENTIALLY MODIFIABLE/ PREVENTABLE RISK FACTORS
Baseline Risk Factors	Age APOE-4 genotype History of hypertension Pre-existing cognitive impairment History of alcohol use History of tobacco use History of depression	Sensory deprivation (i.e., hearing or vision impairment)
Acute Illness-Related Risk Factors	High severity of illness Respiratory disease Medical illness (vs. surgical) Need for mechanical ventilation Number of infusing medications Elevated inflammatory biomarkers High LNAA metabolite levels	Anemia Acidosis Hypotension Infection/sepsis Metabolic disturbances (e.g., hypocalcemia, hyponatremia, azotemia, transaminases, hyperamylasemia, hyperbilirubinemia) Fever
Hospital-Related Risk Factors	Lack of daylight Isolation	Lack of visitors Sedatives/analgesics (e.g., benzodiaze-pines and opiates) Immobility Bladder catheters Vascular catheters Gastric tubes Sleep deprivation

APOE-4, Apolipoprotien-E4 polymorphism; LNAA, large neutral amino acids.
Modified from Brummel NE, Girard TD. Preventing delirium in the intensive care unit. *Crit Care Clin.* 2013;29(1):51-65.

Table 3-2. Mnemonics for Risk Factors for Delirium

I WATCH DEATH	DELIRIUM (S)	
• **I**nfection HIV, sepsis, Pneumonia	**D**	Drugs
• **W**ithdrawal Alcohol, barbiturate, sedative-hypnotic	**E**	Eyes, ears, and other sensory deficits
• **A**cute metabolic Acidosis, alkalosis, electrolyte disturbance, hepatic failure, renal failure	**L**	Low O_2 states (e.g. heart attack, stroke, and pulmonary embolism)
• **T**rauma Closed-head injury, heat stroke, postoperative, severe burns	**I**	Infection
• **C**NS pathology Abscess, hemorrhage, hydrocephalus, subdural hematoma, Infection, seizures, stroke, tumors, metastases, vasculitis, Encephalitis, meningitis, syphilis	**R** **I** **U** **M**	Retention (of urine or stool) Ictal state Underhydration/undernutrition Metabolic causes [DM, Post-operative state, sodium abnormalities]
• **H**ypoxia Anemia, carbon monoxide poisoning, hypotension, Pulmonary or cardiac failure	**(S)**	Subdural hematoma
• **D**eficiencies Vitamin B12, folate, niacin, thiamine		
• **E**ndocrinopathies, Hyper/hypoadrenocorticism, hyper/hypoglycemia, Myxedema, hyperparathyroidism		

Table 3-2. Mnemonics for Risk Factors for Delirium *(Continued)*

I WATCH DEATH	DELIRIUM (S)
• **A**cute vascular Hypertensive encephalopathy, stroke, arrhythmia, shock • **T**oxins or drugs Prescription drugs, illicit drugs, pesticides, solvents • **H**eavy Metals Lead, manganese, mercury	

CHF, Congestive heart failure; *CNS*, central nervous system; *CVA*, cerebrovascular accident; *DM*, diabetes mellitus; *HIV*, human immunodeficiency virus; *MI*, myocardial infarction.

9. How is delirium diagnosed?

   The diagnosis of delirium is primarily clinical and is based on history and physical exam to identify delirium risk factors, including a detailed review of outpatient and inpatient medication records with attention to those drugs whose administration or abrupt withdrawal are associated with delirium.

   A cognitive function assessment using a delirium detection tool, validated for use in ICU populations, is important.

   Delirium assessment is a two-step process. The level of arousal to voice is first assessed using a sedation scale. The Society of Critical Care Medicine (SCCM), in the PAD guidelines recommend the use of the Richmond Agitation-Sedation Scale (RASS) or the Riker Sedation-Agitation Scale (SAS).

   Many tools have been developed and validated for delirium assessment in ICU populations:
   - Confusion Assessment Method ICU (CAM-ICU),
   - Delirium Detection Score (DDS),
   - Intensive Care Delirium Screening Checklist (ICDSC),
   - Cognitive Test for Delirium (CTD),
   - Abbreviated Cognitive Test for Delirium,
   - Neelson and Champagne Confusion Scale (NEECHAM),
   - Nursing Delirium Screening Scale (NuDESC).

   Of these, the CAM-ICU and the ICDSC are the most valid and reliable delirium monitoring tools in adult ICU patients and have been translated into a number of languages. They have shown high inter-rater reliability and high sensitivity and specificity. Another validated tool is the Delirium Rating Scale–Revised 98 (DRS-R 98) that provides a measure of severity of delirium in addition to the ability to diagnose delirium.

10. How can detection of delirium be improved?

    The delirium screening instruments differ in the components of delirium they evaluate, the threshold for diagnosing delirium, and their ability to be used in patients with impaired vision and hearing and in those who have endotracheal tubes and are receiving mechanical ventilation. Hence, it is important to consider the patient population when choosing the instrument.

11. How should the work-up of delirium be pursued?

    The SCCM recommends routine monitoring of delirium with use of validated tools.

    In addition to the cognitive assessment, a physical exam should be performed, including assessment of vital signs and physical examination to rule out life-threatening problems (e.g., hypoxia, self-extubation, pneumothorax, hypotension) or other acutely reversible physiologic causes (e.g., hypoglycemia, metabolic acidosis, stroke, seizure, pain) to identify factors triggering delirium.

12. What studies should be considered in the work-up of delirium?

    Routine laboratory tests are important but not the mainstay of diagnosis. These include a complete blood cell count, electrolytes, blood urea nitrogen, creatinine, glucose, calcium, pulse oximetry or arterial blood gas, urinalysis, urine drug screens, liver function tests with serum albumin, cultures, chest radiograph, and electrocardiogram.

    Cerebrospinal fluid examination should also be considered for cases in which meningitis or encephalitis is suspected. Other tests that need to be considered are venereal disease research laboratory (VDRL), human immunodeficiency virus, B12 and folate, heavy metal screen, antinuclear antibody, ammonia level, thyroid-stimulating hormone, measurement of serum medication levels (e.g., digoxin), and urinary porphyrins.

Electroencephalogram, neuroimaging, and measures of serum anticholinergic have been suggested as possible tools to study the brain in the setting of delirium research. However, at the present time these are not ready for routine use in daily clinical practice.

13. What are the differential diagnoses for delirium?

Dementia can be difficult to distinguish from delirium, particularly when information about baseline cognitive functioning is unavailable, and is the most common differential diagnosis. Memory impairment is common to both delirium and dementia, but the person with dementia alone is alert and does not have the disturbance in consciousness or attention that is characteristic of delirium. In delirium, the onset of symptoms is much more rapid and fluctuates during a 24-hour period.

Delirium that is characterized by vivid hallucinations, delusions, language disturbances, and agitation must be distinguished from psychotic disorder, schizophrenia, schizophreniform disorder, and mood disorder with psychotic features. Finally, delirium associated with fear, anxiety, and dissociative symptoms such as depersonalization must be distinguished from acute stress disorder.

Delirium must also be distinguished from malingering and factitious disorder.

14. How is delirium treated?

The treatment of underlying medical conditions and nonpharmacologic issues like noise, light, sleep, and mobility are cardinal aspects of delirium management.

Once life-threatening causes are ruled out, focus should be on the following:

A. Reorienting patients
B. Improvement of sleep hygiene
C. Visual and hearing aids if previously used
D. Removing medications that can provoke delirium
E. Discontinuing invasive devices not required (e.g., bladder catheters, restraints)
F. Early ambulation

To improve patient outcome, an evidence-based organizational approach referred to as the ABCDEF bundle (**A**ssess for and manage pain, **B**oth Spontaneous Awakening Trials [SAT] & Spontaneous Breathing Trials [SBT], **C**hoice of appropriate sedation, **D**elirium monitoring, and **E**arly mobility and exercise, **F**amily engagement) is presented.

ASSESS FOR AND MANAGE PAIN

Pain assessment is the first step in proper pain relief and could be very important in patients with delirium. Patient self-reporting of pain using a 1 to 10 numerical rating scale (NRS) is considered the gold standard and is highly recommended by Critical Care Societies. If the patient is unable to self-report, observable behavioral and physiologic indicators become important indices for the assessment of pain. The Behavioral Pain Scale (BPS) and the Critical Care Pain Observation Tool (CPOT) are the most valid and reliable BPSs for ICU patients unable to communicate. According to ICU PAD Guidelines, pain medications should be routinely administered in the presence of significant pain (i.e., NRS > 4, BPS > 5, or CPOT > 3) and prior to performing painful invasive procedures.

BOTH SPONTANEOUS AWAKENING TRIALS AND SPONTANEOUS BREATHING TRIALS

Protocolized target-based sedation and daily SATs reduce the number of days of mechanical ventilation. This strategy also exposes the patient to smaller cumulative doses of sedatives. SBTs were shown to be superior to other varied approaches to ventilator weaning. Thus incorporation of SBTs into practice reduced the total time of mechanical ventilation.

The awakening and breathing controlled trial combined the SAT with the SBT and showed shorter duration of mechanical ventilation, a 4-day reduction in hospital length of stay, a remarkable 15% decrease in 1-year mortality, and no long-term neuropsychological consequences of waking patients during critical illness.

CHOICE OF APPROPRIATE SEDATION

The guidelines of the society of Critical Care Med emphasize the need for goal-directed delivery of psychoactive medications to avoid over-sedation, to promote earlier extubation, and the use of sedation scales (SAS, RASS) to help the medical team agree on a target sedation level for each individual patient.

Numerous studies have identified that benzodiazepines are associated with worse clinical outcomes. The Maximizing Efficacy of Targeted Sedation and Reducing Neurological Dysfunction (MENDS) study showed that patients treated with dexmedetomidine had more days alive without delirium or coma (7.0 vs. 3.0 days; $P = .01$), with a lower risk for delirium developing on subsequent days. The SEDCOM trial (Safety and Efficacy of Dexmedetomidine Compared with Midazolam) showed a reduction in the prevalence of delirium (54% vs. 76.6% [95% confidence intervals, 14% to 33%]; $P < .001$) and in the duration of mechanical ventilation in patients sedated with dexmedetomidine compared with midazolam. Few studies have compared dexmedetomidine to propofol. The propofol versus dexmedetomidine (PRODEX) study showed no difference in delirium outcomes, though delirium was measured only at a single time point after discontinuation of sedation. On the other hand, Djaiani et al. recently showed that dexmedetomidine reduced delirium incidence in cardiac surgical patients in the ICU as compared to propofol, while Su et al. showed a reduction in patients treated with dexmedetomidine in non-cardiac surgical patients admitted to the ICU.

DELIRIUM MANAGEMENT

An important third element in the PAD guidelines is monitoring and management of delirium by using validated tools (CAM-ICU, ICDSC). In delirious patients, a search for all reversible precipitants is the first line of action and pharmacologic treatment should be considered when available and not contraindicated.

EXERCISE AND EARLY MOBILITY

Early mobility is an integral part of the ABCDEF bundle and has been the only intervention resulting in a decrease in days of delirium. Morris et al. showed that initiating physical therapy early during the patient's ICU stay was associated with decreased length of stay both in the ICU and in the hospital. Schweickert et al. showed that a daily SAT, plus physical and occupational therapy, from the start of ICU stay, in patients on mechanical ventilation (MV), resulted in an improved return to independent functional status at hospital discharge, shorter duration of ICU-associated delirium, and more days alive and breathing without assistance.

Although all these studies demonstrated feasibility of physical therapy, it may more effective to start physical therapy early in the ICU course.

FAMILY ENGAGEMENT

Family members and surrogate decision-makers must become active partners in multi-professional decision making and care.

A mnemonic can aid clinicians recalling strategies to consider when delirium is present: DR DRE (Disease remediation, Drug Removal, Environmental modifications).

15. Describe the pharmacologic management of delirium

    Multiple classes of pharmacologic agents including benzodiazepines, antipsychotics, central alpha-2 agonists (dexmedetomidine), and cholinesterase inhibitors have been studied in the treatment of ICU delirium. Of these, antipsychotics and dexmedetomidine are frequently used to control the undesired symptoms of ICU delirium. Pharmacologic treatment should be individualized to each patient and their clinical circumstances.

    Evidence for the safety and efficacy of *typical* (e.g., haloperidol) and *atypical* antipsychotics agents (e.g., risperidone, ziprasidone, quetiapine, or olanzapine) in this patient population is lacking; hence, the 2013 PAD Guidelines include no specific recommendations for using any particular medication.

    The Modifying the Incidence of Delirium (MIND) study showed no difference in the duration of delirium between haloperidol, ziprasidone, or placebo when used for prophylaxis and treatment. Effect of intravenous haloperidol on the duration of delirium and coma in critically ill patients (Hope-ICU): a randomised, double-blind, placebo-controlled trial showed that an early treatment with haloperidol did not modify the prevalence or duration of delirium or coma in critically ill patients.

    A smaller study done by Devlin et al. showed that quetiapine was more effective than placebo in resolution of delirium when supplementing ongoing haloperidol therapy.

    Haloperidol, risperidone, aripiprazole, and olanzapine were equally effective in the management of delirium; however, they differed in terms of their side-effect profile. Extrapyramidal symptoms were most frequently recorded with haloperidol, and sedation occurred most frequently with olanzapine.

Table 3-3. Pharmacologic Treatment of Delirium in Hospitalized Patients

Antipsychotic Haloperidol	0.5–1 mg PO twice daily[a], with additional doses every 4 h as needed up to a maximum of 20 mg daily 0.5–1 mg IM; observe after 30–60 min and repeat if needed
Atypical antipsychotics • Risperidone • Olanzapine • Quetiapine • Ziprasidone	0.25–1 mg/day up to a maximum of 6 mg/day 2.5–10 mg once or twice daily 25–50 mg PO once or twice daily 20–40 mg PO once or twice daily
Antidepressant Trazodone	25–150 mg PO at bedtime

[a]Note: See text for more rapid effects with IV/IM dosing.
IM, Intramuscular; IV, intravenous; PO, orally.

Antipsychotic agents should be used with caution in patients with Parkinson Disease or Lewy Body Disease, as the use of antipsychotic agents in these patients can precipitate life-threatening Parkinsonian crisis.

Data from the MENDS study and the SEDCOM trial support the view that dexmedetomidine can decrease the duration and prevalence of delirium when compared with lorazepam or midazolam. Dexmedetomidine showed to be useful as a rescue drug for treating agitated delirium in non-intubated patients in whom haloperidol has failed, as well as in patients receiving mechanical ventilation.

Benzodiazepines remain the drugs of choice for the treatment of delirium tremens (and other withdrawal syndromes) and seizures (Table 3.3), though evidence is mounting that non-benzodiazepine protocols may be efficacious even in alcohol withdrawal.

16. Describe the use of haloperidol in delirium
Haloperidol is a butyrophenone *typical* antipsychotic that works as a DA receptor antagonist by blocking the D_2 receptor, treating the positive symptoms (hallucinations and unstructured thought patterns) of delirium without suppressing the respiratory drive.

Adverse effects include hypotension, acute dystonia, extrapyramidal effects, laryngeal spasm, malignant hyperthermia, glucose and lipid dysregulation, and anticholinergic effects. There is no published evidence that treatment with haloperidol reduces the duration of delirium in adult ICU patients.

17. How are second-generation antipsychotic agents used in delirium?
Newer *atypical* antipsychotic agents (e.g., risperidone, ziprasidone, quetiapine, and olanzapine) may also prove helpful for delirium. They may be able to reduce the duration of delirium in ICU patients. Studies need to be repeated with larger patient populations before any concrete recommendations can be made regarding the efficacy of typical or atypical antipsychotics in delirium.

18. Delirium prevention
Routine monitoring of delirium is recommended in all adult ICU patients. Risk factors for delirium should be identified and modified if possible. Attempt should be made to target the lightest level of sedation possible. Attempts should be made to promote sleep hygiene and ambulate patients as early as possible. Delirium prophylaxis with medications is discouraged in the PAD guidelines. Baseline psychiatric medications should also be restarted if indicated.

ACKNOWLEDGMENT

The authors wish to acknowledge Drs. Pratik Pandharipande, MBBS, MSCI, and Arna Banerjee, MD, for the valuable contributions to the previous edition of this chapter.

KEY POINTS: SEDATION, ANALGESIA, DELIRIUM

1. Delirium is a disturbance in attention, accompanied by a change in cognition or perceptual disturbances that develop over a short period of time and fluctuate over days.

2. Delirium is a strong predictor of increased length of mechanical ventilation, longer ICU stays, increased cost, long-term cognitive impairment, and mortality.
3. Routine monitoring for delirium is recommended for all ICU patients and the diagnosis of delirium is a two-step process. Level of arousal is first measured, and, if the patient is arousable to voice, delirium evaluation is performed with use of validated instruments.
4. Hypoactive delirium is seen more frequently in ICU patients than hyperactive delirium.
5. Psychoactive medications, especially benzodiazepines, and sleep disturbances may be potentially modifiable risk factors of delirium
6. In mechanically ventilated adult ICU patients the ABCDEF bundle (**A**ttention to analgesia, **B**oth awakening and breathing trials, **C**hoosing right sedative, **D**elirium monitoring and management, **E**arly exercise, and **F**amily involvement) is recommended and associated with improved outcomes. Sedatives should be administered only if needed and should be interrupted daily, or a light level of sedation should be routinely targeted.
7. In delirious patients, pharmacologic treatment should be used only after giving adequate attention to correction of modifiable contributing factors.
8. Haloperidol is not recommended for the treatment of delirium. Atypical antipsychotics may have some evidence in reducing the duration of delirium. Dexmedetomidine may reduce delirium incidence and duration.

WEBSITES

ICU Delirium and Cognitive Impairment Study Group: www.icudelirium.org
American Psychiatric Association guidelines (including treatment of delirium): www.psych.org/psych_pract/treatg/pg/prac_guide.cfm

BIBLIOGRAPHY

1. American Psychiatric Association. *Diagnostic and Statistical Manual of Mental Disorders*. 5th ed. Washington, DC: American Psychiatric Association; 2013.
2. Banerjee A, Pandharipande P. Delirium. In: Bope ET, Rakel RE, Kellerman RD, eds. *Conn's Current Therapy 2010*. Philadelphia: Saunders; 2010:1117.
3. Devlin JW, Roberts RJ, Fong JJ, et al. Efficacy and safety of quetiapine in critically ill patients with delirium: a prospective, multicenter, randomized, double-blind, placebo-controlled pilot study. *Crit Care Med*. 2010;38:419–427.
4. Ely E, Shintani A, Truman B, et al. Delirium as a predictor of mortality in mechanically ventilated patients in the intensive care unit. *JAMA*. 2004;291:1753–1762.
5. Ely EW, Inouwe SK, Bernard GR, et al. Delirium in mechanically ventilated patients: validity and reliability of the confusion assessment method for the intensive care unit (CAM-ICU). *JAMA*. 2001;286:2703–2710.
6. Girard TD, Jackson JC, Pandharipande PP, et al. Delirium as a predictor of long-term cognitive impairment in survivors of critical illness. *Crit Care Med*. 2010;38:1513–1520.
7. Girard TD, Kress JP, Fuchs BD, et al. Efficacy and safety of a paired sedation and ventilator weaning protocol for mechanically ventilated patients in intensive care (Awakening and Breathing Controlled trial): a randomised controlled trial. *Lancet*. 2008;371:126–134.
8. Salluh JI, Wang H, Schneider EB, et al. Outcome of delirium in critically ill patients: systematic review and meta-analysis. *BMJ*. 2015;350:h2538.
9. Pandharipande PP, Girard TD, Jackson JC, et al. Long-term cognitive impairment after critical illness. *N Engl J Med*. 2013;369:1306–1316.
10. Klein Klouwenberg PMC, Zaal IJ, Spitoni C, et al. The attributable mortality of delirium in critically ill patients: prospective cohort study. *BMJ*. 2014;349:g6652.
11. Barr J, Fraser GL, Puntillo K, et al. Clinical practice guidelines for the management of pain, agitation, and delirium in adult patients in the intensive care unit. *Crit Care Med*. 2013;41(1):263–306.
12. Brummel NE, Girard TD. Preventing delirium in the intensive care unit. *Crit Care Clin*. 2013;29(1):51–65.
13. Girard TD, Pandharipande PP, Ely EW. Delirium in the intensive care unit. *Crit Care*. 2008;12(suppl 3):S3.
14. Gunther ML, Morandi A, Ely EW. Pathophysiology of delirium in the intensive care unit. *Crit Care Clin*. 2008;24:45–65, vii.
15. Marcantonio ER, Juarez G, Goldman L, et al. The relationship of postoperative delirium with psychoactive medications. *JAMA*. 1994;272:1518–1522.
16. Morris PE, Goad A, Thompson C, et al. Early intensive care unit mobility therapy in the treatment of acute respiratory failure. *Crit Care Med*. 2008;36:2238–2243.
17. Moss M, Nordon-Craft A, Malone D, et al. A randomized trial of an intensive physical therapy program for patients with acute respiratory failure. *Am J Respir Crit Care Med*. 2016;193(10):1101–1110.
18. Pandharipande P, Cotton BA, Shintani A, et al. Motoric subtypes of delirium in mechanically ventilated surgical and trauma intensive care unit patients. Intensive *Care Med*. 2007;33:1726–1731.

19. Pandharipande P, Cotton BA, Shintani A, et al. Prevalence and risk factors for development of delirium in surgical and trauma intensive care unit patients. *J Trauma.* 2008;65:34–41.
20. Pandharipande PP, Morandi A, Adams JR, et al. Plasma tryptophan and tyrosine levels are independent risk factors for delirium in critically ill patients. *Intensive Care Med.* 2009;35:1886–1892.
21. Maldonado JR. Neuropathogenesis of delirium: review of current etiologic theories and common pathways. *Am J Geriatr Psychiatry.* 2013;21(12):1190–1222.
22. Pandharipande PP, Pun BT, Herr DL, et al. Effect of sedation with dexmedetomidine vs lorazepam on acute brain dysfunction in mechanically ventilated patients: the MENDS randomized controlled trial. *JAMA.* 2007;298:2644–2653.
23. Pandharipande PP, Sanders RD, Girard TD, et al. Effect of dexmedetomidine versus lorazepam on outcome in patients with sepsis: a priori–designed analysis of the MENDS randomized controlled trial. *Crit Care.* 2010;14:R38.
24. Pandharipande P, Shintani A, Peterson J, et al. Lorazepam is an independent risk factor for transitioning to delirium in intensive care unit patients. *Anesthesiology.* 2006;104:21–26.
25. Riker RR, Shehabi Y, Bokesch PM, et al. Dexmedetomidine vs midazolam for sedation of critically ill patients: a randomized trial. *JAMA.* 2009;301:489–499.
26. Djaiani G, Silverton N, Fedorko L, et al. Dexmedetomidine versus Propofol Sedation Reduces Delirium after Cardiac Surgery: A Randomized Controlled Trial. *Anesthesiology.* 2016;124(2):362–368.
27. Su X, Meng ZT, Wu XH, et al. Dexmedetomidine for prevention of delirium in elderly patients after non-cardiac surgery: a randomised, double-blind, placebo-controlled trial. *Lancet.* 2016;388(10054):1893–1902.
28. Schweickert WD, Pohlman MC, Pohlman AS, et al. Early physical and occupational therapy in mechanically ventilated, critically ill patients: a randomised controlled trial. *Lancet.* 2009;373:1874–1882.

CHAPTER 4

PAIN MANAGEMENT IN THE INTENSIVE CARE UNIT

Lane Crawford and Brinda B. Kamdar

1. Do critically ill patients require analgesia?

   Intensive care unit (ICU) patients experience pain from underlying medical conditions, noxious stimuli, surgery, and trauma. Insertion and maintenance of monitoring and therapeutic devices (venous and arterial catheters, chest tubes, drains, and endotracheal tubes) and routine bedside care (dressing changes, repositioning, physical therapy, and airway suctioning) may also cause pain and discomfort in ICU patients.

2. What are the main challenges of pain management in critically ill patients?

   Maximizing patient comfort and minimizing adverse effects of treatment strategies can be a difficult balance to achieve in this often frail population. Oversedation has negative consequences such as increasing risk of delirium, thromboembolism, impairment of bowel function, and the need for prolonged ventilatory support. Conversely, undertreatment of acute pain can lead to hypermetabolism, increased oxygen consumption, hyperglycemia, and impaired wound healing as well as long-term consequences such as posttraumatic stress disorder and debilitating chronic pain syndromes.

3. Is pain relief generally adequate in ICU patients?

   The degree of analgesia in critically ill patients is often inadequate. The incidence of moderate to severe pain in both medical and surgical ICU patients has been reported as 50% or higher. In a recent study by Schelling et al., greater than 80% of recently discharged cardiac surgery patients reported pain as the most common traumatic memory of their ICU experience. Undertreatment may be a result of an impaired ability to detect and assess pain in patients who are unable to communicate, as well as difficulty managing competing clinical goals of preserving end-organ function and maintaining hemodynamic stability.

4. How can pain be assessed in critically ill patients?

   Pain should be assessed and documented at regular intervals. Physiologic measures such as heart rate, blood pressure, diaphoresis, and respiratory rate should not solely be relied upon to assess pain as they are not consistent indicators of pain. For patients who are able to communicate, self-report is optimal given the multidimensional and subjective nature of pain. Chanques and colleagues prospectively compared five different self-report pain intensity scales and found the visually enlarged 0 to 10 Numerical Rating Scale (NRS-V) to be the most reliable and preferred pain assessment tool in the critically ill population. Younger patients' pain is assessed by using the faces scale (Fig. 4.1), which is a modified visual analog scale. For nonverbal patients, observational pain scales, such as the Behavioral Pain Scale (BPS) and the Critical-Care Pain Observational Tool (CPOT), are validated and reliable methods for pain assessment. These scales rely on observation of body movements, facial expressions, and compliance with the ventilator.

5. Is pain harmful?

   Through activation of the stress response, pain can result in a series of deleterious physiologic, immunologic, and neuroendocrine effects. Physiologically, the activation of the sympathetic nervous system can lead to hemodynamic changes such as tachycardia, hypertension, and increased myocardial work. An increase in catecholamines can lead to arteriolar vasoconstriction potentially impairing tissue perfusion and wound healing. The neuroendocrine response includes the release of catabolic hormones such as cortisol and glucagon which can promote muscle wasting, hyperglycemia, and impaired immunity. Pain after thoracic or upper abdominal surgery induces an acute restrictive respiratory defect (reflex muscle rigidity, splinting, loss of functional residual capacity) resulting in impaired cough, atelectasis, and pneumonia. Pain can also lead to immobility promoting venous stasis and thrombosis as well as contribute to the development of delirium, which is increasingly recognized as a contributor to poor outcomes and even long-term cognitive dysfunction.

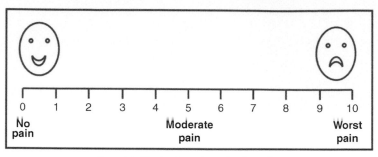

Figure 4-1. Visual analog and numeric rating scales.

6. What are the treatment options for a critically ill patient in pain?
   - **Nonpharmacologic treatment** of pain includes proper positioning of patients, stabilization of fractures, elimination of irritating physical stimulation, attention to bowel/bladder care, and environmental modification such as attention to temperature control and light to promote comfort. Because sleep deprivation as well as anxiety and delirium may diminish the pain threshold, it is important to minimize stimuli that can disturb the normal diurnal sleep pattern (noise, artificial light) and to treat anxiety and delirium promptly. Other behavioral modalities such as relaxation and music therapy may also be employed as opioid-sparing, safe techniques.
   - **Pharmacologic treatment** of pain works by inhibition of the release of local mediators in damaged tissue (nonsteroidal antiinflammatory drugs [NSAIDs], acetaminophen), blocking nerve conduction (regional anesthesia), or altering pain neurotransmission in the central nervous system (opioids, acetaminophen, ketamine, dexmedetomidine).

7. What is the role of opioids in the ICU, and how do they act?
   Opioids are the mainstay of analgesic therapy in the ICU. Long-standing familiarity has fostered relative safety of their use. They are mainly effective against visceral pain of a static nature but relatively ineffective against somatic and dynamic pain; analgesic efficacy tends to dissipate once movement including out-of-bed mobilization and respiratory therapy maneuvers are instituted.

   The term *opioid* refers to any agent with activity at an opioid receptor. There are at least four discrete opioid receptors in the central and peripheral nervous system; the analgesic effects of opioids are mediated mostly via mu (μ) or kappa (κ) receptors. These are G protein–coupled receptors that mediate inhibition of adenyl cyclase.

8. Which opioids are recommended for routine administration in ICU patients?
   Morphine, fentanyl, hydromorphone, and remifentanil are the opioids most commonly recommended for use in the ICU (Table 4.1).

9. How do you decide which opioid to use?
   Appropriate selection of an opioid requires knowledge of the drug's pharmacologic profile including plasma half-life, active metabolites, and adverse effects. Formulating a therapeutic plan often involves balancing comfort to hemodynamic, respiratory, and end-organ goals of care.

   Morphine is a naturally occurring, relatively hydrophilic opioid with a long clinical history and therefore familiarity with its use. The onset of action is slow (effect site equilibration time 15–30 minutes), and duration of action is 2 to 4 hours. The primary metabolism of morphine occurs in the liver, where it undergoes rapid glucuronidation to several metabolites, the most potent being morphine-6-glucuronide. Caution must be taken in patients with renal insufficiency as accumulation of these metabolites can lead to prolonged respiratory depression.

   Fentanyl is a synthetic, potent, and highly lipid-soluble opioid. The lipid solubility is responsible for the rapid onset of action (effect site equilibration time 1–3 minutes), making it a preferable analgesic in the acutely distressed patient. Fentanyl has a short duration of action (30–45 minutes after one bolus); however, repeated dosing may cause accumulation and prolonged action (long context-sensitive half-life). Cardiovascular side effects are minimal.

   Hydromorphone is a semisynthetic opioid that is approximately 5 to 7 times more potent than morphine and has a lipid solubility between morphine and fentanyl. Compared with morphine, its

Table 4-1. Pharmacology of Opioid Analgesics in the Adult Intensive Care Unit[a]

	RELATIVE POTENCY	BOLUS DOSE (IV)	PLASMA HALF-LIFE (H)	CONTINUOUS DOSE (MG/H; IV)	COMMENT
Morphine	1	2–4mg	2–4	2–10	Histamine release. Accumulation of active metabolite (morphine-6-glucuronide), especially in renal insufficiency
Fentanyl	80–100	25–100 mcg	2–4	0.025–0.4	Marked accumulation of parent drug after prolonged infusion
Hydromorphone	5–7	0.2–1 mg	2–3	0.5–3	More potent alternative to morphine
Remifentanil	100–300	NA	3–10 min	0.025–0.2 mcg/kg/min	Hydrolysis by plasma esterases. May cause dose-dependent bradycardia and hypotension
Meperidine[b]	0.1	12.5–50 mg	2.5–4	NA	Effective for treatment of shivering. Accumulation of active, neuroexcitatory metabolite (normeperidine), especially in renal insufficiency. Not to be used with monoamine oxidase inhibitors
Methadone	1	2.5–5 mg (with cautious repeat dosing every 8–12 h)	9–87	NA	May accumulate with repeated dosing causing sedation. May cause QT prolongation.

[a]Doses are approximate for a 70-kg adult patient.
[b]Not recommended for routine use in ICU patients.
IV, Intravenous; NA, not applicable.

onset and duration of action are slightly shorter (effect site equilibration time 10–20 minutes, duration of action 1–3 hours). Hydromorphone is metabolized in the liver and produces the metabolite hydromorphone 3-glucuronide. Metabolite accumulation can occur in patients with renal dysfunction and lead to neuroexcitatory effects such as myoclonus and restlessness.

Remifentanil is a potent ultra-short-acting opioid with the unique pharmacokinetic properties of a rapid predictable onset of action (<3 minutes) as well as a very short context-sensitive half-life (3–10 minutes) even with prolonged infusions. It is metabolized by plasma and tissue esterases, thus providing a potential benefit in patients with hepatic or renal failure. Remifentanil has similar side effects as other opioids as well as a characteristic dose-dependent hypotension and bradycardia. Though a large 2009 meta-analysis did not suggest an improvement in mortality with its use in the ICU, remifentanil may reduce the time to extubation after cessation of sedation and have potential benefits in patients with multi-organ failure.

10. What is the role of methadone in the ICU?
    Methadone is a long-acting mu-opioid agonist with antagonistic properties at the N-methyl-D-aspartate (NMDA) receptor, as well as serotonin reuptake inhibitory activity. These unique properties, as well as

its excellent oral bioavailability and lack of active metabolites, make it a useful drug in the treatment of neuropathic pain as well as in acute and chronic pain states. Methadone has been increasingly used in the ICU setting to facilitate ventilatory weaning as well as to prevent withdrawal symptoms and allodynia in patients with opioid tolerance. However, these benefits must be weighed carefully in the setting of significant adverse reactions associated with methadone. Methadone has a highly variable half-life which, in the hands of the inexperienced clinician, can lead to oversedation and respiratory depression. Electrocardiogram (ECG) monitoring is important given that methadone prolongs the QT interval (time between ventricular depolarization and repolarization) and can induce torsades de pointes ventricular arrhythmia. Finally, methadone is metabolized by the hepatic cytochrome P-450 system, and a risk exists for drug interactions and accumulation after repeated dosing.

11. Which opioids should be avoided in the ICU for routine analgesia?
    - *Mixed agonist-antagonists* (e.g., nalbuphine) are useful in the treatment of opioid-related itching when used in small doses. Larger doses may antagonize other opioids and precipitate a withdrawal syndrome in patients in whom tolerance or dependence has developed.
    - *Meperidine* is useful in the treatment of postoperative shivering and has been demonstrated to be superior to morphine and fentanyl for this indication. A small intravenous (IV) dose of 12.5 to 50 mg is usually sufficient. Postoperative shivering can increase oxygen consumption and may be detrimental if it occurs in patients with ischemic heart disease. However, meperidine is not recommended for repetitive use in ICU patients because its active metabolite normeperidine may cause central nervous system excitation and it has interactions with antidepressants (contraindicated with monoamine oxidase inhibitors, best avoided with selective serotonin reuptake inhibitors).
    - *Codeine* is an opiate prodrug that requires conversion to morphine for its analgesic activity. Given the variability of metabolism depending on genetics, its effects are not predictable, and it is therefore not a suitable treatment drug in this setting.

12. How are opioids most commonly administered for acute pain management in the ICU?
    The IV route is most common because enteral medications are often contraindicated or poorly absorbed in critically ill patients. Regional hypoperfusion due to shock or edema may render the absorption of opioids less reliable via the subcutaneous and intramuscular routes. IV opioids can be delivered in three different modes:
    - *IV bolus injections* are often used for moderate to severe pain that is episodic in nature. Analgesia is prompt, but relatively brief.
    - *Continuous IV infusions* may be considered in clinical situations in which moderate to severe pain is constant or poorly controlled with repeated boluses. In the patient that is not ventilator-dependent, use of this modality requires vigilant respiratory monitoring.
    - *Patient-controlled analgesia (PCA)* is the preferred modality in conscious, cooperative patients with moderate to severe pain.

13. Explain the concept of PCA
    PCA consists of a programmable pump that allows the patient to self-administer IV opioid as needed, within the bounds of dosing limits set by the physician. The doses with PCA are smaller and more frequent than the doses with intermittent nurse-administered boluses. This allows patients to achieve a "steady state" of analgesia with less fluctuation in their level of pain control over time. PCA minimizes the risk of oversedation and respiratory depression because if patients become sedated, they are unable to self-administer further opioid. The following parameters can be set on a PCA pump:
    - *Bolus dose* (dose administered when the patient pushes the button)
    - *Lockout interval* (minimum length of time between two doses)
    - *Maximum hourly dose*
    - *Basal rate* (continuous infusion in addition to the boluses)
      Any IV analgesic may be administered by PCA, but the most commonly used agents are morphine, hydromorphone, and fentanyl.

14. Why should you avoid routinely prescribing basal rate infusions by PCA?
    Adding a continuous opioid infusion to a PCA regimen bypasses the intrinsic safety feature of bolus-only PCA by allowing opioid to be continuously delivered even if sedation is excessive. Studies have demonstrated that surgical patients treated with PCA plus continuous infusion have no improvement in analgesia, but have a significantly greater number of side effects compared with patients receiving bolus-only PCA. Basal rates are best reserved for the treatment of severe refractory pain in very opioid-tolerant patients.

Table 4-2. Side Effects of Opioid Analgesics

Central nervous system	Miosis Euphoria, dysphoria, sedation, delirium Tolerance, dependence, hyperalgesia
Pulmonary	Respiratory depression Muscle rigidity (especially highly lipid-soluble opioids)
Cardiovascular	Bradycardia, hypotension
Gastrointestinal	Nausea, emesis Constipation, ileus
Urogenital	Urinary retention Antidiuretic hormone release (water retention)
Other	Histamine release: flushing, tachycardia, hypotension, bronchospasm Pruritus

15. What are the side effects of opioids? (See Table 4.2.)
    - Opioids can cause *sedation* and *delirium* especially when used in vulnerable patients such as the critically ill, or in conjunction with other central nervous system (CNS)-depressant or psychotropic agents.
    - Although seldom a problem in the euvolemic patient, opioids can cause *hypotension* through reduction in sympathetic tone or histamine release. The latter is more frequent with morphine than with other opioids.
    - Opioids cause central *respiratory depression* by blunting the ventilatory response to elevated arterial carbon dioxide tension. They can also cause hypoventilation or apnea from upper airway obstruction, especially in patients with obstructive sleep apnea. Large bolus doses of opioid may cause muscle rigidity that can impair respiration even in mechanically ventilated patients.
    - Opioid-induced *nausea and vomiting* is common and can be a barrier to progression of enteral feeding. *Decreased gastrointestinal motility* is common in the ICU. Etiologies include splanchnic hypoperfusion, intestinal wall edema, postoperative ileus, lack of enteral feeding, and pain. Opioids exacerbate this problem by causing increased gastrointestinal smooth muscle tone, decreased peristalsis, and increased anal sphincter tone through stimulation of peripheral mm-receptors in the myenteric plexus. Judicious use of laxative, prokinetic, and antiemetic agents is essential whenever opioids are administered. Peripheral opioid antagonists such as methylnaltrexone may be used to treat severe opioid-induced constipation, but are contraindicated in the setting of mechanical bowel obstruction.
    - With increasing duration of opioid therapy, patients develop *tolerance*, often requiring escalation of opioid dose to achieve the same analgesic effect, as well as *dependence*, which places them at risk for withdrawal with cessation of therapy. *Opioid-induced hyperalgesia* (OIH) is a phenomenon in which patients become paradoxically more sensitive to painful stimuli after exposure to opioids, and can occur even after acute opioid administration. Although the mechanism of OIH is not fully understood, it seems to be more common with use of remifentanil compared to other opioids.

16. What is multimodal analgesia and what is its role in the ICU?
    Multimodal analgesia is the strategy of using a variety of analgesics with different mechanisms of action to optimize pain control while decreasing opioid use and the accompanying adverse side effects. Because ICU patients are especially susceptible to opioid-induced side effects such as sedation, delirium, and gastrointestinal dysmotility, multimodal analgesia should be employed for this population whenever possible. Common components of multimodal analgesic regimens include acetaminophen, NSAIDs, neuropathic agents, epidural analgesia, and nerve blocks. Acetaminophen and NSAIDs have been shown to decrease the need for opioids and are particularly effective in reducing muscular and skeletal pain, as well as pain from pleural or pericardial rubs which responds poorly to opioids. Many postsurgical or trauma patients may have a component of neuropathic pain, for which agents such as gabapentin may be useful. Basic pharmacology is summarized in Table 4.3.

17. What are the side effects of nonopioid analgesics?
    - **Acetaminophen** is potentially hepatotoxic, especially in patients with depleted glutathione stores. Therefore acetaminophen should be avoided in acute liver failure, and the drug dosage

Table 4-3. Pharmacology of Selected Nonopioid Analgesics in the Adult Intensive Care Unit

	DOSE RECOMMENDATIONS	HALF-LIFE (H)	COMMENT
Acetaminophen	PO: 325–650 mg every 4–6 h IV: 500–1000 mg every 6–8 h	2–3	Maximum dose ≤4 g daily. Use with caution in hepatic impairment
Ibuprofen	PO: 400–800 mg every 4–6 h	2	Maximum dose 3200 mg daily. Use with caution in renal impairment
Ketorolac	IV: 15–30 mg every 6 h	2–9	Avoid >5 days use. Reduce dose if age >65 or renal impairment
Gabapentin	PO: 300–1200 mg every 8 h	5–7	Reduce dose in renal impairment
Dexmedetomidine	IV infusion: 0.2–0.7 mcg/kg/h	2–3	May cause hypotension or bradycardia at high doses
Ketamine	IV bolus: 0.1–0.5 mg/kg IV infusion: 1–5 mcg/mg/min	2.5	Sympathomimetic and psychotropic effects are common

IV, Intravenous; *PO*, oral.

should be reduced in the elderly and in patients with a significant history of alcohol intake or poor nutritional status.

- **NSAIDs** may cause bleeding as a result of platelet inhibition, gastrointestinal side effects such as ulcers and bleeding, and acute kidney injury (AKI). Risk factors for the development of AKI are patient age, preexisting renal impairment, hypovolemia, and shock. The prolonged use of NSAIDs should be avoided. For example, it has been shown that ketorolac administration for ≥5 days has been associated with a two-fold increased risk of AKI. NSAIDs should be used with caution in patients with asthma.
- *Gabapentin* may cause sedation, cognitive changes, and painful peripheral neuropathy. It is renally excreted and dose reduction is recommended in renal impairment.

18. What are the advantages of dexmedetomidine?
Dexmedetomidine is a highly selective intravenous α_2-agonist that causes sedation and analgesia without respiratory depression. As such it is useful in patients with obstructive sleep apnea or pulmonary disease, or for patients being weaned from mechanical ventilation. Recent research demonstrates a reduction in ventilator days and possibly delirium with dexmedetomidine compared to other sedatives. Although an initial loading dose can be given prior to starting a maintenance infusion, caution is advised in the critically ill patient given its tendency to produce bradycardia and hypotension.

19. How should ketamine be used in the ICU?
Ketamine is a phencyclidine derivative which at various doses causes potent analgesia, sedation, or anesthesia, primarily by NMDA antagonism. Unlike opioids, it does not cause respiratory depression and in fact has bronchodilatory properties. Ketamine's sympathomimetic effects make it a useful option in hypotensive patients, though it can still cause hypotension through myocardial depression in catecholamine-depleted patients. Because ketamine increases cerebral blood flow and metabolic rate, it has traditionally been avoided in patients for whom increases in intracranial pressure would be detrimental (e.g., acute brain injury). Recent studies, however, have failed to validate this concern. Ketamine has psychomimetic effects that can manifest as delirium, hallucinations, or psychosis. Although these effects can be attenuated with gradual dose titration and benzodiazepines, ketamine is best avoided in patients with a history of psychosis or high risk of delirium. In the ICU, ketamine can be used in IV boluses to enhance tolerance of brief but painful procedures such as dressing changes, or as a continuous infusion for analgesia.

20. When should epidural analgesia or nerve blocks be considered for ICU patients?
- Infusion of local anesthetic through an epidural catheter can provide excellent analgesia to the chest, abdomen, pelvis, and lower extremities after surgery or trauma. Benefits of epidural analgesia versus systemic opioid analgesia include superior pain control, decreased incidence

of pulmonary, cardiac, and thromboembolic complications, and improved gastrointestinal motility. It may also provide a mortality benefit in some populations, such as patients with multiple rib fractures. As such, epidural analgesia should be strongly considered for patients undergoing major thoracic or abdominal surgery, or patients with trauma to the chest wall.
- Nerve blocks involve injection or continuous infusion of local anesthetic around peripheral nerves and can be used for opioid-sparing analgesia of a limb or the trunk when epidural analgesia is not possible.
- Infusions for epidural analgesia or nerve block usually consist of a dilute local anesthetic such as 0.1% to 0.125% bupivacaine or ropivacaine. A small amount of opioid (e.g., hydromorphone 10 to 20 mcg/mL) may be added to epidural infusions to augment analgesia.

21. What are the risks of epidural analgesia in ICU patients?
- The most feared complication of epidural analgesia is epidural hematoma, which can require emergency surgery to avoid permanent spinal cord damage. As such, epidural analgesia is contra-indicated in the setting of significant medical or pharmacologic coagulopathy, both of which are common in the ICU. Epidurals may be used safely in patients receiving prophylactic anticoagulation within certain parameters. Practitioners are strongly advised to follow the most recent guidelines of the American Society of Regional Anesthesia and Pain Medicine (www.asra.com) and to monitor closely for new neurologic deficits when utilizing epidural analgesia for any patient who has been receiving anticoagulants. If low-dose unfractionated heparin is being used, needle placement and/or catheter removal should be done ≥2 hours after discontinuing heparin, and reheparinization may be started ≥1 hour after an uncomplicated epidural insertion. If fractionated low-molecular-weight heparin (LMWH) is being used in prophylactic doses, a waiting period of ≥12 hours for any neuraxial technique should be applied after the last dose of LMWH, and the next LMWH dose should be given ≥2 hours after an uncomplicated procedure.
- Due to the risk of infectious complications such as epidural abscess and meningitis, epidural analgesia is contraindicated in ICU patients with infection at the site of catheter insertion, and is probably best avoided in patients with bacteremia or severe immunocompromise.
- Because epidural analgesia causes sympathectomy, it may not be tolerated in hemodynamically unstable patients.
- In adult patients, epidural placement is usually performed with the patient awake or lightly sedated so that the patient can report early symptoms of local anesthetic toxicity, intrathecal placement, or nerve injury. In the ICU however, many patients require deeper sedation that precludes this safety measure. Epidural placement in these patients is controversial, and requires careful risk-benefit analysis by the provider.

ACKNOWLEDGMENT

The authors wish to acknowledge Drs. Philip McArdle, MB, BCh, BAO, FFARCSI, and Jean-François Pittet, MD, for the valuable contributions to the previous edition of this chapter.

KEY POINTS: PAIN MANAGEMENT IN THE INTENSIVE CARE UNIT

1. Adequate analgesia in the critically ill patient is necessary because of the following:
   a. Patient comfort, ethical aspects
   b. Attenuation of potentially deleterious physiologic responses to pain
      i. Sympathetic activation
      ii. Increased myocardial oxygen consumption
      iii. Persistent catabolism
      iv. Hypercoagulability
      v. Immunosuppression
2. Opioids are a mainstay of analgesia in the ICU, but can cause adverse side effects including sedation, respiratory depression, and gastrointestinal dysmotility.
3. Multimodal analgesia is the strategy of using a variety of analgesics with different mechanisms of action to optimize pain control while decreasing the requirement for opioids and the accompanying adverse side effects.
4. Epidural analgesia should be considered for patients with major surgery or trauma of the chest, abdomen, or lower extremities.

BIBLIOGRAPHY

1. Barr J, Fraser GL, Puntillo K, et al. Clinical practice guidelines for the management of pain, agitation, and delirium in adult patients in the intensive care unit. *Crit Care Med.* 2013;41:263-306.
2. Bonnet F, Marret E. Influence of anaesthetic and analgesic techniques on outcome after surgery. *Br J Anaesth.* 2005;95:52-58.
3. Chanques G, Viel E, Constantin JM, et al. The measurement of pain in intensive care unit: comparison of 5 self-report intensity scales. *Pain.* 2010;151:711-721.
4. Chou R, Gordon DB, de Leon-Casasola OA, et al. Management of Postoperative Pain: A Clinical Practice Guideline from the American Pain Society, the American Society of Regional Anesthesia and Pain Medicine, and the American Society of Anesthesiologists' Committee on Regional Anesthesia, Executive Committee, and Administrative Council. *J Pain.* 2016;17(2):131-157.
5. Domino EF. Taming the ketamine tiger. 1965. *Anesthesiology.* 2010;113:678-684.
6. Elefritz JL, Murphy CV, Papadimos TJ, Lyaker MR. Methadone analgesia in the critically ill. *J Crit Care.* 2016;34:84-88.
7. Erstad BL, Patanwala AE. Ketamine for analgosedation in critically ill patients. *J Crit Care.* 2016;35:145-149.
8. Jacobi J, Fraser GL, Coursin DB, et al. Clinical practice guidelines for the sustained use of sedatives and analgesics in the critically ill adult. *Crit Care Med.* 2002;30:119-141.
9. Lee M, Silverman SM, Hansen H, Patel VB, Manchikanti L. A comprehensive review of opioid-induced hyperalgesia. *Pain Physician.* 2011;14(2):145-161.
10. Mehta S, McCullagh I, Burry L. Current sedation practices: lessons learned from international surveys. *Crit Care Clin.* 2009;25:471-488.
11. Pöpping DM, Elia N, Van Aken HK, et al. Impact of epidural analgesia on mortality and morbidity after surgery: systematic review and meta-analysis of randomized controlled trials. *Ann Surg.* 2014;259(6):1056-1067.
12. Rijkenberg S, Stilma W, Endeman H, Bosman RJ, Oudemans-van Straaten HM. Pain measurement in mechanically ventilated critically ill patients: behavioral pain scale versus critical-care pain observation tool. *J Crit Care.* 2015; 30(1):167-172.
13. Riker RR, Shehabi Y, Bokesch PM, et al. Dexmedetomidine vs midazolam for sedation of critically ill patients: a randomized trial. *JAMA.* 2009;301:489-499.
14. Schelling G, Richter M, Roozendaal B, et al. Exposure to high stress in the intensive care unit may have negative effects on health-related quality-of-life outcomes after cardiac surgery. *Crit Care Med.* 2003;31:1971-1980.
15. Tan JA, Ho KM. Use of remifentanil as a sedative agent in critically ill adult patients: a meta-analysis. *Anaesthesia.* 2009;64:1342-1352.

ETHICS AND PALLIATIVE CARE

Caitlin Baran and Prema R. Menon

CHAPTER 5

1. What is palliative care?
   Palliative care is support provided by an interdisciplinary team that focuses on relief of suffering in the physical, emotional, and spiritual domains of health.

2. Name the elements of palliative care that are important in the care of critically ill patients.
   - Communication skills
   - Decisional support
   - Prognostication
   - Symptom management
   - Psychosocial and spiritual support
   - Decisions to withhold or withdraw
   - End-of-life care

3. How can palliative care be utilized in the intensive care unit (ICU)?
   There are two main models for ICU-palliative care integration: The *consultative* model focuses on increasing the involvement and effectiveness of palliative care consultants in the care of ICU patients and their families, particularly those patients with highest risk of death or morbidity. The *integrative* model embeds palliative care principles and interventions into daily practice by the ICU team for all patients and family members dealing with critical illness.

4. Describe the *shared decision-making* paradigm.
   The key to the shared decision-making (SDM) paradigm is communication. Both parties share information: the clinician offers options and describes their risks and benefits, and the patient/surrogate expresses their preferences and values. Each participant is armed with a better understanding of the relevant factors and shares responsibility in the decision about how to proceed.

5. What is a goals-of-care discussion?
   The discussion begins with the patient or surrogate decision maker and the medical team having a shared understanding of the patient's goals of medical therapy. The physician must then also provide a medical prognosis and possible outcomes. With this information, the patient or surrogate can provide information on his or her treatment preferences. The patient values can then be the primary driver of the goals of medical care, weighing burdens of treatments with likelihood of positive benefits or outcomes to make a care plan. Goals are fluid and can change on the basis of the medical condition and prognosis. It is essential to establish the goals of treatment before discussing new treatment options.

6. What are the goals of the ICU family conference?
   - Begin to understand the patient's values.
   - Gain an understanding of the patient's previous functional status.
   - Exchange medical information between the patient, family, and the medical team.
   - Engage in complicated medical decision-making.
   - Make medical recommendations based upon the patient's values, acceptable states of health, and their current medical situation.
   - Provide emotional support to families.

7. How can we improve communication around goals of care?
   Effective strategies to improve decision-making about goals of care are clustered around five themes: patient and family factors, communication between healthcare providers and patients, inter-professional collaboration, education, and resources. Identifying patient and family factors that might inhibit SDM and ensuring communication, collaboration, education, and resources are key steps to improving communication.

8. What are the steps of a family meeting?
   - Pre-meeting
     - Invite family members and care team members. Arrange a time and location.
     - Discuss among team members to reach consensus on goals of the meeting, medical condition, prognosis, and treatment options.
   - Introductions
     - Identify family, team members, roles, and goals of the meeting.
   - Perceptions
     - Ask family members what they hope to have addressed in the meeting.
     - Ask what the family members know about the illness and what they expect or hope for.
   - Explain
     - Provide medical information about condition, prognosis, and treatment options, as well as best and worst-case scenario.
     - Explain aspects of surrogate decision-making.
   - Exploration
     - Elicit questions, concerns, and the patient's values, and explore how these influence decisions.
   - Empathize
     - Recognize the difficult time a family is passing through.
   - Recommendation
     - Provide medical guidance based on stated goals and values and the clinician's professional knowledge and experience.
   - Summary
     - Review goals, medical plan, next steps, and follow-up.

9. What questions can be asked of a surrogate decision maker to help elicit patient values and goals?
   - *Help me understand how things were for your father before he got this sick. What did he enjoy doing? What things are most important to the quality of his life? Is there an outcome or quality of life that would not be acceptable to him?*
   - *If your loved one were here listening to this conversation, what would she be thinking or saying?*
   - *Did your loved one ever talk about his wishes if he were to get sicker and were nearing the end of his life?*

10. Are there components of the family meeting associated with better outcomes?
    Yes. Studies have identified specific elements of family meetings that are associated with increased quality of care, decreased negative psychological symptoms during bereavement, and improved family satisfaction with communication. See Table 5.1.

11. What communication tool has been shown to be beneficial in improving communication in the ICU family meeting?
    Incorporating the **VALUE** mnemonic has been shown to significantly reduce family symptoms of anxiety, posttraumatic stress disorder, and depression measured 3 months after the patient's death:
    - **V**alue what the family says.
      - *"As I listen to you, it sounds like the most important things are x, y, etc."*

Table 5-1. Components of Family Meetings Associated with Better Outcomes

Family meeting within 72 h of ICU admission
Healthcare providers listen more, speak less
Make empathic statements
Make statements of non-abandonment and support for decision-making
Explore patient values and treatment preferences
Explaining principles of surrogate decision-making
Reassure that the patient will be comfortable and not suffer

Modified from Curtis J, White D. Practical guidance for evidence-based ICU family conferences. *Chest.* 2008;134:835-843.

- **A**cknowledge expressed emotions.
  - *"I can see you are concerned about x." "It's hard to deal with all this."*
- **L**isten.
- **U**nderstand the patient as a person.
  - *"What brings John joy?"*
- **E**licit family questions.
  - *"What other questions can I answer for you?" "Does what we have talked about make sense so far?"*

12. What tools can be used to defuse conflicts?
    - Notice the conflict
      - Recognize any of the irritation, anger, or disconnect you might feel.
    - Find a non-judgmental starting point
      - Recognize what the real topic is, rather than the emotions around it. *"I feel like we are talking about the medical options from here" or "I sense we are talking about how hard it is to be in this situation."*
    - Listen to their story first
    - Identify what the conflict is about and recognize it as a shared interest
      - *"I think we are all interested in ensuring that we do right by [the patient]."*
    - Brainstorm options
      - *"Would it be okay to talk about the options and pros and cons of each?"*
    - Seek an option the recognizes interests of all parties
      - *"Perhaps we could consider continuing on this path and monitoring for x over the next x hours/ days and using this to understand if we are moving in the right direction."*
    - Recognize some conflicts cannot be resolved

13. Do palliative care interventions improve outcomes in the ICU?
    Although improved communication in the ICU has shown to lessen the burden of bereavement and may reduce length of stay and costs, there are no data to support early palliative care involvement in the ICU improves mortality or satisfaction with care. There has been no evidence of harm from any intervention.

14. What is the role of the social worker in the ICU?
    Social workers play a critical role in supporting patients and families in the ICU by providing communication, counseling, and assisting with practical needs. When coordinating a family meeting, they can help families anticipate what will be discussed, help clarify their questions for the medical team, and provide emotional support during and after the meeting.

15. What if clinicians disagree with the patient or surrogate?
    After additional clarification of values, goals, prognosis, and treatment options, both parties can try to persuade the other and/or seek common ground. A time-limited trial of continued therapy, followed by reassessment, may bring about resolution. Consider additional supportive services from second-opinion consultations, social services, chaplaincy, ethics consultation, psychiatry, and/or palliative care.

16. What if there is no surrogate decision maker for the patient?
    Gather as much information as possible about the person to best understand the patient's story, lifestyle, functional status, and values. Consider contacting neighbors, work colleagues, clergy, community members, primary care providers, and other outside healthcare providers. Use the information gained to approximate a *substituted judgment* to supplement the "best interests" standard to make decisions. Ethics consultation and advice from hospital legal counsel may be required to complement the plans devised by the attending physician and ICU team.

17. How can dying and end-of-life planning be discussed when prognosis is ambiguous but concerning?
    When recovery is not possible, it can be hard to find the words to convey this in a clear, supportive, and empathetic manner. This involves delivering bad news and reframing hope for what goals can be accomplished. Experts recommend truthful prognostic disclosure, emotional support, tailoring the disclosure strategy to each family's needs, and checking for understanding. In addition, stakeholders (patient, healthcare workers, and other communication experts) suggest showing families radiographic images (to help them "see" the prognosis themselves), not using numeric estimates to convey prognosis, and considering prognostic communication to be an iterative process that is mentioned even early in an ICU stay as a potential outcome.

18. How should the clinician discuss stopping or withholding life-supporting treatments when recovery is not possible?

When goals transition to providing comfort at end of life and the decision is made to stop life-prolonging treatments, family members can feel burdened that decisions they make are the cause of death. They also may worry that stopping or withholding treatments may cause suffering. It is important for providers to be clear that it is the underlying disease that causes death. Clinicians must be ready to provide support for the decisions made and take time to explain in detail how comfort is assessed and maintained.

Although we can't control the disease, we can treat the symptoms of the disease and help Jane feel as comfortable as possible with the time she has left. And when she is at the end of her life, we can assure that she will pass peacefully, comfortably, and on her own terms.

19. Give an example of how you would describe the process of stopping or withholding life-supporting treatments to family members/loved ones.

Unfortunately we have reached the point where John cannot recover, and his life is coming to an end no matter what decisions we make today. Would it be helpful for you to know how we would care for John if the goals of his medical care shifted to focus on comfort and allowing a peaceful death? That would mean that we would aggressively treat pain, anxiety, and shortness of breath with medications like morphine, that once we were sure he was comfortable we would remove the breathing machine, and that we would allow his life to come to an end from his lung disease as peacefully as possible.

20. What is spirituality?

The 2009 Consensus Conference on Quality of Spiritual Care defined spirituality as *"the aspect of humanity that refers to the way individuals seek and express meaning and purpose and the way they experience their connectedness to the moment, to self, to others, to nature, and to the significant or sacred."* (p. 887)

21. Why is understanding and discussing spirituality important in the ICU?

Family members and clinicians consider spirituality an important dimension of end-of-life care. Supporting the expression of various forms of spirituality during the dying process in the ICU can improve the overall experience with death and dying.

22. How should the clinician discuss spiritual and religious issues?

Spiritual support is a fundamental pillar of palliative care. Most patients want their physicians to ask about their religious and spiritual beliefs, though many practitioners feel uncomfortable doing so. Some patients and families may base their preferences for starting or stopping treatment on their religious or spiritual beliefs.

23. What tool has been shown to be an effective and feasible framework for a clinical spiritual assessment?

FICA is as follows.
- **F**aith, belief, meaning
  - *Is spirituality, faith, or religion an important part of your life?*
  - *Do you have spiritual beliefs that help you cope with stress?*
  - *What gives your life meaning?*
- **I**mportance and influence
  - *What role do your beliefs play in your healthcare decisions?*
- **C**ommunity
  - *Are you part of a religious or spiritual community?*
  - *Is this helpful to you and how?*
- **A**ddress in care
  - *How would you like your healthcare providers to use this understanding of your beliefs as they care for you?*

24. What are indicators of spiritual or existential distress?

When facing a life-threatening illness, individuals can experience great distress in psychological, spiritual, and existential domains. Indicators of existential or spiritual suffering include statements of meaninglessness, hopelessness, and guilt. Helpful responses to spiritual or existential distress are statements that acknowledge the pain, provide a nonjudgmental supportive presence, and bear witness to the patient and family. Hospital chaplains are specially trained to provide this type of therapeutic support irrespective of specific faith or belief system of the patient or family member.

25. What is clinical futility?

American Thoracic Society (ATS)/American Association of Critical-Care Nurses (AACN)/American College of Chest Physicians (ACCP)/European Society of Intensive Care Medicine (ESICM)/Society of Critical Care

Medicine (SCCM) issued a recent consensus statement recommending the use of the term "potentially inappropriate" rather than "futile" to describe treatments that clinicians believe have some chance of accomplishing what the patient/surrogate wants but the clinicians believe that competing ethical considerations do not justify providing them. The reasons for this are twofold: First, the word "inappropriate" conveys more clearly than "futile" or "ineffective" that the assertion made by clinicians is based on technical medical expertise and a value-laden claim, not just a technical judgment. Second, the word "potentially" signals the judgments that are preliminary and require review before being acted on.

26. **How do you approach a conflict regarding "potentially inappropriate" treatments?**
    The consensus statement recommends the following approach to manage such cases:
    - Enlist expert consultation to continue negotiation during the conflict resolution process
    - Give notice of the process to surrogates
    - Obtain a second medical opinion
    - Obtain review by an interdisciplinary hospital committee
    - Offer surrogates the opportunity to transfer the patient to an alternate institution
    - Inform surrogates of the opportunity to pursue extramural appeal
    - Implement the decision of the resolution process

27. **How do you manage conflict during time-pressured situations (i.e., urgency of clinical scenario does not allow for above resolution process to occur)?**
    In situations like this, a temporizing treatment plan should be initiated and should not include the requested treatment. Before refusing the treatment, (1) pause to evaluate facts and moral blind spots (Table 5.2), and (2) try to engage other clinicians to ensure consensus. Finally, explain to the surrogates the reasons for refusing to administer the requested treatment. Remember to (1) base judgments on best understanding of professional obligations, (2) have a high degree of certainty that the treatment requested is outside the boundaries of practice, and (3) only enact this strategy if you cannot carry out the entire resolution process above.

28. **How prevalent is conflict in ICUs and what causes conflict?**
    Over 70% of ICU workers report perceived conflicts with over 50% considered as "severe" yet preventable with improved communication. The most common sources of conflict were lack of psychological support (in end-of-life care), absence of staff meeting, and problems with the decision-making process. Factors associated with conflicts include: working more than 40 hours/week, more than 15 ICU beds, caring for dying patients, perception of symptom control, and no routine unit-level meetings.

29. **List means to lessen or resolve moral distress and intra-team or team-family conflicts.**
    Proactive family meetings, open visitation, family presence on rounds, respect of cultural norms, routine unit-level meetings, staff debriefings, collaborative care, spiritual support, relieving patients' distressing symptoms, ethics consultation, and integration of palliative care principles and practices into the ICU.

30. **How can an ethics consultation help in the ICU? Ethics consultations can:**
    - Clarify areas that need elucidation
    - Identify and name the ethical issues
    - Help discern a good process for arriving at decisions
    - Identify relative guidance from policy, literature, and/or case precedent
    - Help formulate justifications for courses of action
    - Help caregivers address moral distress

Table 5-2. Questions to Assist in Understanding Moral Issues in Time-Sensitive Situations

Am I certain this treatment is OUTSIDE of the boundaries of accepted practice?
Am I willing to have my decision-making rationale publicly reviewed in a court?
What are the consequences to the patient, family member/surrogate, team, and institution?
Am I sure that my decision is based on the clinical situations alone (i.e., not related to sex, race, ability to pay, etc.)?

Modified from Bosslet GT, Pope TM, Rubenfeld GD, et al. An official ATS/AACN/ACCP/ESICM/SCCM policy statement: responding to requests for potentially inappropriate treatments in ICUs. *Am J Respir Crit Care Med.* 2015;191(11):1318-1330.

31. Have *ethics interventions* been shown to reduce ICU length of stay or improve other ICU quality indicators?

    Yes. A large multicenter randomized controlled trial of ethics consultation in the ICU showed mitigation of treatment conflicts and, for non-survivors, reduced ICU length of stay by 1.44 days, days of ventilator use by 1.7 days, hospital length of stay by 2.95 days, and costs (range of savings: $3000–$40,000). These reductions were achieved without altering mortality between the intervention and control groups.

32. What is the difference between acceptable end-of-life care in the ICU and active euthanasia?

    Good end-of-life care in an ICU involves focusing on comfort (physical, psychosocial, and spiritual) while withholding or withdrawing life sustaining therapies (LST) from a patient. The focus is on achieving relief of distressing symptoms and on foregoing burdensome therapies.

    On the other hand, the goal of active euthanasia is the death of the patient. Practitioners of active euthanasia usually also intend the comfort of the patient, but one of the means they use to achieve that goal is by killing the patient. Many persons note an ethical difference between "letting die" and "killing."

33. Why is the administration of narcotics and sedatives during the terminal withdrawal of LSTs not considered active euthanasia?

    It is not considered active euthanasia when doses are titrated "to effect," with the intent being the relief of particular distressing symptoms. The foreseen but unintended consequences of lowering blood pressure or slowing respirations are ethically acceptable if it is clear, from the titrating of doses, that the intention is palliation. Such dosing is justifiable under the "doctrine of double effect." One multicenter study found that palliative sedation did not shorten life when used to relieve refractory symptoms in dying patients. However, when doses are given with the intent to cause death, it is considered active euthanasia.

34. My patient has a "Do Not Attempt Resuscitation (DNR)" status, yet needs surgery. Do we need to make him or her "full code" for the operating room?

    No or maybe. It depends on what the patient's goals of care are, what he or she hopes to achieve from the surgery, and what the patient has delineated as unacceptable outcomes. Although a patient's severity of illness may be the reason a patient is not considered for a surgical intervention, it is unethical to deem a person unable to receive surgery or procedures due to their DNR status alone. Thus a thorough discussion must occur before the surgery in the context of discussing the expected benefits and risks of the procedure in light of the patient's condition, values, hopes, fears, and reasonable goals.

ACKNOWLEDGMENT

The authors wish to acknowledge Drs. Alexandra F.M. Cist, MD, Ursula McVeigh, MD, and Allan Ramsay, MD, for the valuable contributions to the previous edition of this chapter.

KEY POINTS: ETHICS AND PALLIATIVE CARE

1. Palliative care focuses on the relief of suffering of patients and helps to relieve surrogate and healthcare provider burden.
2. The foundation of quality end-of-life care in the ICU is early, high-quality, and iterative communication.
3. Structured and thoughtful family meetings help ensure a continued shared-decision making process throughout an ICU stay.
4. Ethics consultations help relieve moral distress and intra-team and team-family conflict.
5. Doctrine of double effect is when the foreseen but unintended consequences of potential death are ethically acceptable if it is clear that the intent of utilizing sedative/analgesic medication is palliation of symptoms.

BIBLIOGRAPHY

1. Alaskson RA, Curtis JR, Nelson JE. The changing role of palliative care in the ICU. *Crit Care Med.* 2014;42(11): 2418-2428.
2. Alaskson R, Cheng J, Vollenweider D, Galusca D, Smith TJ, Pronovost PJI. Evidence-based palliative care in the intensive care unit: a systematic review of interventions. *J Palliat Med.* 2014;17(2):219-235.

3. Anderson WB, Cimino JW, Ernecoff NC, et al. A Multicenter study of key stakeholders' perspectives on communicating with surrogates about prognosis in ICUs. *Ann Am Thorac Soc.* 2015;12(2):142-152.

4. Azoulay E, Timsit JF, Sprung CL, et al. Prevalence and factors of intensive care unit conflicts: the conflicus study. *Am J Respir Crit Care Med.* 2009;180:853-860.

5. Back A, Arnold R, Tulsky J. *Mastering communication with seriously ill patients.* New York: Cambridge Press; 2009:21-137.

6. Borneman T, Ferrell B, Puchalski CM. Evaluation of the FICA tool for spiritual assessment. *J Pain Symptom Manage.* 2010;40:163-173.

7. Bosslet GT, Pope TM, Rubenfeld GD, et al. An Official ATS/AACN/ACCP/ESICM/SCCM policy statement: responding to requests for potentially inappropriate treatments in ICUs. *Am J Respir Crit Care Med.* 2015;191(11):1318-1330.

8. Charles C, Gafni A, Whelan T. Shared decision-making in the medical encounter: what does it mean? *Soc Sci Med.* 1997;44:681-692.

9. Curtis J, White D. Practical guidance for evidence-based ICU family conferences. *Chest.* 2008;134:835-843.

10. Kyremanteng K, Gagnon LP, Thavorn K, Heyland D4, D'Egidio G. The impact of palliative care consultation in the ICU on length of stay: a systematic review and cost evaluation. [published online ahead of print August 31, 2016]. *J Intensive Care Med.* 1-8. DOI: 10.1177/0885066616664329.

11. Lautrette A, Darmon M, Megarbane B, et al. A communication strategy and brochure for relatives of patients dying in the ICU. *N Engl J Med.* 2007;356(5):469-478.

12. Maltoni M, Pitturi C, Scarpi E, et al. Palliative sedation therapy does not hasten death: results from a prospective multicenter study. *Ann Oncol.* 2009;20(7):1163-1169.

13. McCormick AJ, Engelberg R, Curtis JR. Social workers in palliative care: assessing activities and barriers in the intensive care unit. *J Palliat Med.* 2007;10:929-937.

14. Nelson JE, Bassett R, Boss RD, et al. Models for structuring a clinical initiative to enhance palliative care in the ICU: a report from the IPAL-ICU Project. *Crit Care Med.* 2010;38(9):1765-1772.

15. Roze des Ordons AL, Sharma N, Heyland DK, You JJ. Strategies for effective coals of care discussions and decision-making: perspectives from a multi-centre survey of Canadian hospital-based health car providers. *BMC Palliat Care.* 2015;14:38.

16. Schneiderman LJ, Gilmer T, Teetzel HD, et al. Effect of ethics consultations on nonbeneficial life-sustaining treatments in the intensive care setting: a randomized controlled trial. *JAMA.* 2003;290:1166-1172.

17. Swinton M, Giacomini M, Toledo F, et al. Experiences and expressions of spirituality at the end of life in the ICU. *Am J Respir Crit Care Med.* 2017;195(2):198-204.

18. White DB, Curtis JR. Establishing and evidence base for physician-family communication and shared decision making in the ICU. *Crit Care Med.* 2006;34(9):2500-2501.

19. White D, Curtis JR, Wolf LE, et al. Life support for patients without a decision maker: who decides? *Ann Intern Med.* 2007;147:34-40.

CHAPTER 6

FLUID THERAPY

Elizabeth Cox Williams and Keith Baker

1. How is water distributed throughout the body?

   Total body water comprises 60% of body weight in males and 50% of body weight in females. The distribution of this water is 40% in the intracellular space (30% in females because of larger amounts of subcutaneous tissue and smaller muscle mass) and 20% in the extracellular space. The extracellular fluid is broken down into 15% interstitial and 5% plasma. Total body water decreases with age; 75% to 80% of a newborn infant's weight is water.

2. What are sensible and insensible fluid losses? How are maintenance fluid requirements calculated?
   - Insensible losses (nonmeasurable)
     - Skin: 600 mL
     - Lungs: 200 mL
   - Sensible losses (measurable)
     - Fecal: 200 mL
     - Urine: 800 to 1500 mL
     - Sweat: Variable

       These losses account for 2000 to 2500 mL/day, giving a 24-hour fluid requirement of 30 to 35 mL/kg to maintain normal fluid balance.

3. What are fluid maintenance requirements for children?

   Twenty-four-hour fluid requirements for children have been formulated on the basis of weight:
   - **4:2:1 rule:**
     - **4** mL/kg/h for the first 10 kg
     - **2** mL/kg/h for the next 10 kg
     - **1** mL/kg/h for every kilogram after that

   EXAMPLE: For a 34-kg child:

   $$(4 \text{ mL/kg} * 10 \text{ kg}) + (2 \text{ mL/kg} * 10 \text{ kg}) + (1 \text{ mL/kg} * 14 \text{ kg}) = 40 + 20 + 14 = 74 \text{ mL/h}$$

4. Describe the clinical features of volume deficit and volume excess.
   - Deficits (low volume)
     - Central nervous system: decreased mentation in severe cases
     - Cardiovascular: tachycardia, hypotension (in later stages)
     - Skin: decreased turgor in subacute volume loss
   - Excesses (volume overload)
     - Distended neck veins
     - Pulmonary edema
     - Peripheral edema

5. What are the classes of hemorrhagic shock, and what fluid should be administered in each class? See Table 6.1.

6. What is the 3:1 rule in fluid therapy after acute blood loss?

   Three milliliters of crystalloid are given for each milliliter of blood loss. This ratio compensates for administered crystalloid that is lost into the interstitial space. While this is a starting dose, most patients need further resuscitation to restore normovolemia. See Chapter 54 for description of blood replacement in patients who require massive transfusions (greater than 10 U of packed red blood cells).

7. What empiric replacement fluids can be used for fluid losses?
   - **Sweat:** 5% dextrose (D_5) {1/4} normal saline solution with 5 KCl/L
   - **Gastric, colon:** D_5 {1/2} normal saline solution with 30 KCl/L

Table 6-1. Severity of Hemorrhagic Shock for a 70-Kilogram Adult

	I	II	III	IV
Blood loss (mL)	<750	750–1500	1500–2000	>2000
Blood loss (% BV)	<15	15–30	30–40	>40
Pulse rate (beats/min)	<100	>100	>120	>140
Blood pressure	Normal	Normal	Decreased	Decreased
Respiratory rate (respirations/min)	14–20	20–30	30–40	>35
Urine output (mL/h)	>30	20–30	5–15	Negligible
CNS symptoms	Normal	Anxious	Confused	Lethargic
Resuscitation fluid	LR	LR	LR + blood	LR + blood

BV, Blood volume; CNS, central nervous system; LR, lactated Ringer's solution.

- **Bile, pancreas, small bowel:** lactated Ringer's solution
- **Third space (interstitial loss):** lactated Ringer's solution

8. What is the difference between crystalloids and colloids? Give examples of each.
   - **Crystalloids:** Crystalloids are mixtures of sodium chloride and other physiologically active ionic solutes. The distribution of sodium will determine the distribution of the infused crystalloid. Examples are normal saline solution, lactated Ringer's solution, and hypertonic saline solution.
   - **Colloids:** Colloids contain high-molecular-weight molecules that stay in the vascular space and exert an oncotic force. Examples are albumin, dextran, and fresh frozen plasma (FFP).

9. Describe the composition of normal saline and lactated Ringer's solution. Which should be used for acute resuscitation?
   Table 6.2 summarizes the composition of normal saline and lactated Ringer's solution. Lactated Ringer's solution is preferable for acute volume replacement because normal saline solution can result in hyperchloremic metabolic acidosis.

10. What evidence-based data exist to support the use of various resuscitation fluids?
    - **Lactated Ringer's solution:** This remains the least expensive and best fluid for trauma resuscitation.
    - **Albumin and other colloids:** No evidence from randomized controlled trials exists to demonstrate that resuscitation with colloids reduces the risk of death, pulmonary edema, or hospital stay compared with resuscitation with crystalloids in patients with trauma or burns, or after surgery. Because colloids are more expensive, it is difficult to justify their continued use in this setting.
    - **Hypertonic saline solution:** The only benefit is shown in patients with head trauma and cerebral edema causing elevated intracranial pressure.

ACKNOWLEDGMENT

The editors gratefully acknowledge the contributions of James E. Wiedeman, MD, and Mark W. Bowyer, MD, DMCC, COL, USAF, MC, authors of this chapter in prior editions.

Table 6-2. Composition of Crystalloids

FLUID	NA (MMOL/L)	CL (MMOL/L)	K (MMOL/L)	CA (MG/DL)	LACTATE (MMOL/L)	PH
Normal saline solution	154	154	—	—	—	6.0
Lactated Ringer's solution	130	109	4	3	28	6.5

KEY POINTS: FLUID THERAPY

1. Total body water is 60% of body weight (40% intracellular and 20% extracellular). Blood volume is 70 mL/kg.
2. Diagnose volume deficit or excess by clinical examination, not laboratory study results.
3. Avoid fluid and electrolyte abnormalities by measuring and replacing ongoing gastrointestinal losses with appropriate fluids.
4. Use lactated Ringer's solution for acute volume resuscitation.
5. There is no proven benefit to colloid over crystalloid in acute resuscitation.

BIBLIOGRAPHY

1. Roberts I, Blackhall K, Alderson P, Bunn F, Schierhout G. Human albumin solution for resuscitation and volume expansion in critically ill patients. *Cochrane Database Syst Rev.* 2011;(11):CD001208. doi:10.1002/14651858. CD001208.pub4.
2. Fan E, Stewart TE. Albumin in critical care: SAFE but worth the salt? *Crit Care.* 2004;8:297-299.
3. Perel P, Roberts I, Ker K. Colloids versus crystalloids for fluid resuscitation in critically ill patients. *Cochrane Database Syst Rev.* 2013;(2):CD000567. doi:10.1002/14651858.CD000567.pub6.

CHAPTER 7

NUTRITION IN CRITICALLY ILL PATIENTS

Renee D. Stapleton

1. **Why is nutrition therapy in critical illness important?**
   Critical illness is most often accompanied by a catabolic stress state in which patients demonstrate a systemic inflammatory response, hypermetabolism, multiple organ dysfunction, infectious complications, and malnutrition. Malnutrition is associated with impaired immunologic function and increased morbidity and mortality in acutely ill patients. Therefore, nutrition therapy is important to attempt to improve patient outcomes.

2. **What are the goals of nutritional therapy in critically ill patients?**
   Over the past 15 to 20 years, there has been a shift away from the concept of nutrition *support*, where nutrition was provided as a fuel to support patients during a time of critical illness, toward the concept of nutrition *therapy,* where nutritional interventions are focused on modulating the immunologic and inflammatory response of critical illness. Therefore the generally accepted goals of nutritional delivery in critically ill patients are to:
   - Provide nutritional therapy consistent with the patient's condition
   - Prevent nutrient deficiencies
   - Avoid complications related to delivering nutrition
   - Improve patient outcomes

3. **How should the nutritional status of critically ill patients be assessed?**
   Nutritional status assessment in critically ill patients is difficult. For many years, albumin, prealbumin, and anthropometric measurements were used to assess nutritional status. However, these are inaccurate in critical illness because of fluid resuscitation and the acute phase response. The new 2016 American Society for Parenteral and Enteral Nutrition (A.S.P.E.N.) and Society of Critical Care Medicine (SCCM) *Guidelines for the Provision and Assessment of Nutrition Support Therapy in the Adult Critically Ill Patient* recommend using either the Nutrition Risk in the Critically Ill (NUTRIC) Score (Fig. 7.1) or the Nutritional Risk Score (NRS-2002) for nutrition risk assessment, as nonrandomized studies have found that critically ill patients at higher nutritional risk are more likely to benefit from enteral nutrition (EN) initiated early.

4. **What mode of feeding (enteral or parenteral) should be initiated in critically ill patients?**
   Unless an absolute contraindication to EN exists (such as ischemic bowel or bowel obstruction), EN should be initiated preferentially over parenteral nutrition (PN). Several randomized controlled trials (RCTs) have compared EN with PN in critically ill patients with an intact gastrointestinal (GI) tract. When these studies were aggregated in a meta-analysis, no difference in survival was seen. However, EN may be associated with reductions in infectious complications, and it is less expensive than PN. Evidence also suggests that lack of use of the GI tract rapidly results in atrophy of gut luminal mucosa, which may lead to bacterial translocation across the gut wall and into the systemic circulation. Even small amounts of, or trophic, EN increase blood flow to the gut, preserve GI epithelial structures, and maintain villous height. EN also improves immune function by supporting gut-associated lymphoid tissue. EN is therefore recommended over PN unless the patient has an absolute contraindication to enteral feeding (discussed later).

5. **When should enteral nutrition be initiated in critically ill patients?**
   Early EN is usually defined as initiating enteral feedings within 48 hours of intensive care unit (ICU) admission. Many small RCTs have compared early EN versus delayed nutrient intake in critically ill patients receiving mechanical ventilation, and, when these results were aggregated in meta-analyses, early EN was associated with a trend toward mortality reduction and a significant reduction in infectious complications. Starting EN early does not seem to affect the duration of mechanical ventilation or ICU length of stay. The presence of bowel sounds and the passage of flatus are not necessary before the institution of EN.

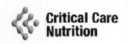

Critical Care Nutrition

NUTRIC Score

The NUTRIC Score is designed to quantify the risk of critically ill patients developing adverse events that may be modified by aggressive nutrition therapy. The score, of 1 to 10, is based on 6 variables that are explained below. The scoring system is shown in Tables 1 and 2

NUTRIC Score variables

Variable	Range	Points
Age	<50	0
	50–<75	1
	≥75	2
Acute Physiology and Chronic Health Evaluation (APACHE) II score	<15	0
	15–<20	1
	20–28	2
	≥28	3
Sequential Organ Failure Assessment (SOFA) score	<6	0
	6–<10	1
	≥10	2
Number of Comorbidities	0–1	0
	≥2	1
Days from hospital to ICU admission	0–<1	0
	≥1	1
Interleukin (IL)-6	0–<400	0
	≥400	1

NUTRIC Score scoring system: if IL-6 available

Sum of points	Category	Explanation
6-10	High Score	• Associated with worse clinical outcomes (mortality, ventilation). • These patients are the most likely to benefit from aggressive nutrition therapy.
0-5	Low Score	• These patients have a low malnutrition risk.

NUTRIC Score scoring system: if no IL-6 available*

Sum of points	Category	Explanation
5-9	High Score	• Associated with worse clinical outcomes (mortality, ventilation). • These patients are the most likely to benefit from aggressive nutrition therapy.
0-4	Low Score	• These patients have a low malnutrition risk.

* It is acceptable to not include IL-6 data when it is not routinely available; it was shown to contribute very little to the overall prediction of the NUTRIC score.

Figure 7-1. Assessing nutritional risk with the NUTRIC Score. (From Heyland DK, Dhaliwal R, Jiang X, Day AG. Identifying critically ill patients who benefit the most from nutrition therapy: the development and initial validation of a novel risk assessment tool. *Crit Care.* 2011;15(6):R268. Available from: http://criticalcarenutrition.com/resources/nutric-score.)

6. How many calories should critically ill patients receive?

Energy expenditure varies with age, sex, body mass, and type and severity of illness. During critical illness, total energy expenditure (TEE) can be measured with indirect calorimetry. However, in clinical practice, resting energy expenditure (REE) is usually estimated by using a variety of available equations and is then multiplied by a *stress factor* of 1.0 to 2.0 to estimate TEE (and therefore caloric requirements). Roughly 25 kcal/kg ideal body weight is often the standard practice, and other equations, such as Harris-Benedict, Ireton-Jones, and Weir, are commonly used (Table 7.1). Unfortunately, predictive equations tend to be inaccurate. The optimal amount of calories to provide critically ill patients is unclear, given the paucity of existing data. New guidelines recommend that patients with high nutrition risk assessed by either the NUTRIC score (Fig. 7.1) or the Nutritional Risk Score [NRS-2002] receive more calories; those at lower risk may not benefit from more calories during their first week in the ICU.

7. What should be the composition of enteral nutrition in critically ill patients?

Few data are available to inform the macronutrient composition of enteral feedings. In general, critically ill patients should receive an amount of protein daily between 1.5 and 2.0 g/kg of ideal body weight, and emerging evidence suggests that receiving more protein, rather than total calories, may be associated with improved patient outcomes. The use of whole protein, or polymeric, formulas is recommended because insufficient data exist to support the routine use of peptide-based formulas in most patients. In most enteral formulas, approximately 25% to 30% of calories are from fat. Similar to the situation with protein, evidence in the literature is insufficient to support the routine use of high-fat or low-fat enteral formulas. In some ICU populations, specific enteral formulas are recommended (discussed later). For example, formulas containing arginine are often considered in patients who have had elective surgery, trauma, or traumatic brain injury, but should not be used in patients with sepsis. Specific formulas designed for patients with renal failure are also available.

8. Should critically ill patients in shock and/or receiving vasopressors receive enteral nutrition?

Ischemic bowel is a very rare complication of EN but has been reported in critically ill patients and can be fatal. Therefore the general recommendation is that EN be avoided in patients who are in shock and in those patients in whom resuscitation is active, vasopressors are being initiated, or vasopressor doses are increasing. Once patients are resuscitated and hemodynamically stable, EN may be initiated, even if they are receiving stable lower doses of vasopressors. However, special attention should be paid to signs of enteral feeding intolerance such as abdominal distention or vomiting.

Table 7-1. Examples of Predictive Equations for Resting Energy Expenditure in Critical Illness

Harris-Benedict	Men: [66.5 + (13.8 × AdjBW) + (5 × Ht) - (6.8 × Age)] × 1.3 Women: [655 + (9.6 × AdjBW) + (1.8 × Ht) - 4.7 × Age)] × 1.3
Owen	Men: 879 + (10.2 × ActBW) Women: 795 + (7.2 × ActBW)
Mifflin	Men: 5 + (10 × ActBW) + (6.25 × Ht) - (5 × Age) Women: 161 + (10 × ActBW) + (6.25 × Ht) - (5 × Age)
Ireton-Jones equation for obesity	Men: 606 + (9 × ActBW) - (12 × Age) + 400 (if ventilated) + 1400 Women: ActBW - (12 × Age) + 400 (if ventilated) + 1444
Ireton-Jones for patients with mechanical ventilation	Men = 2206 - (10 × Age) + (5 × ActBW) + 292 (if trauma) + 851 (if burn) Women = 1925 - (10 × Age) + (5 × ActBW) + 292 (if trauma) + 851 (if burn)
25 kcal/kg	BMI <25: ActBW × 25 BMI ≥25: IBW × 25

ActBW, Actual body weight = weight on admission (kilograms); *AdjBW*, adjusted body weight = ideal body weight + 0.4 (actual body weight - ideal body weight); *BMI*, body mass index; *Ht*, height (centimeters); *IBW*, ideal body weight = 50 + 2.3 per inch >60 inches (men), 45.5 + 2.3 per inch >60 inches (women).

9. Should gastric or small-bowel enteral nutrition be used?

   EN can be delivered through an intragastric gastric (nasogastric or orogastric) or postpyloric (either in the duodenum or jejunum) feeding tube. Enteral tubes may also be surgically placed. Each option has risks and benefits. In patients who have endotracheal tubes in place, nasal tubes can increase the risk of sinusitis. Intragastric feeding tubes can be placed at the bedside, and their position can be immediately confirmed radiographically (it is not sufficient to assess placement with auscultation alone). However, successful placement of a small-bowel feeding tube at the bedside varies from 11% to 93%, depending on technique and operator experience. The use of endoscopy or fluoroscopy for postpyloric feeding tube placement can cause delays in initiating enteral feeding. In a meta-analysis of gastric versus small-bowel feeding in ICU patients, small-bowel feeding was not found to be associated with any improvement in survival but was associated with a reduction in infections, particularly pneumonia. Therefore the routine use of small-bowel enteral feeding is recommended when possible. However, in many ICUs, obtaining access to the small bowel may be logistically difficult and expensive if fluoroscopy or endoscopy is needed. In ICUs where obtaining small-bowel access is less feasible, small-bowel feedings should be considered for patients showing signs of intolerance to intragastric feeding (see later) or at high risk for aspiration (e.g., must remain in supine position).

10. Should enteral nutrition be delivered continuously or in boluses?

    Continuous feeding delivers a small amount of feeding formula continuously over a 24-hour period, whereas bolus feeding delivers a large volume of formula over a short period of time. Because one pseudorandomized study found that aggressive early EN via bolus feeding was harmful, it is generally thought that bolus feeding is less safe than continuous feeding. However, a paucity of evidence is available on this topic.

11. How should enteral feeding tolerance be monitored?

    Patients should be monitored frequently (e.g., every 4–6 hours) for tolerance of EN, especially in the first few days after initiating enteral feedings. This monitoring should include an assessment of pain (often difficult in critically ill patients), abdominal distention, stooling, and vomiting. New guidelines recommend that gastric residual volumes (GRVs) should no longer be measured, as three prospective studies (including two RCTs) have demonstrated that checking GRVs provides no clinical benefit to patients.

12. How should critically ill patients be positioned during enteral feeding?

    Two prior randomized trials have compared semirecumbent with supine positioning in ICU patients. In one study (Drakulovic et al., 1999), the incidence of pneumonia was significantly reduced in patients in the semirecumbent position. The other study (van Nieuwenhoven et al., 2006) did not achieve the target positioning and did not find a reduction in infections. On the basis of these limited data, it is recommended that critically ill patients have the head of their beds raised to 30 to 45 degrees.

13. Should motility agents be used in critically ill patients?

    The use of motility agents is recommended when clinically feasible, especially in patients with signs of enteral feeding intolerance. Motility agents, including erythromycin or metoclopramide, have been found to improve gastric emptying and tolerance of EN but do not seem to change outcomes in critically ill patients. In one study, administration of enteral naloxone (to reverse the side effects of opioid narcotics on the GI tract) resulted in an increased volume of EN infused, decreased GRVs, and decreased incidence of ventilator-associated pneumonia.

14. Should feeding protocols be used in intensive care units?

    Nurse-driven feeding protocols that include early rapid startup of enteral feeding, goal infusion rate, and directions for when to stop and start feedings increase the percentage of goal calories administered. In an effort both to start enteral feedings in the critically ill patient early and to provide an amount of calories close to goal, especially in patients with higher nutrition risk, feeding protocols should be implemented.

15. When is enteral nutrition contraindicated?

    Contraindications to EN include conditions that lead to a nonfunctioning GI tract, such as ischemic bowel, intestinal obstruction, severe malabsorption, and severe short gut syndrome. In general, pancreatitis, enterocutaneous fistulae, and recent GI surgery are not contraindications to enteral feeding.

16. What are some complications of enteral feeding, and how can they be minimized?

    EN is not without risks, and complications can be categorized as GI, mechanical, or metabolic.
    - **GI complications** include diarrhea, nausea, vomiting, constipation, aspiration, and ischemic bowel. Decreased gastric motility occurs in a majority of critically ill patients, and therefore nausea and

vomiting with resultant aspiration are not uncommon. These can be minimized with semirecumbent positioning, placement of a small-bowel feeding tube, and continuous rather than bolus enteral feeding (discussed earlier). Ileus also commonly occurs in a critical care setting, often as a result of opioid administration, and can be treated with small doses of oral naloxone that do not affect the analgesia of opioids. Diarrhea is common in the ICU and may be due to antibiotics or other medications. If diarrhea develops in a patient receiving EN, infectious causes (i.e., *Clostridium difficile*) should first be ruled out. If those tests are negative, stool-bulking agents such as banana flakes can be administered. Alternative strategies to decrease diarrhea include increasing soluble fiber intake or changing to another enteral formula.

- **Mechanical complications** include obstruction of the feeding tube with medications; erosion of the feeding tube into nasal or gastric mucosa with risk of bleeding, infection, or perforation; accidental insertion of the feeding tube into the pulmonary tree with risk of injury; displacement of the tube with risk of aspiration; and sinusitis. To minimize these complications, tubes should be soft and well lubricated for insertion, and tube position should always be verified radiographically before use (auscultation over the stomach alone is not adequate).
- **Metabolic complications** include hyperglycemia, electrolyte derangements, and overfeeding. Monitoring of blood glucose and electrolytes can detect these and lead to appropriate changes in feedings. If overfeeding is a concern, a metabolic cart (indirect calorimetry) can be performed to measure TEE.

17. When should parenteral nutrition be used in critically ill patients?

Three recent high-impact RCTs have found that using PN as a supplement to EN offers no benefits to critically ill patients, and may even be harmful. EN is the preferred method of delivering nutrition therapy in critically ill patients, and measures such as placing a small-bowel feeding tube and starting motility agents should be used in patients who have signs of intolerance to enteral feedings before considering initiating PN. The recent A.S.P.E.N.-SCCM Guidelines recommend that PN be considered in the following two circumstances:

- After 7 to 10 days of hospitalization in critically ill patients who are not malnourished and who have a lower nutritional risk, but in whom enteral feeding has not been feasible or who have only received a fraction of goal calories.
- On admission in critically ill patients who are malnourished, who have higher nutritional risk, and in whom enteral feeding is not feasible.

  Given these recommendations, very few patients in a medical ICU should need PN.

18. What are some complications of parenteral nutrition?

- **Mechanical complications** in patients receiving PN include those related to the catheter used for delivery of PN, such as pneumothorax and venous thromboembolism.
- **Metabolic complications** from PN include hyperglycemia and electrolyte abnormalities. Hyperglycemia can be treated with an appropriate insulin protocol for hyperglycemia associated with critical illness.
- **Infectious complications** from parenteral feeding include central line–associated bloodstream infection and sepsis.
- **Hepatobiliary complications.** PN can occasionally cause elevated hepatic transaminase, alkaline phosphatase, and bilirubin levels, as well as steatosis (i.e., fatty liver), and acalculous cholecystitis may result.

19. Should critically ill patients receive pharmaconutrients or specialized feeding formulas?

- **Antioxidants:** Based on low-quality evidence, new guidelines for the provision of nutrition in critically ill adults recommend administration of antioxidants (such as vitamins E and C) and minerals (such as selenium, zinc, and copper) to ICU patients, especially those with burns or trauma and receiving mechanical ventilation. Very few data are currently available on individual nutrients.
- **Glutamine:** Glutamine has long been felt to play a role in maintaining the integrity of the gut lumen, and prior small studies suggested that supplementation may improve outcomes in critically ill patients. However, recent high-quality evidence suggests that enteral glutamine does not benefit critically ill patients, and parenteral glutamine may even be harmful. Therefore, glutamine should not be administered to ICU patients.
- **Arginine:** Enteral feeding formulas containing arginine should be used in patients with severe trauma or traumatic brain injury, and in postoperative critically ill patients. On the basis of results from prior studies, however, patients with sepsis should not receive arginine because it has been suggested that it may increase mortality.

- **Omega-3 fatty acids:** The use of feeding formulas containing omega-3 fatty acids (fish oil) in patients with acute lung injury and sepsis remains controversial. Three prior trials comparing an enteral formula containing omega-3 fatty acids, borage oil (γ-linolenic acid [GLA]), and antioxidants with placebo found benefit. However, two additional randomized trials (one used a liquid fish oil supplement and another used a twice-daily supplement containing fish oil, GLA, and antioxidants) found no benefit. Given these conflicting data, new guidelines do not make a specific recommendation.

20. What nutrition therapy should patients with acute kidney injury receive?

    Like most other critically ill patients, patients with acute kidney injury (AKI) should receive early EN with standard amounts of protein and calories. Protein restriction should not be used to delay the initiation of dialysis. Specific enteral formulas designed for renal failure that have varying electrolyte compositions (e.g., lower phosphate or potassium) or are calorie dense (i.e., fluid restricted) can be used if needed.

21. What nutrition therapy should patients with acute pancreatitis receive?

    Early EN is now standard of care in patients with acute pancreatitis. In past decades, patients with acute pancreatitis were not allowed any enteral intake and were fed parenterally. Over the last 20 years, however, research has found that these patients have improved outcomes if they receive early EN started within 48 hours of admission, even in cases of severe acute pancreatitis. Trials have also found that outcomes in these patients are not different when they are fed gastrically versus jejunally.

22. How might propofol influence the nutritional support provided to critically ill patients?

    Propofol is a sedative commonly used in an ICU setting that is delivered as a 10% lipid emulsion and provides 1.1 kcal/mL. When patients are receiving propofol for longer periods of time (i.e., more than 3 to 4 days) or in large doses, the calories received from propofol should be taken into account in relation to the overall caloric prescription to avoid excess delivery of calories. Because propofol can also cause hypertriglyceridemia, which can lead to acute pancreatitis, serum triglyceride levels should be measured in patients receiving larger doses of propofol.

KEY POINTS: NUTRITION IN CRITICALLY ILL PATIENTS

1. EN should be used in the vast majority of ICU patients rather than PN.
2. EN should be started within 24 to 48 hours of ICU admission.
3. After patients with shock are resuscitated and hemodynamically stable, they can safely receive EN even if they are receiving stable lower doses of vasopressors.
4. In patients intolerant of EN, measures such as semirecumbent positioning and motility agents should be attempted before starting PN.
5. Patients with acute pancreatitis, even if it is severe, should receive EN, which can be delivered either gastrically or jejunally.
6. Glutamine should not be administered to critically ill patients.

BIBLIOGRAPHY

1. Arabi YM, Aldawood AS, Haddad SH, et al. Permissive Underfeeding or Standard Enteral Feeding in Critically Ill Adults. *N Engl J Med.* 2015;372:2398-2408.
2. Canadian critical care nutrition clinical practice guidelines. https://criticalcarenutrition.com/cpgs. Published May 29, 2015, Accessed January 23, 2017.
3. Casaer MP, Mesotten D, Hermans G, et al. Early versus late parenteral nutrition in critically ill adults. *N Engl J Med.* 2011;365:506-517.
4. Casaer MP, Van den Berghe G. Nutrition in the acute phase of critical illness. *N Engl J Med.* 2014;370:2450-2451.
5. Cerra FB, Benitez MR, Blackburn GL, et al. Applied nutrition in ICU patients. A consensus statement of the American College of Chest Physicians. *Chest.* 1997;111:769-778.
6. Doig GS, Simpson F, Sweetman EA, et al. Early parenteral nutrition in critically ill patients with short-term relative contraindications to early enteral nutrition: a randomized controlled trial. *JAMA.* 2013;309:2130-2138.
7. Drakulovic MB, Torres A, Bauer TT, et al. Supine body position as a risk factor for nosocomial pneumonia in mechanically ventilated patients: a randomised trial. *Lancet.* 1999;354:1851-1858.
8. Harvey SE, Parrott F, Harrison DA, et al. Trial of the route of early nutritional support in critically ill adults. *N Engl J Med.* 2014;371:1673-1684.

9. Heidegger CP, Berger MM, Graf S, et al. Optimisation of energy provision with supplemental parenteral nutrition in critically ill patients: a randomised controlled clinical trial. *Lancet.* 2013;381:385-393.
10. Khalid I, Doshi P, DiGiovine B. Early enteral nutrition and outcomes of critically ill patients treated with vasopressors and mechanical ventilation. *Am J Crit Care.* 2010;19:261-268.
11. McClave SA, Taylor BE, Martindale RG, et al. Guidelines for the Provision and Assessment of Nutrition Support Therapy in the Adult Critically Ill Patient: Society of Critical Care Medicine (SCCM) and American Society for Parenteral and Enteral Nutrition (A.S.P.E.N.). *JPEN J Parenter Enteral Nutr.* 2016;40:159-211.
12. Nicolo M, Heyland DK, Chittams J, et al. Clinical outcomes related to protein delivery in a critically ill population: a multicenter, multinational observation study. *JPEN J Parenter Enteral Nutr.* 2016;40:45-51.
13. Reignier J, Mercier E, Le Gouge A, et al. Effect of not monitoring residual gastric volume on risk of ventilator-associated pneumonia in adults receiving mechanical ventilation and early enteral feeding: a randomized controlled trial. *JAMA.* 2013;309:249-256.
14. Rice TW, Wheeler AP, Thompson BT, et al, NHLBI ARDS Clinical Trials Network. Enteral omega-3 fatty acid, gamma-linolenic acid, and antioxidant supplementation in acute lung injury. *JAMA.* 2011;306:1574-1581.
15. Stapleton RD, Martin TR, Weiss NS, et al. A phase II randomized placebo- controlled trial of omega-3 fatty acids for the treatment of acute lung injury. *Crit Care Med.* 2011;39:1655-1662.
16. van Nieuwenhoven CA, Vandenbroucke-Grauls C, van Tiel FH, et al. Feasibility and effects of the semirecumbent position to prevent ventilator-associated pneumonia: a randomized study. *Crit Care Med.* 2006;34:396-402.

CHAPTER 8

MECHANICAL VENTILATION

Daniel F. Fisher and Robert M. Kacmarek

1. What are the indications for using mechanical ventilation?
   Mechanical ventilation is used to treat apnea, acute or chronic respiratory failure, and impending acute respiratory failure. Respiratory failure can be either hypoxemic, hypercarbic, or a combination of the two. Depending on the type and severity of respiratory failure, the method of mechanical ventilatory support can be either invasive or noninvasive.

2. When to choose between invasive ventilation and noninvasive ventilation (NIV)?
   NIV should be considered if the patient is experiencing hypercarbic respiratory failure, pulmonary edema, or obstructive sleep apnea. A prime factor to consider is can the patient protect their airway. Some have recommended the use of NIV for hypoxemic respiratory failure; however, outcome data is generally poor except for acute pulmonary edema. If NIV is used in the setting of hypoxemic respiratory failure, a low threshold for accepting failure of NIV is essential. If the patient's status has not improved in 1 to 2 hours, patients with hypoxemic respiratory failure should be intubated and invasively ventilated. Invasive ventilation should always be considered if the patient is hemodynamically unstable, has failed previous NIV attempts, is worsening on NIV, or cannot protect their airway.

3. What is the difference between continuous positive airway pressure (CPAP) and bilevel positive airway pressure (BiPAP)?
   CPAP elevates the baseline pressure that patients spontaneously breathe from; no inspiratory assistance is provided. End expiratory airway pressure is maintained at the set CPAP level. This maintains alveolar recruitment and stents open the upper airway. BiPAP provides two levels of positive pressure: inspiratory pressure support and CPAP positive end expiratory pressure (PEEP). CPAP is useful for patients with congestive heart failure, obstructive sleep apnea, or atelectasis. BiPAP is useful when patients are hypoventilating and need to unload their work of breathing.

4. What is the difference between pressure and volume ventilation?
   Both are *methods* for providing ventilatory support; they describe the primary control over the delivery of gas during inspiration. During pressure ventilation, the ventilatory pressure assist is set and flow is provided to meet the patient's inspiratory demand. As a result, the patient controls their tidal volume, being capable of inhaling small or large tidal volumes. However, the set inspiratory pressure is maintained in a square wave pattern. Tidal volume (V_T) is dependent upon the impedance of the lung and chest wall, the set inspiratory airway pressure, and the effort of the patient. With pressure assist/control ventilation, airway pressure and inspiratory time are set but with pressure support, only airway pressure is set. Generally pressure-targeted modes of ventilation are better tolerated than volume-targeted modes of ventilation.

   In volume-controlled ventilation, the V_T is set and the inspiratory airway pressure is allowed to vary. With volume ventilation, the inspiratory flow pattern, maximum flow, and inspiratory time are set. As a result, in patients actively triggering the ventilator because of precise control over Volume, Flow, and Time, patient-ventilator asynchrony is common.

5. Which is better: pressure or volume ventilation?
   During controlled mechanical ventilation, both pressure and volume ventilation can be applied in a lung-protective manner; neither is better.

   During patient-triggered ventilation, the patient's active involvement in gas delivery varies the effects of pressure and volume ventilation. Volume ventilation is considered more lung protective because of tidal-volume limitation, but newer data indicates that pendelluft occurs within the lung, resulting in local overdistention. However, asynchrony is generally greater in volume ventilation than pressure ventilation because of the greater control over the variables associated with gas delivery.

   With pressure-assisted ventilation, synchrony is generally better than with volume ventilation because of less control over the variables defining gas delivery. However, many believe because tidal volume is patient-determined to a great extent with pressure ventilation, that pressure ventilation is less lung protective than volume ventilation. However, there is no definitive data indicating that any mode of ventilation has a greater effect on outcome than any other mode.

6. Is it possible and beneficial to refrain from using mechanical ventilation?

Yes, the use of high-flow nasal cannula (HFNC) in cases of hypoxemic respiratory failure has been shown to avoid the need for NIV or invasive mechanical ventilation in some situations. HFNC is the administration of heated humidified oxygen at extremely high flows (40 and 60 L/min in adults). This rapid gas movement provides a small amount of PEEP and flushes carbon dioxide from the upper airway, reducing the work of breathing. The rapid gas velocity provides a stable inspired oxygen concentration (FIO_2) because it limits air entrainment. However, the same caution that exists with NIV in hypoxemic respiratory failure exists here. If patients do not respond with a marked change in their oxygenation status and clinical presentation within 1 to 2 hours, patients should be intubated.

7. Please explain the various modes of ventilation.

During mechanical ventilation, the ventilator can be programmed to control pressure, flow, volume, or time; the greater the control by the ventilator the less control by the patient. Modes of ventilation go from complete ventilator control of gas delivery to complete patient control of gas delivery where no specific variable is machine-controlled (proportional assist ventilation [PAV] and neurally adjusted ventilatory assist [NAVA]). In addition, mode can be volume-targeted: a set tidal volume is provided each breath; or pressure targeted: a set peak airway pressure is established each breath. Modes of ventilation span a spectrum of ventilation; one end is complete machine control with no patient interaction, for example, "control modes." The opposite end is full patient control with only monitoring in effect, for example, "spontaneous modes." Within the center of this spectrum lie hybrid modes that are a mixture of full machine control and full patient control.

8. Is any mode of ventilation better than the others?

There is no data demonstrating that a specific mode of mechanical ventilation results in better outcome than another mode except regarding patient-ventilator synchrony and the use of high-frequency oscillatory ventilation. High-frequency oscillatory ventilation has been shown to result in greater mortality than conventional modes of mechanical ventilation in adult patients with acute respiratory distress syndrome (ARDS). Regarding patient-ventilator synchrony, the greater control of gas delivery provided by the ventilator, the greater the asynchrony. Volume assist/control results in the greatest amount of asynchrony, and PAV and NAVA the least amount of asynchrony.

9. What is meant by the term "patient-ventilator asynchrony"?

Patient-ventilator asynchrony refers to the phenomenon of the patient's respiratory efforts and the support provided by the ventilator not being in synchrony. Asynchrony has been defined in four categories: flow asynchrony (patient inspiratory efforts demand greater flow than provided by the ventilator), triggering asynchrony (activation of inspiration by the patient is not coordinated with the ventilator), cycle asynchrony (the patient's ending of inspiration and the ventilators ending of inspiration are not synchronous), and mode asynchrony (the modes applied increase the amount of asynchrony; Box 8.1). Managing asynchrony is important because asynchrony has been associated with increased length of mechanical ventilation and intensive care unit (ICU) stay as well as mortality. Minor adjustments of gas delivery with each patient assessment can minimize the level of asynchrony.

Box 8-1. Common Types of Patient-Ventilator Asynchrony

Trigger asynchrony—An inability to sequentially trigger a ventilator-delivered breath

    Delayed triggering—long time delay (>100 ms) between patient development of a negative airway pressure and the ventilator responding with a delivered breath

    Missed triggering—the patient's inspiratory effort fails to trigger a mechanical breath

    Double triggering—the delivery of a second mechanical breath before the patient has normally exhaled

Reverse triggering—A form of double triggering in which the delivery of a controlled mechanical breath results in the initiation of a spontaneous inspiratory effort

Flow asynchrony—The gas flow provided by the ventilator does NOT match the inspiratory demand of the patient

Cycle asynchrony—The termination of the patient's inspiratory time and the ventilator inspiratory time are not in sync

Mode asynchrony—The selection of a specific mode of ventilation is not well-tolerated by a given patient

10. **What is the most common type of patient-ventilator asynchrony?**
The most common type of patient-ventilator asynchrony is ineffective inspiratory efforts (IIE) or missed triggering. Specifically, the patient makes an inspiratory effort but the effort does not trigger a breath. IIE usually occurs when the patient's inspiratory effort starts before exhalation reaches functional residual capacity (FRC), which means that gas is still within the airway (intrinsic PEEP; $PEEP_i$). That is, the patient's effort is insufficient to overcome the $PEEP_i$ and the ventilator fails to respond to the patient effort, increasing the work of breathing and resulting in a "missed trigger."

11. **What is flow asynchrony?**
How asynchrony indicates that the ventilator's delivered gas flow is less than the patient's inspiratory flow demands, markedly increasing the patient's workload and resulting in high transpulmonary pressures potentially inducing lung injury. Flow asynchrony occurs more frequently in modes where the inspiratory flow is fixed. It is less common in modes where inspiratory flow is variable. Flow asynchronies along with double triggering are the forms of asynchrony most likely to negatively affect patient outcome.

12. **What is double triggering?**
Double triggering is the activation of a second ventilator-delivered breath before exhalation of the previous breath is complete. As a result, tidal volume is increased and in volume ventilation, peak airway pressure is increased. Double triggering along with flow asynchrony are the most potentially damaging types of asynchrony since they both tidal volume, transpulmonary pressure and driving pressure are increased, potentially inducing lung injury. If double triggering occurs in volume ventilation before the patients begin exhalation, tidal volume can be doubled. Factors that contribute to double triggering are inadequate mechanical inspiratory flow, too short mechanical inspiratory time, and decreased compliance.

13. **What is reverse triggering?**
This phenomenon was described 30 years ago and relates to the ventilator's flow stimulating the patient to make an inspiratory effort. This occurs during controlled mechanical ventilation and frequently presents in a defined pattern: one, two, or three controlled mechanical breaths followed by a patient-triggered breath. In most circumstances, the spontaneous breath is stacked on top of the controlled breath or a double-triggered type breath. Reverse triggering occurs during volume- or pressure-triggered breaths and commonly results in tidal volumes near twice the set tidal volume. The impact of the reverse triggering is the same as any double-triggered breath.

14. **What is cycle asynchrony?**
Another cause of patient ventilator asynchrony is "cycle asynchrony" in which the patient's inspiratory time and the ventilator's inspiratory time are either of different lengths or out of phase with each other. This phase imbalance results in the patient's inspiratory time being either shorter or longer than the ventilator's inspiratory time. Cycle asynchrony is most commonly identified in pressure ventilation (pressure assist/control or pressure support) and frequently can be corrected by adjustment of inspiratory termination criteria during pressure support or inspiratory time during pressure assist/control.

15. **In which modes of ventilation is asynchrony most common?**
As mentioned previously, patient-ventilator asynchrony can occur regardless of the mode. Proper adjustments to the ventilator settings can minimize the impact of asynchrony. In VCV, flow asynchrony can be lessened by using a higher peak inspiratory flow rate and a shorter inspiratory time, or perhaps a decelerating flow waveform. In PCV, asynchrony can be reduced by adjustment of inspiratory time, flow acceleration, and driving pressure. Expiratory termination criteria or inspiratory time adjustments can improve asynchrony in pressure-support ventilation and PCV, respectively. In general, the greater control the ventilator exerts over a patient's ventilator pattern, the greater the likelihood for asynchrony.

16. **What does the term *lung protective mechanical ventilation* (LPMV) mean?**
LPMV is a term used to define an approach to mechanical ventilatory support that minimizes the likelihood of inducing lung injury by the process of mechanical ventilation. The concept was originally described in patients with acute respiratory distress syndrome, but today it is a concept that is applied to all patients acutely requiring ventilatory support. It should be implemented as soon as a patient is intubated and continued until the patient is weaned from ventilatory support. The components of an LPMV strategy include the following: (1) a tidal volume of 4 to 8 mL/kg predicted body weight (PBW), (2) a plateau pressure (P_{PLAT}) of less than 28 cm H_2O, (3) a driving pressure of less than 15 cm H_2O, (4) a PEEP level that sustains the lung open at end exhalation, and (5) an FIO_2 that maintains the PaO_2 between 55 and 80 mm Hg or a SpO_2 between 88% and 95% (Box 8.2).

Box 8-2. Components of a Lung Protective Ventilatory Strategy

A tidal volume of 4–8 mL/kg predicted body weight (PBW),
    A plateau pressure of less than 28 cm H_2O,
    A driving pressure of less than 15 cm H_2O,
    A positive end expiratory pressure (PEEP) level that sustains the lung open at end exhalation
        An inspired oxygen concentration (FIO_2) that maintains the PaO_2 between 55 and 80 mm Hg or a SpO_2 between 90% and 95%.

---

17. **Why should a small tidal volume be set when ventilating a patient?**
At rest, all mammals breathe with a tidal volume of about 6 mL/kg PBW. Generally, patients requiring an acute application of ventilatory support have reduced lung volume and as a result, a tidal volume that is less than 6 mL/kg PBW with minute ventilation sustained by an increase in the respiratory rate. Randomized controlled trials have shown better survival if patients are ventilated with a tidal volume in the range of 4 to 8 mL/kg PBW than with larger tidal volumes. This range should be applied throughout the course of ventilatory support, although some patients nearing the time of extubation may demand larger tidal volume to 10 mL/kg PBW, which generally is acceptable if ventilator discontinuance is imminent.

18. **Why should I be concerned with the plateau pressure?**
P_{PLAT} is the end inspiratory equilibration pressure or the mean peak alveolar pressure. In patients receiving controlled ventilation, it is the closest noninvasive estimate of the mean maximum end inspiratory transpulmonary pressure. It should be noted that during controlled mechanical ventilation, the P_{PLAT} is ALWAYS greater than the end inspiratory transpulmonary pressure. However, this is not true during assisted ventilation because of active inspiratory efforts by the patient. A reasonable estimate of P_{PLAT} can be made in most patients actively triggering the ventilator, but a number of measurements should be made and the closer the values obtained, the more reliable the measurement. During mechanical ventilation the goal is to keep the P_{PLAT} less than 28 cm H_2O to avoid inducing lung injury. However, in morbidly obese patients, patients with a stiff chest wall, and those with abdominal compartment syndrome, a higher P_{PLAT} may be necessary. It is in these patients that esophageal pressure should be measured to directly determine the transpulmonary pressure to insure the risk of induced lung injury is minimized.

19. **What is meant by driving pressure and why it is important?**
Driving pressure is the amount of pressure necessary to sustain a volume of gas in a given patient's lungs. It is defined as End Inspiratory P_{PLAT} minus PEEP. At a constant tidal volume, it is an expression of the compliance of the lung. Driving pressure has been associated with patient survival. The cut point seems to be about 15 cm H_2O. That is, a driving pressure greater than 15 cm H_2O increases the risk of mortality and a driving pressure less than 15 cm H_2O decreases the risk of mortality.

20. **What is positive end expiratory pressure and how should I set it in acute hypoxemic respiratory failure?**
PEEP is the elevation of the end expiratory pressure during mechanical ventilation to a specific level above atmospheric. The goal of PEEP is to sustain open alveolar units at end expiration. There are a number of approaches to setting PEEP, but the approaches that make the most physiologic sense are to set PEEP based on the best compliance during a decremental PEEP trial or the PEEP level that sustains a positive (1 to 4 cm H_2O) end expiratory transpulmonary pressure. Remember the transpulmonary pressure is the pressure across the lung (airway opening to pleural space). If the transpulmonary pressure is negative at end exhalation, the lung will collapse if positive lung units are kept open.

21. **What is a lung recruitment maneuver?**
A lung recruitment maneuver (Box 8.3) is the application of a higher than normal pressure for a short period of time to open lung units that are normally closed at end inspiration. Following a recruitment maneuver, PEEP is selected and set by a decremental best-compliance PEEP trial, or the PEEP level that sustains the end expiratory transpulmonary pressure positive (Box 8.4).

22. **What is the correct setting of FIO_2 during mechanical ventilation?**
The human body never evolved to tolerate hyperoxia; if anything, it evolved to tolerate hypoxemia. A recent randomized controlled trial indicated that patients maintained with normoxia have better

---

Box 8-3. Performing a Recruitment Maneuver

Place the patient in pressure-control ventilation, FIO$_2$ 1.0:
  Set pressure control level 15 cm H$_2$O
  Set inspiratory Time: 3 s, Rate: 10/min
  Increase positive end expiratory pressure (PEEP) 3–5 cm H$_2$O every five breaths until the maximum peak airway pressure (PIP) is achieved
    Maximum applied PEEP between 25 and 35 cm H$_2$O dependent upon the targeted maximum PIP

  Maximum PIP is between 40 and 50 cm H$_2$O based on the patient hemodynamic stability
    Once at maximum, PIP continue to ventilate for 1 min
    Then perform a decremental PEEP trial or set PEEP to insure a positive end expiratory transpulmonary pressure

---

Box 8-4. Performing a Decremental Best Compliance Positive End Expiratory Pressure Trail

Ventilate in volume control ventilation (VCV)
  Set PEEP at 20–25 dependent on patient severity of lung injury
  Set V$_T$ 4–6 mL/kg PBW
  Set flow to allow normal inspiratory time (0.6–0.8 s)
  Adjust respiratory rate to a rate that DOES NOT result in the development of autoPEEP (20–30 breaths/min)
  Measure dynamic compliance (it only takes 30–45 s for compliance to stabilize once PEEP is set)
  Decrease PEEP 2 cm H$_2$O; reassess dynamic compliance

  Continue to decrease PEEP by 2 cm H$_2$O reassessing dynamic compliance until a clear pattern indicates what is the best compliance PEEP
    Initially, compliance will increase as PEEP is decreased, but then as the lung begins to derecruit, compliance will decrease. Once it is obvious that compliance is decreasing the decremental trail can be stopped
    Recruit the lung and set PEEP at the best compliance decremental PEEP plus 2 cm H$_2$O. The best compliance decremental PEEP underestimates the best oxygenation decremental PEEP by about 2 cm H$_2$O

PBW, Predicted body weight; *PEEP*, positive end expiratory pressure.

---

survival than patients maintained with hyperoxia. Thus FIO$_2$ and the resulting PaO$_2$ and SpO$_2$ must be considered part of a lung-protective ventilatory strategy. Patients acutely requiring mechanical ventilation should be maintained with a PaO$_2$ of 55 to 80 mm Hg or a SpO$_2$ of 88% to 95%.

23. **What does the term *transpulmonary pressure* actually mean?**
Transpulmonary pressure (P$_{TP}$) is the pressure across the respiratory system during ventilation. It can be measured during spontaneous unsupported breathing or during mechanical ventilation. Specifically, the P$_{TP}$ is calculated as the airway opening pressure minus the pleural pressure. It is commonly measured at end inspiration as end inspiratory P$_{PLAT}$ minus pleural pressure and at end expiration as PEEP minus pleural pressure. Pleural pressure is estimated by measurement of the esophageal pressure.

24. **Explain the concepts of alveolar stress and alveolar strain.**
Both alveolar stress and strain are factors related to ventilator-induced lung injury. Alveolar stress is measured by transpulmonary pressure; the greater the P$_{TP}$ the greater the stress. The maximum sustainable alveolar stress without causing lung injury is not known, but many believe it is a transpulmonary pressure between 15 and 20 cm H$_2$O. Alveolar strain is the volume of deformation of the lung by the addition of lung volume. All volume increase above the patient's baseline FRC is considered contributing to alveolar strain; thus, the larger the tidal volume the larger the strain. The process of repeated opening and collapse of alveolar units also contributes to stress and strain.

25. **Why should we consider prone positioning to improve oxygenation?**
Changing patient position from supine to prone recruits lung, improves ventilation/perfusion match, and allows for drainage of secretions. Prone positioning has been shown to improve outcome in severe ARDS (P/F ratio less than 100 mm Hg). However, there are considerable side effects of prone positioning. Prone positioning should be used in patients with severe hypoxemia (P/F ratio less than 100 mm Hg) when the application of all aspects of an LPMV strategy have failed. The specific components of an LPMV strategy as a whole are less likely to result in complications than prone positioning.

ACKNOWLEDGMENT

The authors wish to acknowledge Dr. Manuel Pardo, Jr., MD, for the valuable contributions to the previous edition of this chapter.

KEY POINTS: MECHANICAL VENTILATION

1. All patients' should be ventilated with a lung protective ventilator strategy from the time of intubation to extubation-
   - Tidal volume 4 to 8 ml/kg PBW
   - Plateau pressure < 28 cm H_2O
   - Driving pressure < 15 cm H_2O
   - PEEP sufficient to prevent end expiratory alveolar collapse
   - F_1O_2 titrated to maintain pO_2 55 to 80 and SpO_2 88% to 95%.
2. The greater the control over the process of ventilation the greater the level of asynchrony.
3. The forms of asynchrony most likely to cause ventilator induced lung injury are flow asynchrony and double triggering.

BIBLIOGRAPHY

1. Goligher EC, Ferguson ND, Brochard LJ. Clinical challenges in mechanical ventilation. *Lancet.* 2016;387:1856-1866.
2. Ferrer M, Esquinas A, Arancibia F, et al. Noninvasive ventilation during persistent weaning failure: a randomized controlled trial. *Am J Respir Crit Care Med.* 2003;168:70-76.
3. Ferguson ND, Cook DJ, Guyatt GH, et al. High-frequency oscillation in early acute respiratory distress syndrome. *N Engl J Med.* 2013;368:795-805.
4. Young D, Lamb SE, Shah S, et al. High-frequency oscillation for acute respiratory distress syndrome. *N Engl J Med.* 2013;368:806-813.
5. Murias G, Lucangelo U, Blanch L. Patient-ventilator asynchrony. *Curr Opin Crit Care.* 2016;22:53-59.
6. Amato MB, Meade MO, Slutsky AS, et al. Driving pressure and survival in the acute respiratory distress syndrome. *N Engl J Med.* 2015;372:747-755.
7. Guérin C, Reignier J, Richard JC, et al. Prone positioning in severe acute respiratory distress syndrome. *N Engl J Med.* 2013;368:2159-2168.
8. Santiago VR, Rzezinski AF, Nardelli LM, et al. Recruitment maneuver in experimental acute lung injury: the role of alveolar collapse and edema. *Crit Care Med.* 2010;38:2207-2214.
9. Kallet RH. A comprehensive review of prone position in ARDS. *Respir Care.* 2015;60:1660-1687.
10. Protti A, Cressoni M, Santini A, et al. Lung stress and strain during mechanical ventilation: any safe threshold? *Am J Respir Crit Care Med.* 2011;183:1354-1362.
11. Graves C, Glass L, Laporta D, Meloche R, Grassino A. Respiratory phase locking during mechanical ventilation in anesthetized human subjects. *Am J Physiol.* 1986;250:R902-R909.

CHAPTER 9

NONINVASIVE RESPIRATORY SUPPORT

Dean Hess

1. **Are there benefits for high-flow nasal cannula (HFNC) beyond oxygen administration?**
   The equipment used for HFNC is shown in Fig. 9.1. The major benefit for HFNC is the high flow, which minimizes room air dilution. This allows administration of precise high oxygen concentrations. Because the oxygen administration is by nasal prongs rather than by face mask, there are fewer interruptions of therapy due to removal of the device. The high flow into the nose effectively flushes the upper airway, which is a dead-space lowering effect. This reduction in anatomic dead space reduces the minute ventilation requirement, and studies have consistently reported a lower breathing frequency when HFNC is applied. The high flow into the pharynx opposes expiratory flow, thus producing a continuous positive airway pressure (CPAP) effect. With the mouth closed, there is an increase in CPAP of about 1 cm H_2O for each 10 L/min increase in flow. Much of this CPAP effect might be lost, however, if the mouth is opened. The high flow provided through the upper airway also decreases inspiratory resistance, and this may reduce the work of breathing.

2. **When should HFNC be used?**
   The available evidence supports the use of HFNC for selected patients with acute hypoxemic respiratory failure. It can also be used to prevent hypoxemic respiratory failure, such as postextubation and during intubation. Frat et al. randomized patients with acute hypoxemic respiratory failure to receive HFNC, standard oxygen therapy by face mask, or noninvasive positive pressure ventilation (NIV). With HFNC, 28-day intubation rate was 38% for HFNC, 47% for conventional oxygen therapy, and 50% for NIV. The subgroup with a PaO_2/FIO_2 $\leq$200 had a lower intubation rate with HFNC than with the other two methods ($P = .009$). The hazard ratio for death at 90 days was 2.01 (95% CI 1.01–3.99) with standard oxygen versus HFNC and 2.50 (1.31–4.78) with NIV versus HFNC.

3. **Should HFNC be used postextubation?**
   Maggiore et al. compared the use of an air-entrainment mask with HFNC in 105 patients after extubation who had PaO_2/FIO_2 $\leq$300 immediately before extubation. Fewer re-intubations were needed (4% versus 21%; $P = .01$), and the need for any form of ventilator support in the HFNC group was lower than in the conventional oxygen group. With HFNC, PaO_2/FIO_2 was higher, discomfort associated with the interface and airway dryness was lower, fewer displacements of the interface were noted, and fewer desaturations were reported. Current evidence does not support routine application of HFNC postextubation, suggesting that the therapy should be reserved for patients with demonstrated hypoxemia. Futier et al. found that preventive application of HFNC directly after extubation, compared with standard oxygen therapy, was not effective in reducing the incidence of hypoxemia following abdominal surgery; there were also no differences in pulmonary complications and length of hospital stay.

4. **What is a practical approach to the clinical use of HFNC?**
   A practical approach to the use of HFNC is shown in Fig. 9.2. HFNC should be initiated at a flow of 50 L/min. That flow is maintained and FIO_2 is decreased, provided that SpO_2 is more than 90%. Note that the FIO_2 is decreased rather than the flow. If the FIO_2 reaches $\leq$0.4, consideration can be given to a change to conventional oxygen therapy. Some patients will be uncomfortable with a flow of 50 L/min and a lower flow might be necessary to promote patient tolerance. When HFNC is initiated, it is important to monitor the patient closely. If SpO_2 cannot be maintained at a flow of 50 L/min and $FIO_2 = 1$, serious consideration should be given to escalation of care (e.g., intubation). Unsuccessful use of HFNC might cause delayed intubation and worse clinical outcomes in patients with respiratory failure.

5. **How do CPAP and NIV differ?**
   With mask CPAP, a pressure greater than atmospheric is applied to the airway (Fig. 9.3). However, the patient's spontaneous breathing effort is necessary for ventilation. With NIV, a pressure is applied

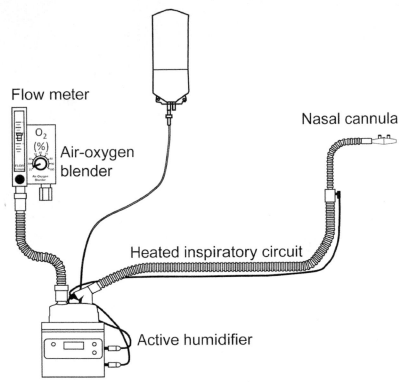

Figure 9-1. High-flow nasal cannula system. (From Nishimura M. High-flow nasal cannula oxygen therapy in adults: physiological benefits, indication, clinical benefits, and adverse effects. *Respir Care*. 2016;61:529.)

during inspiration that is greater than the expiratory pressure. Thus, with NIV, respiratory assistance is provided. The tidal volume is typically determined by the combination of pressure applied to the mask and the inspiratory effort of the patient. With NIV, the inspiratory pressure is often called inspiratory positive airway pressure (IPAP) and the expiratory pressure is called expiratory positive airway pressure (EPAP).

6. When should CPAP be used?

Mortality is reduced when CPAP is applied in patients with acute cardiogenic pulmonary edema. In a meta-analysis, risk ratio for mortality was 0.64 (95% CI 0.44–0.92) for CPAP compared to conventional therapy alone. For acute cardiogenic pulmonary edema, outcomes are similar for CPAP and NIV. Benefits from the use of CPAP have also been reported for post-operative patients with hypoxemic respiratory failure and in the setting of hypoxemic respiratory failure in patients with hematologic malignancy.

7. Should NIV be used for hypoxemic respiratory failure?

The use of NIV for de novo hypoxemic respiratory failure without hypercapnia is controversial. Its use is warranted for acute cardiogenic pulmonary edema and postoperative hypoxemic respiratory failure. However, caution should be exercised for the use of NIV for acute respiratory distress syndrome (ARDS), particularly for $PaO_2/FIO_2 < 200$. NIV may decrease the inspiratory effort, but tidal volume can also be significantly higher during NIV; this is particularly true if the applied inspiratory pressure is high. Thus, lung protective ventilation, an important tenant in the management of ARDS, might be difficult with NIV. Of note, one single-center study did report better outcomes for NIV with the helmet interface compared to oronasal mask in patients with ARDS, but this study needs to be replicated before widespread adoption of this practice.

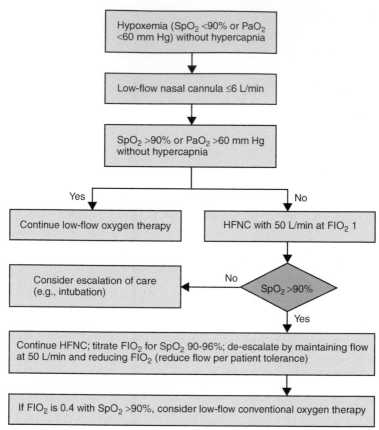

Figure 9-2. Flow diagram of use of high-flow nasal cannula for hypoxemic acute respiratory failure. *HFNC,* High-flow nasal cannula; *SpO2,* oxygen saturation measured by pulse oximetry; *PaO2,* partial pressure of oxygen in arterial blood; *FIO2,* fraction of inspired oxygen. (From Levy SD, Alladina JW, Hibbert KA, et al. High-flow oxygen therapy and other inhaled therapies in intensive care units. *Lancet.* 2016;387:1867.)

8. When should NIV be used postextubation?
   NIV has been shown to reduce the risk of reintubation (risk ratio 0.46, 95% CI 0.25–0.84) and to provide a survival benefit in patients at risk for extubation failure (relative risk 0.63, 95% CI 0.40–0.99). Risk factors for failed extubation include hypercapnia, failed previous extubation, history of chronic obstructive pulmonary disease (COPD) or congestive heart failure, and co-morbid conditions. In this setting, patients should be extubated directly to NIV following a successful spontaneous breathing trial (SBT). NIV should be used cautiously in patients who successfully complete an SBT, but develop respiratory failure within 48 hours postextubation. In this setting, NIV is indicated only in patients with hypercapnic respiratory failure.

9. When should HFNC versus NIV be used postextubation?
   Generally, HFNC is used in the setting of hypoxemic respiratory failure and NIV is used in the setting of hypercapnic respiratory failure. There are exceptions, however, such as the use of NIV rather than HFNC for hypoxemic respiratory failure related to congestive heart failure. Evidence does not support routine postextubation use of NIV or HFNC.

10. Are there contraindications to the use of NIV for acute respiratory failure?
    NIV should not be used in patients who require urgent intubation (respiratory arrest, severely depressed consciousness), who require an endotracheal tube for airway protection, or who wish not to receive NIV.

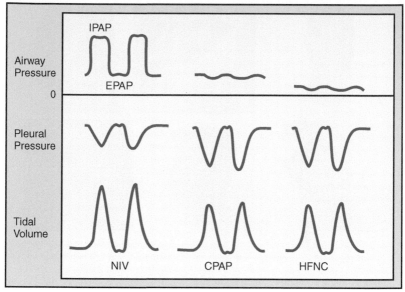

Figure 9-3. Comparison of noninvasive ventilation (NIV), continuous positive airway pressure (CPAP), and high-flow nasal cannula (HFNC). Note that NIV provides respiratory assistance, whereas CPAP and HFNC do not. Also note that HFNC provides a small amount of CPAP. *IPAP*, Inspiratory positive airway pressure; *EPAP*, expiratory positive airway pressure. (From Hess DR, MacIntyre NR, Galvin WF, et al. *Respiratory Care: Principles and Practice*. 3rd ed. Burlington, MA: Jones & Bartlett Learning; 2015.)

11. What interface should be used for NIV?
    A variety of interfaces are available for application of NIV (Fig. 9.4). In the setting of acute respiratory failure, an interface that fits over the nose and mouth (e.g., oronasal mask, total face mask, helmet) if preferable to minimize mouth leak. It is important that the interface chosen fits well to minimize leaks and is comfortable to enhance adherence.

12. How can skin breakdown be avoided during NIV?
    Skin breakdown can be avoided by proper strap tightening, use of barrier tape or cushioning between mask and face, selection of an appropriate size and type of interface, and rotating interfaces. The risk of skin breakdown might be lower with a total facemask compared to an oronasal mask. A common mistake is tightening of the straps in an attempt to control leaks. This is often not successful, it may increase patient discomfort and tolerance, and it will frequently contribute to facial skin breakdown. Tape, such as hydrocolloid dressing, can be applied to the bridge of the nose to prevent breakdown, but this is less effective after substantial skin breakdown has occurred.

13. Which ventilator should be used for NIV?
    Bilevel ventilators use a blower and a single-limb circuit to generate inspiratory and expiratory pressures, usually with a single-limb circuit. These ventilators typically demonstrate good leak compensation. With the single-limb circuit of bilevel ventilators, there is no exhalation valve, but rather an exhalation port in the circuit near the patient, or in the interface, that exhausts CO_2. In the past, critical care ventilators, with dual-limb circuits and an exhalation valve, were intolerant of leaks. However, newer generation critical care ventilators have NIV modes with leak compensation. As a group, bilevel ventilators outperform critical care ventilators for NIV for leak compensation and patient-ventilator synchrony. However, the NIV modes on some, but not all, critical care ventilators, is as good as that of bilevel ventilators. For acute care applications, it is also desirable to use a ventilator with a blender allowing precise FIO_2 delivery from 0.21 to 1.0, which is not possible for some bilevel ventilators.

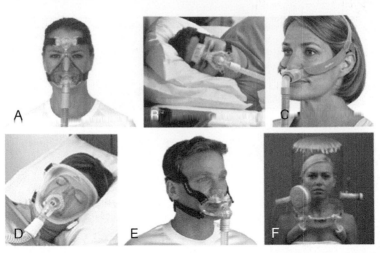

Figure 9-4. Interfaces for noninvasive ventilation. (A) Oronasal mask. (B) Nasal mask. (C) Nasal pillows. (D) Total face mask. (E) Hybrid mask. (F) Helmet. (From Hess DR, Kacmarek RM. *Essentials of Mechanical Ventilation.* 3rd ed. New York: McGraw-Hill; 2014.)

14. What mode should be used for NIV?

Pressure support is most commonly used for NIV. On bilevel ventilators, this is achieved by setting IPAP and EPAP; the level of pressure support is the difference between the IPAP and EPAP levels. Adaptive pressure modes, like average volume-assured pressure support (AVAPS), are available. However, these modes are not recommended because they reduce the level of support if patient effort causes the tidal volume to exceed what is set. Pressure control can be used, and offers the benefits of a back-up rate and fixed inspiratory time in the presence of a large leak. On bilevel ventilators, spontaneous/timed (S/T) mode is commonly used. In S/T, the patient receives pressure support, but the ventilator delivers pressure control if the patient's breathing frequency drops below the rate set on the ventilator. Proportional assist ventilation (PAV) and neurally adjusted ventilatory assist (NAVA) are not commonly used for NIV, but have the advantage of better patient-ventilator synchrony.

15. How does one know when NIV is failing?

Even with proper patient selection, some patients will fail NIV due to progression of the disease process. Clinical signs that are equivocal at the time of NIV initiation become more definitively predictive of failure if they persist after 2 hours of NIV. Thus, it is important to assess clinical trajectory after 1 to 2 hours of initiation of NIV to identify response. If gas exchange and symptoms fail to improve within several hours of NIV initiation, escalation of care is appropriate (e.g., intubation). An issue of concern is inappropriate use of NIV for too long when the therapy is failing, which may increase mortality due to excessive delay of intubation.

16. What are some practical approaches to synchrony during NIV?

Good NIV tolerance has been associated with success of NIV, and improved comfort has been associated with better synchrony. Asynchrony is commonly associated with leaks. Thus, reducing the leak related to the interface and using a ventilator with good leak compensation should reduce the degree of asynchrony. Asynchronies can also be related to the underlying disease process and respiratory drive. Manipulation of ventilator settings might address asynchrony in some patients, such as inspiratory and expiratory pressure levels, trigger sensitivity, rise time, flow cycle criteria, and back-rate. Modes such as PAV and NAVA might help for some patients. The best solution for asynchrony in an individual patient is often determined by trial and error.

17. Is humidification necessary during NIV?

Adequate humidification during NIV is necessary to improve comfort and tolerance. Although either active or passive humidification can be used, active humidification is more effective and does not introduce additional dead space into the circuit. Use of passive humidification was shown to result in decreased CO_2 elimination during NIV, despite increased minute ventilation, in hypercapnic subjects. However, in a randomized controlled trial, no difference in intubation rate was found between subjects receiving NIV with active or passive humidification.

18. Can aerosols be administered during NIV and HFNC?

 Available evidence supports the delivery of aerosols during NIV. Either a nebulizer or metered dose inhaler with spacer can be used, provided that the device is positioned between the circuit leak port and mask. Clinical studies on aerosol delivery during HFNC are needed, but the available in vitro evidence suggests that aerosols can be delivered during HFNC.

19. How does one go about initiating NIV?

 Suggestions for initiation of NIV are listed in Box 9.1.

20. Should NIV always be managed in the ICU?

 Although it has been argued that all acute care NIV should be initiated in the ICU, this is often not practical due to ICU bed availability. Choice of an appropriate site for NIV requires consideration of the patient's need for monitoring, the monitoring capabilities of the unit, the technical and personnel resources available (physicians, nursing, and respiratory therapy), and the skill and experience of the staff. NIV is commonly initiated in the emergency department, after which the patient is transferred to the ICU. Stepdown units can be good locations for NIV. Due to lack of availability of ICU beds, many hospitals are forced to manage some patients receiving NIV on general wards. This can be done safely with more stable patients, provided that suitable monitoring and adequately trained staff are available.

Box 9-1. Practical Suggestions for Initiation of Noninvasive Ventilation

- Select appropriate patient who is likely to benefit from NIV, such as those with COPD exacerbation or acute cardiogenic pulmonary edema.
- Choose a ventilator that meets the patient's needs and one that has a good leak compensation algorithm. The most common mode is pressure-support ventilation.
- Choose the correct interface. For acute respiratory failure, an oronasal mask is commonly used. Avoid a mask that is too large. If the patient is intolerant of an oronasal mask, try a total face mask.
- Explain NIV to the patient. It can be extremely frightening for a patient in acute respiratory failure to have a mask strapped over the face. Explain the goals of NIV and the alternatives.
- Silence alarms and begin with low settings, even if the settings are sub-therapeutic, which helps the patient acclimate to the mask and the pressure.
- Initiate NIV while holding the mask in place. This helps the patient acclimate to the mask.
- Secure the mask. A common mistake is to strap the mask too tightly. Strapping the mask too tightly decreases patient tolerance and increases the risk of facial skin breakdown.
- Titrate the pressure support to patient comfort. For some ventilators, the difference between the inspiratory pressure and expiratory positive determines the level of pressure support. Gradually increase the inspiratory pressure while observing accessory muscle use and respiratory rate. Avoid tidal volume >8 mL/kg ideal body weight.
- Titrate the FIO_2 to achieve an SpO_2 >90%.
- Avoid inspiratory pressure >20 cm H_2O, which decreases patient comfort and increases the risk of gastric insufflation.
- Titrate expiratory pressure (PEEP) per trigger effort (to counter-balance auto-PEEP with COPD exacerbation) and SpO_2.
- Continue to coach and reassure the patient. Make adjustments per patient comfort and adherence to therapy. It is acceptable to give the patient a break from NIV if the patient does not acutely decompensate when the mask is removed. HFNC can be used during breaks from NIV.
- Evaluate NIV success. If signs of improvement are absent 1–2 h after initiation of NIV, consider alternative therapies (e.g., intubation).

COPD, Chronic obstructive pulmonary disease; *HFNC*, high-flow nasal cannula; *NIV*, noninvasive ventilation.
Modified from Hess DR. How to initiate a noninvasive ventilation program: bringing the evidence to the bedside. *Respir Care*. 2009; 54:232.

21. How is NIV weaned?

There is usually no formal approach to weaning patients from NIV. The interface will typically be removed as requested by the patient, to provide facial hygiene, or to administer oral medications. If the patient deteriorates when NIV is interrupted, the therapy is resumed. Otherwise NIV is discontinued.

22. What complications are associated with NIV?

Minor complication of NIV include mask discomfort, mild asynchrony due to leaks, upper airway discomfort due to inadequate humidification, and mild gastric insufflation. More serious complications include facial skin breakdown, gastric distention, regurgitation and aspiration, and the hemodynamic effects of the positive intrathoracic pressure. Serious complications are uncommon.

ACKNOWLEDGMENT

The authors wish to acknowledge Dr. Manuel Pardo, Jr., MD, for the valuable contributions to the previous edition of this chapter.

KEY POINTS: NONINVASIVE RESPIRATORY SUPPORT

1. HFNC is used for patients with acute hypoxemic respiratory failure.
2. In addition to delivery of precise high oxygen concentration, HFNC flushes dead space from the upper airway, reduces inspiratory resistance, and produces a small level of CPAP.
3. Mask CPAP is used for the treatment of cardiogenic pulmonary edema, post-operative hypoxemia, and for hypoxemic respiratory failure in patients with hematologic malignancy.
4. The primary indications for NIV are COPD exacerbation, acute cardiogenic pulmonary edema, post-operative respiratory failure, and prevention of extubation failure.
5. An interface that fits over the nose and mouth is recommended for application of NIV for acute respiratory failure.
6. Skin breakdown is an important avoidable complication of NIV.
7. Leak compensation is the most important consideration when selecting a ventilator for NIV.
8. Aerosol therapy can be combined with NIV and HFNC.

BIBLIOGRAPHY

1. Cabrini L, Landoni G, Oriani A, et al. Noninvasive ventilation and survival in acute care settings: a comprehensive systematic review and metaanalysis of randomized controlled trials. *Crit Care Med.* 2015;43:880.
2. Carteaux G, Millán-Guilarte T, De Prost N, et al. Failure of noninvasive ventilation for de novo acute hypoxemic respiratory failure: role of tidal volume. *Crit Care Med.* 2016;44:282.
3. Esquinas Rodriguez AM, Scala R, Soroksky A, et al. Clinical review: humidifiers during non-invasive ventilation—key topics and practical implications. *Crit Care.* 2012;16:203.
4. Frat JP, Thille AW, Mercat A, et al. High-flow oxygen through nasal cannula in acute hypoxemic respiratory failure. *N Engl J Med.* 2015;372:2185.
5. Futier E, Paugam-Burtz C, Godet T, et al. Effect of early postextubation high-flow nasal cannula vs conventional oxygen therapy on hypoxaemia in patients after major abdominal surgery: a French multicentre randomised controlled trial (OPERA). *Intensive Care Med.* 2016;42:1888.
6. Hess DR. Aerosol Therapy During Noninvasive Ventilation or High-Flow Nasal Cannula. *Respir Care.* 2015;60:880-891. [discussion: 891-893].
7. Hess DR. Noninvasive ventilation for acute respiratory failure. *Respir Care.* 2013;58:950.
8. Hess DR. Patient-ventilator interaction during noninvasive ventilation. *Respir Care.* 2011;56:153.
9. Hess DR. The role of noninvasive ventilation in the ventilator discontinuation process. *Respir Care.* 2012;57:1619.
10. Levy SD, Alladina JW, Hibbert KA, et al. High-flow oxygen therapy and other inhaled therapies in intensive care units. *Lancet.* 2016;387:1867.
11. Maggiore SM, Idone FA, Vaschetto R, et al. Nasal high-flow versus Venturi mask oxygen therapy after extubation. Effects on oxygenation, comfort, and clinical outcome. *Am J Respir Crit Care Med.* 2014;190:282.
12. Nishimura M. High-flow nasal cannula oxygen therapy in adults: physiological benefits, indication, clinical benefits, and adverse effects. *Respir Care.* 2016;61:529.
13. Papazian L, Corley A, Hess D, et al. Use of high-flow nasal cannula oxygenation in ICU adults: a narrative review. *Intensive Care Med.* 2016;42:1336.
14. Patel BK, Wolfe KS, Pohlman AS, Hall JB, Kress JP. Effect of noninvasive ventilation delivered by helmet vs face mask on the rate of endotracheal intubation in patients with acute respiratory distress syndrome: a randomized clinical trial. *JAMA.* 2016;315:2435.
15. Yamaguti WP, Moderno EV, Yamashita SY, et al. Treatment-related risk factors for development of skin breakdown in subjects with acute respiratory failure undergoing noninvasive ventilation or CPAP. *Respir Care.* 2014;59:1530.

WEANING FROM MECHANICAL VENTILATION, AND EXTUBATION

Ryan Clouser

1. **What proportion of patients can be readily removed from mechanical ventilation?**
   The majority of patients (75%) supported with mechanical ventilation are able to resume unsupported breathing within 7 days of intubation if the illness that resulted in respiratory failure resolves or improves. One of the clinician's challenging tasks is to determine when the patient is ready for ventilator discontinuation. Continuing mechanical ventilation beyond the time that is necessary exposes the patient to risks for nosocomial infection and ventilator-induced lung injury. Conversely, removing ventilator support from a patient prematurely can lead to severe stress from respiratory and cardiovascular decompensation and exposes the patient to the risks associated with reintubation including increased mortality rate, increased time in the intensive care unit (ICU), and need for long-term care in a rehabilitation facility.

2. **When should patients receiving mechanical ventilation be assessed for ventilator discontinuation?**
   Every patient receiving mechanical ventilation should be assessed for ventilator discontinuation on a *daily* basis as long as his or her medical status meets the following criteria:
   - Lung injury stable or resolving
   - Adequate gas exchange with low positive end-expiratory pressure (PEEP) and fraction of inspired oxygen (FiO_2) requirements (e.g., PEEP < 5–8 cm H_2O, $FiO_2 < 0.4$–0.5)
   - Hemodynamic stability (e.g., not requiring pressors, or weaning, and no serious arrhythmias)
   - Patient capable of initiating inspiratory efforts

   Evidence indicates that systematic daily weaning assessments improve patient outcomes, reduce the number of days patients are dependent on the ventilator, and reduce the number of patients who require tracheostomies.

3. **How, exactly, should this assessment be done?**
   As of yet, no systematic weaning protocol has been agreed on. However, most protocols have a stepwise assessment that varies in the details. The above criteria should be assessed daily as a *wean screen*. For the patients who pass the daily wean screen, there is first an initial brief trial or *readiness assessment* during which patients are closely observed for 1 to 5 minutes while receiving minimal or no support (continuous positive airway pressure [CPAP] ≤ 5 cm H_2O), to assess their ability to undergo a formal spontaneous breathing trial (SBT). If the patient does well during the readiness assessment, an SBT is performed for roughly 30 minutes. During this time patients are closely monitored for signs of respiratory insufficiency, hemodynamic deterioration, problems with gas exchange, or patient discomfort. Full ventilator support is promptly reinitiated if problems develop. Successfully completing an SBT is highly predictive of successful ventilator discontinuation. These steps are illustrated in Fig. 10.1.

4. **To which mode should the ventilator be set during the SBT?**
   The specific ventilator mode during the SBT is not critical; however, in general, most ventilator weaning protocols are carried out using pressure support mode of ventilation. Pressure support levels during SBTs are typically set between 5 to 8 cm H_2O and 0 to 5 cm H_2O of PEEP. For patients with a tracheostomy on prolonged mechanical ventilation, tracheostomy collar trials with supplemental oxygen have been shown to decrease time to liberation from mechanical ventilation.

5. **What are the traditional weaning parameters, and how are they used?**
   Traditional weaning parameters include maximal inspiratory pressure, minute volume, vital capacity, maximum voluntary ventilation, thoracic compliance, and respiratory resistance. In the past, they were used to predict the likelihood of success with weaning trials. It is now known that they do not discriminate well between patients who will have success and those who will have failure after

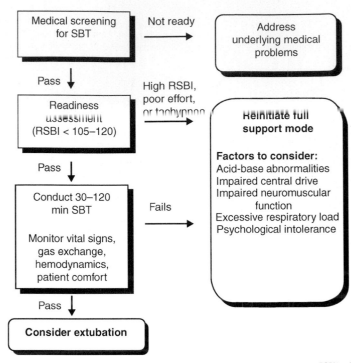

Figure 10-1. A protocol for daily assessment for extubation. *PEEP*, positive end expiratory pressure; *RSBI*, rapid shallow breathing index; *SBT*, spontaneous breathing trial.

extubation. Assessment during a carefully monitored SBT appears to provide the most clinically useful information regarding ventilator discontinuation. Measurement of traditional weaning parameters is generally not necessary.

6. How should sedation and analgesia be managed in mechanically ventilated patients?
   Patients are often medicated with sedatives and analgesics while receiving mechanical ventilation to reduce patient pain and discomfort and to limit patient movements that could lead to accidental extubation or other injuries. Continuous sedation may provide a more constant level of sedation, but this has been associated with a longer duration of mechanical ventilation, ICU stay, and hospitalization compared with intermittent sedation protocols. Patients randomly assigned to undergo a planned interruption of continuous sedation on a daily basis as well as aggressive early attempts at mobilization had reduced days of mechanical ventilation and days in the ICU compared with those who were randomly assigned to receive continuous sedation. No adverse effects of interruption of sedation were apparent. The optimal method of providing sedation and analgesia for these patients is not known. However, minimizing sedatives to the level that achieves a specified sedation target and attempting to awaken the patient daily appear to be important aspects of patient management during mechanical ventilation. It is also important to have the daily sedation vacation correspond with the weaning trial to ensure an accurate assessment of the patient's ability to breathe. Systematic improvements in sedation practice are associated with improvements in outcomes including shorter ICU and hospital length of stay, duration of mechanical ventilation, and costs.

7. What do you do with patients who have failed the SBT?
   Two actions are necessary:
   - Return the patient to a full ventilator support mode (e.g., assist/control).
   - Perform a comprehensive review of potential contributing factors to the failure.
     To sustain spontaneous ventilation successfully, patients must have an intact respiratory center drive and adequate neuromuscular function and not have excessive loads on the respiratory muscles.

Box 10.1 provides one method of systematically reviewing possible causes of failure during an SBT. Patients often have more than one cause for failure to wean, and correction of these factors may require multiple interventions. In general, it is recommended to wait 24 hours before attempting another SBT.

8. What criteria are important when considering removal of an artificial airway?

Successful completion of an SBT does not necessarily indicate that the patient is ready for extubation. Reintubation for respiratory failure occurs in approximately 10% to 15% of patients in most well-run ICUs. This rate is higher among those who have had endotracheal tubes in place for longer than 48 hours, who are older, or who have increased severity of illness, anemia, or cardiac failure. Unfortunately, reintubation is associated with a significantly increased mortality compared with patients not requiring reintubation, even when controlling for the severity of illness among these patients. Patients should be able to protect their airway, should demonstrate good cough effort, and should not have copious secretions. Patients should be responsive and able to follow commands. The difficulty of reintubating the patient's airway should be taken into account; the threshold for extubation in someone with a difficult airway should be higher. A cuff leak test can be performed if there is concern about postextubation upper airway obstruction. Though the presence of a leak is reassuring, the absence of a leak does not necessarily predict stridor or laryngeal edema after extubation. A helpful pneumonic for extubation evaluation is noted below.

CAALMS

CNS: Is mental status clear? Is the patient able to follow commands?

Airway: Do you suspect the patient will maintain a patent airway? Was the patient a difficult intubation? Do you suspect patient is at risk for laryngeal edema? Is there a cuff leak?

Box 10-1. Factors to Consider When Tests of Inspiratory Efforts or Spontaneous Breathing Trials Fail in Patients

The patient has an increasing partial pressure of carbon dioxide ($PaCO_2$) without increases in respiratory effort or rate.
  (a) Inadequate respiratory center drive because of excessive narcotics, sedatives, hypothyroidism, or brain injury
  (b) Appropriate compensation for metabolic alkalosis because of excessive diuresis or nasogastric suctioning
  (c) Return to a chronic hypercapnic state after inappropriate overventilation in patients with COPD or sleep apnea
The patient has tachypnea, tachycardia, or distress.
Impaired neuromuscular function
  • Fatigue due to prolonged high loads, inadequate rest, or ventilator asynchrony
  • Hypothyroidism
  • Electrolyte deficiencies (e.g., hypokalemia, hypophosphatemia, hypomagnesemia)
  • Critical illness myopathy or polyneuropathy
  • Steroid myopathy
  • Effects of drugs (e.g., aminoglycosides, neuromuscular antagonists)
  • Diaphragmatic paresis or paralysis due to phrenic nerve injury resulting from cold cardioplegia or thoracic or neck surgery
  • Prolonged malnutrition
Excessive respiratory load
  • Increased airway resistance (e.g., asthma, COPD, excessive secretions, small endotracheal tube)
  • Air trapping and increased threshold load due to positive residual pressures (particularly in patients with COPD)
  • Decreased respiratory system compliance (e.g., pulmonary edema, fibrosis, pneumonia, abdominal distention, thoracic cage abnormalities, pleural effusions)
  • High minute ventilation requirements (e.g., fever, sepsis, metabolic acidosis, high physiologic dead space, excessive caloric intake, pulmonary embolism)
Impaired left ventricular function
Psychological dependence: a diagnosis of exclusion but not rare in patients in ICUs

COPD, Chronic obstructive pulmonary disease.

Abdomen: Does the patient have normal abdominal compliance? Is the stomach decompressed? Are tube feedings off?

Lungs: Is oxygenation better? Has the pulmonary cause of acute respiratory failure resolved?

Meds: Is the patient receiving any medications that could suppress respiratory drive? (opiates, benzodiazepines, etc.)

Secretions: Does the patient have difficult-to-clear copious secretions with weak cough?

9. **What about using noninvasive ventilation (NIV) for patients who have respiratory failure after extubation?**

   The initial use of NIV—ventilators that interface with the patient through a full face or nasal mask rather than an endotracheal tube—has been found to improve outcomes in subsets of patients with acute respiratory failure, particularly patients with chronic obstructive pulmonary disease (COPD) and cardiogenic pulmonary edema. A Cochrane review found that in patients with COPD in whom extubation failed, NIV may be a reasonable option. In this patient population, NIV had a positive effect on mortality and ventilator-associated pneumonia, length of stay in the ICU and hospital, and total duration of ventilation. NIV may also be useful as a prophylactic measure in patients who are thought to be high reintubation risks. The full utility of NIV after failure of extubation needs to be further elucidated. The majority of positive trials enrolled exclusively or predominately patients with COPD.

10. **What is prolonged mechanical ventilatory support (PMV)?**

    PMV is defined as requiring at least 6 h/day of ventilator support for ≥ 21 days. These patients generally require a tracheostomy for optimal care. It is estimated that approximately 3% to 7% of patients receiving mechanical ventilator support meet this definition. One-year survival rates among these patients range from 23% to 76%, with older age and poor functional status before the acute illness predicting a worse prognosis. In patients receiving PMV, the criteria used in the weaning protocols previously described for acutely ill patients do not apply. Many of these patients are managed in long-term acute care units (LTACs) outside the ICU.

11. **Should these patients be managed with different modes of ventilation?**

    Patients who are ventilator dependent after 14 to 21 days despite improvement in disease state may require different management strategies. Multidisciplinary rehabilitation with focus on ventilator support, nutrition, physical therapy, and psychosocial support are all important aspects of care. Gradual reduction in ventilator support may be used in PMV patients. Many clinicians wean patients to approximately 50% of their maximal support levels without using SBTs. Once at the 50% level, daily SBTs are started. Ventilator support should be withdrawn gradually during the day, with progressively longer SBTs, allowing rest and sleep on full support modes at night. Once the patient tolerates spontaneous ventilation throughout the day, withdrawal of nocturnal ventilation may proceed relatively quickly. The success rate of ventilator discontinuation is only 50% to 60%. A recent trial showed that the simple use of tracheostomy collar trials, where a patient is removed from mechanical ventilation and allowed to breathe spontaneously, resulted in faster liberation from mechanical ventilation than standard slow-pressure support weaning. For patients in whom ventilator liberation remains elusive, clinicians should continue efforts to identify and correct physiologic reasons for the patient's inability to resume spontaneous ventilation (see Box 10.1).

12. **Why is there such an emphasis on protocols?**

    Protocols to guide ventilator weaning and minimize or interrupt sedation have been associated with improved patient outcomes and reductions in the cost of care because they reduce variability in patient care. These protocols are often driven by nurses and/or respiratory therapists and have been shown to result in faster liberation from the ventilator. A recent Cochrane review found that protocolized weaning in critically ill adults resulted in a reduced shorter duration of mechanical ventilation by 25%, weaning duration was reduced by 78%, and ICU length of stay was reduced by 10%.

13. **Does the use of high-flow nasal cannula (HFNC) oxygen decrease postextubation respiratory failure?**

    HFNC provides humidified oxygen at flow rates up to 60 L/min and FiO_2 of up to 100%. The rate of flow can decrease dead space and can decrease the work of breathing of a patient and humidification can make it easier to clear secretions. A recent multicenter study in Spain randomized patients to HFNC versus conventional oxygen therapy and examined reintubation rates. With the use of HFNC, reintubation rates within 72 hours from extubation were lower (4.9% vs. 12%) than in the conventional oxygen group. For patients who did require reintubation, HFNC did not significantly affect time to intubation.

ACKNOWLEDGMENT

The authors wish to acknowledge Drs. Theodore W. Marcy, MD, MPH, and Jenny L. Martino, MD, MSPH, for the valuable contributions to the previous edition of this chapter.

KEY POINTS: WEANING FROM MECHANICAL VENTILATION, AND EXTUBATION

1. Daily systematic assessments of patients receiving mechanical ventilation for the ability to breathe spontaneously are important in achieving timely discontinuation of ventilator support and reducing complications related to artificial airways and mechanical ventilation.
2. A respiratory therapist–driven or nurse-driven protocol for this daily assessment can safely reduce the duration of mechanical ventilation and performs better than standard physician assessments.
3. Sedation and analgesia should be minimized or interrupted on a daily basis.
4. Before removing the artificial airway, patients should be able to protect their airway, follow commands, should demonstrate good cough effort, and should not have copious secretions. (Remember **CAALMS**.)
5. Systematic attention to medical conditions that impair spontaneous breathing, such as left-ventricular dysfunction, muscle fatigue, and metabolic abnormalities, should be part of daily patient assessment. This can guide the medical care for those patients in whom a spontaneous breathing trial fails or who require prolonged ventilator support.

WEBSITE

Institute for Healthcare Improvement (IHI) Knowledge Center: Implement the IHI Ventilator Bundle. http://www.ihi.org/knowledge/Pages/Changes/ImplementtheVentilatorBundle.aspx

BIBLIOGRAPHY

1. Blackwood B, Alderdice F, Burns KE, Cardwell CR, Lavery G, O'Halloran P. Protocolized versus non-protocolized weaning for reducing the duration of mechanical ventilation in critically ill adult patients. *Cochrane Database Syst Rev.* 2010;(5): CD006904. doi:10.1002/14651858.CD006904.pub2.
2. Burns KE, Adhikari NK, Keenan SP, Meade MO. Noninvasive positive pressure ventilation as a weaning strategy for intubated adults with respiratory failure. *Cochrane Database Syst Rev.* 2010;(8):CD004127. doi:10.1002/14651858. CD004127.pub2.
3. El-Khatib MF, Bou-Khalil P. Clinical review: liberation from mechanical ventilation. *Crit Care.* 2008;12:221.
4. Ely E, Meade M, Haponik E, et al. Mechanical ventilator weaning protocols driven by nonphysician health-care professionals: evidence-based clinical practice guidelines. *Chest.* 2001;120(suppl 6):S454-S463.
5. Epstein SK, Ciubotaru RL, Wong JB. Effect of failed extubation on the outcome of mechanical ventilation. *Chest.* 1997; 112:186-192.
6. Esteban A, Anzueto A, Frutos F, et al. Characteristics and outcomes in adult patients receiving mechanical ventilation: a 28-day international study. *JAMA.* 2002;287:345-355.
7. Jackson DL, Proudfoot CW, Cann KF, Walsh T. A systematic review of the impact of sedation practice in the ICU on resource use, costs and patient safety. *Crit Care.* 2010;14:R59. http://ccforum.com/content/14/2/R59. Accessed 04.02.12.
8. Jubran A, Grant B, Duffner L, et al. Effect of pressure support versus unassisted breathing through a tracheostomy collar on weaning duration in patients requiring prolonged mechanical ventilation. A randomized controlled trial. *JAMA.* 2013;309:671-677.
9. Kress J, Pohlman A, O'Connor M, Hall JB. Daily interruption of sedative infusions in critically ill patients undergoing mechanical ventilation. *N Engl J Med.* 2000;342:1471-1477.
10. Krishan J, Moore D, Robeson C, Rand CS, Fessler HE. A prospective, controlled trial of a protocol-based strategy to discontinue mechanical ventilation. *Am J Respir Crit Care Med.* 2004;169:673-678.
11. MacIntyre N. Discontinuing mechanical ventilatory support. *Chest.* 2007;132:1049-1056.
12. MacIntyre N, Epstein S, Carson S, et al. Management of patients requiring prolonged mechanical ventilation: report of a NAMDRC consensus conference. *Chest.* 2005;128:3937-3954.
13. MacIntyre NR, Cook DJ, Ely EW, et al. Evidence based guidelines for weaning and discontinuing mechanical ventilation: a collective task force facilitated by the American College of Chest Physicians; the American Association for Respiratory Care; and the American College of Critical Care Medicine. *Chest.* 2001;120 (suppl 6):S375-S395.

14. Patel KN, Ganatra KD, Bates JH, Young MP. Variation in the rapid shallow breathing index associated with common measurement techniques and conditions. *Respir Care*. 2009;54:1462-1466.
15. Tobin M. Advances in mechanical ventilation. *N Engl J Med*. 2001;344:1986-1996.
16. Yang KL, Tobin MJ. A prospective study of indexes predicting the outcome of trials of weaning from mechanical ventilation. *N Engl J Med*. 1991;324:1445-1450.
17. Hernández G, Vaquero C, González P, et al. Effect of postextubation high flow nasal cannula vs. convention oxygen therapy on reintubation in low risk patients: a randomized clinical trial. *JAMA*. 2016;315(13):1354-1361.

QUALITY ASSURANCE AND PATIENT SAFETY IN THE INTENSIVE CARE UNIT

Nitin Puri and Antoinette Spevetz

CHAPTER 11

1. **Why is quality and patient safety such a "hot" topic?**
   In the late 1990s the Institute of Medicine released a report highlighting important patient safety concerns. In the years that have passed, significant improvement has not occurred. Although the United States spends a large sum on healthcare, its outcomes are not commensurate with spending. The Accreditation Council for Graduate Medical Education (ACGME), among other organizations, has patient safety and quality improvement as two of the six focus areas of its Clinical Learning Environment Review (CLER) program. The hope is that as newly trained physicians are specifically trained in these areas and understand the importance of patient safety and quality improvement, we will see changes in outcomes.

2. **How is quality assessed?**
   The definition of *quality* encompasses many things but clearly involves meeting the expectations of the consumer. In healthcare, this standard usually involves the satisfaction of patients, physicians, and payers as well as good clinical outcomes, appropriate resource use, cost containment, and attention to patient safety. Reimbursement is now attached to quality indicators, further emphasizing the need for high-quality care.

3. **What is benchmarking?**
   Benchmarking is the process of comparing one's own performance in a variety of outcomes with a standard. The Joint Commission requires that hospitals benchmark with other hospitals. Common quality indicators are available online and now allow consumers to choose a high-performing healthcare organization for their own care. Private companies such as Healthgrades.com and the government on Medicare.gov enable patients to compare hospitals using publicly reported data. A commonly used benchmarking tool is the incidence of healthcare-associated infections (HAIs).

4. **What is the relationship between the intensive care unit (ICU) organization and quality of care?**
   Evidence continues to accumulate that the structure and organization of an ICU influences patient outcomes. A full-time intensivist presence is recommended, but the need for 24-hour staffing remains an active area of exploration. A multidisciplinary approach to the care of the critically ill improves patient outcomes, with data supporting a team-based approach, including critical care nurses, pharmacists, and respiratory therapists. The use of non–physician-driven clinical protocols has led to an improvement of care in the critically ill, including earlier liberation of patients from mechanical ventilation and a reduction in ICU length of stay. Early mobility protocols in the ICU have led to decreased ICU length of stay, hospital length of stay, and decreased need for post–acute care services. Implementation has occurred in less than half of American ICUs, partly due to concerns about patient safety. This concern is not substantiated by review of the medical literature, and the loss of benefits by the lack of implementation can be substantial. Resistance to change in the practice of critical care medicine is reflective of a broader problem in medicine, since studies suggest that 30% to 40% of patients do not receive care consistent with current medical knowledge.

5. **List the uses to which severity-of-illness scoring systems are commonly applied**
   Stratification: Multiple scoring systems exist to stratify the severity or acuity of illness of critically ill patients. Examples of such classification systems are as follows:
   - Acute Physiology and Chronic Health Evaluation (APACHE)
   - Simplified Acute Physiology Score (SAPS)
   - Sequential Organ Failure Assessment (SOFA)
   - Multiple Organ Dysfunction Score (MODS)

These systems allow comparison of outcomes related to differing therapeutic approaches and attempt to match patients for severity of illness. The multiple scoring systems have not been compared in a prospective manner. Disease-specific scoring systems allow for standardized assessment, enabling uniformity for research.

Decision making in clinical management: Decision making may be aided by considering the information provided by scoring systems, as these models allow physicians to stratify patients into cohorts. However, clinicians must be cognizant that scoring systems provide population illness overview, not specific patient prognosis. Individual patient data must be used when providing prognostic information for patients and their families.

6. How is performance improvement carried out in the ICU?
   Members of the multidisciplinary critical-care team should identify performance improvement opportunities in the ICU and engage their leadership in developing solutions. A formal process to address performance improvement measures must exist. Common systems used are the **PDSA** process (**p**lan, **d**o, **s**tudy, **a**ct) or **PDCA** process (**p**lan, **d**o, **c**heck, **a**ct). Another system that has been used to improve performance in healthcare is the Lean Six Sigma Process. Originally it was used in industry to improve quality by eliminating variability. The process involves the DMAIC framework (Define, Measure, Analyze, Improve, and Control) and, under the guidance of experts in the Lean Process, improvements have been achieved in surgical-site infections and catheter-related infections. Performance improvement programs should be institution-specific and initiatives addressed by multidisciplinary teams.

7. List a number of observations on which to base assessment of outcome.
   Although a variety of indicators can be used to assess outcome, the following usually provide a reasonable database and can be used for benchmarking when similar data are available from other institutions:
   - **Patient satisfaction:** Hospital Consumer Assessment of Healthcare Providers and Systems (HCAHPS) surveys provide patient or family feedback on patients' experiences while they are hospitalized. The results of these surveys are tied to hospital reimbursement. However, they do not provide an isolated view of patients' experiences in the ICU. The 24-question Family Satisfaction Intensive Care Unit (FS-ICU) questionnaire provides a more granular view of family experiences in ICUs. A recent checklist assessing respect and dignity in the ICU showed that significant room for improvement exists, with 75% of respondents saying that physicians were not compassionate toward their loved one when they were in the ICU.
   - **Length of stay:** The length of stay both in the hospital and in the ICU for patients who were stratified by diagnosis, acuity, and comorbidities on admission provides valuable insight into outcomes and an excellent database for benchmarking if studied consistently over a reasonable period.
   - **Mortality indexed to severity of illness:** Although this information can provide a simple benchmarking tool, the data should be critically analyzed, as mortality is not the only indicator of the quality of care provided to a patient. This has been seen in the field of cardiac surgery, as a focus on mortality and public reporting has created the unintended consequence of making some surgeons risk-averse. Additionally, patients who are listed as hospice at the time of death may not count in mortality statistics. Hence mortality alone may not be the best predictor of quality.
   - **Incidence of unanticipated returns to the ICU during the same hospital stay:** This indicator may yield important information if examined in some detail. In addition to the actual incidence (which can be used for benchmarking), the individual cases should be reviewed. This may reveal a need to review the criteria for transferring patients from the unit or the compliance with the same. Alternatively, it may stimulate consideration of the adequacy of the care capabilities of the environments receiving the patients on discharge from the unit.
   - **Incidence of complications:** Complications may be linked to procedures (e.g., line placement, endotracheal intubation) or to general management (e.g., nosocomial infection, medication errors). Of major importance are those that have a clear impact on patient welfare. The criteria for identifying these and the methodology for data collection and analysis should be defined and consistently applied. Outcomes outside of the expected norm should be thoroughly investigated.

8. Are clinical pathways applicable to the critically ill?
   Although the development of clinical pathways has had considerable success in reducing costs while maintaining or improving standards of care and clinical outcomes, this methodology appears to be applicable mainly to patients with diagnoses wherein there is a fairly homogeneous group of patients who run broadly similar courses. Good examples of these diagnoses are acute coronary syndromes and hip fractures. In the case of the patient population in a mixed adult medical-surgical ICU,

---

Box 11-1. Surgical Time-Out Checklist

- All team members have been introduced by name and role.
- Confirmation of the patient's identity, surgical site, and procedure.
- Review of anticipated critical events.

- Confirmation that prophylactic antibiotics have been administered ≤60 min before incision is made or antibiotics not indicated.
- Confirmation that all essential imaging results for the correct patient are displayed in the operating room.

---

however, there is no such homogeneity, and it is often virtually impossible to describe an average course for a given diagnosis. Such a diversity of progression exists that relates primarily to the individual patient circumstances that it is of little value to compare the course of an individual patient with the clinical pathway. A much better approach in the ICU is to write treatment algorithms applicable to discrete segments of the patient's care within the continuum of the entire illness (e.g., weaning with use of therapist-driven protocols or use of the ventilator bundle, Centers for Disease Control and Prevention line insertion bundle, or sepsis bundle; Box 11.1). The use of this approach maintains all the advantages of getting groups together to discuss and agree on a unified approach toward aspects of care (thus reducing expensive diversity) without wasting time and energy on trying to define nonexistent average courses of these illnesses.

9. Is patient safety a concern in ICUs?

Patient safety remains a significant concern, with up to 58% of patients affected by medical error during their stay in an ICU. The high frequency of medical errors exists due to a multitude of reasons. A significant amount of research has gone into human factors research aimed at understanding the organizational reasons for safety events. One reason is suboptimal communication in ICUs with significant heterogeneity in patient handoff among attending intensivists. The use of the IPASS mnemonic (Illness severity, Patient summary, Action list, Situation awareness and contingency plans, and Synthesis by receiver) was found to have a 30% relative reduction in the rate of preventable adverse events in a multicenter trial.

10. How can patient safety be improved?

Medical errors remain too frequent, with some ascribing it as the third leading cause of death in the United States. Patient safety can be improved by embracing a zero tolerance for errors. This does not mean creating an environment of blame and recrimination, but instead fostering a culture of safety. Three simple recommendations have been made:

1. Make errors more visible
2. Respond to error
3. Make errors less frequent

If errors are committed, there must be a process to understand their root causes and rectify them. Innovative strategies from other high-risk professions have helped physicians understand that safety can be improved. For example, although there are significant differences between the airline industry and the delivery of critical care medicine, there is one glaring similarity, which is that mistakes can have horrendous consequences. The use of checklists in aviation has led to increased safety, and the similar use of checklists has dramatically decreased surgical complications (Box 11.2).

11. Can you give an example of a patient safety project that dramatically improved patient care in critically ill patients?

Multiple examples exist in the medical literature, but among the most dramatic was the Michigan Health & Hospital Association Keystone ICU project, which addressed central line–associated bloodstream infections (CLABSI). Catheter-related bloodstream infections cause close to 30,000 deaths in ICUs annually, and each infection leads to accrued cost over $40,000. The safety project used five proven techniques to reduce CLABSI (Box 11.3). After 18 months of intervention, CLABSI decreased by 60%, and in a follow-up study the results were sustained at 36 months.

Box 11-2. Five Components of the Ventilator Bundle

- Elevation of the head of the bed to at least 30 degrees
- Daily sedation vacation

- Daily assessments of readiness to extubate
- Peptic ulcer disease prophylaxis
- Deep vein thrombosis prophylaxis

> **Box 11-3.** Five Components of the Keystone Safety Project
>
> - Hand hygiene
> - Maximal barrier precautions
> - Chlorhexidine skin antisepsis
> - Avoid femoral site when possible
> - Remove unnecessary catheters

12. What are common barriers to improvements in patient safety?

    Introducing change into any complex organization is fraught with difficulty. Healthcare is not unique to this difficult process; common barriers to change include lack of knowledge and concerns about loss of autonomy. Most importantly, a culture of safety needs to be embraced and resources allocated to educate the healthcare team about safety. All members of the healthcare team need to report near misses and errors so that systems can be analyzed and improved.

ACKNOWLEDGMENT

The authors wish to acknowledge Dr. Carolyn E. Bekes, MD, MHA, FCCM, for the valuable contributions to the previous edition of this chapter.

KEY POINTS: QUALITY ASSURANCE AND PATIENT SAFETY IN THE INTENSIVE CARE UNIT

1. Quality assurance in the ICU means meeting the expectations of patients and payers.
2. The presence of intensivists in the ICU improves common quality indicators.
3. Medical errors are frequent and a culture of safety needs to be created.
4. Multiple processes exist to improve patient safety, including PDSA, PDCA, and Lean Six Sigma.
5. Healthcare is undergoing rapid change, and providers must be willing to adapt to the new culture of safety even if it means losing autonomy.

BIBLIOGRAPHY

1. Kim MM, Barnato AE, Angus DC, Fleisher LF, Kahn JM. The effect of multidisciplinary care teams on intensive care unit mortality. *Arch Intern Med*. 2010;170(4):369-376.
2. Weled BJ, Adzhigirey LA, Hodgman TM, et al. Critical care delivery: the importance of process of care and ICU structure to improved outcomes: an update from the American College of Critical Care Medicine Task Force on Models of Critical Care. *Crit Care Med*. 2015;43(7):1520-1525.
3. Corcoran JR, Herbsman JM, Bushnik T, et al. Early rehabilitation in the medical and surgical intensive care units for patients with and without mechanical ventilation: an interprofessional performance improvement project. *PM&R*. 2016;9(2):113-119.
4. Mason SE, Nicolay CR, Darzi A. The use of Lean and Six Sigma methodologies in surgery: a systematic review. *Surgeon*. 2015;13(2):91-100.
5. Wright SE, Walmsley E, Harvey SE, et al. *Family-Reported Experiences Evaluation (FREE) study: a mixed-methods study to evaluate families' satisfaction with adult critical care services in the NHS*. Southampton (UK): NIHR Journals Library; 2015. (Health Services and Delivery Research, No. 3.45.) Available from: https://www.ncbi.nlm.nih.gov/books/NBK333190/. doi:10.3310/hsdr03450.
6. Delgado MM, de Cos PM, Rodríguez GS, et al. Analysis of contributing factors associated to related patients safety incidents in Intensive Care Medicine. *Med Intensiva (English Edition)*. 2015;39(5):263-271.
7. Lane-Fall MB, Collard ML, Turnbull AE, Halpern SD, Shea JA. ICU attending handoff practices: results from a national survey of academic intensivists. *Crit Care Med*. 2016;44(4):690-698.
8. Makary MA, Daniel M. Medical error—the third leading cause of death in the US. *BMJ*. 2016;353:i2139.
9. Bota PD, Melot C, Ferreira FL, Ba VN; Vincent JL. The multiple organ dysfunction score versus the Sequential Organ Failure Assessment (SOFA) score in outcome prediction. *Intensive Care Med*. 2002;28:1619-1624.
10. Pronovost PJ, Goeschel CA, Colantuoni E, et al. Sustaining reductions in catheter related bloodstream infections in Michigan intensive care units: observational study. *BMJ*. 2010;340:c309.

II

MONITORING

PULSE OXIMETRY, CAPNOGRAPHY, AND BLOOD GAS ANALYSIS

Paul H. Alfille

CHAPTER 12

PULSE OXIMETRY

1. What is pulse oximetry?
    Pulse oximetry is a noninvasive use of the change of hemoglobin absorption spectrum to determine the relative amount of arterial blood saturated with oxygen. The technique was first developed in the late 1970s and is now in widespread use. It is part of the American Society of Anesthesiologists (ASA) standards for monitoring and one of three initiatives promulgated by the World Health Organization to improve global operating room safety.
    Pulse oximetry is used in many clinical settings, including the operating room, emergency department, and intensive care unit (ICU).
    a. Pulse oximeters can monitor for impaired oxygenation.
    b. Pulse oximeters can also be used to assess therapeutic interventions, such as adjustments to ventilator settings.
    c. Pulse oximetry is also useful for assessing the presence of pulsatile circulation and effective ventilation.

2. How does pulse oximetry work?
    In its simplest form, a pulse oximeter comprises a light source at two frequencies (red 660 nm and infrared 940 nm) that is shone through a tissue bed, such as a fingertip. Oxyhemoglobin (saturated) and deoxyhemoglobin (unsaturated) absorbs the two light frequencies differently, and the ratio corresponds to the amount of saturated hemoglobin. Because the tissue bed absorbs as well, only the change in absorption with each pulse is analyzed, separating the capillary inflow from tissue myoglobin (Fig. 12.1).
    In practice, pulse oximeters emit light at each of the wavelengths and add a pause to measure ambient light. By measuring the ratio of absorption at each of the two wavelengths, a ratio of oxyhemoglobin to deoxyhemoglobin can be determined.

3. How accurate are pulse oximeters?
    Pulse oximeter accuracy can be separated into:
    a. Inherent measurement accuracy (Fig. 12.2)
    Although accuracy is manufacturer-specific, most pulse oximeters are calibrated to the clinically relevant range. For instance, the General Electric (GE) Solar 8000 specifies pulse oximeter accuracy of 1.4% above 90% saturation, 2.4% above 60% saturation, and is "unspecified" below that. Studies on humans have shown similar variability between manufacturers, with better accuracy at higher saturations.
    b. Skin color and dyes
    Skin pigmentation does not seem to cause problems in pulse oximetry, but there are varying reports of surface dyes (henna, and nail polish) causing inaccuracies. A number of injected vital dyes interfere with pulse oximetry readings, including Patent Blue, indocyanine green, indigo carmine, methylene blue, and isosulfan blue (Lymphazurin); all cause factitiously decreased pulse oximetry readings, as well as causing worrying changes in skin color that can mimic cyanosis.
    c. Dyshemoglobin
    Although oxyhemoglobin and deoxyhemoglobin are the primary hemoglobin species participating in oxygen delivery, hemoglobin can exist as methemoglobin and carboxyhemoglobin if poisoned by nitric oxide or carbon monoxide, respectively. These forms do not carry oxygen but have absorption spectra that can interfere with conventional two-wavelength pulse oximetry. Carboxyhemoglobin readings are falsely elevated, while methemoglobin tends to 85% saturation reading. Sickle hemoglobin and fetal

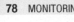

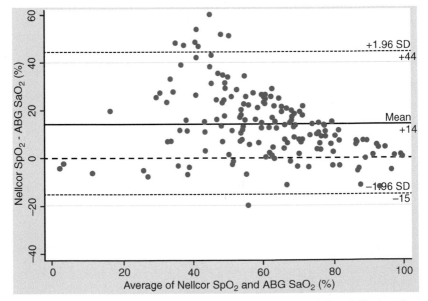

Figure 12-1. Oxyhemoglobin (HbO₂) and deoxyhemoglobin (Hb) absorption spectra. Pulse oximeters measure at 660 nm and 940 nm. (From Prahl S. Optical absorption of hemoglobin. Available at: <http://omlc.ogi.edu/spectra/hemoglobin/index.html>; 1999 Accessed 01.06.17.)

Figure 12-2. Comparison of pulse oximetry and arterial saturation in an animal model. *ABG*, Arterial blood gas. (From Dawson JA, Bastrenta P, Cavigioli F, et al. The precision and accuracy of Nellcor and Masimo oximeters at low oxygen saturations (70%) in newborn lambs. *Arch Dis Child Fetal Neonatal Ed.* 2014;99:F278-F281.)

hemoglobin have only minor effects on pulse oximeter readings. Use of multi-wavelength pulse oximeters can pick up these alternate hemoglobin forms, as well as measure total hemoglobin.

4. **What interferes with pulse oximetry?**
   Pulse oximetry can be confused by patient movement, ambient light, and light paths around the tissue bed (badly positioned probe). Peripheral vasoconstriction from hypovolemia, hypothermia, or vasoconstrictor administration can make fingertip reading fail. Other tissue beds, like the earlobe, seem to be more reliable in low-flow states. Different manufacturers use various signal processing techniques to improve reliability.

   Nonpulsatile flow from cardiopulmonary bypass, ventricular assist devices, artificial hearts, or aortic balloon counterpulsation also make pulse oximetry readings impossible or inaccurate.

5. **What advanced technologies are based on pulse oximetry?**
   a. Hemoglobin concentration
   Advanced oximeters with multiple waveforms can measure total hemoglobin levels, potentially saving delays and blood draws for lab testing. Actual clinical outcomes have not yet borne out the utility in trauma patients or ICU patients.
   b. Pulse contour
   Cardiac output and fluid balance have been studied noninvasively using the delay (transit time) from the electrocardiogram (ECG) to the peripheral pulse oximetry impulse. On the other hand, using the plethysmographic waveform variability with respiration was not found to be a reliable intraoperative fluid status monitor.
   c. Organ perfusion
   There is considerable interest in measuring specific tissue oxygen levels. Most advanced is cerebral oximetry, where advanced signal processing and multiple light paths are used to distinguish surface perfusion from deeper cortex. In addition, regional perfusion of tissue flaps, reimplanted limbs, or esophagus or bowel can be assessed with reflection pulse oximetry.
   d. Population and global health
   At the other end of the complexity spectrum, there is considerable interest in low-tech methods of pulse oximetry. Lifebox is an initiative to supply pulse oximetry to medically underserved areas to improve patient safety. It is accurate to US Food and Drug Administration (FDA) standards. Using consumer smartphones to monitor oxygenation is available, either with added hardware or using the built-in camera and photo light. One study found that the added hardware–based pulse oximeter was a relatively low-tech way of monitoring for sleep apnea in children. A test of the built-in phone pulse oximeter was not very accurate.

6. **What is capnography?**
   Capnography is the measurement of CO_2 in the airway gas. Capnography can be sidestream or in-line. In both cases, infrared light absorption is used. More sophisticated systems measure at multiple wavelengths and can distinguish between CO_2 and anesthetic gases.
   a. Sidestream capnography continuously removes gas from the airway into an analyzer. It suffers from the delay of gas transit in the sample line but allows more flexibility in sensor design, up to gas spectroscopy. The sampled gas can either be returned to the circuit (in a semiclosed anesthesia system) or accounted for as an intentional leak.
   b. In-line capnography has the respiratory gas to pass directly through a light sensor. It has the fastest response time but adds weight and complexity to the breathing apparatus.
   c. A colorimetric sensor is a chemical-based device that shows color change in the presence of CO_2. The color change varies with each breath, but the device usually does not function reliably for long periods. It is not a quantitative device but is inexpensive and has the advantage of easy deployment in a remote or emergency environment, since it requires no power source. New technology is being developed that can give reliable quantitative information from the colorimetric sensor.

7. **What are the uses for capnography?**
   a. Confirmation of endotracheal intubation
   Capnography, specifically the presence of CO_2 in the exhaled gas, is considered the standard of care in confirmation of proper endotracheal tube placement. It is also used to assess effective laryngeal mask airway (LMA) placement. Expiratory CO_2 requires gas movement, metabolism, and circulation. Although some CO_2-containing gas can be forced into the stomach with ineffective mask ventilation, the end-expiratory level will rapidly decrease. Ingested carbonated beverages can prolong the period of CO_2 presence, especially if nonquantitative sensing is used and the tube is uncuffed.

b. Confirming nontracheal placement of feeding tubes
Using capnography to guide the placement of feeding tubes has been frequently reported. It has the advantage of continuous feedback rather than placing a tube deeply in the airway and risking bronchial injury. Other methods include fluoroscopy and self-inflating bulbs.
c. Guiding resuscitation
End-tidal CO_2 has been long used as a method of assessing the effectiveness of resuscitation and is increasingly emphasized in advanced cardiac life support (ACLS) guidelines. Adequate end-tidal levels guide the placement of an endotracheal tube, the adequacy of chest compressions and circulation, and the return of spontaneous circulation. Poor end-tidal levels can also be used as a guide to cessation of resuscitation efforts, or the need for artificial support of circulation.
d. Assessing ventilation
Monitoring expiratory CO_2 is an effective way of monitoring for apnea and is used in procedural sedation and sleep studies.

8. How do end-tidal CO_2 ($ETCO_2$) and arterial CO_2 ($PaCO_2$) differ?
   See Fig. 12.3.

9. The expiratory CO_2 levels follow a predictable pattern. Starting from end-inspiration, which should show the CO_2 of the inspired gas, to end-expiration, which should show the alveolar gas CO_2 concentration, there is considerable information in the tracing.
   a. Inspiratory concentration should be near zero unless there is rebreathing—usually an indication of inadequate gas flow or faulty valves.
   b. Expiratory level should reach a near plateau unless the respiratory rate is too rapid, tidal volumes are too shallow, or there is considerable inhomogeneity in the lung (e.g., emphysema), leading to differing emptying rates for different classes of alveoli.
   c. The gradient between the end-tidal levels and the arterial CO_2 level is caused by dilution from non-perfused alveoli. This can be a marker for low cardiac output (increased west zone I) or pulmonary emboli.

10. Volumetric capnography
    A conventional capnogram measures the concentration of CO_2 in the gas stream versus time. If a measure of instantaneous flow is also obtained, volumetric capnography can be achieved, allowing measurement of total CO_2 production. This has been used in metabolic studies and assessment of nutritional support in the ICU care setting. Volumetric capnography has also been found to be an accurate way to measure dead space without requiring arterial sampling.

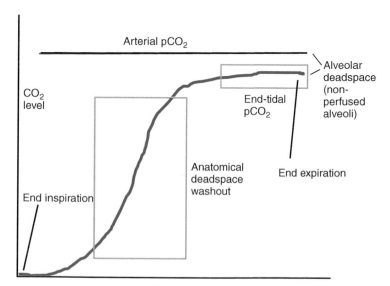

Figure 12-3. Capnogram.

11. What is an arterial blood gas (ABG)?

ABG is a laboratory measure of O_2 partial pressure, CO_2 partial pressure, and pH in an arterial blood sample. A number of measurement technologies can be used, typically half-cell electrodes or pH-sensitive enzymatic reactions. The ABG has the unique advantage of identifying acid-base status.

Many blood gas laboratory machines will also measure electrolytes such as Ca^{2+}, K^+, and Cl^- as well as BUN and creatinine. The overall intent is to monitor and identify alterations in renal function and acid production.

12. What interferes with ABG measurements?

a. Temperature

Gas solubility and H^+ dissociation are sensitive temperature changes. ABG is usually measured in a sample that is heated to 37°C, and then values can be adjusted to actual body temperature.

b. Continued metabolism

A syndrome variously labeled "pseudohypoxemia" or "leukocyte larceny" occurs when high leukocyte levels continue metabolism in the sample between time of acquisition and measurement. Falsely low O_2 levels will be found. Placing the sample on ice to slow metabolism or measuring immediately will confirm the cause.

13. Why measure PaO_2 if pulse oximetry is so good?

Pulse oximetry gives a faster response and a relatively accurate measurement, at least in the range of 70% to 99% hemoglobin saturation. When supplemental oxygen is supplied, PaO_2 above 100 torr will continue to read 100% by pulse oximetry. If accurate measurements in this range are needed (perhaps to assess early lung dysfunction), only ABGs will be accurate. There is some evidence that avoiding hyperoxia is advantageous in critically ill patients and can reduce mortality.

An ABG measurement that is discordant with the clinical picture or measured saturation can also indicate the need to look for methemoglobin or carboxyhemoglobin toxicity.

14. What is the relationship between the saturation and partial pressure of oxygen?

Oxygen in the blood is either freely dissolved or bound to hemoglobin. Hemoglobin is well designed to bind and release oxygen at partial pressures encountered on earth, with small effects from pH and CO_2. Fully saturated blood, with a normal hemoglobin concentration will have over 95% of its oxygen bound to hemoglobin (Fig. 12.4).

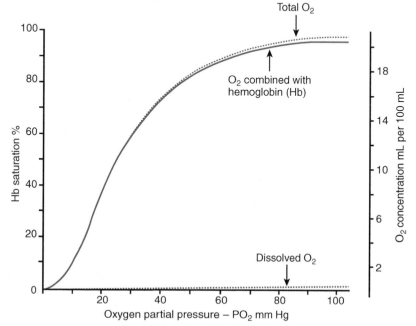

Figure 12-4. Oxyhemoglobin dissociation curve.

ACKNOWLEDGMENT

The authors wish to acknowledge Dr. Philip E. Bickler, MD, PhD, for the valuable contributions to the previous edition of this chapter.

KEY POINTS: PULSE OXIMETRY, CAPNOGRAPHY, AND BLOOD GAS ANALYSIS

1. Pulse oximetry is a continuous measure of oxygen saturation. It can be confused by vital dyes, nail polish, and movement. More advanced machines are needed to distinguish other hemoglobin types.
2. Capnography is a continuous measurement of expiratory CO_2. Its presence can ascertain respiration and circulation. It is useful in guiding resuscitation, and advanced waveform analysis can guide ventilation.
3. Arterial blood gases are a sporadic measure of oxygen and carbon dioxide. It is most useful in determining acid-base status in critical illness.

BIBLIOGRAPHY

1. Van Meter A, Williams U, Zavala A, et al. Beat to beat: a measured look at the history of pulse oximetry. *J Anesth Hist*. 2017;3:24-26.
2. Healthcare GE. Solar 8000M/I patient monitor Service Manual Software Version 5, page A-11. 2008. http://www3. gehealthcare.com/en/Services/Equipment_Services/Support_Center/~/media/Downloads/us/Services/Equipment%20 Services/Support-Center/Daylight-Savings-Time/Patient-Monitoring/Monitors/GEHC-Service-Manual_Solar-8000M-i-Patient-Monitor-v5-2008.pdf. Accessed 12/12/2017.
3. Yang S, Hu PF, Anazodo A, et al. Trends of hemoglobin oximetry: do they help predict blood transfusion during trauma patient resuscitation? *Anesth Analg*. 2016;122:115-125.
4. Marques NR, Kramer GC, Voigt RB, Salter MG, Kinsky MP. Trending, accuracy, and precision of noninvasive hemoglobin monitoring during human hemorrhage and fixed crystalloid bolus. *Shock*. 2015;44(suppl 1):45-49.
5. Phillips JP, Kyriacou PA, Jones DP, Shelley KH, Langford RM. Pulse oximetry and photoplethysmographic waveform analysis of the esophagus and bowel. *Curr Opin Anaesthesiol*. 2008;21:779-783.
6. Dubowitz G, Breyer K, Lipnick M, et al. Accuracy of the Lifebox pulse oximeter during hypoxia in healthy Volunteers. *Anaesthesia*. 2013;68:1220-1223.
7. Siobal MS. Monitoring exhaled carbon dioxide. *Respir Care*. 2016;61:1397-1416.
8. Hwang WS, Park JS, Kim SJ, Hong YS, Moon SW, Lee SW. A system-wide approach from the community to the hospital for improving neurologic outcomes in out-of-hospital cardiac arrest patients. *Eur J Emerg Med*. 2017;24:87-95.
9. Wagner PD. The physiological basis of pulmonary gas exchange: implications for clinical interpretation of arterial blood gases. *Eur Respir J*. 2015;45:227-243.
10. Damiani E, Adrario E, Girardis M, et al. Arterial hyperoxia and mortality in critically ill patients: a systematic review and meta-analysis. *Crit Care*. 2014;18:711-725.
11. Collins JA, Rudenski A, Gibson J, Howard L, O'Driscoll. Relating oxygen partial pressure, saturation and content: the haemoglobin–oxygen dissociation curve. *Breathe (Sheff)*. 2015;11:194-201.

HEMODYNAMIC MONITORING

Bryan Simmons

CHAPTER 13

1. **What is the purpose of hemodynamic monitoring?**

   Adequate tissue perfusion delivers substrates necessary for cellular metabolism and removes byproducts. The primary objective of hemodynamic monitoring is to assess the performance of the cardiovascular system in maintaining adequate tissue perfusion. It is important to mention that normal hemodynamic parameters do not ensure adequate tissue perfusion and hemodynamic monitoring offers data to guide therapy, but is not therapeutic by itself.

2. **How do automated blood pressure cuffs work?**

   Unlike manual blood pressures cuffs that rely upon Korotkoff sounds to determine systolic and diastolic pressures, most automated blood pressure cuffs utilize oscillometry. As automated blood pressure cuffs deflate, the monitor senses oscillations produced by the arterial pulse. The maximum oscillation amplitude occurs at the mean arterial pressure. The systolic and diastolic blood pressures are not measured directly; they are derived from the rate of change in the oscillation amplitude based upon proprietary algorithms. Errors in measurement may occur with inappropriate cuff size, motion artifact, arrhythmias, and extremes of blood pressure.

3. **What is the dynamic response of a pressure monitoring system?**

   Dynamic response refers to the ability of a pressure monitoring system to respond to, and accurately portray, changes in the system being measured. Two components of the dynamic response are the *natural frequency* and *dampening coefficient*. Natural frequency describes how quickly the system oscillates and is determined by the components of the system. A system with a low natural frequency (<24 Hz) will be unable to oscillate fast enough to portray an accurate waveform; thus a higher natural frequency is better. The dampening coefficient quantifies the frictional forces that absorb energy and determine how quickly a signal decays back to baseline. A low dampening coefficient will result in an *underdampened* signal characterized as exaggerated systolic and diastolic pressures, while a high dampening coefficient will result in an *overdampened* signal with a factiously narrowed pulse pressure and loss of detail in the arterial waveform. Regardless of the degree of dampening, the mean arterial pressure remains relatively unaffected. Overdampening occurs with additional tubing, stopcocks, air bubbles, or blood clots in the system. The natural frequency and dampening coefficient can be assessed with a bedside flush test (for more information, see reference 4).

4. **When is arterial catheterization indicated?**

   Arterial catheterization and continuous blood pressure monitoring is commonly performed for established or anticipated hemodynamic instability, need for strict blood pressure control, inability to obtain noninvasive blood pressure measurements, or when frequent blood sampling is required. The radial artery is most commonly cannulated, given the good collateral circulation to the hand, accessibility, and relatively low complication rate. Usually, radial artery pressures offer good approximations of aortic root pressure; however, in instances of severe vasoconstriction, femoral or axillary artery pressures may more accurately reflect central arterial pressures.

5. **How are pressure monitoring systems zeroed and leveled?**

   After assembly of the pressure monitoring system, it must be referenced to atmospheric pressure by *zeroing the transducer*. This is done by exposing the transducer to atmospheric pressure (usually by opening the stopcock of the transducer) and pressing the zero button on the monitor. *Leveling the transducer* aligns the plane of measurement with the area of interest, thereby accounting for effects of hydrostatic pressure. By convention, the transducer is leveled to the phlebostatic axis (midaxillary line in the fourth intercostal space) or to the point 5 cm posterior to the sternal notch, which approximates the right atrium. It is important to remember that, once zeroed and leveled, changes in transducer height relative to this axis will affect measurements (e.g., for each 10 cm the transducer is lowered in reference to this axis, the measurement will increase by roughly 7.5 mm Hg, and vice versa). Of note, *calibrating the transducer*, which references pressure measurements to known standards, is no longer required of transducers used today.

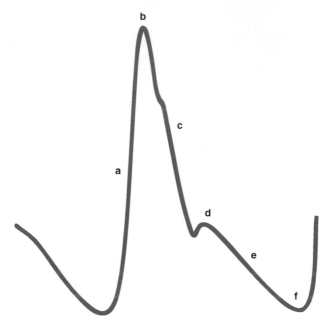

Figure 13-1. Six components of a normal arterial waveform: (a) systolic upstroke, (b) peak systolic pressure, (c) systolic decline, (d) dicrotic notch, (e) diastolic runoff, and (f) end-diastolic pressure.

6. What are the components of a normal arterial waveform and how does the location of measurement within the arterial system affect these components?
   There are six components of the arterial waveform (Fig. 13.1). The *systolic upstroke* occurs as the left ventricle ejects blood into the arterial system. The upstroke continues until the *peak systolic pressure*, which is followed by the *systolic decline*. The systolic upstroke, peak pressure, and decline are all systolic events that correlate with left ventricular (LV) ejection. The *dicrotic notch*, or incisura, represents the closure of the aortic valve and beginning of diastole. This is followed by the *diastolic runoff* and finally the *end-diastolic pressure*. Due to changes in arterial compliance, pressure wave propagation, and wave reflection, the arterial waveform is different between central and more peripheral locations (Fig. 13.2). In comparison with the aortic root, peripheral locations have a higher systolic pressure, a lower diastolic pressure, and a delay in the dicrotic notch along with a very small decrease in the mean arterial pressure.

7. How do aortic stenosis and aortic regurgitation affect the arterial waveform?
   The arterial waveform with aortic stenosis is characterized by a delayed systolic upstroke, disappearance of the dicrotic notch, and occasionally a narrowed pulse pressure (Fig. 13.3). On the other hand, aortic regurgitation features a low diastolic pressure and a widened pulse pressure as diastolic runoff occurs back into the left ventricle as well as the periphery. Due to the large stroke volumes (SVs) common to aortic insufficiency, there is occasionally a *bisferiens pulse* characterized by two systolic peaks; the second peak represents a reflected pressure wave from the initial systolic peak.

8. What are the indications for central venous catheter (CVC) placement?
   CVCs are indicated for frequent venous blood sampling, infusion of concentrated vasoactive or irritating medications, total parenteral nutrition, aspiration of entrained air in situations with high risk of air embolism (e.g., sitting craniotomy), monitoring of central venous pressure (CVP), and inadequate peripheral venous access.

9. Name the components of the CVP waveform.
   The CVP waveform consists of two major positive deflections (*a* and *v waves*) and two major negative deflections (*x* and *y descents*) (Fig. 13.4). The *a* wave is the result of atrial contraction, which is followed by the *x descent*, which represents relaxation of the atria and downward displacement of the tricuspid annulus with ventricular systole. A *c wave* occasionally interrupts the *x descent*, which

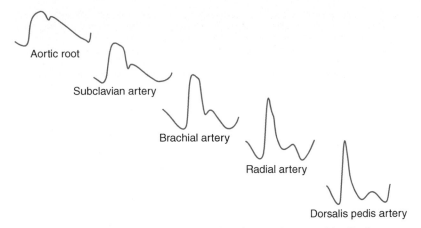

Figure 13-2. Comparison of arterial pressure waveforms from central to more peripheral locations.

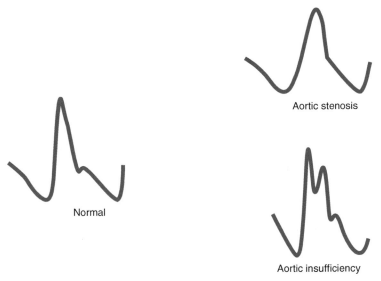

Figure 13-3. Characteristic waveforms of aortic stenosis and aortic insufficiency. Aortic stenosis yields a delayed systolic upstroke, disappearance of the dicrotic notch, and a narrowed pulse pressure, whereas aortic insufficiency produces a low diastolic pressure, widened pulse pressure, and occasionally two systolic peaks (bisferiens pulse).

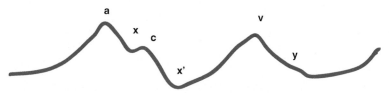

Figure 13-4. Components of a normal central venous pressure waveform: *a wave* (atrial contraction), *v wave* (venous filling), *c wave* (ventricular contraction with tricuspid bowing into the right atrium), *x and x' descents* (atrial relaxation and downward displacement of tricuspid annulus), *y descent* (opening of the tricuspid valve).

results from bulging of the tricuspid leaflets into the right atrium during ventricular systole. When a *c wave* is present, the portion of the *x descent* following the *c wave* is referred to as the *x' descent*. During ventricular systole, the atrium fills passively, increasing atrial pressure and producing the *v wave*. At the beginning of diastole, the tricuspid valve opens to allow ventricular filling; this corresponds with the *y descent*. In estimating right ventricular (RV) preload, right atrial pressure should be measured at the end of the *a wave* (beginning of the *c wave*), corresponding to end-diastole. Measurements should be made at end-expiration to minimize effects of intrathoracic pressure.

10. List the indications for pulmonary artery catheter (PAC) placement.
    Clinical uses and possible indications for placement of a PAC include monitoring right sided pressures, particularly with pulmonary hypertension or RV failure; estimating LV filling pressures; measuring cardiac output (CO) in shock states; and measuring mixed venous oxygenation to assess global oxygen delivery.

11. What complications are associated with central venous and PACs?
    Complications of CVCs can arise from cannulation or the catheter itself. Cannulation complications include pneumothorax, hemothorax, nerve injury, arterial puncture, air embolism, arrhythmias, and atrial puncture. Complications of maintaining central venous access include infection, thrombosis, thromboembolism, and air embolism. In addition to the aforementioned complications, PACs are associated with additional mishaps; however, major complications are fortunately rare. These include arrhythmias (most common), balloon rupture, catheter entrapment, pacemaker lead dislodgement, valvular damage, complete heart block in the setting of preexisting left bundle branch block, ventricular rupture, pulmonary artery rupture, and pulmonary infarction. The mortality associated with pulmonary artery rupture, the most feared complication, is roughly 50%.

12. Describe the placement of a PAC and the pressure waveforms as it is advanced into position.
    The PAC is inserted via an introducer, commonly from the right internal jugular (IJ) vein. The pressure is transduced from the distal port to identify the cardiac chambers as the PAC is advanced. After inserting the PAC to 20 cm, a CVP waveform should be present. The balloon at the tip of the catheter is inflated, a CVP waveform is again verified, and the catheter is advanced. From the right IJ position, the right ventricle is reached at around 30 cm, the pulmonary artery at 40 cm, and the wedge position at 50 to 55 cm. During advancement, the RV pressure waveform is recognized by a prominent systolic component with a low (1–6 mm Hg), *flat or gradually increasing* diastolic component (Fig. 13.5). Upon entrance into the pulmonary artery, a diastolic step-up is seen, with a diastolic component that *decreases* toward a trough of 5 to 12 mm Hg. Further advancement yields a pulmonary artery occlusion pressure (PAOP) waveform, which is analogous to the CVP; however, when referenced to the EKG, the waveform lags slightly behind.

13. How will the following pathologic states affect the CVC and PAC waveforms: tricuspid regurgitation, mitral regurgitation, RV failure, pericardial tamponade, pericarditis, and LV ischemia?
    On the CVP waveform, tricuspid regurgitation produces a large *v wave*, sometimes termed a *c–v wave*, with a steep *y descent* and loss of the *x descent* (Fig. 13.6). In an analogous fashion, mitral regurgitation is associated with a tall *v wave* and loss of the *x descent* on the PAOP tracing. This can also be appreciated on the pulmonary artery pressure tracing as a bifid (two-peaked) pattern (Fig. 13.7). There are, however, other causes of a prominent *v wave* on the PAOP waveform, such as poor left atrial compliance, hypervolemia, congestive heart failure, and LV ischemia. LV ischemia can also be accompanied by a prominent *a wave* and an elevated PAOP due to diastolic dysfunction. RV failure, pericarditis, and restrictive cardiomyopathy are hallmarked by an increased CVP with elevated *a* and *v waves* and prominent *x* and *y descents*, referred to as a "M" or "W" pattern (Fig. 13.8). Isolated RV failure can be distinguished from pericardial disease and restrictive cardiomyopathy by the presence of a low pulmonary artery pressures and PAOP.

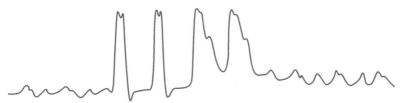

Figure 13-5. The characteristic pressure waveforms encountered as a pulmonary arterial catheter is advanced: central venous, right ventricular, pulmonary artery, and then pulmonary artery occlusion pressures.

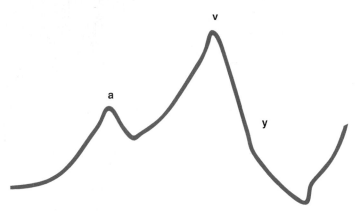

Figure 13-6. Central venous pressure waveform in tricuspid regurgitation features a large *v (c–v) wave*, steep *y descent*, and loss of the *x descent*.

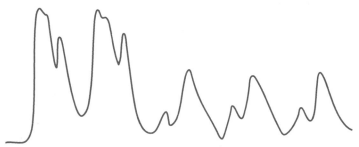

Figure 13-7. Pulmonary artery and pulmonary artery occlusion pressure waveforms in mitral regurgitation. Note the *c-v wave* with loss of the *x descent* on the pulmonary artery occlusion pressure waveform and bifid appearance of the pulmonary artery pressure tracing.

14. What factors influence the ability of the CVP and the PAOP to estimate right and LV preload (end-diastolic volume [EDV]), respectively?

    SV increases in direct proportion to end-diastolic sarcomere length, known as the Frank-Starling principle (Fig. 13.9). Clinically, EDV is used in place of sarcomere length; however, a measure of EDV is usually not readily available and cardiac filling pressures are used as a surrogate. This becomes problematic because the relationship between intracardiac volumes and pressures (i.e., ventricular compliance) is not linear and differs among patients. For instance, patients with chronic hypertension, aortic stenosis, myocardial ischemia, or diastolic dysfunction have decreased ventricular compliance with higher filling pressures for a given EDV. Valvular pathology, such as tricuspid regurgitation, can also profoundly affect measurements.

    With a PAC in the wedged position, a static column of blood is created in the corresponding pulmonary artery, capillary bed, and vein. The pressure obtained reflects the pressure at the end of this static column of blood in the pulmonary vein, which accurately reflects left atrial pressure under normal circumstances. This system may lead to erroneous measurements in a number of situations, such as incorrect PAC tip placement, pulmonary vascular disease (pulmonary hypertension), left-side valvular disease, or any situation where alveolar pressure exceeds pulmonary capillary pressure (e.g., chronic obstructive pulmonary disease, high levels of positive end-expiratory pressure or positive pressure ventilation).

15. How does the PAC measure CO and what are sources of error?

    The PAC measures blood flow through the right side of the heart using the thermodilution method. A known amount of saline (10 mL) of known temperature is injected into the central venous port. A thermistor near the tip of the catheter measures the temperature, which is displayed as a function of time. CO is then calculated using the modified Stewart-Hamilton equation and integrating the change in blood temperature over time.

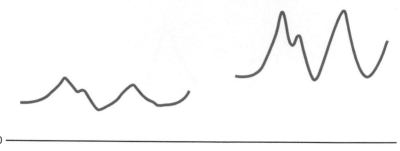

Figure 13-8. A normal *(left)* and "M or W pattern" *(right)* central venous pressure waveform that can be seen in right ventricular failure, pericarditis, and restrictive cardiomyopathy.

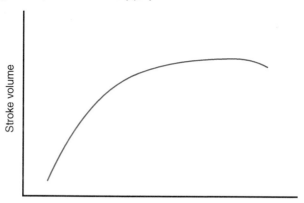

End-diastolic volume

Figure 13-9. The Frank-Starling principle describing the relationship between stroke volume (and cardiac output) and end-diastolic volume.

V = volume of injectate
T_B = initial blood temperature
T_I = initial injectate temperature
K_1 = density factor
K_2 = computation constant

$\int_0^\infty (\Delta T_B t)dt$ = area under the curve (AUC) from temperature versus time

$$CO = \frac{V(T_B - T_I) \times K_I \times K_2}{\int_0^\infty (\Delta T_B t)dt}$$

CO is inversely proportional to the AUC; thus, the temperature returns to baseline quickly with high CO, while the opposite is true with low CO. Inaccuracies occur with inaccurate injectate volume, simultaneous rapid infusion of fluids, pulmonic or tricuspid regurgitation, and intracardiac shunts.

16. Describe other methods to measure CO.
    Transpulmonary thermodilution determines CO in a manner analogous to the PAC; but it requires only a CVC through which cold saline is injected and a central arterial (femoral or axillary) line equipped with a thermistor to measure changes in blood temperature. The CO is derived from the change in blood temperature over time. Other measurements obtained include extravascular lung water and intra-thoracic blood volume, which are surrogate measures of pulmonary edema and preload, respectively.
    Transpulmonary lithium dilution is an indicator dilution method of calculating CO in which a small dose of lithium is injected via an intravenous (IV) catheter. The change in lithium concentration

over time is measure at a peripheral arterial catheter equipped with a means of measuring lithium concentration. Similar to the thermodilution method, integrating the AUC of the change in lithium concentration over time allows derivation of CO.

Pulse contour analysis relies on the concept that pulsatility of an arterial waveform is proportional to SV, from which CO can be easily calculated. Although it can be easily measured by different methods, pulsatility is determined not only by SV but also arterial resistance and compliance as well as wave reflection. To account for this, some systems use an alternative method (transpulmonary thermodilution or lithium dilution) for calibration, while other systems incorporate additional proprietary waveform analysis to account for these variables.

Transesophageal aortic Doppler utilizes ultrasound and the Doppler principle to measure the velocity of red blood cells (RBCs). Integration of the RBCs velocity over time (velocity-time integral, or VTI) and multiplying this value by the cross-sectional area (CSA) at the point of measurement will yield the SV. CO is then easily derived. In this method, an esophageal probe measures RBC velocity in the descending aorta and either estimates or measures the descending aorta CSA. Only the CO delivered to the descending aorta is measured; however, this is circumvented by multiplying CO obtained by a constant to approximate whole-body CO. Errors can be introduced with redistribution of blood flow, inaccurate CSA measurements, and probe malposition.

Bioimpedance cardiac output monitoring measures CO by detecting decreases in thoracic impedance that occurs with increases in intrathoracic blood volume. Electrodes are placed around the chest and neck that emit and sense low-amplitude electric current and measure thoracic impedance. Changes in impedance due to respirations are filtered out, leaving a pulsatile waveform that is analyzed to yield a CO.

The *Fick method* is derived from the concept that oxygen consumption must equal oxygen delivery to the tissues, as expressed in the following formula:

$$VO_2 = (CaO_2 - CvO_2) \times CO$$

CO can be calculated if the arterial oxygen content *(CaO_2)*, mixed venous oxygen content *(CvO_2)*, and oxygen consumption *(VO_2)* are known. *CaO_2* and *CvO_2* are measured from an arterial and mixed venous blood sample, respectively. *VO_2* is measured by calorimetry using inspired and expired oxygen contents. Measurements must be taken at steady state, making it difficult to apply in dynamic, critically ill patients. Another limitation relates to the difficulty measuring oxygen consumption.

17. **What is volume responsiveness?**
The concept of volume responsiveness refers to the ability to augment SV (and CO) with IV fluid administration in a patient with evidence of end-organ malperfusion. In essence, the location of a patient on the Frank-Starling curve is being sought (see Fig. 13.9). Patients on the steep portion of the curve will improve CO with administration of IV fluids via preload augmentation, whereas those on the flat portion of the curve will not benefit. A fluid challenge involves administration of IV fluids (e.g., 500 mL of crystalloid over 10 to 15 minutes) and assessing SV or CO. Patients are generally accepted to be volume responsive if their SV increases 10%–15%. Ideally, volume responsiveness would be predictable without having to administer IV fluids, thus avoiding potential volume overload. Static measurements, such as CVP or PAOP, have performed poorly in this regard; however, dynamic measures such as pulse pressure variation, SV variation, and the passive leg raise test have proven to be more reliable.

18. **How can an arterial catheter be used to predict volume responsiveness?**
Variations in pulse pressure (PPV), systolic pressure (SPV), and stroke volume (SVV) during the respiratory cycle can be used to predict a patient's location on the Frank-Starling curve. During positive-pressure ventilation, inspiration decreases venous return and RV preload while increasing RV afterload; this ultimately decreases RV stroke volume. Within a few cardiac cycles, the lower RV stroke volume decreases LV preload, leading to a drop in LV stroke volume. This is reflected by cyclic decreases in SV, systolic pressure, and pulse pressure in cadence with the respiratory rate. Those with greater variation have larger changes in SV with changes in preload, correlating to the steep portion of the Frank-Starling curve. These patients benefit from fluid therapy. Variation greater than 12% to 13% predicts volume responsiveness. PPV, SPV, and SVV can all be obtained from arterial waveform or pulse contour analysis. Of note, the following must be present for these measures to be valid: positive-pressure ventilation using 8 to 10 mL/kg tidal volumes without patient–ventilator interactions and no arrhythmias (sinus rhythm).

19. **How can bedside ultrasound be used in the ICU as a hemodynamic monitor?**
Point-of-care bedside ultrasound has become increasingly popular in acute care settings. Transthoracic (TTE) and transesophageal (TEE) echocardiography assist in distinguishing cardiogenic from

noncardiogenic causes of hemodynamic instability. Although TEE offers better resolution and image quality, TTE is preferred, if feasible, given that it is less invasive. Bedside echocardiography is used to assess global LV and RV function, gross valvular function, and volume status. Cardiogenic causes of hemodynamic instability—such as RV failure from pulmonary embolus, pulmonary hypertension, or pericardial tamponade—can be diagnosed quickly. Other uses for ultrasound include abdominal ultrasonography to assess for intraabdominal bleeding and lung ultrasonography to evaluate pulmonary edema, consolidation, or pleural effusions. As with all ultrasound, acquisition and interpretation of ultrasound data is operator-dependent.

20. Are there direct measures of tissue perfusion?

Common indices to assess resuscitation, such as lactate, mixed venous oxygen saturation, and arterial pH, reflect global perfusion. More direct measures of tissue perfusion and the microcirculation may be more sensitive in assessing perfusion. Methods used to measure tissue perfusion are not widely employed but include tissue pCO_2, tissue oxygenation, and videomicroscopy.

Tissue pCO_2 ($PtCO_2$) measures CO_2 concentration of tissue beds, usually in the stomach or sublingual area. With hypoperfusion, CO_2, a byproduct of cellular metabolism, accumulates and is released from the mucosa, where it is detected by specialized probes. There is some evidence to suggest that resuscitation guided by gastric pCO_2 improves outcome.

Tissue oxygenation measures the balance between oxygen delivery and consumption at the tissue level. Near-infrared spectroscopy (NIRS) measures all oxy- and deoxyhemoglobin in the sample volume (i.e., arterial and venous blood). At the tissue level, most of the hemoglobin is found in the venous system. During episodes of hemorrhage, the portion of venous blood decreases relative to arterial blood, and tissue oxygenation reflects more of the arterial component. In such cases, the ability of NIRS to reflect oxygen consumption (venous component) is poor.

Videomicroscopy utilizes various microscopic methods to directly image the microcirculation, most commonly in the sublingual region or nail bed. Irregular patterns of perfusion can be visualized and quantified using indices such as the microvascular flow index that scores the perfusion and heterogeneity of a vascular bed. Currently this is used for research purposes.

ACKNOWLEDGMENT

The authors wish to acknowledge Drs. Daniel Saddawi-Konefka, MD, MBA, and Jonathan E. Charnin, MD, for the valuable contributions to the previous edition of this chapter.

KEY POINTS: HEMODYNAMIC MONITORING ✓

1. Hemodynamic monitoring assesses the adequacy of tissue perfusion and oxygenation; it provides data to guide therapy but is not by itself therapeutic.
2. Arterial, central venous, and pulmonary artery pressure waveforms have signature morphologies. Pathologic conditions, such as valvular abnormalities, produce characteristic changes to these waveforms.
3. Point-of-care transthoracic echocardiography is becoming increasingly utilized in the ICU for assessing global LV and RV function, gross valvular function, and volume status.
4. "Fluid responsiveness" is defined as an increase in stroke volume by 10% to 15% resulting from a fluid bolus (fluid challenge). The passive leg raise test can be used in spontaneously ventilated patients to predict fluid responsiveness, whereas in fully ventilated patients, systolic pressure, pulse pressure, or stroke volume variation can be used.

BIBLIOGRAPHY

1. Chatterjee K. The Swanz-Ganz catheters: past, present, and future. A viewpoint. *Circulation*. 2009;119:147-152.
2. Cholley B, Payen D. Noninvasive techniques for measurements of cardiac output. *Curr Opin Crit Care*. 2005;11: 424-429.
3. Esper SA, Pinsky MR. Arterial waveform analysis. *Best Pract Res Clin Anaesthesiol*. 2014;28:363-380.
4. Gardner RM. Direct blood pressure measurement—dynamic response requirements. *Anesthesiology*. 1981; 54:227-236.
5. Jensen MB, Sloth E, Larsen KM, Schmidt MB. Transthoracic echocardiography for cardiopulmonary monitoring in intensive care. *Eur J Anesthesiol*. 2004;21:700-707.
6. Leatherman JW, Marini J. Interpretation of hemodynamic waveforms. In: Hall JB, Schmidt GA, Kress JP, eds. *Principles of Critical Care*. 4th ed. China: McGraw-Hill; 2015:186-201.
7. Marik PE, Monnet X, Teboul JL. Hemodynamic parameters to guide fluid therapy. *Ann Intensive Care*. 2011;1:1.
8. Schroeder B, Barbeito A, Bar-Yosef S, et al. Cardiovascular monitoring. In: Miller R, ed. *Miller's Anesthesia*. 8th ed. Philadelphia: Saunders; 2015:1345-1295.

CHAPTER 14

NEUROMONITORING

Ryan Clouser

1. **When should critically ill patients receive advanced neuromonitoring?**
   Any critically ill patient with severe neurologic disease should be considered for advanced neuro-monitoring modalities. The American Neurocritical Care Society recommends that neurologically in-jured patients receive multimodal neuromonitoring in an intensive care unit (ICU) setting. Examples of neurologic injury where neuromonitoring might be appropriate include ischemic stroke, intracra-nial hemorrhage, seizures, coma, and bacterial meningitis. Monitoring techniques can include contin-uous electroencephalography (EEG), intracranial pressure (ICP) monitoring, transcranial Doppler ultrasound, and neurologic exams. The physical exam is the most important neuromonitoring tool and should be performed serially to look for sudden changes that could indicate an acute neurologic deterioration or emergency.

2. **What is the difference between an extraventricular drain and an ICP monitor?**
   Both devices can be used to measure ICP. An EVD is typically used when there is an obstruction of cerebrospinal fluid (CSF) flow through the ventricular system, as in cases of intracerebral hemorrhage with extension into the ventricles, causing obstructive hydrocephalus. An EVD allows drainage of ob-structed CSF, blood, or pus and can also be used to measure ICP; it is therefore both therapeutic and diagnostic. An ICP monitor placed on the surface of the brain and can measure only pressure and potentially may reflect only regional pressure differences within the brain parenchyma. An ICP monitor can be used to manage acute elevations in ICP through maneuvers that either lower ICP or raise cerebral perfusion pressure (CPP).

3. **How would ICP monitoring change management of a critically ill patient?**
   Prolonged periods of raised ICP can severely impair cerebral blood flow and lead to irreversible neuro-logic injury. In patients with neurologic disease and elevated ICP (greater than 20 to 25 mm Hg), an ICP monitor is useful in guiding management. For example, the effectiveness of lowering ICP by sedation, hyperventilation, administration of mannitol, or hyperosmolar therapy can rapidly be observed. ICP measurement can also be used to accurately target CPP. Maintenance of an adequate CPP is critically important in the care of a neurologically injured patient. When CPP is significantly impaired, secondary brain injury and further complications may ensue. CPP is the difference between the mean arterial pressure (MAP) and the ICP. It is imperative to ensure adequate brain perfusion by maintaining a CPP of at least 55 to 60 mm Hg by either lowering ICP, raising MAP, or both.

4. **Is there a role for continuous EEG monitoring in the ICU?**
   Continuous EEG monitoring is a useful tool in evaluating patients with acute encephalopathy, coma or seizures. Patients admitted to the ICU with seizures and altered mental status should be considered candidates for EEG monitoring to ensure that they are not exhibiting subtle findings of nonconvulsant status epilepticus (NCSE), which would require more aggressive antiepileptic therapy. EEG can also be useful in patients who have suffered a recent cardiac arrest, as evidence suggests that EEG patterns of burst suppression, nonreactivity to stimuli, and NCSE obtained shortly after return of spontaneous circulation can aid in prognostication.

5. **Should patients be monitored for acute delirium while in the ICU?**
   Acute ICU delirium is a common manifestation of critical illness and should be considered a form of brain dysfunction. It is heralded by acute alteration in baseline mental status and the inability to focus, with the key feature of inattention. The incidence of acute delirium is directly related to patient factors such as age, severity of illness, metabolic derangements, and effects of medications. The presence of delirium directly impacts both the morbidity and mortality of critically ill patients, and prevention may be the best way to handle this aspect of critical illness.

   Screening for acute ICU delirium is best carried out by using the validated Confusion Assessment Method for the Intensive Care Unit (CAM-ICU; Fig. 14.1). CAM-ICU is easily performed at the bedside and can be completed within minutes. CAM-ICU positive delirium should prompt the clinician to evaluate for

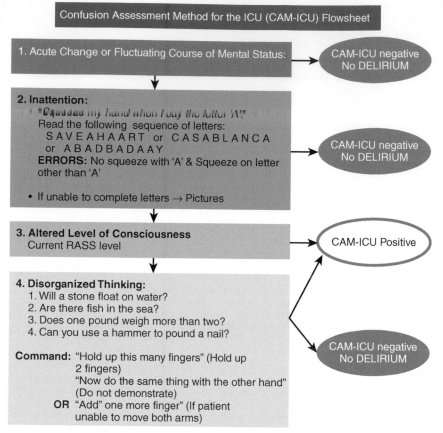

Figure 14-1. Confusion Assessment Method for the Intensive Care Unit tool. RASS, Richmond agitation-sedation scale. (From www.icudelirium.org, Vanderbilt University.)

evidence of infection, medication effects, and metabolic problems that can be corrected. It is recommended that CAM-ICU screening should be routinely done several times throughout the day.

6. **How should continuous sedation be monitored and adjusted in the ICU?**
Critically ill patients, especially those that require invasive mechanical ventilation or other invasive forms of life support, often require continuous infusions of sedating medications in order to provide comfort and tolerance. Monitoring aids such as the validated Richmond Agitation and Sedation Scale (Fig. 14.2) are useful tools that allow healthcare providers to judge level of sedation or arousal and target the level of sedation while titrating sedative agents. In general it is best to aim for a mild level of sedation if necessary.

7. **Can EEG predict cerebral ischemia from vasospasm after subarachnoid hemorrhage (SAH)?**
SAH from a ruptured cerebral aneurysm can have devastating neurologic consequences. One of the feared complications of SAH is delayed cerebral ischemia from arterial vasospasm. Vasospasm following SAH occurs more frequently in large SAHs and can occur between 2 days and roughly 2 weeks after initial presentation. Vasospasm leads to underperfused areas of brain and can cause secondary ischemic stroke and worse neurologic outcomes. Traditionally, screening for vasospasm following SAH is conducted with serial transcranial Doppler ultrasound. Recent evidence suggests that EEG may be able to more rapidly detect early ischemic changes from vasospasm and allow time for rapid treatment to prevent secondary stroke.

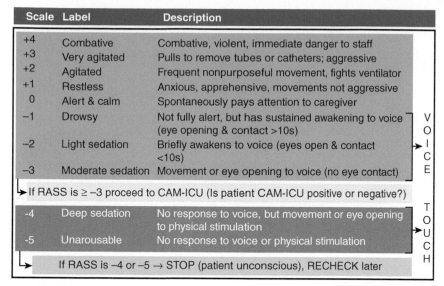

Scale	Label	Description	
+4	Combative	Combative, violent, immediate danger to staff	
+3	Very agitated	Pulls to remove tubes or catheters; aggressive	
+2	Agitated	Frequent nonpurposeful movement, fights ventilator	
+1	Restless	Anxious, apprehensive, movements not aggressive	
0	Alert & calm	Spontaneously pays attention to caregiver	
−1	Drowsy	Not fully alert, but has sustained awakening to voice (eye opening & contact >10s)	V O I C E
−2	Light sedation	Briefly awakens to voice (eyes open & contact <10s)	
−3	Moderate sedation	Movement or eye opening to voice (no eye contact)	

→ If RASS is ≥ −3 proceed to CAM-ICU (Is patient CAM-ICU positive or negative?)

−4	Deep sedation	No response to voice, but movement or eye opening to physical stimulation	T O U C H
−5	Unarousable	No response to voice or physical stimulation	

↳ If RASS is −4 or −5 → STOP (patient unconscious), RECHECK later

Figure 14-2. Richmond Agitation and Sedation Scale. *CAM-ICU,* Confusion Assessment Method for the Intensive Care Unit. RASS, Richmond Agitation-Sedation Scale. *(Courtesy of Curtis N. Sessler, M.D.)*

8. How do you diagnose brain death?
Brain death is a clinical diagnosis that requires a vigorous exam in order to establish. Most institutions have strict policies that must be followed to meet the clinical criteria for brain death declaration. In general, a patient must have a clinical scenario and neurologic imaging that could precipitate brain death, such as diffuse cerebral edema, and a physical exam that affirms the absence of all brain stem reflexes. Patients being evaluated for brain death also must be normothermic, lack severe metabolic abnormalities, and have no evidence of intoxicants or drugs in their systems that could blunt brain stem reflexes. If all these criteria are met, a clinician would proceed with an apnea test. An apnea test is performed while providing a patient supplemental oxygen, removing mechanical ventilation, and observing for spontaneous respirations. If no respirations are observed and the partial pressure of carbon dioxide increases by 20 mm Hg from baseline, the patient may be declared brain dead. Remember, brain death is a legal definition of death, and time of death should be documented as the time of the completion of the apnea test.

9. Do you need to perform confirmatory tests to confirm brain death?
A confirmatory test/ancillary test for brain death declaration is only required in cases of clinical uncertainty, when a patient cannot tolerate an apnea test due to hypoxemia, hypotension, or arrhythmia or when there is significant concern over intoxication or prolonged effects of drug-induced coma. Ancillary tests that are recommended by the American Academy of Neurology include EEG, cerebral angiography, nuclear scan, and transcranial Doppler.

10. What methods are useful in neuroprognostication after cardiac arrest?
Cardiac arrest is very common and can lead to devastating neurologic complications due to severe anoxic brain injury. Routinely following cardiac arrest, patients are treated with targeted temperature management with control of body temperature at either 33°C or 36°C using automated cooling blankets or intravascular cooling catheters. Prognostication of neurologic recovery is a best done with a multitiered approach including regular physical exam, continuous EEG monitoring, somatosensory evoked potentials in which an electrical stimulus is applied to the median nerve and electrical activity is measured over the cortex of the brain, and magnetic resonance imaging (MRI). Caution should be used when prognosticating for patients who have received temperature management at 33°C, as evidence suggests that return of neurologic function could be significantly delayed. Despite this warning, review of physical exam findings in patients treated with therapeutic hypothermia at 33°C has shown

that patients with absence of corneal reflexes and pupillary reflexes at 72 hours postarrest did not have good neurologic outcomes.

KEY POINTS: NEUROMONITORING

1. Patients with severe neurologic disease should be considered candidates for multimodal neuro-monitoring in an intensive care unit setting. Neuromonitoring techniques include serial physical exams, EEG, and intracranial pressure monitoring.
2. Continuous EEG monitoring should be considered when patients remain comatose or have exhibited evidence of seizure activity in order to rule out continued nonconvulsant status epilepticus.
3. Extraventricular drains are useful as a therapeutic and diagnostic tool in patients with obstructive hydrocephalus and infectious processes.
4. Brain death is diagnosed clinically by an exam with absence of all brain stem reflexes and a failed apnea test.
5. In dealing with a patient with acute intracranial hypertension and high risk for cerebral herniation, it is imperative to perform maneuvers to lower ICP to less than 20 mm Hg and maintain a cerebral perfusion pressure of 55 to 60 mm Hg.

BIBLIOGRAPHY

1. Ely EW, Margolin R, Francis J, et al. Evaluation of delirium in critically ill patients: Validation of the Confusion Assessment Method for the Intensive Care Unit (CAM-ICU). *Crit Care Med.* 2001;29(7):1370-1379.
2. Greer D, Yang J, Scripko P, et al. Clinical exam for prognostication in comatose cardiac arrest patients. *Resuscitation.* 2013;84(11):1546-1551.
3. Kondziella D, Friberg C, Wellwood I, Reiffurth C, Fabricius M, Dreier JP. Continuous EEG monitoring in aneurysmal subarachnoid hemorrhage: a systematic review. *Neurocritical Care.* 2015;22:450-461.
4. Le Roux P, Menon D, Citerio G, et al. Consensus summary statement of the international multidisciplinary consensus conference on multimodality monitoring in neurocritical care. *Neurocritical Care.* 2014;21:S1-S26.
5. Lee K, ed. *The Neuro ICU Book.* 1st ed. New York: Mcgraw Hill; 2012.
6. Rossetti A, Urbano L, Delodder F, Kaplan PW, Oddu M. Prognostic value of continuous EEG monitoring during therapeutic hypothermia after cardiac arrest. *Crit Care.* 2010;14:R173.
7. Rossetti A, Oddo M, Logroscino A, Kaplan PW. Prognostication after cardiac arrest and hypothermia: a prospective study. *Ann Neurol.* 2010;67(3):301-307.
8. Sessler C, Gosnell M, Grap MJ, et al. The Richmond agitation-sedation scale: validity and reliability in adult intensive care unit patients. *Am J Respir Crit Care Med.* 2002;166(10):1338-1344.
9. Wijdicks EFM, Hijdra A, Young GB, Bassetti CL, Wiebe S; Quality Standards Subcommittee of the American Academy of Neurology. Practice parameter: prediction of outcome of comatose survivors after cardiopulmonary resuscitation (an evidenced based review): report of the Quality Standards Subcommittee of the American Academy of Neurology. *Neurology.* 2006;67(2):203-210.
10. Wijdicks EF, Varelas P, Gronseth G, Greer DM. Evidence based guideline update: determining brain death in adults. Report of the quality standards subcommittee of the American Academy of Neurology. *Neurology.* 2010;74(23):1911-1918.

III
PROCEDURES

CARDIOPULMONARY RESUSCITATION

Ala Nozari and Sten Rubertsson

The information provided in this chapter can be reviewed in greater detail by referring to specific guidelines published by the American Heart Association (AHA) in conjunction with the European Resuscitation Council and the International Liaison Committee on Resuscitation (ILCOR). The 2010 guidelines provide a comprehensive review of evidence-based recommendations for cardiopulmonary resuscitation (CPR), while the 2015 update focuses on topics with significant new science or controversy.

1. **What is the definition and incidence of out-of-hospital and in-hospital cardiac arrest?**
   Cardiac arrest is defined as a sudden cessation of cardiac mechanical activity, rendering the victim unresponsive without signs of circulation and breathing. There are large variations in the reported incidence of cardiac arrest. The 2009 Resuscitation Outcomes Consortium Cardiac Epistry data reported the incidence of out-of-hospital cardiac arrest to be 126.5 per 100,000 adults, with a survival rate of 4.5%. Survival rate was greater after emergency medical services (EMS)–treated and bystander-initiated CPR. The 2011 adult in-hospital cardiac arrest rate was reported by the Get With The Guidelines–Resuscitation Investigators to be 0.92 per 1000 bed days, translating to about 192,000 in-hospital cardiac arrests per year throughout the United States.

2. **Name common factors that affect survival rates and outcomes of patients experiencing cardiac arrest.**
   There are regional and patient-related differences in survival to hospital discharge, varying from about 3%–16.3% for out-of-hospital cardiac arrest and up to 23.9% for adults and 40.2% for children after in-hospital cardiac arrest. Factors that are known to affect outcome include the etiology of sudden cardiac arrest (0%–2% survival to hospital discharge for asystole versus 25%–40% after ventricular fibrillation [VF]), age, gender (men have a higher incidence of VF as the initial rhythm and a higher survival rate), preexisting comorbidities, bystander CPR and time to resuscitation, duration and quality of CPR, timing of defibrillation, time to return of spontaneous circulation (ROSC), and body temperature. The Good Outcome Following Attempted Resuscitation (GO-FAR) score was derived from the Get With The Guidelines-Resuscitation registry to predict survival with good neurologic outcome and provides higher likelihood of survival scores to younger patients with normal baseline neurologic function and fewer comorbidities.

3. **Name the most important elements of basic life support (BLS).**
   With the exception of cardiac arrest following asphyxiation, the most important steps for adult patients in cardiac arrest are:
   1. Immediately recognize unresponsiveness.
   2. Check for apnea or lack of normal breathing.
   3. Activate emergency response system and retrieve an automated external defibrillator (AED).
   4. Check for a pulse (no more than 10 seconds).
   5. Start cycles of 30 chest compressions followed by two breaths.
   This applies to all adult cardiac arrest victims regardless of location (in hospital or out of hospital). Rescue breaths are not prioritized over chest compressions during the first few minutes of resuscitation, as respiratory attempts can reduce CPR efficacy due to—among others—interruption in chest compressions. Therefore it is recommended that a lone rescuer should not interrupt chest compressions for ventilation. Moreover, it is important to ensure that placement of an advanced airway (intubation) does not delay the initiation of effective CPR. Once the AED or defibrillator arrives, it should be attached without delay, so that an electrical shock can be delivered to improve the likelihood of ROSC. Electrode pad or paddle placement on the chest wall should be to the right of the upper sternal border below the clavicle and to the left of the nipple, with the center in the midaxillary line.

4. **What are the compressions, airway, and breathing (CAB) of resuscitation?**
   The 2010 AHA and ILCOR guidelines were changed to underscore the importance of early and effective chest compressions. These changes stem from evidence supporting the importance of chest

compressions and the need to quickly restore blood flow to improve the likelihood of ROSC. Therefore the *CAB* of resuscitation has replaced the *ABCD* of resuscitation to emphasize that the initial resuscitation should now begin with closed-chest compressions once it has been established that the patient is unresponsive, is not breathing, and has no pulse. After 30 chest compressions, the airway is opened and two breaths are delivered. Thus the sequence is CAB, emphasizing quality chest compressions as early as possible with the goal to

- Minimize interruptions in chest compressions
- Allow complete chest recoil
- Provide 100 to 120 compressions per minute
- Provide compression depth of at least 5 cm (2 in) in adults and 4 cm (1.5 in) in infants
- Maintain compression/ventilation ratio of 30:2 for adults and children (15:2 in children when two or more rescuers are present). In the presence of an advanced airway, that is, an endotracheal tube, chest compressions should be provided continuously at a rate of 100 to 120/min, with 1 breath every 6 seconds.
- Avoid excessive ventilation (>8–10 breaths/min or large tidal volumes)

5. How does blood flow during closed-chest compressions?
   Two basic models derived from animal studies explain the movement of blood during closed-chest compressions:
   - In the **cardiac pump** model, the heart is squeezed between the sternum and the spine. Systole occurs when the heart is compressed; the atrioventricular valves close and the pulmonary and aortic valves open, ensuring ejection of blood with unidirectional, antegrade flow. Diastole occurs with the release of the squeezed heart, resulting in a fall in intracardiac pressures; the atrioventricular valves open while the pulmonary and aortic valves close. Blood is subsequently drawn into the heart from the venae cavae and lungs.
   - In the **thoracic pump** model, the heart is considered a passive conduit. Closed-chest compression results in uniformly increased pressures throughout the thoracic cavity. Forward flow of blood occurs with each squeeze of the heart and thorax because of the relative noncompliance of the arterial system (i.e., they resist collapse) and the one-way valves preventing retrograde flow in the venous system. Both of these models probably contribute to blood flow during CPR.

6. List the main determinants of a successful ROSC.
   - Effective and early initiation of high-quality chest compressions.
   - Early defibrillation: For most adults, the primary cause of sudden, normovolemic nontraumatic cardiac arrest is VF or pulseless ventricular tachycardia (pVT), for which the recommended treatment is electrical defibrillation.
   - Duration of no-flow (cardiac arrest with no chest compressions) and low-flow (ongoing CPR) circulatory arrest, as well as the quality of CPR and hence cerebral and coronary perfusion pressures. Survival from a VF arrest decreases by 7% to 10% for each minute of delay.

7. What is the role of pharmacologic therapy during advanced cardiac life support (ACLS)?
   The immediate goals of pharmacologic therapy are to improve cerebral and myocardial blood flow, increase ventricular inotropy, and terminate life-threatening arrhythmias, thereby maximizing the perfusion of the vital organs and restoring spontaneous circulation. Combined α/β-adrenergic agonists, such as epinephrine, and smooth-muscle V_1 agonists, such as vasopressin, augment the mean aortic-to-ventricular end-diastolic pressure gradient (coronary perfusion pressure) by increasing arterial vascular tone. Despite physiologic benefits and an increased rate of ROSC, however, rigorous clinical trials have failed to consistently show outcome benefits from epinephrine in these patients. Phenylephrine and norepinephrine also increase arterial pressure and myocardial blood flow, but neither has been shown to be superior to epinephrine. Clinically, vasopressin does not offer any outcome benefits over epinephrine, nor does the combined use of vasopressin and epinephrine. Therefore, vasopressin was removed in the 2015 AHA guidelines to simplify the algorithm.

   In addition to improving or maintaining myocardial blood flow, pharmacologic therapy during ACLS is also aimed at terminating or preventing arrhythmias, which can further damage an already severely ischemic heart. VF and pVT markedly increase myocardial oxygen consumption at a time when oxygen supply is tenuous because of poor delivery. Intracellular acidosis only causes the myocardium to be more dysfunctional and irritable, which makes the heart more vulnerable to arrhythmias. Amiodarone, a class III antiarrhythmic agent, or alternatively lidocaine (class Ib), may be considered for the treatment of VF or pVT that is unresponsive to CPR with vasopressors and defibrillation.

8. Is sodium bicarbonate indicated in the routine management of cardiopulmonary arrest?
   No! The primary treatment of metabolic acidosis from tissue hypoperfusion and hypoxia during a cardiac arrest is adequate chest compressions and ventilations. Shortly after circulatory arrest, a mixed metabolic and respiratory acidosis starts to develop. Studies have shown that severe acidosis can lead to depression of myocardial contractile function, ventricular irritability, and a lowered threshold for VF. In addition, a markedly low pH interferes with the vascular and myocardial responses to adrenergic drugs and endogenous catecholamines, reducing cardiac chronotropy and inotropy. Although it is appealing to administer sodium bicarbonate in this situation, the clinician must keep in mind that the bicarbonate ion, after combining with a hydrogen ion, generates new carbon dioxide. Cell membranes are highly permeable to carbon dioxide (more so than bicarbonate); therefore administration of sodium bicarbonate causes a paradoxical intracellular acidosis. The resultant intracellular hypercapnia can lead to a decline in cardiac contractile function and worsening chance of ROSC. The generated carbon dioxide also needs to be eliminated to prevent worsening of an already present respiratory acidosis. Other non-CO_2-generating buffers such as trometamol; tris-hydroxymethyl aminomethane (THAM), tribonate, or carbicarb may be considered to minimize some adverse effects of sodium bicarbonate. It should be noted, nevertheless, that severe systemic alkalosis during cardiac arrest is also associated with worse outcome, although it could be a consequence of poor tissue perfusion with suboptimal clearance and washout of cellular acidosis (or a result of poor quality CPR) rather than the cause of the poor outcome. Routine administration of sodium bicarbonate is currently not recommended.

9. What are common arrhythmias associated with cardiopulmonary arrests?
   The initial rhythm in many nontraumatic cardiac arrests in adults is VF or pVT, often caused by myocardial ischemia or infarct. The incidence of cardiac arrest with an initial rhythm of VF is, nevertheless, decreasing, possibly as a result of an increasing and more comprehensive management of patients with advanced coronary artery disease, including pharmacologic, interventional or surgical treatments, the use of implantable cardioverter-defibrillators or simply an increasing response time by the EMS team in highly populated urban or remote suburban areas. Electrolyte disturbances (hypokalemia or hypomagnesemia), prolonged hypoxemia, and drug toxicity can also be important inciting factors in patients with preexisting medical problems. Also not uncommon are bradyasystolic arrests (as many as 50% of in-hospital arrests). One cause of this arrhythmia could be unrecognized hypoxemia or acidemia. Other causes include heightened vagal tone precipitated by medications, an inferoposterior myocardial infarction (Bezold–Jarisch reflex), or invasive procedures. A third common arrest rhythm seen is pulseless electrical activity (PEA). A common etiology is prolonged arrest itself. Typically, after 8 minutes or more of VF, electrical defibrillation induces a slow, wide-complex PEA that tends to be terminal and is known as a pulseless idioventricular rhythm. On most occasions of an unsuccessful resuscitation, VF degrades to pulseless idioventricular rhythm before the patient becomes asystolic. The rhythm of PEA can also be narrow and fast, which accompanies other reversible life-threatening conditions rather than just representing a terminal rhythm. Examples are cardiac tamponade, hypovolemia, pulmonary embolus, or tension pneumothorax.

10. What are the most common, immediately reversible causes of cardiopulmonary arrest?
    The "H"s and "T"s that can lead to cardiopulmonary arrest should always be ruled out, and if present, treated immediately:
    - **Hypovolemia:** should be suspected in all cases of arrest associated with rapid blood loss. Common etiologies include trauma, gastrointestinal hemorrhage, and nontraumatic rupture of major arteries such as an aortic aneurysm. *Relative* hypovolemia can be the clinical manifestation of other underlying conditions such as severe sepsis or anaphylaxis leading to vasodilation and extensive capillary leak. Regardless of the type, a large amount of fluid (crystalloid, colloid, blood) should be rapidly administered and the cause of the hypovolemia corrected (e.g., through surgical control of the bleeding).
    - **Hypoxia:** Hypoxia is a more common cause of cardiac arrest in the pediatric population. Tracheal intubation with the delivery of a high concentration of oxygen is often required while the cause of the hypoxia is determined and definitive management instituted.
    - **Hydrogen ions (acidosis):** These can lead to myocardial failure resulting in cardiogenic shock and arrest. The high hydrogen ion concentration also increases myocardial irritability and arrhythmia formation. Known preexisting severe acidosis can be partially compensated for by hyperventilation, but sodium bicarbonate may still need to be administered. The underlying cause of the acidosis should be diagnosed and corrected.
    - **Hyperkalemia:** This condition is encountered in patients with renal insufficiency, diabetes, and profound acidosis. Peaked T waves and a widening of the QRS complex, with the electrical activity eventually deteriorating to a sinus-wave pattern, herald hyperkalemia. Treatment includes the

administration of calcium chloride, sodium bicarbonate, insulin, and glucose. *Hypokalemia* and other electrolyte disturbances leading to a cardiac arrest are much less common. Treatment of the abnormality should help restore spontaneous circulation.

- **Hypothermia:** This condition should be easily detected on examination of the patient. The electrocardiogram (ECG) may reveal Osborne waves, which are pathognomonic. All resuscitation efforts should be continued until the patient is euthermic. Extracorporeal circulation and warming may be needed.

- **Tablets or toxins:** Ingestion of these items should be considered primarily in younger patients with an out-of-hospital cardiac arrest. Some of the more common intoxications include carbon monoxide poisoning after prolonged exposure to smoke or exhaust fumes from incomplete combustion, cyanide poisoning during fires involving synthetic materials, and drug overdoses (intentional or unintentional). High-flow, high-concentration, and, if possible, hyperbaric oxygen, along with the management of acidosis, are the cornerstones of treatment for carbon monoxide and cyanide poisonings. In addition, intravenous (IV) sodium nitrite and sodium thiosulfate can be used to help remove cyanide from the circulation. Tricyclic antidepressant drugs act as a type Ia antiarrhythmic agent and cause slowing of cardiac conduction, ventricular arrhythmias, hypotension, and seizures. Alkalinization of blood and urine, in addition to seizure control, can aid in controlling toxicity. An opiate overdose causes hypoxia from hypoventilation, whereas an overdose of cocaine can lead to myocardial ischemia. Naloxone reverses the effects of opioids and should be administered immediately if an opioid overdose is suspected.

- **Cardiac tamponade:** Cardiac tamponade presents with hypotension, a narrowed pulse pressure, elevated jugular venous pressure, distant and muffled heart sounds, and low-voltage QRS complexes on the ECG. Trauma patients and patients with malignancies are at greatest risk. Pericardiocentesis or subxiphoid pericardiorrhaphy can be lifesaving.

- **Tension pneumothorax:** This condition must be recognized immediately and can occur in trauma patients and those receiving positive-pressure ventilation. The signs of a tension pneumothorax are rapid-onset hypotension, hypoxia, and an increase in airway pressures. Subcutaneous emphysema and reduced breath sounds on the affected side with tracheal deviation toward the unaffected side are commonly noted. The placement of a 14- or 16-gauge IV catheter into the second intercostal space at the midclavicular line or into the fifth intercostal space at the anterior axillary line for immediate decompression is imperative for restoration of circulation. A chest tube can be placed after the tension pneumothorax is converted to a simple pneumothorax, which does not pose a similar immediate threat to patient's life.

- **Thrombosis of a coronary artery:** This condition can lead to myocardial ischemia and infarct. Reperfusion is a vital determinant of eventual outcome. Cardiac catheterization is the primary choice if it is immediately available; thrombolysis is an alternative when this is not readily available.

- **Thrombosis of the pulmonary artery:** Thrombosis of the pulmonary artery can be devastating. Some patients may be seen initially with dyspnea and chest pain, similar to acute coronary syndromes, but those who are seen in cardiac arrest have a minimal chance of survival. Management can include activation of a multidisciplinary response team for immediate thrombolysis or surgery to unload the right ventricle while restoring pulmonary blood flow.

11. How should VF be treated?

Early defibrillation with a single nonsynchronized electrical shock is recommended to minimize myocardial damage. Biphasic defibrillators are recommended because of their greater efficacy at lower energy levels. In employing a biphasic defibrillator, the initial dose of energy recommended by the manufacturer (120–200 J) should be delivered; but if this dose is not known, the maximal dose may be used. Recommended shock energy for monophasic defibrillators remains at 360 J. It may be helpful to continue chest compressions while charging the defibrillator, thus minimizing any interruptions in coronary perfusion before defibrillation. Chest compressions should be resumed immediately after defibrillation without rechecking for a pulse and should not be interrupted to assess the rhythm. Rhythm checks and additional shocks should be performed no more frequently than every 2 minutes.

　　If the initial single shock is not successful and VF or pVT persists after 2 minutes of CPR, epinephrine should be administered (1 mg IV every 3 to 5 minutes) without interruption of high-quality CPR. Although antiarrhythmic drugs provide little survival benefit in refractory VF or pVT, they may be considered after a second unsuccessful defibrillation attempt in anticipation of a third shock. Amiodarone is administered as a single dose of 300 mg IV with a repeat dose of 150 mg IV as indicated. Alternatively, lidocaine 1 to 1.5 mg/kg IV, then 0.5 to 0.75 mg/kg can be administered every 5 to 10 minutes if amiodarone is unavailable. Magnesium sulfate is not recommended for routine use during CPR but should be considered in patients with polymorphic ventricular tachycardia consistent with torsade de pointes.

12. **Is pulseless idioventricular rhythm treatable?**
Delayed electrical defibrillation or prolonged VF frequently results in a pulseless idioventricular rhythm or asystole. In the majority of cases, the idioventricular rhythm is not amenable to treatment and results in death. In animal experiments, high-dose epinephrine (0.1–0.2 mg/kg) has helped to restore cardiac contractility and pacemaker activity. However, several clinical studies have shown no benefit in long-term survival or neurologic outcome, and it is therefore not recommended.

13. **How is asystole treated?**
Given the grim prognosis for successful resuscitation, the clinician should rapidly determine whether evidence exists that resuscitation should not be attempted in approaching a patient in asystole. Management of both asystole and PEA includes rapid institution of high-quality CPR and reversal of underlying causes such as hypoxia, hyperkalemia, and hemorrhage. Defibrillation is not required for either condition, as asystole has no electrical activity and PEA is an organized electrical rhythm without cardiac pump function. It is important to note that fine-wave VF can sometimes be mistaken for asystole. Rotate the monitoring leads 90 degrees (if using paddles), and maximize the amplitude to rule out fine VF (if present, defibrillation should be performed immediately). If using the pads and ECG leads, cycle through the various leads (I, III, III).

Contrary to asystole, PEA has a more favorable outcome. However, the underlying cause must be addressed for the resuscitation to be successful. High-quality CPR with epinephrine administration should be continued until ROSC or a shockable rhythm is achieved.

14. **What are the appropriate routes of administration of drugs during resuscitation?**
The preferred choice is by the IV route. If a central venous catheter is in place, this should be used over a peripheral venous line. Administration of drugs through a peripheral venous line will result in a slightly delayed onset of action, although the peak drug effect is similar to that achieved via the central route. Drugs administered peripherally should be followed with at least 20 mL of normal saline solution to ensure central delivery. Intracardiac administration should not be performed. Virtually every resuscitation drug can be administered in conventional doses via the intraosseous route. Because of the ease of insertion via readily available kits, this method is preferred in all patients when an IV line cannot be readily obtained. Endotracheal administration of drugs should be considered only when attempts at obtaining an IV or intraosseous line have failed. The *NAVEL* drugs (i.e., naloxone, atropine, vasopressin, epinephrine, lidocaine) are absorbed systemically after endotracheal administration. Although pulmonary blood flow, and hence systemic absorption, is minimal during CPR, recent animal studies suggest that comparable hemodynamic responses can occur. Two to three times the standard IV doses are recommended for the endotracheal route.

15. **How can mechanical chest compression devices improve the quality of CPR, and why is the standard use of these devices not yet included in the AHA/ILCOR CPR guidelines?**
A key factor that improves survival in victims of cardiac arrest is good-quality chest compressions. The quality of CPR delivered at out-of-hospital cardiac arrest is often suboptimal, due, among others things, to provider fatigue and the need for them to attend to other important tasks during chest compressions. Mechanical chest compression devices can provide compressions with a standard depth and frequency for prolonged periods, enabling the provider to focus on other aspects of patient care. The main technologies employed include piston devices (e.g., the LUCAS device), which compresses the chest in a similar way to manual chest compressions using a piston mounted on a frame that fits around the patient's chest, and load-distributing bands (e.g., the Auto pulse device), which provide rhythmic chest compressions with an alternately shortened and lengthened wide band around the chest. Despite their theoretical advantages, however, randomized trials of out-of-hospital cardiac arrest have failed to prove survival benefits or improved neurologic outcome with current versions of mechanical chest compression devices as compared with manual chest compressions. Therefore routine use of these devices is yet not recommended by the AHA or ILCOR, although they may be reasonable alternatives to conventional CPR in specific settings where the delivery of high-quality manual compressions would be challenging for the provider. These conditions may include prolonged CPR with a limited number of providers and CPR in a moving ambulance or in the angiography suite.

16. List the important goal-oriented postresuscitation interventions.

The main objectives of the postresuscitation interventions are to optimize blood flow and oxygenation to vital organs and to prevent organ system dysfunction and secondary injury. Hypotension may worsen the initial insult and the neurologic outcome, but overzealous hemodynamic goals may also overstress a decompensated heart with risk for worsening hemodynamics and multiorgan failure. Accordingly, a mean arterial blood pressure goal of greater than 65 mm Hg, if tolerated, may be targeted to minimize secondary tissue injury and may include appropriate titration of inotropic and vasoactive agents in addition to maintaining adequate volume status and urine output greater than 0.5 mL/kg. Active control of temperature should be initiated as soon as possible. Many earlier laboratory and clinical studies have shown beneficial effects of therapeutic hypothermia of 32°C to 33°C after resuscitation from cardiac arrest, but a recent study failed to confirm outcome benefits in survivors of in-hospital cardiac arrest. Consequently many centers no longer employ therapeutic hypothermia of 32°C to 33°C but instead are using temperature control to 36°C in these patients. It has been argued that therapeutic hypothermia may need to be tailored to the individual patient's clinical exam, such that uncomplicated patients may be considered for treatment to a target temperature of only 36°C (active temperature control avoiding fever); whereas those with deep coma or loss of motor response/brain stem reflexes can be treated to a target temperature of 32°C to 34°C (mild therapeutic hypothermia). Needless to say, acute coronary syndrome should be managed quickly and appropriately, and emergent coronary catheterization or reperfusion therapy must be considered in patients with ECG evidence of ST-segment elevation myocardial infarction or in those with persistent hemodynamic instability.

ACKNOWLEDGMENT

The authors wish to acknowledge Dr. David Shimabukuro, MDCM, for the valuable contributions to the previous edition of this chapter.

KEY POINTS: CARDIOPULMONARY RESUSCITATION

1. High-quality chest compressions and early defibrillation are the main determinants of successful return of spontaneous circulation in cardiac arrest victims.
2. Reversible causes of cardiac arrest include hypovolemia, hypoxia, hydrogen ions (acidosis), hyperkalemia, toxins, tamponade, tension pneumothorax, coronary thrombosis, and pulmonary thrombosis.
3. If intravenous access is not readily available, then move to the intraosseous route.

BIBLIOGRAPHY

1. Field JM, Hazinski MF, Sayre MR, et al. Part 1: executive summary: 2010 American Heart Association Guidelines for Cardiopulmonary Resuscitation and Emergency Cardiovascular Care. *Circulation.* 2010;122:S640-S656.
2. Neumar RW, Shuster M, Callaway CW, et al. 2015 American Heart Association Guidelines Update for Cardiopulmonary Resuscitation and Emergency Cardiovascular Care. *Circulation.* 2015;132:S315-S367.
3. Gueugniaud PY, David JS, Chanzy E, et al. Vasopressin and epinephrine vs. epinephrine alone in cardiopulmonary resuscitation. *N Engl J Med.* 2008;359:21-30.
4. Soar J, Nolan JP, Böttiger BW, et al. European Resuscitation Council Guidelines for Resuscitation 2015 Section 3. Adult advanced life support. *Resuscitation.* 2015;95:100-147.

CHAPTER 16

ARTERIAL AND CENTRAL VENOUS CATHETERS

Hovig V. Chitilian

1. What are the indications for intra-arterial blood pressure monitoring?
   - Inability to obtain noninvasive blood pressure measurements (i.e., burn or multitrauma patient with all extremities affected; during cardiopulmonary bypass; in patients with left ventricular assist devices)
   - Continuous blood pressure monitoring due to patient's underlying condition
   - Frequent intraoperative blood sampling for laboratory testing

2. Which are the common sites for intra-arterial catheter placement? What is the effect of the catheter site on the measured blood pressure?
   The common sites are the radial, brachial, axillary, femoral, and dorsalis pedis arteries. As the monitoring site is moved further distally in the arterial tree, the systolic blood pressure increases and the diastolic blood pressure decreases when compared with central arterial pressure. The mean arterial pressure, however, remains the same between peripheral and central arterial sites of measurement.

3. What additional data can be determined from the intra-arterial pressure waveform?
   In addition to direct pressure measurements, the arterial pressure waveform can be used to determine a patient's fluid responsiveness as well as cardiac output. Changes in the arterial pressure waveform during positive pressure ventilation have been shown to predict fluid responsiveness (a measurable increase in stroke volume with the administration of fluid). Goal-directed intraoperative fluid management based on arterial waveform changes has been shown to improve outcome in patients undergoing high-risk surgery. In addition, a number of commercially available devices exist that allow the continuous measurement of cardiac output with use of arterial pressure waveform analysis.

4. What are the most common complications of arterial catheterization?
   Vascular insufficiency (3%–5%), bleeding (1.5%–2.5%), and infection (<1%)

5. What are the risk factors for vascular complications in patients with intra-arterial catheters?
   Concomitant use of vasopressors, prior arterial injury, duration of cannulation longer than 48 or 72 hours, hematoma formation, presence of disseminated intravascular coagulation, reduced cardiac output, and female gender.

6. What is the risk of permanent distal ischemic damage?
   Studies have suggested that the rate of arterial occlusion is lower in axillary and femoral catheters compared with radial artery catheters; however, the rate of permanent distal ischemic damage is comparable at 0.1% to 0.2%. The incidence of permanent ischemic damage to the hand after radial artery catheterization has been reported to be 0.09%.

7. Is the modified Allen test useful?
   The modified Allen test is a test of circulatory supply to the hand based on alternating occlusion of the radial and ulnar arteries. There is no evidence that it can predict hand ischemia with radial artery cannulation.

8. What is the risk of arterial catheter–related bloodstream infection (BSI)?
   The incidence of BSIs associated with arterial catheters is 0.8% or 1.7 per 1000 catheter days. Data are conflicting regarding the association of the site of catheterization with risk of infection, with some studies suggesting that radial or dorsalis pedis arterial sites are associated with a decreased incidence of BSI when compared with the femoral artery.

9. What measures can be taken to reduce the risk of BSI associated with intra-arterial catheters?
   The Centers for Disease Control and Prevention do not recommend routine replacement of peripheral arterial catheters at fixed time intervals as a method for preventing catheter-related BSIs. The use of

full-barrier sterile precautions (chlorhexidine skin preparation, mask, hat, sterile gloves, gown, and sheet) has not been shown to reduce the risk of bacterial colonization or BSI when compared with the use of hand washing, chlorhexidine preparation, and sterile gloves for the placement of radial or dorsalis pedis arterial catheters.

10. What are the indications for central venous cannulation?
    - Monitoring of cardiac filling pressures
    - Rapid administration of fluid
    - Intravenous administration of medications or fluids that are potentially damaging to peripheral veins or tissues (vasoactive medications, parenteral nutrition)
    - Insertion of pulmonary artery catheter or transvenous pacing wires
    - Aspiration of air embolus
    - Access for hemodialysis or hemofiltration
    - Venous access in the instance of difficult peripheral venous access

11. Which veins are commonly used? How are they accessed?
    The most commonly accessed central veins are the internal jugular, the subclavian, and the femoral veins. With use of either anatomic landmarks or ultrasound guidance, the vein is accessed percutaneously with a *finder* needle of a gauge smaller than the catheter. A guidewire is then passed through the needle and into the vein. The needle is removed, and a dilator is passed over the wire and into the vein to dilate the tissue tract and venous entry point. The dilator is removed, and the catheter is then passed over the wire and into the vein.

12. What are the complications associated with central venous catheterization?
    It is estimated that more than 15% of patients who receive central venous catheters have complications. Significant complications include arterial puncture, hematoma, pneumothorax, hemothorax, air embolus, and BSI. The risk of each complication varies with the location of the vein that is cannulated. The most common mechanical complications are arterial puncture, hematoma, and pneumothorax. Internal jugular venous catheterization and subclavian venous catheterization carry similar risks of mechanical complications. Subclavian venous cannulation carries the highest risk of pneumothorax (1.5%–3%). Femoral venous cannulation carries the highest risk of arterial puncture (9%–15%), followed by internal jugular venous cannulation (6%–9.5%).

13. Is there any benefit to the use of ultrasound guidance?
    The use of ultrasound guidance for central venous catheterization has been shown to reduce the number of cannulation attempts, as well as the incidence of a number of mechanical complications, including arterial puncture, hematoma, pneumothorax, brachial plexus injury, and infection. The data showing the benefit of ultrasound guidance of central venous catheterization has prompted regulatory agencies in both the United States and Europe to recommend the routine use of ultrasound guidance for establishing central venous access.

14. How can ultrasound be used to establish central venous access?
    Ultrasound-guided vascular access should be conducted with a linear probe using a 7- to 12-MHz frequency range. In general, imaging with higher ultrasound frequencies yields greater resolution but lower penetration. The use of lower ultrasound frequencies yields greater penetration but reduced resolution. Blood vessels can be visualized in the long axis (ultrasound beam parallel to the vessel) or in the short axis (ultrasound beam perpendicular to the vessel). Likewise, the needle can be visualized in the plane of the ultrasound beam and parallel to it (*in-plane* visualization) or perpendicular to the plane of the ultrasound beam *(out-of-plane* visualization*)*. During imaging, the ultrasound probe should always be held perpendicular to the skin. The relevant ultrasound anatomy should be identified in the short axis, and the vein of interest should be examined for evidence of thrombosis or aberrant anatomy. The vessel of interest should be centered on the screen, and its depth should be noted. Veins can be distinguished from arteries based on their thinner walls, compressibility, and nonpulsatile flow.

15. What is the risk of central venous catheter–related bloodstream infection (CRBSI)?
    It is estimated that approximately 72,000 CRBSIs occur in intensive care and dialysis units in the United States each year. These infections are associated with increased mortality, greater length of hospital stay, and excess costs of $45,000 per episode.

16. What are the risk factors for CRBSI in patients with central venous catheters?
    - Prolonged hospitalization before catheterization
    - Prolonged duration of catheterization

- Heavy microbial colonization at the insertion site
- Heavy microbial colonization of the catheter hub
- Internal jugular venous catheterization
- Neutropenia
- Total parenteral nutrition through the catheter
- Substandard care of the catheter
     The subclavian site of insertion is associated with the lowest risk of CRBSI.

17. **What is the pathogenesis of CRBSI?**
CRBSI arises from bacterial colonization of the central venous catheter. The four methods of colonization are:
- Migration of bacteria along the skin-catheter interface
- Contamination of a catheter access port
- Seeding of the catheter through the bloodstream from another focus of infection
- Infusion of a contaminated solution
     Common bacterial pathogens in hospital-acquired CRBSI include coagulase-negative *Staphylococcus aureus*, *S. aureus*, *Enterococcus* species, *Candida* species, *Escherichia coli*, and *Klebsiella* species.

18. **How is a CRBSI diagnosed?**
CRBSI should be suspected in patients who have evidence of a BSI (such as fever) and an indwelling central venous catheter. The Infectious Diseases Society of America (IDSA) guidelines recommend that the diagnosis be confirmed with simultaneous quantitative blood cultures drawn through the central venous catheter (or a culture of the catheter tip) and a peripheral vein with at least a threefold greater colony count from the central line sample. If a peripheral venous sample cannot be drawn, samples should be drawn from each lumen of the central venous catheter. A threefold greater colony count from one lumen compared with the others indicates a possible CRBSI.

19. **How is a CRBSI treated?**
Once cultures have been obtained, treatment of CRBSI consists of the removal of the catheter and the initiation of systemic antibiotics. Empiric therapy with vancomycin is recommended in institutions with an increased prevalence of methicillin-resistant staphylococci until culture results and sensitivities are obtained. Empiric coverage should include antibiotics with activity against gram-negative bacilli and *Candida* species in patients who receive total parenteral nutrition, are taking a prolonged course of broad-spectrum antibiotics, have a hematologic malignancy, have had stem cell or solid organ transplantation, or have had femoral catheterization.

20. **What steps are recommended to prevent CRBSI?**
Recommendations by the IDSA to prevent CRBSI include
- Performance of hand hygiene prior to catheter insertion
- Centralization of central venous catheter insertion supplies in a line cart or kit
- Use of maximal sterile barrier precautions
- Skin preparation with 2% chlorhexidine-based antiseptic
- Preferential use of the subclavian vein and avoidance of the femoral vein
- Disinfection of catheter ports before access
- Evaluation of the need for continued central catheter use on a daily basis
     The use of ultrasound guidance for central venous catheter insertion has also been shown to reduce the risk of CRBSI.

KEY POINTS: ARTERIAL AND CENTRAL VENOUS CATHETERS

1. Indications for intra-arterial blood pressure monitoring: inability to obtain noninvasive blood pressure measurements, need for continuous blood pressure monitoring, need for frequent intraoperative blood sampling for laboratory testing.
2. Common complications of intra-arterial catheter placement: vascular insufficiency, hematoma, and infection.
3. Common indications for central venous cannulation: monitoring of cardiac filling pressures, central administration of drugs, rapid administration of fluid, and insertion of pulmonary artery catheter.
4. Prevention of central venous CRBSIs includes performance of hand hygiene before catheter insertion, use of maximal sterile barrier precautions, preferential use of the subclavian vein, and skin preparation with 2% chlorhexidine-based antiseptic.

BIBLIOGRAPHY

1. Brzezinski M, Luisetti T, London MJ. Radial artery cannulation: a comprehensive review of recent anatomic and physiologic investigations. *Anesth Analg.* 2009;109:1763-1781.
2. Chew MS, Aneman A. Hemodynamic monitoring using arterial waveform analysis. *Curr Opin Crit Care.* 2013;19:234-241.
3. de Waal EE, Wappler F, Buhre WF. Cardiac output monitoring. *Curr Opin Anesthesiol.* 2009;22:71-77.
4. Fragou M, Gravvanis A, Dimitriou V, et al. Real-time ultrasound-guided subclavian vein cannulation versus the landmark method in critical care patients: a prospective randomized study. *Crit Care Med.* 2011;39:1607-1612.
5. Frezza EE, Mezghebe H. Indications and complications of arterial catheter use in surgical or medical intensive care units: analysis of 4932 patients. *Am Surg* 1998;64:127 131.
6. Karakitsos D, Labropoulos N, De Groot E, et al. Real-time ultrasound-guided catheterisation of the internal jugular vein: a prospective comparison with the landmark technique in critical care patients. *Crit Care.* 2006;10:R162.
7. Lipira AB, Mackinnon SE, Fox IK. Axillary arterial catheter use associated with hand ischemia in a multi-trauma patient: case report and literature review. *J Clin Anesth.* 2011;23:325-328.
8. Maki DG, Kluger DM, Crnich CJ. The risk of bloodstream infection in adults with different intravascular devices: a systematic review of 200 published prospective studies. *Mayo Clin Proc.* 2006;81:1159-1171.
9. Mark JB, Barbeito A. Arterial and central venous pressure monitoring. *Anesthesiol Clin.* 2006;24:717-735.
10. McGee DC, Gould MK. Preventing complications of central venous catheterization. *N Engl J Med.* 2003;348:1123-1133.
11. Mermel LA, Allon M, Bouza E, et al. Clinical practice guidelines for the diagnosis and management of intravascular catheter-related infection: 2009 Updates by the Infectious Diseases Society of America. *Clin Infect Dis.* 2009;49:1-45.
12. Michard F. Stroke volume variation: from applied physiology to improved outcomes. *Crit Care Med.* 2011;39:402-403.
13. O'Grady NP, Alexander M, Burns LA, et al. Guidelines for the prevention of intravascular catheter–related infections. *Am J Infect Control.* 2011;39:S1-S34.
14. Rupp ME, Majorant D. Prevention of vascular catheter-related bloodstream infections. *Infect Dis Clin North Am.* 2016; 30:853-868.
15. Scheer BV, Perel A, Pfeiffer UJ. Clinical review: complications and risk factors of peripheral arterial catheters used for hemodynamic monitoring in anaesthesia and intensive care medicine. *Crit Care.* 2002;6:199-204.

CHAPTER 17

CRITICAL CARE ULTRASOUND

Lydia Miller and Kenneth Shelton

QUESTIONS/ANSWERS

1. **Why is learning critical care ultrasonography important?**

   Point-of-care ultrasound by intensivists is a vital tool in the rapid assessment of critically ill patients presenting with hemodynamic instability or respiratory failure. Incorporating ultrasound imaging of the heart, lung, vasculature, and abdomen with other clinical findings helps identify the etiology of shock or respiratory failure and guides treatment. Critical care ultrasonography (CCUS) increases the safety of commonly performed intensive care unit (ICU) procedures including central line placement, thoracentesis, and paracentesis. CCUS can be performed and interpreted immediately, does not expose the patient to radiation or contrast dyes, and can be repeatedly performed to assess response to interventions. The Society for Critical Care Anesthesiologists strongly recommends that critical care training programs include formal teaching in CCUS and has published learning goals and competencies for critical care trainees in cardiac, thoracic, abdominal, and vascular ultrasound.

2. **Is there evidence supporting the use of critical care ultrasonography?**

   Studies have examined the sensitivity and specificity of point-of-case ultrasound compared to other imaging techniques. An expert panel of intensivists recently evaluated these studies and incorporated them into evidence-based guidelines for the use of critical care ultrasonography. Indications for CCUS that received strong recommendation on the basis of high or moderate quality evidence are listed in Box 17.1.

3. **What precautions should be taken when performing or interpreting point-of-care ultrasound?**

   The quality of point-of-care ultrasound images and interpretation is user-dependent. Image quality may be limited by patient positioning, edema, bandages, obesity, or mechanical ventilation. Thorough cleaning of probes and machines is important to prevent spread of infection.

Box 17-1. Strongly Recommended Indications for Thoracic, Vascular, and Cardiac Ultrasound in the Intensive Care Unit

Thoracic Ultrasound

Diagnosis of pleural effusion

Diagnosis of pneumothorax

Vascular Ultrasound

Diagnosis of lower extremity proximal DVT

Internal jugular and femoral vein central line placement

Echocardiography

Undifferentiated hemodynamic instability

Measurement of IVC collapsibility in mechanically ventilated patients to assess volume responsiveness

Assessment of LV systolic function

Assessment of RV function

Evaluation for wall-motion abnormalities after ROSC in ventricular fibrillation arrest

Evaluation of patients with suspected acute coronary syndrome

Diagnosis and treatment of pericardial effusion and cardiac tamponade

New murmurs

Hemodynamically stable patients with penetrating chest trauma

IVC, inferior vena cava; *LV*, left ventricle; *ROSC*, return of spontaneous circulation; *RV*, right ventricle.

Modified from Frankel H, Kirkpatrick A, Elbarbary M, et al. Guidelines for the appropriate use of bedside general and cardiac ultrasonography in the evaluation of critically ill patients—part I: general ultrasonography. *Crit Care Med.* 2015;43:11 and Levitov A, Frankel H, Blaivas M, et al. Guidelines for the appropriate use of bedside general and cardiac ultrasonography in the evaluation of critically ill patients—part II: cardiac ultrasonography. *Crit Care Med.* 2016;44:6.

4. How do ultrasound waves create images of tissues?

Ultrasound waves are inaudible sound waves of very high frequency. For the ultrasound machines used in the ICU, probes emit frequencies in the range of 2 to 15 MHz, far above the audible limit of 20 kHz. When ultrasound waves contact different tissues, the waves are reflected back to the probe as "echoes" of varying intensities. The intensity of the echo corresponds to the brightness of the image. Bright areas of the image are called hyperechoic and dark areas are called hypoechoic. Increasing the gain of an image will increase its brightness.

5. How do liquid, air, and bone appear on ultrasound?

Liquids do not reflect ultrasound waves, appear black or anechoic, and allow waves to pass to tissues beneath them (so called "good acoustic windows"). In contrast, gas-filled structures block transmission of ultrasound waves, which is why lung ultrasound is actually based on interpretation of artifacts. Bones and other calcified structures strongly reflect ultrasound waves, appear very bright, and cast a dark "acoustic shadow" behind them. Muscles, other soft tissues, and solid organs have moderate brightness.

6. What are the different probes available for critical care ultrasonography, and when would you use each probe?

Ultrasound probes contain piezoelectric crystals that convert electrical energy to sound waves of a particular range of frequencies (Fig. 17.1). In general, higher frequency ultrasound waves produce greater resolution of tissues but penetrate poorly, while lower frequency waves penetrate deeper structures but give less resolution. Phased array probes (also called sector array or "cardiac" probe) are low-frequency probes (2–4 MHz) that image over a small area and are therefore well suited for imaging between rib spaces in cardiac and thoracic ultrasound. Curved array probes (also called convex array) are also low frequency (2–6 MHz) but image over a wider area and are ideal for abdominal or pelvic imaging. Linear array probes have the highest frequency (7–15 MHz) and therefore offer the highest resolution and are best for vascular imaging. Either the phased array ("cardiac") or curved array probe can be used for lung ultrasound.

7. Describe the imaging modes most commonly used in critical care ultrasonography

B-mode stands for "brightness" mode and is the standard imaging mode. M-mode stands for "motion" mode and depicts the motion of tissues over a single point in the image. In CCUS, M-mode is most commonly used for analysis of inferior vena cava (IVC) collapsibility and lung sliding (Fig. 17.2). Doppler measures velocity of moving objects. Red color on Doppler imaging indicates blood flow toward the probe, while blue color indicates blood flow away from the probe.

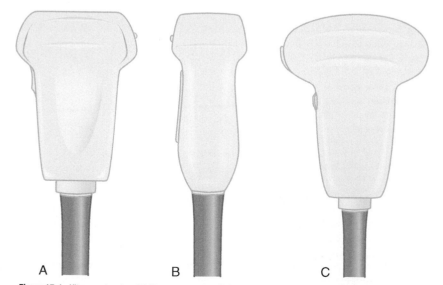

A   B   C

Figure 17-1. Ultrasound probes. (A) Linear array probe. (B) Phased array ("cardiac") probe. (C) Curved array probe.

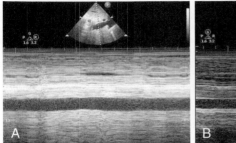
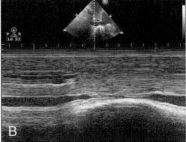

Figure 17-2. Assessment of inferior vena cava (IVC) collapsibility by M-mode. (A) Thick IVC with minimal respiratory variation as might be seen in obstructive shock. (B) Thin IVC with marked respiratory variation in diameter suggestive of hypovolemia. *(Images courtesy of Abraham Sonny, M.B.B.S.)*

8. How does normal lung appear on ultrasound?
   Because air blocks transmission of ultrasound waves, evaluation of lung parenchyma relies on interpretation of artifacts. A low-frequency probe is best for evaluation of deep lung parenchyma (the cardiac probe is a good choice for viewing between rib spaces), while a high-frequency (vascular) probe may be preferable for close examination of the pleura to rule out pneumothorax. The probe should be positioned with the marker pointing toward the patient's head. The ribs will create acoustic shadows throughout the image. Identify a bright horizontal line near the top of the image; this is the pleura. Beneath the pleura, you may see horizontal lines called A-lines; these are reverberation artifacts cast by the pleura and are markers of normal lung (Fig. 17.3A). You should see subtle motion within the bright pleural line; this is lung sliding, which confirms normal contact of parietal and visceral pleura. Applying M-mode will reveal a grainy pattern beneath the bright pleura known as the seashore sign.

9. Describe the characteristic ultrasound findings in pneumothorax, pulmonary edema, lung consolidation, pleural effusion, and acute pulmonary embolism.
   CCUS is very useful in the rapid bedside assessment of patients presenting with acute respiratory failure, perhaps more so compared with portable chest x-ray (CXR). Ultrasound findings should be always interpreted along with other clinical findings when making a diagnosis.
   1. *Pneumothorax:* Identifying lung sliding on ultrasound rules out pneumothorax. Six to eight interspaces on each side of the anterior chest in a supine patient should be scanned. In M-mode, the absence of lung sliding creates the "barcode" or "stratosphere" sign. Importantly, the absence of lung sliding is not specific for pneumothorax, but suggests any process that interferes with normal pleural motion, including acute respiratory distress syndrome (ARDS), pneumonia, effusion, endobronchial intubation, hyperinflation, or atelectasis. Identifying a lung point—an area with lung sliding next to an area lacking lung sliding—confirms a pneumothorax.

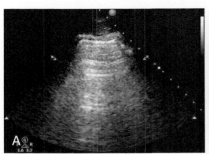
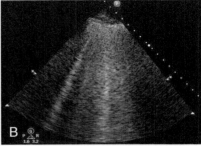

Figure 17-3. Lung ultrasound. (A) B-mode image of normal lung with A-lines. (B) B-mode image of pulmonary edema with B-lines. *(Images courtesy of Abraham Sonny, M.B.B.S.)*

2. *Pulmonary edema:* Pulmonary edema appears as B-lines, which are hyperechoic vertical artifacts that extend from the pleural line to the bottom of the screen (Fig. 17.3B). The density of B-lines correlates with severity of pulmonary edema, with severe edema appearing as a white lung. B-lines are not specific for pulmonary edema and can be seen with other interstitial pathologies including contusion, pneumonitis, and fibrosis.
3. *Pleural effusion:* Pleural effusion appears as an anechoic area flanking a hyperechoic diaphragm.
4. *Consolidation:* Consolidated lung takes on the appearance of liver, often called "hepatization" of lung tissue. Air bronchograms may appear as hyperechoic streaks. Distinguishing pneumonia from atelectasis on ultrasound is more advanced
5. *Acute pulmonary embolism:* Lung and pleura may appear normal with A-lines and lung sliding as described above. Finding a deep vein thrombosis (DVT) and/or evidence of right heart strain on transthoracic echocardiography (TTE) is key to making the diagnosis.

10. What are the five standard views of basic critical care transthoracic echocardiography?
Fig. 17.4 shows the five standard images of point-of-care transthoracic echocardiography. If possible, the parasternal and apical four-chamber views should be performed in the lateral decubitus position.
1. *Parasternal long axis:* Place cardiac probe in the left third to fifth intercostal spaces next to the sternum with marker facing the right shoulder. This view is good for evaluation of ventricle size and function, the pericardium, and mitral and aortic valves. Apply Color Doppler to evaluate for severe mitral and aortic regurgitation. Manipulate the probe until you gain the fullest view of the left ventricle (LV) possible; LV filling could be underestimated depending on where it is imaged. Obliteration of the LV cavity in systole suggests severe hypovolemia.
2. *Parasternal short axis:* From the parasternal long view rotate the probe 90 degrees to point toward left shoulder; this produces a cross-sectional view of the ventricles at the papillary muscle level. This view allows comparison of ventricle size and function and septal motion. Normally the septum bows into the right ventricle (RV) throughout the cardiac cycle due to higher LV pressures. Flattening of the septum creating a D-shaped LV is concerning for RV overload. This view is also good for evaluation for wall motion abnormalities, as all three major coronary artery territories are visible in this view.

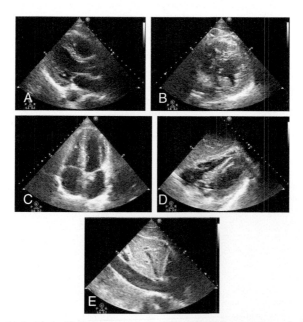

Figure 17-4. Five standard views of basic transthoracic echocardiography. (A) Parasternal long axis. (B) Parasternal short axis. (C) Apical four-chamber. (D) Subcostal. Liver is visualized closest to the probe. (E) IVC. To confirm correct identification of the IVC, follow the vessel until it is seen draining into the right atrium. *(Images courtesy of Abraham Sonny, M.B.B.S.)*

3. *Apical four-chamber:* Move the probe to lower lateral chest wall with the marker facing the left shoulder. This view is also good for comparison of ventricular size and function and identification of pericardial effusion. The RV/LV ratio should be less than 0.6; a higher ratio suggests RV dilation.

4. *Subcostal:* Place the probe below the xiphoid with the marker pointing to 3 to 4 o'clock. This may be the best image possible in patients receiving mechanical ventilation or cardiopulmonary resuscitation (CPR).

5. *IVC:* From the subcostal view, rotate the probe until the marker points toward the patient's head. Be careful not to mistake the aorta for the IVC. Identifying the IVC feeding into the right atrium can help distinguish the vessels. Applying M-mode will allow for calculation of respiratory variation in IVC diameter, which can be used to assess volume responsiveness in mechanically ventilated patients as described below (Fig. 17.2A).

11. How can critical care ultrasonography be used to assess fluid responsiveness?
Determining volume status is often challenging yet crucial in critically ill patients. CCUS has been proposed as a means to assess fluid responsiveness, but intensivists need to be careful to select the appropriate method.

1. *IVC collapsibility:* This is most accurate in patients receiving positive-pressure ventilation, ideally synchronous on volume control ventilation with 8 mL/kg tidal volumes and normal RV function. The IVC is imaged in the subcostal view with M-mode to calculate changes in diameter with respiration (Fig. 17.2). Change in IVC diameter with respiration greater than 15% suggests fluid-responsiveness. Guidelines recommend also examining ventricular filling and function when assessing volume status and repeating the ultrasound exam after fluid administration.

2. *Passive leg raise:* Unlike IVC collapsibility, passive leg raise (PLR) can be used to assess fluid re-sponsiveness in both spontaneously breathing and mechanically ventilated patients. PLR provides an approximately 300 mL fluid bolus. Fluid responsiveness can be assessed by calculating change in stroke volume on TTE; increase in stroke volume greater than 12% to 15% during PLR suggests fluid responsiveness. Echocardiography, pulse contour analysis, and Esophageal Doppler have been shown to be better predictors of fluid responsiveness during PLR compared with measuring pulse pressure variation on the arterial line.

12. How can critical care ultrasonography be used to determine the etiology of shock?
Multiple organs should be examined with CCUS in a patient presenting with shock of unclear etiology. Ultrasound findings in each type of shock are described below.

1. *Obstructive:* Lung ultrasonography can quickly rule out massive pneumothorax based on the pres-ence of lung sliding. The presence of DVT and right heart failure on TTE is very concerning for pul-monary embolism. Signs of right heart failure include abnormal septal flattening (D-shaped LV) on parasternal short axis view (Fig. 17.5A) and increased RV/LV ratio (>0.6) on four-chamber view. Pericardial effusion with collapse of right-sided chambers is concerning for tamponade (Fig. 17.5B). IVC plethora is consistent with obstructive shock (Fig. 17.2A).

2. *Distributive/hypovolemic:* TTE usually reveals a hyperdynamic heart with underfilled LV; severe hypo-volemia appears as "kissing walls." In patients with sepsis, increasing afterload with vasopressors and fluid may reveal septic cardiomyopathy. Frequent reassessment of ventricular function in sepsis is therefore recommended. IVC will show large respirophasic variation in diameter (most accurate

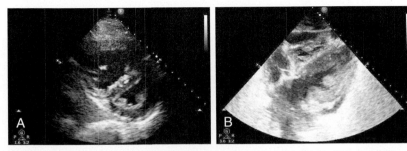

Figure 17-5. Bedside transthoracic echocardiography findings in different types of shock. (A) D-shaped LV and dilated RV on parasternal short axis in a patient with pulmonary embolism. (B) Collapse of right ventricle and pericardial effusion on subcostal view in a patient with cardiac tamponade. *(Images courtesy of Abraham Sonny, M.B.B.S)*

in mechanically ventilated patients) (Fig. 17.2B), and the PLR test is positive as described above. Abdominal or pelvic bleeding can be rapidly assessed with focused assessment by sonography for trauma (FAST) exam.

3. *Cardiogenic:* Ventricles are dilated with minimal systolic wall thickening. Regional wall motion abnormalities suggest myocardial ischemia. The parasternal short axis view is particularly useful in evaluation for wall motion abnormalities, as territories of all major coronary arteries are visible. Severe mitral or aortic regurgitation can be identified on parasternal long axis. Thoracic ultrasound may reveal B-lines suggestive of pulmonary edema and pleural effusions.

13. What are the standard abdominal and pelvic views in the Focused Assessment by Sonography for Trauma exam?
The FAST exam is used to rapidly evaluate for pericardial effusion, abdominal or pelvic bleeding. Fluid appears anechoic.

1. *Hepatorenal:* Probe is applied longitudinally to the right 10th or 11th intercostal space (right costophrenic angle) to identify the diaphragm, liver, and right kidney. Pleural effusion may be seen.
2. *Suprapubic:* Probe is applied transversely in the suprapubic area to look for pelvic fluid.
3. *Perisplenic:* Probe is applied longitudinally to left 10th or 11th intercostal space to identify the spleen and left kidney.

14. How can critical care ultrasonography be used to evaluate for DVT?
B-mode imaging of vessels in cross-section with the vascular probe is sufficient in a bedside exam; Color Doppler (Duplex) is usually not necessary. The femoral and popliteal veins should be examined at several levels. First identify the circular, pulsatile, less compressible artery. The vein next to it is usually oval-shaped and should be fully compressible. Lack of full compressibility is concerning for DVT. Thrombus appears as echogenic material within a vein. Acute thrombi may not be echogenic and can only be identified by compression study.

15. How can critical care ultrasonography facilitate central line placement?
Ultrasound guidance is strongly recommended for internal jugular and femoral central line placement. There is currently insufficient evidence to recommend use of ultrasound guidance in subclavian vein catheterization. A preliminary scan before sterile preparation is important for vessel selection, particularly in patients with previous central lines who could have vessel stenosis or thrombosis. Out-of-plane imaging is currently recommended over in-plane imaging because it allows simultaneous visualization of surrounding structures, namely the carotid or femoral artery. The challenge of out-of-plane technique is to correctly identify the needle tip. Inability to track the needle tip increases the risk of puncturing the posterior vein wall and surrounding structures. Ultrasound should be used to confirm correct guidewire placement prior to dilating the vessel and to rule out pneumothorax following line placement by identifying lung sliding.

ACKNOWLEDGMENT

The authors wish to acknowledge Dr. Daniel W. Johnson, MD, for the valuable contributions to the previous edition of this chapter.

KEY POINTS: CRITICAL CARE ULTRASOUND

1. Point-of-care lung ultrasonography can diagnose pneumothorax, pleural effusion, consolidations, and pulmonary edema, and may be more useful in the evaluation of patients presenting with acute respiratory failure compared with portable CXR.
2. Point-of-care transthoracic echocardiography combined with lung, abdominal and vascular ultrasound can help identify the etiology of shock.
3. Critical care ultrasonography can be used to assess fluid responsiveness based on IVC collapsibility in mechanically ventilated patients and changes in stroke volume with passive leg raise in spontaneously breathing patients.
4. Intensivists can accurately diagnose DVT by ultrasonography with a vascular compression study.
5. Ultrasound guidance improves the safety of internal jugular and femoral central line placement.

BIBLIOGRAPHY

1. Ahmad S, Eisen LA. Lung ultrasound: the basics. In: Lumb P, Karakitsos D, eds. Critical Care Ultrasound. Philadelphia: Elsevier; 2015:105-110.
2. Cardenas-Garcia J, Mayo PH. Bedside ultrasonography for the intensivist. Crit Care Clin. 2015;31(1):43-66.
3. Cherpanath TG, Hirsch A, Geerts BF, et al. Predicting fluid responsiveness by passive leg raising: a systematic review and meta-analysis of 23 clinical trials. *Crit Care Med.* 2016;44(5):981-991.
4. Corradi F, Brusasco C, Pelosi P. Chest ultrasound in acute respiratory distress syndrome. *Curr Opin Crit Care.* 2014;20(1):98-103.
5. Fagley RE, Haney MF, Beraud AS, et al. Critical care basic ultrasound learning goals for American anesthesiology critical care trainees: Recommendations from an expert group. Anesth Analg. 2015;120(5):1041-1053.
6. Frankel HL, Kirkpatrick AW, Elbarbary M, et al. Guidelines for the appropriate use of bedside general and cardiac ultrasonography in the evaluation of critically ill patients—part I: general ultrasonography. *Crit Care Med.* 2015;43(11):2479-2502.
7. Guérin L, Vieillard-Baron A. The use of ultrasound in caring for patients with sepsis. *Clin Chest Med.* 2016;37(2):299-307.
8. Lee FC. Lung ultrasound-a primary survey of the acutely dyspneic patient. *J Intensive Care.* 2016;4:57.
9. Levitov A, Frankel HL, Blaivas M, et al. Guidelines for the appropriate use of bedside general and cardiac ultrasonography in the evaluation of critically ill patients—part II: cardiac ultrasonography. *Crit Care Med.* 2016;44(6):1206-1227.
10. Mok KL. Make it SIMPLE: enhanced shock management by focused cardiac ultrasound. *J Intensive Care.* 2016;4:51.
11. Sargsyan AE, Blaivas M, Lumb P, et al. Fundamentals: essential technology, concepts, and capability. In: Lumb P, Karakitsos D, eds. *Critical Care Ultrasound.* Philadelphia: Elsevier; 2015:1-23.

CHAPTER 18

VENTRICULAR ASSIST DEVICE

Tao Shen and Michael N. Andrawes

1. **What is a ventricular assist device?**
   Ventricular assist devices (VADs) are mechanical devices inserted to assist cardiac function by offloading part or all of the pumping responsibilities from the ventricle. Placement of a VAD can be done on the left side of the heart to assist in left ventricular function (LVAD) or on the right side of the heart to help with the right ventricle (RVAD). The presence of both an LVAD and an RVAD is referred to as biventricular support (BiVAD). A number of different VAD constructs exist, with major differentiators being pulsatile versus continuous flow, extracorporeal versus intracorporeal, degree of assistance provided, ability to help the left or right sides, and the length of time it can be used (Table 18.1). Some VADs are intended to be used for only 7 to 10 days, whereas others have supported patients over a 7-year period.

2. **What are the end goals of ventricular assist device therapy?**
   When deciding the appropriateness of the placement of a VAD, multiple potential end points can be considered. A "bridge to recovery" implies temporary VAD support with the goal of removal once native heart function has returned to baseline. A "bridge to transplant" refers to the use of a VAD in a patient who ultimately will be best served by cardiac transplantation but needs temporary assistance until a heart becomes available. The term "destination therapy" means that the VAD itself is the end goal of therapy. These patients have irreversible heart conditions and, for a variety of reasons, are not eligible for transplantation. Patients initially ineligible for a transplant may, in certain cases, become eligible for transplant after physiologic improvement of end organs with VAD therapy. As such, placement of a VAD can sometimes be a "bridge to decision" in patients with initially equivocal end-points, such as bridge to transplant verses destination therapy.

3. **What is the Randomized Evaluation of Mechanical Assistance for the Treatment of Congestive Heart Failure study?**
   The REMATCH (Randomized Evaluation of Mechanical Assistance for the Treatment of Congestive Heart Failure) study refers to a landmark *New England Journal of Medicine* article from Columbia University in 2001, entitled "Long-term Use of a Left-Ventricular Assist Device for End-stage Heart Failure." The article described a 3-year study in 129 patients with end-stage heart failure who were ineligible for cardiac transplantation and were randomly assigned to two groups: optimal medical management or LVAD therapy. Data showed significant increases in 1- and 2-year survival rates of the LVAD cohort over the medical therapy cohort (52% vs. 25% and 23% vs. 8%, respectively), as well as an improved quality of life.

4. **What are common insertion sites for left ventricular assist devices and right ventricular assist devices?**
   The VAD inflow cannula carries blood to the VAD pump while the outflow cannula carries blood from the pump back to the patient. An LVAD has an inflow cannula in the left ventricle and an outflow cannula in the ascending aorta. An RVAD typically has an inflow cannula in the right atrium and outflow in the main pulmonary artery.

5. **What is the difference between extracorporeal membrane oxygenators and a ventricular assist device?**
   Extracorporeal membrane oxygenators (ECMO) can be similar to a VAD in terms of function and placement. The major difference is that a VAD requires that lung function be adequate, because it only helps with cardiac function, relying on the lungs to oxygenate the blood. ECMO incorporates an oxygenator that maintains gas exchange and is often used in clinical situations in which the lungs are no longer effective in maintaining oxygenation or ventilation. In addition, unlike ECMO, many VADs are created with portability in mind. The degree of hemodynamic support with ECMO varies from primarily oxygenation/ventilation up to complete cardiopulmonary replacement.

Table 18-1. Specific Types of Ventricular Assist Devices

DEVICE	PROPULSION	LOCATION	DURATION	RV/LV/BIV	FLOWS (L/min)	ANTICOAGULATION
First Generation						
Thoratec PVAD	Pneumatic pulsatile	Extracorporeal	Long	RV/LV/BiV	6.5	Yes
Thoratec IVAD	Electric pulsatile	Intracorporeal	Long	RV/LV/BiV	6.5	Yes
Thoratec HeartMate I	Electric pulsatile	Intracorporeal	Long	LV	10	Low dose
Abiomed BVS5000/AB5000	Pneumatic pulsatile	Extracorporeal	Short	RV/LV/BiV	5	Yes
Second Generation						
Abiomed Impella LP 2.5/CP/5.0/LD/RP	Microaxial continuous	Intravascular	Short	LV/RV/BiV	2.5–5	Yes
Levitronix CentriMag	Centrifugal continuous	Extracorporeal	Short	RV/LV/BiV	9	Yes
TandemHeart Percutaneous VAD	Centrifugal continuous	Extracorporeal	Short	LV/RV/BiV	5–8	Yes
Thoratec HeartMate II	Axial continuous	Intracorporeal	Long	LV	10	Yes
Jarvik 2000 Flowmaster	Axial continuous	Intracorporeal	Long	LV	7	Yes
MicroMed HeartAssist 5 (DeBakey)	Axial continuous	Intracorporeal	Long	LV	5	Yes
Third Generation						
Ventracor VentrAssist	Centrifugal continuous	Intracorporeal	Long	LV	5	Yes
HeartWare HVAD	Centrifugal continuous	Intracorporeal	Long	LV (RV off-label)	10	Yes
Thoratec HeartMate III	Centrifugal continuous	Intracorporeal	Long	LV	10	Yes

BiV, biventricular; HVAD, HeartWare ventricular assist device; IVAD, implantable ventricular assist device; LV, left ventricle; PVAD, paracorporeal ventricular assist device; pVAD, The TandemHeart percutaneous ventricular assist device; RV, right ventricle.

6. **What are the indications for ventricular assist device placement?**

   No consensus criteria exist for placement of a VAD. As a result, indications may vary from institution to institution. However, guidelines exist to assist in optimizing patient selection. Examples of parameters for consideration include the following:
   - Cardiac index (CI) index less than 2.0 L/min/m^2
   - Systemic hypotension with mean arterial pressure less than 60 mm Hg
   - Cardiac filling pressures of either right or left atrium greater than 20 mm Hg
   - Persistent inotropic dependence
   - VO_2 less than 12 mL/kg/min, all despite maximal medical therapy

   Consideration may also be given to patients with cardiac function that is better than the parameters listed above but who have unpredictable, life-threatening ventricular arrhythmias.

7. **Are there any contraindications for ventricular assist device placement?**

   Absolute contraindications include abdominal aortic aneurysm greater than 5 cm, active systemic infection or high chronic risk of infection, severe pulmonary dysfunction (FEV$_1$ [Forced expiratory volume (first second)] <1 L or fixed pulmonary hypertension), impending or actual renal or hepatic failure (including portal hypertension), inability to tolerate anticoagulation, and neurologic or psycho-social inability to manage the device. Clearly, a coexisting terminal condition contraindicates VAD placement. Relative contraindications include age greater than 65 years (unless minimal other risk factors); chronic kidney disease; severe chronic malnutrition; morbid obesity; or uncorrected aortic regurgitation, mitral regurgitation, or mitral stenosis. Unrecognized patent foramen ovale or atrial septal defects can lead to hypoxemia or paradoxical emboli due to right-to-left shunting after LVAD implantation. The presence of these shunts should be assessed preoperatively or intraoperatively, and repair should be performed during LVAD implantation.

8. **What are the differences between pulsatile and continuous systems?**

   VADs can be divided into two classes based on how they eject blood from the pump: in a pulsatile or continuous manner. First-generation VADs use pneumatically or electrically driven pulsatile pumps that aim to work like the native heart by displacing a given volume of blood with every beat. The Thoratec paracorporeal VAD (Thoratec, Pleasanton, CA) is a versatile first-generation pulsatile device that can be used as an RVAD, LVAD, or BiVAD for short- to medium-term therapy in instances of bridge to transplant or recovery. Second and third generation VADs are continuous flow systems that have quickly developed over the last two decades, mainly due to its small pump size and durability. Currently, continuous flow VADs are valveless pumps that use a magnetic field to rapidly spin a single impeller supported by mechanical or, more recently, magnetic or hydrodynamic bearings. Currently available in the United States are the Heartmate II (Thoratec, Pleasanton, California), a second-generation pump with the impeller outflow parallel to the axis of rotation (axial pump), and the HVAD (HeartWare, Framingham, Massachusetts), a third-generation pump with impeller outflow directed perpendicular from the axis of rotation (centrifugal pump). While continuous flow VADs have been demonstrated to offer improved survival and device durability in patients requiring long-term hemodynamic support, speculation has been raised regarding the physiologic impact of nonpulsatile flow. In addition to increased hemolysis, continuous flow pumps are thought to negatively affect nitric oxide production, inflammatory biomarkers, endothelial function, and gas exchange.

9. **What are some key parameters associated with continuous flow ventricular assist devices?**
   - Pump speed—measured in revolutions per minute and relates to how fast the impeller is spinning. This is the only variable programmed by the operator.
   - Flow—measured in liters per minute. This correlates with pump speed, and is dependent on the pressure differential (also known as head pressure) across the pump. This pressure differential is in turn dependent on the ventricular chamber pressure (i.e., preload), vascular tone (i.e., afterload), and factors affecting blood viscosity (e.g., hematocrit).
   - Power—the amount of power the VAD consumes to continuously run at a set speed. A sudden or gradual increase in the power can indicate obstruction or thrombus inside the VAD.
   - Pulsatility Index (PI)—a measure of the pressure differential within the VAD pump and indicates the proportion of cardiac output provided by the native heart versus the device. In addition to the left ventricular contractility, the PI of an LVAD is affected by the patient's volume status and right ventricular function.

10. **What are the significant potential complications that arise in patients with ventricular assist devices?**

Complications are not infrequent and can be life-threatening. They include infection, thromboembolic events, and bleeding. As model design has improved, complication rates have decreased. Sepsis is the leading cause of mortality in long-term VAD support; driveline and device pocket infections occur in up to 40% of these patients, the majority of which may be managed with chronic antibiotic therapy. Fortunately, infection rates have decreased with alternative implantation options, sometimes eliminating the need for external or peritoneal device components. Pump thrombosis is associated with all circulatory assist devices, and systemic anticoagulation is crucial. Signs of pump thrombosis include hemolysis, thromboembolic events, heart failure, end-organ hypoperfusion, and increased pump power requirements. With adherence to a higher international normalized ratio (INR) target (2.0–2.5) on top of antiplatelet therapy, the incidence of pump thrombosis has decreased from 12% in 2012 to 1% to 2% currently. Also, sintered (ridged) titanium materials, which promote pseudointimal layer formation on device components, as well as optimization of pump flow mechanics, have helped to decrease the incidence of thromboembolic events. Bleeding is a foreseeable complication in the setting of anticoagulation therapy. The incidence of major bleeding requiring transfusion is over 40% in patients in whom a VAD was placed within 4 months. Early bleeding is usually from the mediastinum, followed by the pleural space, chest wall, gastrointestinal tract, and the brain. Intracerebral hemorrhage can result from hemorrhagic conversion of ischemic strokes (embolic complication), trauma, and spontaneous intracranial hemorrhage. Gastrointestinal bleeding is especially common in patients with a VAD. This is thought to be due to mechanical damage of von Willebrand multimers within the pump leading to impaired platelet aggregation, as well as the formation of arteriovenous malformations from continuous flow perfusion.

11. **Why is it that some patients who have a left ventricular assist device placed subsequently require a right ventricular assist device?**

Placement of an LVAD offloads some or all of the work from the left ventricle (LV). It can increase cardiac output and, as a result, can increase the venous return to the right side of the heart. This increase in right ventricular preload, along with relative emptying of the LV, can result in right ventricle (RV) distention, worsening RV contractility, and increased tricuspid regurgitation, all of which decrease RV performance. In addition, significant cytokine release can take place during the perioperative period. These cytokines can mediate pulmonary vasoconstriction, placing further stress on the RV. It is important to monitor vigilantly for impending right-sided heart failure, because appropriate pharmacologic intervention may help avoid additional surgical intervention.

12. **List the major considerations for intensive care unit management of a patient directly after a left ventricular assist device placement.**

In the immediate postoperative period, hemodynamic management is based on the patient's mean arterial pressure, cardiac index, ventricular filling pressures, and function. A pulmonary artery catheter is an important monitoring tool used to guide therapy. A combination of inotropes, vasopressors, vasodilators, and fluid therapy are used to optimize pump flow, in addition to adjustments in pump speed. Hypotension in association with low pump output can indicate hypovolemia, tamponade, RV failure, or device-related issues. Hypotension in the setting of high VAD flow suggests vasodilation and can be an early sign of sepsis.

Optimization of right-sided heart function is critical after LVAD placement. Inotropic support should be provided as needed to assure optimal right-sided heart functionality. In addition, decreasing pulmonary vascular resistance can assist in RV performance. Milrinone, epoprostenol, and nitric oxide all have their roles in decreasing pulmonary vascular resistance in the postoperative period. In patients who are receiving positive pressure ventilation, the consequence of intrathoracic pressure, ventilation-perfusion mismatch, and hypoxic pulmonary vasoconstriction on RV performance should be considered.

With continuous-flow LVADs, it is also important to understand the concept of suction events. These events can occur when the LVAD motor speeds are high and LV venous return is low, with resultant collapse of the ventricle. Suction events can precipitate ventricular arrhythmias. Treatment may be reducing the LVAD rotational speed or increasing LV preload.

13. **How is weaning attempted with a ventricular assist device?**

When a VAD is used as a bridge to recovery, intermittent assessments of cardiac function are performed to determine the necessity of continued VAD use. Methods of assessment include echocardiography, radionucleotide studies, and exercise stress testing. As cardiac function returns, the amount of support, defined by the VAD flow rate, can gradually be reduced. As VAD flows are decreased, the RV is allowed to fill with blood. Indicators of successful weaning include ability to maintain cardiac output without increases in central venous or pulmonary artery pressures. Once VAD support is weaned to 1 to 1.5 L/min, patients can usually tolerate discontinuation of the device.

14. Do percutaneous options exist for ventricular assist systems?

Several percutaneous VADs (pVAD) can be inserted by cardiologists in the catheterization laboratory or by cardiac surgeons in the operating room. These are typically used for temporary support as a bridge to recovery or bridge to bridge therapy.

One such device is the catheter-based Impella (Abiomed, Inc., Danvers, MA), which sits across the aortic valve and functions via a nonpulsatile axial flow mechanism. The cannulas and pump are integrated into the catheter, with the inflow at the tip and the outflow several centimeters proximal. The pump sits between these two ports. Maximum flow rates range from 2.5 to 5.0 L/min, depending on the size of the device inserted. Insertion sites include the femoral artery, subclavian artery, and directly into the ascending aorta. A right-sided Impella RP was approved by the Food and Drug Administration (FDA) in 2015. The primary differences with this device are reversal of the inflow and outflow ports and a unique shape to pass through the right ventricle. It is typically inserted via the femoral vein, into the right atrium, across the tricuspid and pulmonic valves, and into the pulmonary artery.

Another is the TandemHeart (Cardiac Assist, Inc., Pittsburgh, PA), whose inflow cannula is placed through the femoral vein, and then, via transseptal puncture, the tip of the cannula is positioned in the left atrium. Blood taken from the left atrium is pumped by an external centrifugal pump back into circulation via an outflow cannula placed in the femoral artery. The TandemHeart may also be used for right-sided support by placing the inflow cannula in the right atrium and the outflow in the pulmonary artery. Flow rates up to 5 L/min can be achieved. In addition, an oxygenator may be inserted in-line with a right-sided TandemHeart, making this an option for venovenous (VV) ECMO.

15. What is the future direction of ventricular assist device therapy?

Pulsatility, further miniaturization, and remote monitoring capabilities are leading the trends in the evolving technology of current VAD therapy. Low arterial pulsatility has contributed to the development of arteriovenous malformations. Continuous LV unloading reduces the frequency of aortic valve opening, which leads to commissural fusion and eventually aortic insufficiency. The lack of aortic valve opening may also contribute to thrombosis due to low flow in the aortic root. Recent efforts have been directed at methods to generate more pulsatility and intermittent aortic valve opening, for example, through pump speed modulation, by having periods of lower-speed pump, and allowing the native ventricle to pump during conditions of increased ventricular loading. The HeartMate 3 (Thoratec, Pleasanton, California) is a new LVAD that allows such pump speed modulation, and was recently approved by the FDA for use in heart failure. In the future, speed modulation algorithms may respond to different physiologic demands, such as exercise, arrhythmias and catecholamine changes.

ACKNOWLEDGMENT

The authors wish to acknowledge Drs. Joseph L. Weidman, MD, and Michael G. Fitzsimons, MD, FCCP, for the valuable contributions to the previous edition of this chapter.

KEY POINTS: VENTRICULAR ASSIST DEVICE

1. VADs are placed for three reasons:
   a. As a bridge to recovery
   b. As a bridge to cardiac transplantation
   c. As a therapeutic means in and of itself (destination therapy)
2. A VAD can be used to augment the left ventricle (LVAD), the right ventricle (RVAD), or both ventricles (BiVAD), but does not help with blood oxygenation or ventilation.
3. With the incidence in the United States of new patients with cardiac failure each year being around 40,000 and the number of available donor hearts at only 2300, the role of VADs continues to increase, as does the pressure for technologic and industrial advances that will increase device effectiveness and improve the safety profile.

BIBLIOGRAPHY

1. Campbell LJ. Circulatory assist devices. In: Parsons PE, Wiener-Kronish JP, eds. *Critical Care Secrets*. 4th ed. Philadelphia: Mosby; 2007.
2. Cohn LH. Perioperative/intraoperative care. In: Cohn LH, ed. *Cardiac Surgery in the Adult*. 3rd ed. New York: McGraw-Hill; 2008:507-533.
3. Fitzsimons MG, Ennis S, MacGillivray T. Devices for cardiac support. In: Sandberg WS, Urman R, Ehrenfeld J, eds. *The MGH Textbook of Anesthetic Equipment*. 1st ed. Philadelphia: Saunders; 2010:247-262.
4. Mancini D, Colombo PC. Left ventricular assist devices – a rapidly evolving alterative to transplant. *J Am Coll Cardiol*. 2015;65:2542-2555.
5. Mitter N, Sheinberg R. Update on ventricular assist devices. *Curr Opin Anaesthesiol*. 2010;23:57-66.
6. Nicolosi AC, Pagel PS. Perioperative considerations in the patient with a left ventricular assist device. *Anesthesiology*. 2003;98:565-570.
7. Pratt AK, Shah NS, Boyce SW. Left ventricular assist device management in the ICU. *Crit Care Med*. 2014;42: 158-168.
8. Rose EA, Gelijns AC, Moskowitz AJ, et al. Long-term use of a left ventricular assist device for end-stage heart failure. *N Engl J Med*. 2001;345:1435-1443.
9. Sajgalik P, Grupper A, Edwards BS, et al. Current status of left ventricular assist device therapy. *Mayo Clin Proc*. 2016;91:927-940.
10. Slaughter MS, Rogers JG, Milano CA, et al. Advanced heart failure treated with continuous-flow left ventricular assist device. *N Engl J Med*. 2009;361:2241-2251.
11. Thunberg CA, Gaitan BD, Arabia FA, Cole DJ, Grigore AM. Ventricular assist devices today and tomorrow. *J Cardiothorac Vasc Anesth*. 2010;24:656-680.
12. Wilson SR, Mudge Jr GH, Stewart GC, Givertz MM. Evaluation for ventricular assist device: selecting the appropriate candidate. *Circulation*. 2009;119:2225-2232.

CHAPTER 19

PERCUTANEOUS ASSIST DEVICES

Eva Litvak and Michael G. Fitzsimons

1. **What is a percutaneous ventricular assist device?**
   Mechanical cardiac assist devices have traditionally been bulky and required surgical intervention for appropriate placement. More recently, mechanical cardiac assist devices for use in the setting of acute decompensated heart failure (from a variety of etiologies) have evolved to include a sub-set that are smaller, easier, and more rapid to place, and provide reliable support. These devices are designed primarily for percutaneous insertion or through a small surgical incision. The assist devices most commonly used in the United States include the Impella and the TandemHeart.

2. **What are conditions where a percutaneous ventricular assist device may be used?**
   In general terms, percutaneous ventricular assist devices (PVADs) are indicated in the setting of high-risk percutaneous coronary intervention (PCI), acute cardiogenic shock, and decompensated heart failure. The goal of this type of mechanical circulatory support is to unload the failing ventricle and support systemic perfusion pressure to maintain adequate end-organ perfusion. These nondurable devices are most commonly used as a "bridge to recovery," when there is an expectation that the myocardium will recover and the device will be removed. Potential indications for a PVAD include cardiogenic shock due to myocardial infarction, myocarditis, and postcardiotomy cardiogenic shock (Table 19.1). Newer devices provide specific support to either the left or right ventricle. These devices do not support ventilation (either oxygenation or CO_2 removal) and are not indicated for respiratory compromise or failure. There are a growing number of reports of elective device use.

3. **How does an Impella device work?**
   Impella technology is based on an intracardiac miniaturized axial flow rotary blood pump with a flexible cannula for temporary mechanical support of the left or right heart. The Impella devices are the only percutaneous mechanical circulatory support devices that are FDA approved in both high-risk PCI and cardiogenic shock.

Table 19-1. Potential Uses of Percutaneous Assist Devices

EMERGENT OR URGENT USES	ELECTIVE USE
Cardiogenic shock after myocardial infarction	High-risk PCI
Myocarditis	Support during off-pump CABG
Left ventricular decompression associated with aortic insufficiency and use of ECMO	Support during high-risk ventricular tachycardia ablation
Rescue during transcatheter aortic valve replacement	
Takosubo cardiomyopathy	
Cardiogenic shock after atenolol, lisinopril, overdose	
Support of failing Fontan physiology	
Postpartum heart failure	
Management of unstable arrhythmias	
Bridge to cardiac transplant	
Right ventricular support after heart transplantation	
Support after acute heart transplant rejection	
Heart failure associated with acute mitral regurgitation	
Support for acute ventricular septal rupture	
Support after coronary artery dissection	

CABG, coronary artery bypass grafting; ECMO, extracorporeal membrane oxygenation; PCI, percutaneous coronary intervention.

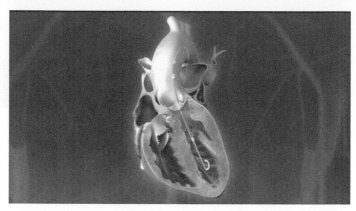

Figure 19-1. Impella device in position. *(Used with permission from Abiomed Inc. [Danvers, Massachusetts]).*

The left-sided Impella devices include the 2.5, CP (cardiac power), 5.0, and LD (left direct). The left-sided devices directly unload the left ventricle (LV) and propel blood antegrade from the left ventricle into the aorta. The Impella 2.5 and the CP are placed percutaneously most commonly through the femoral artery and may deliver flows from 2.5 L/min (Impella 2.5) to 3.5 L/min (Impella CP). Higher levels of support are achievable with the Impella 5.0 (5 L/min) and the Impella LD ("Left Direct"; 5 L/min). The Impella 5.0 requires a surgical cut down (via the femoral or axillary artery) with placement of a graft to the ascending aorta through which the device is delivered. The Impella LD is a direct surgical placement into the aorta.

The Impella RP (right percutaneous) is the first percutaneous device that is designed to support the right ventricle. It is placed via the femoral vein into the pulmonary artery. The RP delivers blood from the inlet, which sits in the inferior vena cava, to the outlet, which sits in the pulmonary artery.

All Impella devices require imaging for placement (fluoroscopy) and repositioning (fluoroscopy and/or echocardiography) (Fig. 19.1 and Table 19.2).

4. How does the TandemHeart work?

The TandemHeart is another percutaneous left ventricular support device that works by aspirating oxygenated blood from the left atrium and returning it to the systemic circulation via the femoral or

Table 19-2. Different Types of Impella Devices

DEVICE	USE	PLACEMENT	CATHETER DIAMETER/ MOTOR SIZE	FLOW RATE
Impella Recover LP 2.5	Support of the left ventricle	Percutaneous through femoral artery	9 Fr/21 Fr	2.5 L/min
Impella CP 3.5	Support of the left ventricle	Percutaneous through the femoral artery	9 Fr/21 Fr	3.5 L/min
Impella Recover 5.0	Support of the left ventricle	Femoral or axillary artery cutdown	9 Fr/21 Fr	5.0 L/min
Impella LD	Support of the left ventricle	Inserted into the left ventricle via an open chest procedure	9 Fr/21 Fr	5.0 L/min
Impella RP	Percutaneous support of the right ventricle	Inserted through the femoral vein across the tricuspid and pulmonary valves	11 Fr/22 Fr	>4 L/min

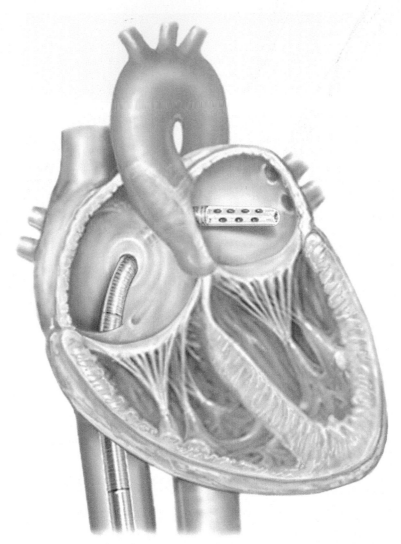

Figure 19-2. TandemHeart in position across interatrial septum. *(Used with permission CardiacAssist, Inc.)*

iliac arterial vessels (Fig. 19.2). A cannula is placed through a percutaneous approach via the femoral vein (21 French). The cannula is advanced to the right atrium and across the interatrial septum into the left atrium. Positioning is generally confirmed by fluoroscopy, but transesophageal echocardiography may also be used. Oxygenated blood is aspirated from the left atrium and then returned to the femoral or iliac arterial vessels (15 or 17 Fr cannula) by a continuous centrifugal flow pump. Its support relies upon acceptable function of the right ventricle as well as the lungs. The TandemHeart can generate an augmented cardiac output of 3.5 to 4.5 L/min.

The TandemHeart has been utilized for treatment of cardiogenic shock after myocardial infarction and support for high-risk PCI. It can also be used for right ventricular support in the setting of right ventricular infarction or right ventricular failure after left ventricular assist device (LVAD) placement. Right-sided cannulation is either percutaneously or surgically implanted. Percutaneous access is through the femoral vein (or the right internal jugular vein), to the right atrium (inflow), and to the pulmonary artery (outflow). Surgical access allows for direct cannulation to the right atrium and pulmonary artery.

5. How does a percutaneous ventricular assist device physiologically improve heart failure?
   PVADs provide support to the failing heart through several mechanisms. Their goal is to increase end-organ perfusion pressure and reduce ventricular workload. Left ventricular wall stress is immediately reduced by removal of blood from the ventricle. This results in a decrease in pulmonary capillary wedge pressure (PCWP). Myocardial oxygen consumption is reduced, and there is some indication that coronary blood flow is increased. However, if the device is only supporting the left ventricle, it does rely upon the efficient filling of the left ventricle by an effective right ventricle.

6. Is there any data to demonstrate survival benefit with percutaneous ventricular assist devices as compared with other nondurable mechanical circulatory support (MCS)?
   There are currently a small number of randomized clinical trials demonstrating hemodynamic improvements by many indices (including improved filling pressures, increased cardiac output, and decreased lactate). Many factors, including study design, patient characteristics, and difficulty in enrollment, limit the ability of current data to demonstrate clear survival benefit of one device over another.
   A randomized multicenter trial (TandemHeart trial) to evaluate safety and efficacy of the TandemHeart versus conventional therapy with an intraaortic balloon pump (IABP) in cardiogenic shock demonstrated that the TandemHeart did improve hemodynamics in as far as increases in cardiac index and mean arterial pressure and a reduction in PCWP, but no difference in 30-day survival was noted.
   A randomized trial to evaluate the safety and efficacy of the Impella 2.5 device versus conventional management with an IABP in cardiogenic shock after myocardial infarction was also performed. Cardiac index was increased more with the Impella compared with IABP, which was the primary endpoint. Although 30-day survival was the same in both groups, this trial was not powered for this endpoint.

7. What are the contraindications of percutaneous ventricular assist devices?
   Major contraindications would include do not resuscitate and/or intubate status, a poor prognosis in the setting of terminal illness, the length and/or difficulty of preceding cardiopulmonary resuscitation, severe multiorgan dysfunction including neurologic disability, and the patient's wishes regarding quality of life.
   Certain structural heart issues may prove problematic. Use in the setting of a ventricular septal defect (VSD) may result in right to left shunt and hypoxemia. Severe aortic insufficiency may result in ventricular distension and pulmonary edema or worse heart function. Right ventricular infarction or severe right heart dysfunction would not be appropriate for a left-sided support device.
   Other considerations include contraindication to systemic anticoagulation, presence of widespread infection or bacteremia, and severe peripheral vascular disease.

8. What are the complications of percutaneous ventricular assist devices?
   Complications of percutaneous assist devices are generally cardiac or other (Table 19.3).

9. How is a percutaneous ventricular assist device weaned from the patient?
   PVADs may be weaned at the bedside or in the operating room. This process should occur under echocardiographic guidance to evaluate ventricular function as support is weaned and the device is decannulated.

Table 19-3. Potential Complications of Percutaneous Assist Devices

CARDIAC COMPLICATIONS	OTHER
Arrhythmias	Hemolysis
Tamponade	Bleeding
Mitral leaflet perforation	Von Willebrand syndrome
Severe aortic insufficiency	Access artery dissection
Functional mitral stenosis	Debris embolization
Paradoxical air embolism	
Intracardiac shunt	

KEY POINTS: PERCUTANEOUS ASSIST DEVICES

1. The goal of percutaneous ventricular circulatory support is to unload the failing ventricle and support systemic perfusion pressure to maintain adequate end-organ perfusion.
2. The Impella and TandemHeart do not assist in ventilation (either oxygenation or CO_2 removal) and are not indicated if there is evidence of respiratory compromise or failure in the setting of the primary cardiogenic insult.
3. If the percutaneous assist device is only supporting the left ventricle, it does rely upon the filling of the left ventricle by an effective right ventricle. Otherwise, a separate device to support the right ventricle may be indicated as well.
4. Studies to date have shown improvement in several hemodynamic indices, though none have conclusively demonstrated improved short- and long-term survival benefit, as compared with other mechanical assist devices (most notably intra-aortic balloon pumps).

BIBLIOGRAPHY

1. Kapur NK, Esposito M. Hemodynamic support with percutaneous devices in patients with heart failure. *Heart Fail Clin.* 2015;11:215-230.
2. Lawson WE, Koo M. Percutaneous ventricular assist devices and ECMO in the management of acute decompensated heart failure. *Clin Med Insights Cardiol.* 2015;9(suppl 1):41-48.
3. Seyfarth M, Sibbing D, Bauer I, et al. A randomized clinical trial to evaluate the safety and efficacy of a percutaneous left ventricular assist device versus intra-aortic balloon pumping for treatment of cardiogenic shock caused by myocardial infarction. *J Am Coll Cardiol.* 2008;52(19):1584-1588.
4. Thiele H, Sick P, Boudriot E, et al. Randomized comparison of intra-aortic balloon support with a percutaneous left ventricular support device in patients with revascularized acute myocardial infarction complicated by cardiogenic shock. *Eur Heart J.* 2005;26:1276-1283.

INTRA-AORTIC BALLOON PUMP

Adam A. Dalia and Michael G. Fitzsimons

CHAPTER 20

1. **What is an intra-aortic balloon pump?**

   An intra-aortic balloon pump (IABP) is a device that is placed in the aorta in order to improve coronary perfusion during diastole and facilitate ejection during systole. The balloon is inflated during the diastolic phase of the cardiac cycle, displacing blood towards the aortic root and coronary arteries and increasing diastolic coronary perfusion. The balloon is deflated at the onset of systole, allowing easier ejection of blood and a reduction in myocardial work.

2. **What are the components of an Intra-Aortic Balloon Pump System?**

   The IABP system contains a signal processor including an amplifier and display, infusion flushing system, helium gas pump, a pressure transducer, and an intra-arterial cannula with an attached polyethylene balloon. The balloon comes in various sizes chosen based on patient height with filling volumes ranging from 25 to 50 mL. The vascular access sheath ranges in size from 7 to 9 Fr.

3. **What gas is used for intra-aortic balloon pump inflation and why?**

   Helium is less dense than oxygen at room temperature (0.164 kg/m^3 vs. 1.33 kg/m^3). The decreased density allows the rapid inflation of the balloon to occur under laminar flow conditions by decreasing the Reynolds number, and has the advantage that if flow within the balloon becomes turbulent, the lower density helium is preferred. Concurrently, if the balloon becomes damaged or leaks in vitro, helium is absorbed rapidly into blood.

4. **How is proper placement of an intra-aortic balloon pump performed and confirmed?**

   The most common placement site for placement of an IABP is the femoral artery. Other sites have been described including the iliac, subclavian, axillary, and even brachial artery. A percutaneous Seldinger technique is most common to place a vascular sheath. The IABP is then advanced through the sheath until the balloon tip is just distal to the left subclavian artery and above the renal arteries. IABPs can be placed blind, under live fluoroscopy, or in the operating room with transesophageal echocardiography (TEE) guidance. Confirmation is generally made via chest x-ray. The appropriate position of the tip is 1.5 to 2.0 cm below the aortic knob.

5. **What is the mechanism of action behind an intra-aortic balloon pump?**

   The IABP works to improve diastolic blood pressure by increasing myocardial oxygen supply (increased coronary perfusion pressure) while decreasing myocardial oxygen consumption (decreased work through decreased afterload during systole). This is accomplished through a counter-propulsion mechanism. The IABP is triggered to inflate after aortic valve closure, which improves blood flow in the aortic root, thereby raising diastolic pressure resulting in increased coronary perfusion pressure. Balloon deflation occurs immediately preceding aortic valve opening resulting in a lower end-diastolic pressure. The pressure the ventricle must generate in order to open the aortic valve in systole is reduced.

6. **Name the four ways an intra-aortic balloon pump is triggered and factors which may impair triggering.**

   Triggering of the IABP refers to the specific indicator for the IABP to inflate and deflate. There are four "triggers", the electrocardiogram (EKG), arterial waveform, synchronized with a pacing device, or an asynchronous mode. The most commonly used trigger is the EKG. The balloon is inflated with the onset of diastole occurring in the middle of the T-wave and deflates at the onset of systole which is roughly the peak of the QRS complex. Triggering utilizing an arterial waveform is another common method; balloon inflation is timed in accordance with the dicrotic notch (Fig. 20.1). Triggering may be impaired by arrhythmias, tachycardia, poor quality EKG, and electrical magnetic interference.

7. **What are the clinical indications for an intra-aortic balloon pump?**

   General clinical indications for an IABP are to improve myocardial oxygen supply while reducing demand through improved coronary perfusion and reduction in afterload. Many potential clinical uses of the IABP have been reported (Table 20.1).

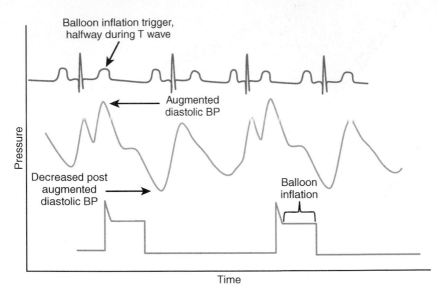

Figure 20-1. Intra-aortic balloon pump electrocardiogram and arterial waveform tracing.

Table 20-1. Clinical Scenarios Where an Intra-Aortic Balloon Pump Has Been Used
• Cardiogenic shock secondary to acute myocardial ischemia (AMI) refractory to medical therapy
• Acute mitral regurgitation from papillary muscle rupture
• Ischemic ventricular septal defect (VSD)
• Refractory ventricular arrhythmia
• Refractory unstable angina
• Decompensated heart failure (as a bridge to definitive therapy)
• Failure to wean from cardiopulmonary bypass
• Low cardiac output syndrome following cardiac surgery
• Perioperative support for high risk CABG
• Decompensated severe aortic stenosis
• Sepsis
• Prophylactic use during high risk PCI

CABG, Coronary artery bypass grafting; PCI, percutaneous coronary intervention.

8. What are the absolute and relative contraindications for an intra-aortic balloon pump?
   There are few absolute contraindications for an IABP. Aortic dissection, severe aortic insufficiency, and patient refusal are generally accepted as situations where an IABP should never be used. Most contraindications are relative and should be considered on a patient-by-patient basis (Table 20.2).

9. How and when are patients weaned from an intra-aortic balloon pump?
   Consideration to wean a patient from an IABP should occur after hemodynamic stability has been established. The weaning process is done gradually over 6 to 12 hours. Baseline hemodynamic data should be established (Table 20.3). Sufficient organ perfusion is generally reflected by a cardiac output (CO) ≥ 2.0 L/min/m^2), normal central venous pressure (CVP), normal serum level lactate, adequate urine output (>0.5 mL/kg/min), acceptable mixed venous saturation SVO$_2$, and the absence of acid-base disturbances or significant cardiac arrhythmias. When these parameters are met the weaning process begins. An incremental decrease of the ratio of IABP-supported heartbeat to unassisted heartbeat. Initially the ratio is 1:1. IABP support is decreased to 1:2, 1:4, and 1:8. Hemodynamic parameters, pharmacologic support, and organ perfusion are monitored with each decrease. The IABP is removed and support ceased when the ratio is 1:8 to prevent thrombosis formation.

Table 20-2. Contraindications for an Intra-Aortic Balloon Pump

Absolute Contraindications
- Severe aortic regurgitation
- Aortic dissection
- Patient or proxy refusal

Relative Contraindications
- Iliac artery stents
- Iliofemoral grafts/stents
- Abdominal aortic aneurysm
- Structural pathologies of the aorta (major reconstructive surgery)
- Septic shock
- Severe bleeding disorder
- Severe bilateral peripheral vascular disease.

Table 20-3. Physiologic Effects of IABP

PARAMETER	EFFECT
Diastolic blood pressure	Increase
Cardiac output	Increase
Cerebral perfusion	Increase
Urine output	Increase
Skin temperature	Increase
Systolic blood pressure	Decrease
Heart rate	Decrease
Wedge pressure	Decrease
LV wall stress	Decrease
Pulmonary blood volume	Decrease

10. **How can improper timing of intra-aortic balloon pump inflation or deflation be harmful?**
   There are four variations of ill-timed balloon inflation/deflation: early inflation, late inflation, early deflation, late deflation. *Early inflation* occurs when the balloon inflates while the heart is still in the systolic phase and the aortic valve is open. Early inflation results in a forced closure of the aortic valve and impairs ventricular ejection. *Late inflation* occurs well after the closure of the aortic valve. Blood in the root of the aorta has run off and inflation does not increase diastolic perfusion as effectively. *Early deflation* occurs when the balloon is deflated early in diastole and full advantage of increased diastolic perfusion does not occur. *Late deflation* occurs when the balloon remains inflated into the early systolic phase of the cardiac cycle. Ventricular work and myocardial oxygen consumption are increased as isovolumic contraction is prolonged.

11. **What are potential complications of the intra-aortic balloon pump?**
   Complications associated with the IABP are generally either vascular or hematologic. Vascular complications include vessel or aortic dissection, limb ischemia, or peripheral embolization of aortic debris. Risk factors for vascular complications include hypertension, diabetes, peripheral vascular disease, smoking, and female sex. Hematologic complications with include thrombocytopenia and bleeding. Improper IABP positioning may compromise blood flow to the renal, splanchnic, or hepatic vessels. Additional complications included infection.

12. **What is the current literature consensus on intra-aortic balloon pump?**
   The true efficacy of the IABP is difficult to study due to variable practices, bias, different placement times, and frequency of some potential indications. The most common traditional use of the IABP is in management of myocardial infarction complicated by cardiogenic shock. Recent studies do not

support the generalized use of an IABP in this setting over percutaneous coronary intervention (PCI). Data does not support the generalized use of an IABP for high-risk PCI or prior to coronary artery bypass grafting (CABG). Very limited data mostly in the form of case reports and small case series indicate that the IABP may be useful to help stabilize patients with mechanical complications of myocardial infarction such as papillary muscle rupture and acute mitral regurgitation or post-myocardial infarction ventricular septal defect associated with hemodynamic instability or shock. There is also limited but supporting observational data that an IABP may help stabilize intractable ventricular arrhythmias.

ACKNOWLEDGEMENT

The authors wish to acknowledge Drs. Joseph L. Weidman, MD, and Michael N. Andrawes, MD, for the valuable contributions to the previous edition of this chapter.

KEY POINTS: INTRA-AORTIC BALLOON PUMP

1. IABP decreases myocardial demand by decreasing afterload during systole and improves myocardial oxygen supply by increasing diastolic blood pressure, thereby increasing coronary perfusion pressure.
2. IABP is absolutely contraindicated in severe aortic regurgitation, aortic dissection, and competent patient or proxy refusal.
3. The most common complications of IABP are vascular, limb ischemia having the highest incidence.

BIBLIOGRAPHY

1. Barnett MG, Swartz MT, Peterson GJ, et al. Vascular complications from intraaortic balloons: risk analysis. *J Vasc Surg.* 1994;19(1):81-87.
2. Davidson J, Baumgariner F, Omari B, et al. Intra-aortic balloon pump: indications and complications. *J Natl Med Assoc.* 1998;90(3):137-140.
3. Ohman EM, Nanas J, Stomel RJ, et al. Thrombolysis and counterpulsation to improve survival in myocardial infarction complicated by hypotension and suspected cardiogenic shock or heart failure: results of the TACTICS Trial. *J Thromb Thrombolysis.* 2005;19(1):33-39.
4. Parissis H. Haemodynamic effects of the use of the intraaortic balloon pump. *Hellenic J Cardiol.* 2007;48(6):346-351.
5. Krishna M, Zacharowski K. Principles of intra-aortic balloon pump counterpulsation. *Contin Educ Anaesth Crit Care Pain.* 2009;9(1):24-28.
6. Ranucci M, Castelvecchio S, Biondi A, et al. A randomized controlled trial of preoperative intra-aortic balloon pump in coronary patients with poor left ventricular function undergoing coronary artery bypass surgery*. *Crit Care Med.* 2013;41(11):2476-2483.
7. Rihal CS, Naidu SS, Givertz MM, et al. 2015 SCAI/ACC/HFSA/STS Clinical Expert Consensus Statement on the Use of Percutaneous Mechanical Circulatory Support Devices in Cardiovascular Care: Endorsed by the American Heart Association, the Cardiological Society of India, and Sociedad Latino Americana de Cardiologia Intervencion; Affirmation of Value by the Canadian Association of Interventional Cardiology-Association Canadienne de Cardiologie d'intervention. *J Am Coll Cardiol.* 2015;65(19):e7-e26.
8. Santa-Cruz RA, Cohen MG, Ohman EM. Aortic counterpulsation: a review of the hemodynamic effects and indications for use. *Catheter Cardiovasc Interv.* 2006;67(1):68-77.
9. Thiele H, Zeymer U, Neumann FJ, et al. Intraaortic balloon support for myocardial infarction with cardiogenic shock. *N Engl J Med.* 2012;367(14):1287-1296.
10. Thiele H, Zeymer U, Neumann FJ, et al. Intra-aortic balloon counterpulsation in acute myocardial infarction complicated by cardiogenic shock (IABP-SHOCK II): final 12 month results of a randomised, open-label trial. *Lancet.* 2013;382(9905):1638-1645.

EXTRACORPOREAL MEMBRANE OXYGENATION

Michael G. Fitzsimons and Michael N. Andrawes

CHAPTER 21

1. **What is extracorporeal membrane oxygenation?**

   Extracorporeal membrane oxygenation (ECMO) is a means to provide peripheral oxygenation, ventilation, and circulation to a variety of patients with diseases of the heart and/or lungs for periods of days or weeks. The lungs of patients with severe respiratory failure have an impaired ability to perform the necessary functions of the thoracic cavity, primarily oxygenation, and ventilation. Data show that patients with respiratory failure who cannot be oxygenated or ventilated adequately with low tidal volumes and without high plateau pressures can often be treated with ECMO successfully. Certain patients with hemodynamic failure who lack the ability to meet the metabolic demands of the organs of the body despite pharmacologic support may also benefit from ECMO. There are also a growing number of indications for elective ECMO to support thoracic functions during elective surgical and interventional procedures.

2. **What is the history of extracorporeal membrane oxygenation?**

   ECMO was developed as an extension of cardiopulmonary bypass. The first reported use of ECMO for respiratory failure in an adult patient was in 1972 for a young man with adult respiratory distress syndrome (ARDS) after a motor vehicle accident. This was followed in 1976 by the first use of ECMO in neonatal patients. Since its development ECMO has been shown to improve survival in neonates with respiratory failure from a variety of causes compared with more traditional therapy. The benefits in adult patients are more controversial.

3. **How is extracorporeal membrane oxygenation different from cardiopulmonary bypass?**

   Cardiopulmonary bypass was developed as a means to provide short-term support to patients undergoing cardiac surgery. Cardiopulmonary bypass is also designed to accomplish several other tasks in addition to those provided by the thoracic cavity, including administration of cardioplegia, suction of the surgical field, and venting of the cardiac chambers (Table 21.1). The presence of a fluid reservoir on the cardiopulmonary bypass circuit allows one to add additional fluids and collect fluids suctioned or drained from the surgical field.

Table 21-1. Differences and Similarities Between Extracorporeal Membrane Oxygenation and Cardiopulmonary Bypass

PARAMETER	ECMO	CARDIOPULMONARY BYPASS
Oxygenation	Yes	Yes
Ventilation	Yes	Yes
Circulatory support	Yes	Yes
Venous reservoir	No	Yes
Ability to deliver cardioplegia	No	Yes
Ability to administer medications into circuit	No	Yes
Supplemental pumps (e.g., suction, vent)	No	Yes
Heating and cooling	Yes	Yes
Ability to adjust oxygenation	Yes	Yes
Ability to add fluids directly to circuit	No	Yes
Ability to administer anesthetics in line	No	Yes

ECMO, Extracorporeal membrane oxygenation.

Table 21-2. Clinical Uses of Extracorporeal Membrane Oxygenation

RESPIRATORY FAILURE	CARDIAC FAILURE	RESCUE	ELECTIVE
ARDS	Bridge to heart transplant	Hypothermia	High-risk PCI
Bridge to lung transplant	Massive PE	Drug overdose	Mediastinal surgery
Status asthmaticus	Graft failure after transplant	Pheochromocytoma crisis	Liver resection
Viral infection	Left heart failure	Traumatic brain injury	Liver transplant
Burn associated respiratory failure	Right heart failure	Septic shock	Tracheal surgery
Near drowning	Low cardiac output after bypass	Cardiopulmonary arrest	
Congenital diaphragmatic hernia	Myocarditis		
Re-expansion pulmonary edema			
Pancreatitis			
Fat emboli			

ARDS, Adult respiratory distress syndrome; *PCI*, percutaneous coronary intervention; *PE*, pulmonary emboli.

4. What are clinical situations where extracorporeal membrane oxygenation may be beneficial?
   ECMO has been used for short-term hemodynamic and respiratory support for numerous conditions (Table 21.2). There are four primary categories of ECMO uses: respiratory failure, cardiac failure, acute cardiothoracic "rescue," and elective.

5. Are there any diagnostic modalities that help determine when emergent extracorporeal membrane oxygenation is indicated?
   Transesophageal echocardiography (TEE) allows real-time assessment of cardiac function. Acute pulmonary thromboemboli, amniotic fluid embolism, and air emboli cause an acute pressure overload on the right ventricle. Acute right ventricular pressure overload results in right ventricular dilatation and failure, tricuspid regurgitation, and a shift of the interventricular septum toward the left, further impairing filling of the left ventricle and a reduction in cardiac output. The septal shift also results in further enlargement of the right ventricle and worsening function. TEE may also be used to guide proper positioning of the venous return cannula into the right atrium when ECMO is initiated.

6. What does the literature show regarding extracorporeal membrane oxygenation?
   Dr. Warren Zapol performed the first randomized study to evaluate the effectiveness of ECMO in adult patients with severe acute respiratory failure. This study, from 1979, determined that ECMO could support respiratory gas exchange, but did not increase long-term survival. Subsequent studies have generally demonstrated survival rates of approximately 50% for patients with primary respiratory failure. Older patients, those having complications while on ECMO, and those having prolonged ventilation before ECMO were less likely to survive. Survival for patients with primary cardiac failure also tends to be lower. The use of ECMO for cardiogenic shock after cardiopulmonary bypass has a survival rate of approximately 33%.

7. Are there any contraindications to extracorporeal membrane oxygenation?
   Few absolute contraindications to ECMO exist. Patient or proxy refusal is an absolute contraindication. Patients with "do not resuscitate" orders should not be subjected to ECMO. Irreversible respiratory failure in patients who are not candidates for lung transplantation should preclude the use of ECMO. Severe bleeding and peripheral vascular disease increase the risk of complications with ECMO. Some have argued against the use in elderly patients, although one study demonstrated that 41.7% of patients older than 75 years with cardiogenic shock treated with ECMO survived to discharge.

8. What are the components of an extracorporeal membrane oxygenation circuit?
   An ECMO circuit contains several key components including the vascular access (cannulae and tubing) driving force (pump), gas exchange unit (oxygenator-ventilator), and the interface or console. Peripheral vascular access is most commonly established in the femoral artery and veins. The venous or *drainage* cannulas are sized between 21 F and 28 F for adults and smaller for newborns and children. The venous cannula should be positioned at the junction of the superior vena cava and right atrium. The

Table 21-3. Cannulation Sites for Extracorporeal Membrane Oxygenation

CANNULATION TECHNIQUE	SITE OF VENOUS DRAINAGE	SITE OF BLOOD RETURN	BENEFITS	DOWNSIDE
Peripheral VV	Drainage from IVC/SVC or right atrium via femoral vein	Return via percutaneous access to right atrium or SVC	No arterial cannulation, easy to establish	No hemodynamic support. Susceptible to shunt
Central VV	Drainage from the right atrium	Return to the pulmonary artery	Very effective. Provides right ventricular support	Requires a sternotomy
Peripheral VA	Drainage from the IVC and right atrium via femoral vein	Femoral artery or axillary artery; the carotid artery has been used in neonates	Hemodynamic support, decreased pulmonary blood flow, ability to rest lungs and heart, does not require a sternotomy	Requires arterial cannulation; lower flows will not distribute blood above diaphragm; risk of limb ischemia
Central VA	Drainage from the right atrium	Return to the aorta or graft to the axillary artery	Effective flows, no risk of limb ischemia	Requires sternotomy

IVC, Inferior vena cava; SVC, superior vena cava; VA, venoarterial; VV, venovenous.

cannula is directed away from the interatrial septum under echocardiography or fluoroscopic guidance. The arterial or *return* cannula is placed in the other femoral vein (venovenous [VV] ECMO) or femoral artery (venoarterial [VA] ECMO). Central cannulation is most commonly used for postcardiotomy cardiogenic shock when the chest is already open (Table 21.3). Central VV ECMO is most commonly from the right atrium to the pulmonary artery, a configuration that also provides right ventricular support. Central VA ECMO is usually from the right atrium to the aorta or a graft attached to the axillary artery.

Most ECMO circuits have a membrane gas exchange unit. This gas exchange unit consists of a series of hollow fibers through which the blood passes. Gas is passed in a countercurrent manner allowing exchange across the membranes. The pump system may be either a centrigular system or a roller system. Centrifugal pumps contain a magnetically driven impeller that cycles at several thousand rotations per minute (RPM), generating a pressure gradient across the pump head and propelling blood forward. It is preload- and afterload-dependent. If flow into the pump is decreased, then flow and pressure will be decreased. The Thoratec CentriMag blood pump is a magnetically levitated centrifugal device that produces unidirectional flow and may generate flows up to 10 L/min (Figs. 21.1 and 21.2). A roller pump, which is less commonly used, consists of flexible tubing in a track. The roller compresses the tubing and forces blood forward with each turn. Such flow is independent of systemic vascular resistance, and high pressures can develop.

9. How does one monitor and assess the physiologic impact of extracorporeal membrane oxygenation?
Monitoring patients subject to ECMO is a multidisciplinary task. Surgeons, intensivists, perfusionists, anesthesiologists, respiratory therapists, and nurses may all be involved in the care of these patients. The *flow* is the amount of blood moved by the circuit and is equivalent to the cardiac output. The *sweep speed* is the amount of gas passed across the membrane oxygenator and is similar to the minute ventilation. The transmembrane gradient is the pressure drop across the membrane oxygenator. Maintenance of normal physiologic parameters is the goal (Table 21.4). Flow rates, sweep speed, and fraction inspired oxygen (FiO_2) are adjusted to attain such measure.

10. How is ventilation managed while a patient is receiving extracorporeal membrane oxygenation?
The avoidance of barotrauma is a prime benefit of ECMO. Most patients will be given *rest* settings to avoid complications associated with high volume and high-pressure ventilation. Inspiratory pressures are often limited to 20 to 25 cm H_2O with a positive end-expiratory pressure of 10 to 15 cm H_2O and

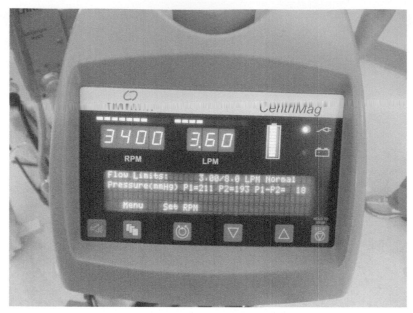

Figure 21-1. CentriMag extracorporeal membrane oxygenation console.

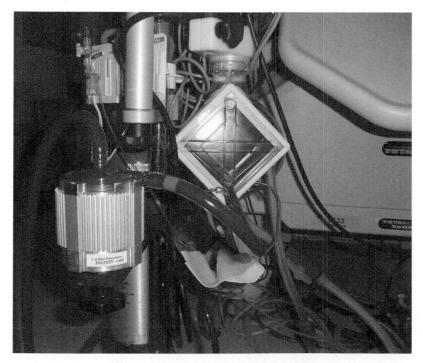

Figure 21-2. CentriMag pump and gas exchange system.

Table 21-4. Goals for Management During Extracorporeal Membrane Oxygenation

PARAMETER	GOAL
Flow rates	50–80 mL/kg/min
Mean arterial pressure (adult)	65–95 mm Hg
Sweep speed (gas flow)	50–80 mL/kg/min
Transmembrane gradient	$<$50 mm Hg
FiO_2 (%)	100% at initiation, wean based on FiO_2
pH	7.35–7.45
$PaCO_2$	35–45 mm Hg
SpO_2 (arterial or return cannula)	100%
SpO_2 (VA ECMO)	$>$95%
SpO_2 (VV ECMO)	85%–92%

ECMO, Extracorporeal membrane oxygenation; *VA,* venoarterial; *VV,* venovenous.

a low respiratory rate. Terragni demonstrated that ECMO allows tidal volumes less than 6 mL/kg (ideal body weight) to be used. An improvement in morphologic markers of lung protection and a reduction in pulmonary cytokines are observed.

11. **What problems are commonly encountered during the clinical management of extracorporeal membrane oxygenation?**
Acute problems tend to fall into three categories:
1. Inadequate flow, commonly due to either hypovolemia or malposition of the drainage cannula. This is indicated by "chatter" or rattling of the venous line. Inadequate flow may also be caused by excessive afterload, inadequate RPMs, or obstruction.
2. Poor oxygenation, maybe due to an inadequate FiO_2, shunt of blood through the lungs, or oxygenator failure.
3. Inadequate ventilation due to malfunction of the gas exchange assembly or low *sweep speed.*

12. **How does one wean a patient from extracorporeal membrane oxygenation?**
The technique of weaning a patient from ECMO support depends on the type of ECMO (VV or VA) and the purpose of the support. In general the lungs and heart assume more and more responsibility for oxygenation, ventilation, and circulation as support is weaned. Sidebotham et al. describe their technique for weaning ECMO (Table 21.5).

13. **What are complications of extracorporeal membrane oxygenation?**
Most adult ECMO is established with peripheral cannulation of the femoral vessels. Lower limb ischemia may occur because of occlusion of arterial inflow and may be treated with decannulation or supplemental cannulation of the superficial femoral artery which supplies perfusion below the cannulation site. Neither body mass index, body surface area, nor cannula size predicts limb ischemia. Abdominal compartment syndrome may occur in both adult and pediatric patients receiving ECMO and is likely due to massive fluid resuscitation in an effort to achieve adequate ECMO flows. Other complications include bleeding, clot formation, stroke, renal failure, and nosocomial infection. Mechanical mishaps such as failure of the pump and oxygenator must be considered in planning support. Transport and movement are times where monitoring and vigilance are especially critical as cannulae can be dislodged.

14. **How does one transfer a patient receiving extracorporeal membrane oxygenation?**
The transfer of patients with severe respiratory failure and hemodynamic failure to large medical centers is increasingly common. The University of Michigan reviewed all patients transferred between 1990 and 1999 while receiving ECMO. Patients were transferred over a range of 2 to 790 miles. No patients died during transport. Complications included power failure, circuit tubing leakages, circuit rupture, membrane lung thrombosis, membrane lung leakage, and hyperventilation.

Table 21-5. Weaning a Patient from Extracorporeal Membrane Oxygenation Support

MEASURE	VV ECMO	VA ECMO
Purpose of support	Oxygenation-ventilation	Hemodynamic support
Measure of improvement	Increased SpO_2 and PaO_2 Decreased $PaCO_2$ Improved CXR Increased lung compliance	Return of pulsatile arterial waveform Improved cardiac function by echo-cardiography
Technique	Provide full ventilatory support Reduce gas "sweep" Reduce flows to 1–2 L/min	Adjust inotropic support to provide acceptable hemodynamics Reduce flows to 1–2 L/min
Monitoring during weaning	Maintenance of SpO_2/PaO_2	Echocardiography (cardiac function) Blood pressure Cardiac output Central venous pressure Pulmonary artery pressure
When to discontinue	Acceptable ABG 2–3 h after weaning and tolerance of flow reduction to zero	Acceptable hemodynamics after 1–2 h of minimal or no hemodynamics support

ABG, Arterial blood gases; CXR, chest radiograph; ECMO, extracorporeal membrane oxygenation; VA, veno-arterial; VV, venovenous.

Modified from Sidebotham D, McGeorge A, McGuinness S, et al. Extracorporeal membrane oxygenation for treating severe cardiac and respiratory failure in adults: part 2—technical considerations. *J Cardiothorac Vasc Anesth.* 2010;24:164–172.

KEY POINTS: EXTRACORPOREAL MEMBRANE OXYGENATION

1. ECMO is a means to provide peripheral oxygenation, ventilation, and circulation to a variety of patients with diseases of the heart and/or lungs for periods of days or weeks.
2. ECMO does not provide several supporting features that cardiopulmonary bypass does such as a reservoir for fluid volume, additional pumps for administration of cardioplegia, the ability to vent the heart, or ability to suction blood from a surgical field directly into the circuit.
3. VA ECMO primarily supports cardiopulmonary failure while VV ECMO only supports the failing lungs.

BIBLIOGRAPHY

1. Augustin P, Lasocki S, Dufour G, et al. Abdominal compartment syndrome due to extracorporeal membrane oxygenation in adults. *Ann Thorac Surg.* 2010;90:e40-e41.
2. Aziz TA, Singh G, Popjes E, et al. Initial experience with CentriMag extracorporeal membrane oxygenation for support of critically ill patients with refractory cardiogenic shock. *J Heart Lung Transplant.* 2010;29:66-71.
3. Brogan TV, Thiagarajan RR, Rycos PT, et al. Extracorporeal membrane oxygenation in adults with severe respiratory failure: a multi-center database. *Intensive Care Med.* 2009;35:2105-2114.
4. Foley DS, Pranikoff T, Younger JG, et al. A review of 100 patients transported on extracorporeal life support. *ASAIO J.* 2002;48:612-619.
5. Hill JD, O'Brien TG, Murray JJ, et al. Prolonged extracorporeal oxygenation in severe acute respiratory failure (shock lung syndrome). Use of the Bramson membrane lung. *N Engl J Med.* 1972;286:629-634.
6. Meilck F, Quintel M. Extracorporeal membrane oxygenation. *Curr Opin Crit Care.* 2005;11:87-93.
7. Peek GJ, Mugford M, Tiruvoipai R, CESAR trial collaboration, et al. Efficacy and economic assessment of conventional ventilator support versus extracorporeal membrane oxygenation for severe adult respiratory failure (CESAR): a multi-center randomized controlled trial. *Lancet.* 2009;374:1351-1363.
8. Saito S, Nakatani T, Kobayashi J, et al. Is extracorporeal life support contraindicated in elderly patients? *Ann Thorac Surg.* 2007;83:140-145.
9. Sidebotham D, McGeorge A, McGuinness S, et al. Extracorporeal membrane oxygenation for treating severe cardiac and respiratory failure in adults: part 2—technical considerations. *J Cardiothorac Vasc Anesth.* 2010;24:164-172.

10. Terragni PP, Del Sorbo L, Mascia L, et al. Tidal volume lower than 6 mL/kg enhances lung protection. Role of extracorporeal carbon dioxide removal. *Anesthesiology.* 2009;111:826-835.
11. Zapol WM, Snider MT, Hill JD, et al. Extracorporeal membrane oxygenation in severe acute respiratory failure. A randomized prospective study. *JAMA.* 1979;242:2193-2196.
12. Zapol WM, Snider MT, Schneider RC. Extracorporeal membrane oxygenation for acute respiratory failure. *Anesthesiology.* 1977;46:272-285.

CHAPTER 22

TRACHEAL INTUBATION AND AIRWAY MANAGEMENT

Rodger White

1. **What is the airway?**
   The airway is the conduit through which air and oxygen must pass before reaching the lungs. It includes the anatomic structures extending from the nose and mouth to the larynx and trachea.

2. **What is airway management?**
   Airway management is the procedure for ensuring that the airway remains patent. It is the first step in the ABCs of basic resuscitation (A, airway; B, breathing; C, circulation).

3. **Why does airway management generally precede management of breathing and circulation?**
   If the airway is completely obstructed, no oxygen can reach the lungs, and the heart and circulation will have no oxygen to distribute to the body's vital organs. However, the 2010 American Heart Association (AHA) *Guidelines for Cardiopulmonary Resuscitation and Emergency Cardiovascular Care* now recommend beginning cardiopulmonary resuscitation with 30 chest compressions before delivering two rescue breaths. Although there is no proven mortality benefit to managing the airway after the circulation, the AHA rationale is that blood flow to vital organs depends on chest compressions.

   Note: In addition, the AHA recommends "hands-only" chest compressions (i.e., no rescue breathing at all) for the untrained lay rescuer of a victim in cardiac arrest.

4. **Describe the ways to manage the airway.**
   The airway may remain patent without any intervention and can be managed with or without tracheal intubation. Airway management without intubation can involve a variety of maneuvers. In unconscious patients, the tongue commonly obstructs the airway. Techniques to open the airway include the head tilt–chin lift maneuver and the jaw thrust maneuver. Placement of oral or nasal airways may also help to maintain a patent airway. The use of a face mask with a bag-valve device (e.g., Ambu bag) is the usual next step in airway management. In the majority of patients, it is possible to maintain a patent airway without tracheal intubation. If tracheal intubation is required, it can be accomplished through surgical or nonsurgical techniques.

5. **What are the indications for tracheal intubation?**
   There are five main indications:
   - Upper airway obstruction
   - Inadequate oxygenation
   - Inadequate ventilation
   - Elevated work of breathing
   - Airway protection

6. **Explain why upper airway obstruction is an indication for tracheal intubation.**
   If the upper airway is obstructed and cannot be opened with the previously described maneuvers, the trachea must be intubated to avoid life-threatening hypoxemia. Although intubation will bypass the anatomic area of obstruction, the cause should be determined to evaluate appropriate timing of extubation or need for further treatment.

7. **Explain how to evaluate hypoxemia as an indication for tracheal intubation.**
   If the patient's oxygen saturation is consistently less than 90% despite the use of high-flow oxygen delivered through a face mask, tracheal intubation should be considered. One hundred percent oxygen can be delivered reliably only with an endotracheal tube (ETT). Other factors to consider are the adequacy of cardiac output, blood hemoglobin concentration, presence of chronic hypoxemia, and reason for the hypoxemia. For example, patients with hypoxemia due to intracardiac right-to-left shunts may have chronic hypoxemia. In these patients, the administration of 100% oxygen with an ETT may not be effective in raising the oxygen saturation level.

8. Explain how to evaluate hypoventilation as an indication for tracheal intubation.

   With hypoventilation, the blood PCO_2 progressively rises, which also lowers the blood pH level (respiratory acidosis). With increasing CO_2 levels, patients eventually become unconscious (CO_2 narcosis). Low systemic pH may be associated with abnormal myocardial irritability and contractility. The exact level of pH or PCO_2 that requires assisted ventilation must be determined for each patient. Chronic respiratory acidosis (e.g., in a patient with severe chronic obstructive pulmonary disease) is usually better tolerated than acute respiratory acidosis.

9. Explain how to evaluate elevated work of breathing as an indication for tracheal intubation.

   Normally, the respiratory muscles account for less than 5% of the total body oxygen consumption. In patients with respiratory failure, this can increase to as much as 40%. It can be difficult to assess the work of breathing by clinical examination. However, patients who have rapid shallow breathing, use of accessory respiratory muscles, or paradoxic respirations have a predictably high work of breathing. The results of an arterial blood gas analysis (i.e., pH, PCO_2, and PO_2) may be initially normal in such patients. Eventually, the respiratory muscles fatigue and fail, causing inadequate oxygenation and ventilation. Mechanical ventilation can sometimes be done without tracheal intubation (see Chapter 8) but is more reliably accomplished with intubation.

10. Explain airway protection as an indication for tracheal intubation.

    In an awake patient, protective airway reflexes normally prevent the pulmonary aspiration of gastric contents. Patients with altered mental status from a variety of causes may lose these protective reflexes, increasing the risk of aspiration pneumonia. Tracheal intubation with a cuffed tube can decrease the risk of aspiration. However, liquids can still leak around the ETT cuff, and the glottic barrier is bypassed, which plays a role in bacterial colonization of the lower airways.

11. What are the surgical techniques for tracheal intubation?

    Surgical techniques include cricothyroidotomy or tracheotomy, which involves placing an ETT directly into the trachea through the cricothyroid membrane or between two tracheal rings.

12. What are the commonly used nonsurgical techniques for tracheal intubation?

    Nonsurgical techniques can be divided into techniques that incorporate direct vision and *blind* techniques. The most commonly used direct vision intubation technique is direct laryngoscopy (DL). The laryngoscope is placed in the mouth and manipulated to expose the larynx. An ETT is then placed through the larynx into the trachea. Another direct vision technique uses the flexible fiberoptic bronchoscope. An ETT is loaded onto the bronchoscope, which is advanced through the larynx via the nose or mouth. Once the bronchoscope is in the trachea, the ETT is advanced into position. Blind intubation is generally performed through the nose because the nasopharynx guides the ETT toward the larynx. Some laryngoscopes incorporate a video screen to allow improved vision of glottic structures via a small camera at the tip of the laryngoscope blade.

13. Which drugs can be given to facilitate tracheal intubation?

    Sedative or analgesic agents are given to reduce the discomfort of laryngoscopy and to blunt the hemodynamic response. Muscle relaxants can make DL easier to perform. The main risks of sedative or analgesic drugs in this setting are hypotension and respiratory depression. The muscle relaxants cause paralysis of all skeletal muscle, including the respiratory muscles. If the trachea cannot be intubated, the patient may not resume spontaneous breathing if sedatives, analgesics, or muscle relaxants have been given.

14. What equipment should be prepared before direct laryngoscopy is attempted?

    Before laryngoscopy is attempted, all equipment should be checked for proper function. This includes laryngoscope blades, laryngoscope handle, suction source, suction catheter, oxygen source, self-inflating bag or breathing circuit, face mask, oral airways, nasal airways, sedative agents, muscle relaxants, intravenous line, and patient monitors.

15. How is direct laryngoscopy accomplished?

    The technique varies slightly depending on the type of blade used (Figs. 22.1 and 22.2). First, the head is placed in the *sniffing* position with cervical spine in flexion and atlanto-occipital joint in extension. The blade is inserted into the right side of the mouth. Then the tongue is moved to the left. With a curved (Macintosh) blade, the tip is inserted between the base of the tongue and the superior surface of the epiglottis, an area called the *vallecula*. If a straight (Miller or Wisconsin) blade is used, the tip is manipulated to lift the epiglottis. With both blade types, once the tip is in position, the blade is moved forward and upward to expose the larynx. An ETT is then inserted into the trachea. Gentle downward pressure on the thyroid cartilage may help to improve the view of the larynx.

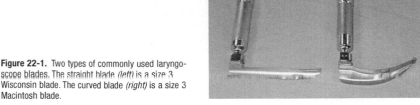

Figure 22-1. Two types of commonly used laryngoscope blades. The straight blade *(left)* is a size 3 Wisconsin blade. The curved blade *(right)* is a size 3 Macintosh blade.

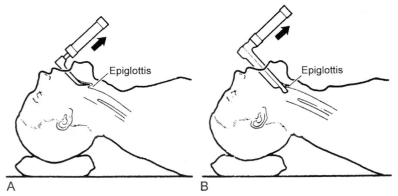

Figure 22-2. Procedure for direct laryngoscopy. (A) A curved laryngoscope blade is placed in the vallecula. Lifting the blade forward and upward exposes the larynx. (B) A straight blade is used to lift the epiglottis directly and expose the larynx. (From Gal TJ. Airway management. In: Miller RD, ed. *Miller's Anesthesia.* 6th ed. New York: Churchill Livingstone; 2005:1634.)

16. What maneuver can be performed to minimize the risk of aspiration during direct laryngoscopy?
Cricoid pressure consists of firm manual pressure on the cricoid cartilage. This maneuver can occlude the esophagus and reduce the chance of gastric distention from mask ventilation. It can also prevent regurgitation of gastric contents into the pharynx. However, controversy exists about the effectiveness of this maneuver.

17. What is a difficult airway? What is a difficult intubation?
A difficult airway is a clinical situation in which an anesthesiologist or other specially trained clinician has difficulty with mask ventilation or tracheal intubation. Difficult intubation can be defined as one requiring more than three attempts at laryngoscopy or more than 10 minutes of laryngoscopy. Although the definitions are arbitrary, the inability to maintain a patent airway (with or without intubation) may be associated with anoxic brain injury and death.

18. How do you evaluate the airway for potential difficulty?
The history should address the ease of prior tracheal intubations. Patients who have general anesthesia for surgery frequently undergo tracheal intubation. The anesthetic record for the procedure should document the ease of intubation and the equipment used. On examination, one must evaluate four anatomic features: mouth opening, pharyngeal space, neck extension, and submandibular compliance.

19. How do you evaluate mouth opening and pharyngeal space to predict difficult intubation?
In the adult, a mouth opening of two to three fingerbreadths is usually adequate. One measure of pharyngeal space is the Mallampati class (Fig. 22.3). The patient is asked to sit upright with the head in a neutral position. Then he or she is asked to open the mouth as widely as possible and protrude the tongue as far as possible. The classification is based on the pharyngeal structures seen.
- **Class I:** The soft palate, fauces, entire uvula, and tonsillar pillars are visible.
- **Class II:** The soft palate, fauces, and part of the uvula are visible.

Class I   Class II   Class III   Class IV

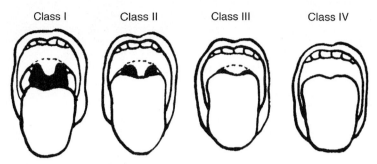

Figure 22-3. The Mallampati classification to evaluate pharyngeal space.

- **Class III:** The soft palate and base of the uvula are visible.
- **Class IV:** The soft palate is not visible at all.
   Intubation is generally easier in patients with class I airways than in patients with class IV airways. However, this test addresses only one of the four anatomic features required for easy DL.

20. How do you evaluate neck extension and submandibular compliance to predict difficult intubation?
   A normal adult has approximately 35 degrees of extension at the atlanto-occipital joint. A decrease in extension may make it impossible to view the larynx with DL. It can be difficult to assess the submandibular compliance by physical examination. Assessment of the mandibular space can be attempted by measuring the distance from the chin to the thyroid cartilage, the *thyromental distance*. An adult with less than 6.5 cm of thyromental distance may have a greater chance of difficult intubation than one with greater than 6.5 cm. Combining the various physical examination tests improves the ability to predict a difficult intubation, but no combination is foolproof.

21. How do you manage a potentially difficult intubation?
   Three types of plans must be made when managing a difficult airway. The first is the primary approach to the intubation. The second is the plan for an emergency nonsurgical airway. Finally, a plan should exist for an emergency surgical airway (cricothyroidotomy or tracheotomy). Many factors affect the management plan for a potentially difficult airway. These factors include the indication for intubation, the urgency of the intubation, the availability of skilled personnel, and the availability of special equipment. Because an awake, cooperative, spontaneously breathing patient normally has a patent airway, an awake intubation may be the safest. Topical or local anesthetics can be used to decrease airway sensation and patient discomfort.

22. What are the ways to provide an emergency nonsurgical airway?
   If tracheal intubation and mask ventilation are not possible and the airway is not patent, an emergency airway must be provided. The options for providing an emergency nonsurgical airway include laryngeal mask ventilation, transtracheal jet ventilation, or esophageal-tracheal Combitube ventilation. The laryngeal mask is the most widely available of the three options. It is inserted into the posterior pharynx and lies opposite the larynx. In elective situations, it has a success rate of more than 90%. It is less successful in emergencies, but its widespread availability makes it a valuable option in managing the difficult airway. Special versions of the laryngeal mask incorporate features designed to facilitate blind passage of an ETT into the trachea.
   Note: Emergency intubations are associated with up to a 2% mortality because of the underlying conditions of the patient and the difficulties associated with the intubations. The risks are increased by performing DL more than twice.

23. How is tracheal intubation confirmed?
   Auscultation for bilateral breath sounds and absence of stomach inflation should be done after each intubation attempt. However, these signs may still be present with an esophageal intubation. Carbon dioxide capnography is one of the most reliable methods to confirm placement. The laryngoscopic view may be useful. If an experienced clinician clearly sees the tube between the vocal cords, this is definitive confirmation. The ETT itself commonly blocks sight of the vocal cords, and inexperienced clinicians may insert the tube in the esophagus despite having a good view of the larynx. Other confirmation methods include fiberoptic bronchoscopy or an esophageal detector device.

24. **What are the immediate, short-term complications of tracheal intubation?**
Immediate complications of intubation include dental injury, cervical spine injury, pharyngeal trauma, laryngeal injury, aspiration of gastric contents, and tracheal rupture. Nosebleed is a risk with nasal intubations. The most common injuries are minor lip trauma and dental injury.

25. **How does video laryngoscopy differ from direct laryngoscopy?**
DL uses patient position and intraoral tissue manipulation to create a line of sight from the clinician's eye to the patient's glottic opening. Often this is quite stimulating to the patient and requires a fair bit of force to move intraoral tissues out of the way.

Video laryngoscopy (VL) uses a video camera placed near the tip of the laryngoscope blade to look around the corner of the oral pharynx without the need to create a direct line of sight. This generally is less stimulating to the patient and requires less force from the clinician.

The techniques for DL have been extensively described in various anesthesia textbooks.

The techniques for VL depend on the blade shape. Blades resembling DL blades can be used with DL techniques. Blades with channels to hold the ETT are manipulated to align the ETT tip with the glottic opening. Nonchanneled, angled blades are most effectively used with a rigid stylette to allow manipulation of the ETT into the glottic opening.

26. **What are common challenges to video laryngoscopy?**
Blades resembling DL blades present the same challenges as regular DL blades in visualizing anterior airways. Channeled blades rely on the ability to align the channel containing the ETT with the glottic opening.

Nonchanneled angled blades combined with rigid stylettes pose a special challenge to clinicians experienced in DL. Clinicians on the steep end of this learning curve often describe easy visualization of the vocal cords but difficulty aligning the ETT tip with the glottic opening. This usually occurs because the VL blade is inserted further into the mouth than necessary and the glottic view is taking up more screen space than needed. Withdrawing the blade until the glottic view is positioned in the upper third of the video screen and slightly left of center will optimize space near the glottis to manipulate the ETT tip. Unlike DL, the tongue should not be swept into the left side of the mouth because the blade often needs to be shifted left to make manipulation of the ETT easier. When using a rigid stylette, the ETT should be held with the finger tips of the right hand as close to the patient's mouth as possible. This allows the ETT tip to be manipulated with precision. Once the ETT cuff is passed the patient's teeth, the ETT should be placed beside the VL blade and advanced along the curvature of the tongue. Once the ETT tip comes into view on the video screen, if the tip is below the glottic opening, the ETT can be lifted with the right hand using the same motion the left hand would use if lifting with a DL blade. If the tip is to the right of the glottic opening, the ETT tip can be rotated left taking care not to fold the right arytenoid into the glottic opening.

Alternatives to inserting the blade followed by the ETT include holding the ETT beside the blade and inserting both at the same time or inserting the ETT first and following it with the blade.

Regardless of the insertion technique, it is vital to take one's gaze from the video screen and look directly into the patient's mouth whenever the blade or ETT is being inserted into the mouth. Failure to do so risks injury to the patient.

27. **How are patients injured by video laryngoscopy?**
Most injuries are caused by a rigidly styletted ETT being pushed against resistance when the ETT tip is out of the clinician's view. One reason for this is looking at the video screen instead of at the patient's mouth while inserting the ETT into the mouth. But even if the clinician looks into the patient's mouth until the ETT tip disappears around the base of the patient's tongue, there will generally be a brief interval between losing direct vision of the ETT tip and seeing the ETT tip come into view on the video screen. At this point it is critical to not push the ETT against resistance if you cannot see the ETT tip. If you encounter resistance at this point, withdraw the blade until the ETT tip is visible on the screen then advance both the ETT and the blade together keeping the ETT tip in view on the screen.

To avoid injury to the vocal cords/trachea, do not advance the ETT tip beyond the plane of the vocal cords with the rigid stylette fully inserted. Once the ETT tip has passed the plane of the arytenoids, an assistant should begin withdrawing the rigid stylette while the intubating clinician advances the ETT tip through the vocal cords.

28. **What if it is difficult to advance the endotracheal tube when the tip is visible on the screen?**
If adjusting the blade (withdrawing slightly and shifting left) does not work, then the ETT is likely pinched between the right molars. (This happens often if the ETT is inserted in the right corner of the mouth instead of midline.) Moving the ETT to the middle of the mouth and hugging the tongue should fix this.

ACKNOWLEDGMENT

The authors wish to acknowledge Dr. Manuel Pardo, Jr., MD, for the valuable contributions to the previous edition of this chapter.

KEY POINTS: TRACHEAL INTUBATION AND AIRWAY MANAGEMENT

For Video Laryngoscopy
Airway management in patients in the intensive care unit
1. In most patients, it is possible to maintain a patent airway without tracheal intubation.
2. Before managing a patient's airway, confirm the availability and function of all equipment that may be used.
3. The five main indications for tracheal intubation are upper airway obstruction, inadequate oxygenation, inadequate ventilation, elevated work of breathing, and airway protection.
4. To predict a difficult intubation, evaluate four anatomic features on physical examination: mouth opening, pharyngeal space, neck extension, and submandibular compliance.
5. Confirm ETT placement immediately with a reliable method such as carbon dioxide capnography.
6. VL: Look in the mouth while inserting the blade midline. Do not sweep the tongue left. Once the light is between the teeth, you can look at the screen and rotate the blade along the curve of the palate following the Median Palatine Raffe to the uvula. Continue rotating until the glottic structures come into view. Only at this point should any lift force be needed on the blade. Lift only enough to maintain a workable view.
7. VL: Ideally the glottic view will be in the upper left corner of the screen to allow screen space to the right of and below the glottic opening to allow early visualization and effective manipulation of the ETT tip.
8. VL: Look back in the mouth to insert the ETT (midline, hugging the tongue) and watch until the ETT tip disappears around back of the tongue. Hold the ETT in the finger tips of the right hand as close to the patient's mouth as possible to make precise control of ETT tip movement easier.
9. VL: Look back at the screen and advance the ETT tip between the arytnoids.
10. VL: Withdraw the rigid stylette before the ETT tip goes between the vocal cords.

BIBLIOGRAPHY

1. American Society of Anesthesiologists. Practice guidelines for management of the difficult airway. Available at: http://ecommerce.asahq.org/p-177-practice-guidelines-for-management-of-the-difficult-airway.aspx. Accessed 13.10.11.
2. Berg RA, Hemphill R, Abella BS, et al. Part 5: adult basic life support: 2010 American Heart Association guidelines for cardiopulmonary resuscitation and emergency cardiovascular care. *Circulation.* 2010;122:S685-S705.
3. El-Orbany M, Connolly LA. Rapid sequence induction and intubation: current controversy. *Anesth Analg.* 2010;110: 1318-1325.
4. Henderson J. Airway management in the adult. In: Miller RD, ed. *Miller's Anesthesia.* 7th ed. New York: Churchill Livingstone; 2010:1573-1610.

CHAPTER 23

TRACHEOSTOMY AND UPPER AIRWAY OBSTRUCTION

Jacqueline C. O'Toole and C. Matthew Kinsey

1. What are some common etiologies of upper airway obstruction?
   Table 23.1

2. How do you approach and initiate management of an upper airway obstruction?
   - Assess urgency: Is emergent airway indicated or is there time for temporizing therapies? Although an emergent airway can be obtained via rapid sequence intubation, awake fiberoptic intubation is, in general, a safer choice. Cricothyrotomy is a life-saving emergent surgical airway.
   - Temporizing therapies include elevation of the head of the bed, inhaled racemic epinephrine, heliox (80% helium and 20% oxygen), and intravenous corticosteroids.
   - Once the airway is secured, evaluation of the etiology of obstruction includes computed tomography (CT) imaging, laryngoscopy, bronchoscopy.

3. What are some novel approaches to upper airway obstruction in the setting of lung cancer or extrinsic airway compression?
   - Immediate response: Balloon dilation, stent placement, laser photoresection, electrocautery, argon plasma coagulation, cryodebridement
   - Delayed response: Cryotherapy, brachytherapy, external beam radiation

4. What are the different techniques for a surgical airway?
   - A *standard surgical tracheostomy* is an open surgical procedure that allows insertion of a tracheostomy tube into the trachea between cartilaginous rings.
   - A *percutaneous dilatational tracheostomy* refers to various procedures that have in common either a modified Seldinger technique for placing a modified tracheostomy tube or a forceps technique to cannulate and dilate tracheal tissue between cartilaginous rings.

Table 23-1. Common Etiologies of Upper Airway Obstruction

LOCATION	ETIOLOGY	SIGNS
Supraglottic	Epiglottitis Ludwig's angina Retropharyngeal abscess Angioedema Chemical injury Neoplasm Foreign body aspiration Extrinsic soft tissue compression	Hoarseness Wheeze Stridor Aphonia
Infraglottic	Chemical injury Neoplasm Foreign body aspiration Inflammation Infection Laryngotracheobronchitis Vocal cord paralysis Retropharyngeal abscess papillomatosis Trauma: postintubation stenosis	Difficult expiration Increased dyspnea with supine positioning Stridor Wheeze

- A *cricothyrotomy* is a technique for placement of an airway into the trachea through the cricothyroid space. A cricothyrotomy can be performed as a surgical procedure through an incision, as a percutaneous procedure by Seldinger technique, or as a needle cricothyrotomy for emergency airway access.
- A *minitracheostomy* allows percutaneous placement of a 7 F cannula through the tracheal rings to allow suctioning for patients with difficulty clearing airway secretions.

5. What is the role for ultrasound guidance in tracheostomy?
   Ultrasound evaluation of the landmarks associated with tracheostomy can be helpful before and during tracheostomy, particularly in obese patients and those with potentially anomalous vascular structures. While there is a paucity of randomized control trials, there have been observations supporting its role in landmarking, structure identification, measuring for tracheostomy tube size, and allowing for visualization of needle penetration through soft tissue structures to the trachea. Ultrasound cannot evaluate posterior tracheal wall structures or possible injuries due to obscuration by intraluminal air. As of now, ultrasound guidance for tracheostomy can be used safely as an adjunct to bronchoscopic guidance and current techniques.

6. What are the indications for a tracheostomy?
   - Maintenance of an airway for patients with upper airway obstruction
   - Airway access for suctioning retained secretions
   - Prevention of aspiration for patients with glottic dysfunction
   - Provides a stable airway support for patients who require long-term mechanical ventilation, which limits damage otherwise incurred by long-term translaryngeal intubation

7. Is emergency tracheostomy the surgical procedure of choice in patients with apnea and acute upper airway obstruction when intubation fails?
   No. Tracheostomy is acceptably safe when performed electively under controlled clinical conditions; however, risks of surgical complications increase significantly when done in an emergency situation. In comparison, the superficial location of the cricothyroid membrane allows for rapid reliable insertion of an airway, thus providing the greatest likelihood of success.

8. How is a cricothyrotomy performed and why is it not done electively?
   A scalpel is used to incise the overlying skin and stab the cricothyroid membrane. This membrane is approximately 1 to 2 cm below the thyroid notch, inferior to vocal cords, within the subglottic larynx. The resultant opening into the airway is enlarged with a spreader, allowing placement of a tracheostomy tube. For a percutaneous cricothyrotomy, commercially available instruments designed for emergency situations allow puncture of the membrane and introduction of an airway cannula in one maneuver or following the placement of a bougie, over which a cuffed tracheal tube can be placed. For long-term airway access, cricothyrotomy has a proposed higher incidence of delayed airway damage such as subglottic stenosis.

9. What are the complications of tracheostomy?
   Table 23.2

Table 23-2. Complications of Tracheostomy

INTRAOPERATIVE COMPLICATIONS	EARLY POSTOPERATIVE COMPLICATIONS	LATE COMPLICATIONS
Cardiorespiratory arrest	Hemorrhage	Tracheal stenosis
Cardiopulmonary arrest	Subcutaneous emphysema	Subglottic stenosis
Hemorrhage	Inadvertent decannulation	Tracheoesophageal fistula
Pneumothorax and pneumomediastinum	Wound infection	Tracheoinnominate fistula
Recurrent laryngeal nerve injury	Pneumonia	Tracheocutaneous fistula
Tracheoesophageal fistula	Tube obstruction	
Tracheal ring fracture and herniation		

10. What is the most lethal complication of tracheostomy in the perioperative period and what do you do?

    Inadvertent decannulation of a tracheostomy tube prior to tract maturation, which can take up to 10 days. One must perform endotracheal or nasotracheal intubation emergently because the stomal tract is not yet mature. Attempts to reinsert the tracheostomy tube may result in the creation of a false tissue tract and the inability to ventilate the patient.

11. Can patients with mechanical ventilation and a tracheostomy speak?

    Yes. Patients with low to moderate minute ventilation requirements can whisper intelligibly if the tracheostomy tube cuff is deflated to allow a small cuff leak. If patients have limited or no mechanical ventilatory requirements, a one-way speaking valve can be placed in-line with the tracheostomy tube allowing inhalation through the tracheostomy tube and exhalation past a deflated cuff through the native airway and the vocal cords. The tracheostomy tube may need to be downsized to facilitate speech.

12. Can patients with a tracheostomy eat?

    If the patient can tolerate the cuff being down they can eat. The inflated cuff causes the posterior trachea to obstruct the esophagus, limiting ability to swallow and increasing aspiration risk. The tracheostomy can also prevent elevation of the larynx which is necessary for swallowing so a swallow evaluation is still recommended prior to advancing the diet.

13. Why is it important to monitor intracuff pressures?

    - Cuff pressures in excess of mucosal capillary perfusion pressures (usually 25 mm Hg) can cause mucosal ischemia and resultant tracheal stenosis.
    - If a tracheostomy tube is underinflated (<18 mm Hg) in a patient undergoing mechanical ventilation, the risks for aspiration and nosocomial pneumonia increase.
    - Injury is less common with the use of low pressure, high volume cuffs.
    - Intracuff pressures can vary with barometric pressure; monitoring for elevation in pressure with flight is important.

14. What should the clinician consider in any patient with airway hemorrhage after the first 48 hours of insertion of a tracheostomy tube?

    - Less than 48 hours: Incisional wound
    - More than 48 hours: Tracheoarterial fistula
      - Requires immediate evaluation by a thoracic surgeon capable of performing an emergency sternotomy for ligation of the innominate artery because massive hemorrhage often develops after an initial herald episode of mild to moderate bleeding.

15. When should you suspect development of tracheoesophageal fistula?

    Patient presents with cough and shortness of breath about 2 months following removal of tracheostomy. Recurrent aspiration of esophageal secretions may manifest as nosocomial pneumonia. A tracheoesophageal fistula is related to pressure necrosis by the tube cuff or tube tip and occurs as a complication of tracheostomy in fewer than 1% of patients. Suspicion of a tracheoesophageal fistula should be pursued by endoscopic evaluation by either tracheoscopy or bronchoscopy, which can establish the location and extent of the fistula.

16. Is there an optimal time to perform tracheostomy?

    Tracheostomy is generally performed at around 10 to 14 days of intubation. Randomized controlled trials have failed to demonstrate a consistent benefit earlier to this time point. However, select patients with additional considerations such as anticipated prolonged respiratory failure, a difficult airway, or difficulty with airway clearance may benefit from tracheostomy performed earlier. The potential benefits of tracheostomy over prolonged translaryngeal intubation include improved comfort, enhanced ability to communicate, and greater mobility.

17. Variations of tracheostomy tubes in the intensive care unit.

    - Cuffed versus Uncuffed Tracheostomy tubes: Cuffed tubes allow inflation to facilitate positive pressure ventilation and maximal airway protection. Uncuffed tubes are appropriate in those with minimal ventilator support and intact airway protection.
    - Fenestrated versus Unfenestrated Tracheostomy tubes: Fenestrated tubes have an additional opening in the posterior portion of tube to facilitate airflow through vocal cords. However, fenestrated tubes may become obstructed with secretions. Fenestration also promotes the

formation of granulation tissue resulting in bleeding during tracheostomy change and, potentially, tracheal stenosis.

- Speaking valve: Occludes tracheostomy tube opening in exhalation and allows for speaking. Permits easier swallowing as well because cuff must be down.

18. Why do patients aspirate after removal of a tracheostomy tube?
Scarring at the stoma site may interfere with the rostrocaudal excursion of the larynx during swallowing, which is necessary for glottic closure. In addition, prolonged diversion of ventilation away from the glottis causes attenuation of the vocal cord adductor response that is important in aspiration prevention.

19. When should you look for upper airway obstruction after decannulation of a tracheostomy tube?
Patients may have upper airway obstruction immediately after decannulation, or obstruction may develop months to years later. Causes of delayed upper airway obstruction after decannulation include subglottic or tracheal stenosis, and tracheomalacia. These complications may progress slowly with a gradual narrowing of the airway causing exercise-induced dyspnea, which may be ascribed to the patient's underlying respiratory condition. Stridor or dyspnea at rest is generally a late finding so a high index of suspicion should be maintained. Late presentations with the sudden onset of stridor may result from acute illnesses, such as bronchitis or pneumonia that unveil the underlying airway narrowing, and may be life threatening.

20. What is the role for tracheostomy in obstructive sleep apnea (OSA)?
Tracheostomies can be helpful in obese and nonobese individuals who fail continuous positive airway pressure (CPAP) usage for treatment of obstructive sleep apnea (OSA). Compared with no treatment, tracheostomies can decrease apnea index, mortality, and sleepiness in individuals with OSA.

ACKNOWLEDGMENT

The authors wish to acknowledge Dr. John E. Heffner, MD, for the valuable contributions to the previous edition of this chapter.

KEY POINTS: TRACHEOSTOMY AND UPPER AIRWAY OBSTRUCTION

3 to 5 Facts
- Upper airway obstruction may be a life-threatening condition if not addressed immediately.
- Cricothyrotomy is the procedure of choice in an emergency, while tracheostomy is a better airway for prolonged mechanical ventilation needs.
- Tracheostomy allows for more patient comfort, ability to eat and speak while maintaining a patent airway.

BIBLIOGRAPHY
1. Al-Qadi MO, Artenstein AW, Braman SS. The "forgotten zone": acquired disorders of the trachea in adults. *Respir Med.* 2013;107:1301-1313.
2. Alansari M, Alotair H, Al Aseri Z, et al. Use of ultrasound guidance to improve the safety of percutaneous dilational tracheotomy: a literature review. *Crit Care.* 2015;19:229.
3. Allan JS, Wright CD. Tracheoinnominate fistula: diagnosis and management. *Chest Surg Clin North Am.* 2003;13: 331-341.
4. Camacho M, Certal V, Brietzke SE, et al. Tracheotomy as treatment for adult obstructive sleep apnea: a systematic review and meta-analysis. *Laryngoscope.* 2013;124:803-811.
5. Clec'h C, Alberti C, Vincent F, et al. Tracheotomy does not improve the outcome of patients requiring prolonged mechanical ventilation: a propensity analysis. *Crit Care Med.* 2007;35:132-138.
6. Diaz-Reganon G, Minambres E, Ruiz A, et al. Safety and complications of percutaneous tracheotomy in a cohort of 800 mixed ICU patients. *Anaesthesia.* 2008;63:1198-1203.
7. Engels PT, Bagshaw SM, Meier M, et al. Tracheotomy: from insertion to decannulation. *Can J Surg.* 2009;52(5): 427-433.
8. Ernst A, Feller-Kopman D, Becker HD, et al. Central airway obstruction. *Am J Respir Crit Care Med.* 2004;169: 1278-1297.
9. Frerk C, Mitchell VS, McNarry AF, et al. Difficult airway society 2015 guidelines for management of unanticipated difficult intubation in adults. *Br J Anaesth.* 2015;115(6):827-848.
10. Francois B, Clavel M, Desachy A, et al. Complications of tracheotomy performed in the ICU: subthyroid tracheotomy vs surgical cricothyroidotomy. *Chest.* 2003;123:151-158.

11. Heffner JE. Toward leaner tracheotomy care: first observe, then improve. *Respir Care*. 2009;54:1635-1637.
12. Hess DR. Tracheotomy tubes and related appliances. *Respir Care*. 2005;50:497-510.
13. Higgins KM, Punthakee X. Meta-analysis comparison of open versus percutaneous tracheotomy. *Laryngoscope*. 2007;117:447-454.
14. Mooty RC, Rath P, Self M, et al. Review of tracheo-esophageal fistula associated with endotracheal intubation. *J Surg Educ*. 2007;64:237-240.
15. Pierson DJ. Tracheotomy and weaning. *Respir Care*. 2005;50(4):526-533.
16. Putensen C, Theuerkauf N, Guenther U, et al. Percutaneous and surgical tracheotomy in critically ill adult patients: a meta-analysis. *Crit Care*. 2014;18:544.
17. Scales DC, Ferguson ND. Early vs late tracheotomy in ICU patients. *JAMA*. 2010;303:1537-1538.
18. Wain JC, Jr. Postintubation tracheal stenosis. *Semin Thorac Cardiovasc Surg*. 2009;21:284-289.
19. Young D, Harrison DA, Cuthbertson BH, et al. Effect of early vs late tracheotomy placement on survival in patients receiving mechanical ventilation, The TracMan Randomized Trial. *JAMA*. 2013;309(20):2121-2129.

CHAPTER 24

CHEST TUBES AND PNEUMOTHORAX

Cornelia Griggs and Peter J. Fagenholz

1. What is a chest tube?

   A chest tube, or tube thoracostomy, is used to evacuate the pleural space of air, blood, serum, bile, chyle, purulent, or other fluid. The goal of evacuating this material is to allow re-expansion of the lung and re-apposition of the visceral and parietal pleura.

2. What are the indications to place a chest tube?

   Common indications to place a chest tube include pneumothorax, hemothorax, and pleural effusions. However, each of these diagnoses does not necessarily require a chest tube. Small pneumothoraces (typically less than 2 cm) may not require intervention if the patient is clinically and hemodynamically stable. Spontaneous pneumothoraces may require chest tube placement when the pneumothorax is large, progressive, or if the patient is clinically unstable. Tension pneumothorax and pneumothorax caused by penetrating chest trauma are indications for chest tube placement. Esophageal rupture with leak into the pleural space requires chest tube placement. Large pleural effusions, chylothorax, parapneumonic effusions, and empyema are other indications for chest tube placement. Many patients will require chest tube drainage as part of routine postoperative care, for example, after coronary artery bypass, thoracotomy, or lobectomy.

3. How do you choose the type of chest tube to place?

   There are many varieties of chest tubes, but usually the basic choice is between a small chest tube (e.g., 14 Fr) placed by Seldinger technique or a larger traditional chest tube (28 Fr or larger) placed by open technique. The choice to place a smaller Seldinger technique tube versus a larger traditional chest tube is usually driven by the material you need to evacuate. Air is evacuated easily by both small lumen tubes (14 F or smaller) and large lumen tubes. Larger chest tubes (28 F–40 F) have traditionally been considered more effective for removal of thicker and more viscous fluid (e.g., hemothorax or parapneumonic effusion), though this has not generally been borne out in studies. Small or loculated collections are best drained using some form of image guidance (ultrasound or computed tomography [CT]). Empirically placed chest tubes such as are occasionally placed in trauma when it is unknown if the lung is collapsed or not are probably best done using open technique, since the Seldinger needle will injure the lung on entry if it is not collapsed. Smaller tubes are more comfortable for patients and should be used when appropriate.

4. Describe the steps of a tube thoracostomy:
   - Prepare and drape the skin around the area of insertion. Use sterile technique including gown, mask, gloves, and draping of the whole patient as for central line placement. A common and safe choice for placement is along the anterior axillary or midaxillary line between the fourth and fifth intercostal space. Consider using ultrasound to identify the point of insertion.
   - Administer local anesthesia (1% lidocaine) if the patient is not otherwise sedated.
   For "open" technique:
   - Make a 2-cm incision over the rib, just below the site chosen for insertion.
   - Create a subcutaneous tunnel, using blunt dissection, and spread the muscle using a Kelly clamp.
   - Gently enter the pleural space using the Kelly clamp. The process of entering the pleural space is commonly accompanied by a gush or air or fluid.
   - Explore the space digitally to make sure you are in the pleural cavity and that no adhesions exist between the visceral and parietal pleura.
   - Insert the tube (clamped at the insertion end with the Kelly clamp), and place apically and anteriorly for a pneumothorax or superiorly and posteriorly for a hemothorax or pleural effusion.
   - After placement, secure the tube to the skin of the chest wall and connect to a sealed container with controlled negative pressure suction.

For Seldinger technique:
- Make a skin incision slightly larger than the anticipated tube.
- Insert the guide needle into the pleural space tracking over the superior border of the nearest rib until fluid or air is aspirated.
- Pass the guidewire into the pleural space. It should pass with minimal resistance.
- Dilate the tract with dilator placed over the wire.
- Insert the chest tube over the wire.
- Remove the wire and secure the chest tube as above.

5. What is the "triangle of safety"?

The triangle of safety refers to a common, safe location for placement of a chest tube. A chest tube is placed in the anterior axillary or midaxillary line in the **fifth** *to* **sixth** intercostal space. The triangle of safety is bounded by the anterior border of the latissimus dorsi, the lateral border of the pectoralis major muscle, the apex just below the axilla, and the inferior line just above the level of the nipple: the triangle of safety. This is a safe anatomic location because it lies above the diaphragm in an area where the chest wall musculature is thin, allowing rapid and minimally painful insertion with minimal risk to surrounding structures.

6. Define *occult pneumothorax.*

An occult pneumothorax occurs when a small amount of air is trapped within the pleural space. Typically an occult pneumothorax is not obvious on chest radiograph but may be identified on a CT. Occult pneumothoraces can be caused by blunt and/or penetrating trauma, ruptured bleb, or may occur spontaneously. Approximately 2% to 10% of trauma patients will be diagnosed with an occult pneumothorax. There are generally no associated clinical findings. Work up of an occult pneumothorax typically includes reimaging to evaluate progression but usually does not require treatment. The need for positive-pressure ventilation (PPV; i.e., a trip to the operating room for nonthoracic injury) is *not* an indication for pleural space decompression of an occult pneumothorax.

7. What is a hemothorax and how is it treated?

When blood accumulates in the pleural cavity it is called a hemothorax. A hemothorax becomes radiographically detectable on a standard chest radiograph once 200 to 300 mL of blood collects within the pleural space. Up to one liter of blood may accumulate before systemic signs of shock and hypoperfusion are manifested. Large chest tubes (32 F–40 F) should be used to evacuate a large-volume hemothorax. In 85% of patients, hemorrhage will spontaneously cease and the lung will re-expand. Large amounts of undrained clotted blood (loculated hemothorax) should be evacuated via operative drainage (video-assisted thoracoscopic surgery). Thoracotomy is required only rarely. Traumatic hemothorax with initial chest tube output of 1500 mL of blood (massive hemothorax), or persistent drainage of 200 to 300 mL/hr is an indication for thoracotomy.

8. What are some possible complications associated with chest tubes?

Chest tube complications are typically insertional or positional. Malposition is the most common complication, especially when chest tubes are placed in traumatic or suboptimal situations. In critically ill patients, roughly 20% of tubes are place in a fissure and 9% in the lung parenchyma. On insertion, it is essential to avoid intercostal vessel laceration by dissecting directly on top of the rib, thereby avoiding the intercostal neurovascular bundle. Perforation of other visceral organs (heart, diaphragm, and intra-abdominal organs) can best be avoided using the triangle of safety (described above). In addition, chest tubes can be ineffective in certain settings, such as loculated empyema or retained hemothorax. In these instances, larger tubes and lysis with TPA and/or dornase may be useful for more complete evacuation of retained clot or fluid.

If a previously functional chest tube stops working, check for kinking or dislodgement. Avoid postremoval pneumothorax by removing the tube during forced expiration which can be achieved by having the patient hum, pulling the tube swiftly, and using an occlusive dressing over the site. Ongoing or long-term pain after chest tube removal is usually related to intercostal neuralgia. Avoiding the intercostal neurovascular bundle on insertion is the best way to prevent this complication.

9. What is an "air leak"?

Many chest tube drainage collection systems use an underwater seal that allows air to escape through chest tube without re-entering the thoracic cavity. Persistent bubbling of air through the water chamber of the collection system indicates an air leak from the lung or thoracic cavity. Ongoing air leak (whether continuous or "large"—or only evident on Valsalva/cough, i.e., "small") suggests a persistent pneumothorax or an unhealed injury to the lung or bronchus. An air leak that persists when the tube is clamped at the patient's skin is due to a leak in the collection system.

10. **How do you treat a chronic air leak or a pneumothorax that does not resolve with initial chest tube placement?**
Persistent air leak or recurrent pneumothorax warrants consultation with a thoracic surgery or interventional specialist. Pleurodesis, endobronchial valve placement, up-sizing/replacement of existing chest tubes, or surgical resection may be required, depending on the underlying cause of the air leak.

11. **When can you remove a chest tube?**
Before chest tube removal, the following criteria generally should be met:
    1. The lung must be fully expanded again (a final chest radiograph can be helpful here).
    2. During Valsalva maneuver or coughing, there must be no air leak in the water seal chamber.
    3. The daily amount of fluid drainage should be less than 200 mL.
    4. The fluid should be serous.
    5. The patient's clinical status has improved.

12. **How long does a trial of water seal need to be before chest tube removal?**
For chest tubes placed for a traumatic pneumothorax, a prospective randomized trial demonstrated that a short 6-hour trial of water seal is adequate to allow occult air leaks to become clinically or radiographically apparent. Therefore, chest tubes placed for a traumatic pneumothorax may safely be removed after 6 hours on water seal.

13. **Do you need to give the patient antibiotics before placing a chest tube?**
Much controversy exists as to whether prophylactic antibiotics should be administered before placing a chest tube. Some trials show a reduction in infections (especially in patients with penetrating chest trauma), but most trials showed no benefit. Generally, a single dose of gram-positive coverage should be given before chest tube placement if the tube is being placed for trauma. Otherwise, no antibiotics are indicated. Antibiotics should not be continued while the chest tube is in.

14. **What is a tension pneumothorax or hemothorax?**
Tension pneumothorax occurs when a chest wall injury allows the entry of a large amount of air or blood resulting in lung collapse, mediastinal shift, and tracheal deviation. This in turn results in compression of the contralateral lung and decreased venous return to the heart, hypotension, and respiratory distress. Tension pneumothorax requires decisive and emergent intervention.

15. **Should I perform needle decompression or tube thoracostomy for tension pneumothorax?**
Needle decompression is an effective first-line treatment option for a tension pneumothorax, especially if a chest tube is not immediately available or if you are not facile with rapid placement of a chest tube. Needle decompression can rapidly decompress the pleural space. A large-bore needle is inserted in the second intercostal space in the midclavicular line. Subsequently, a regular chest tube should be placed.
    For spontaneous pneumothoraces, two recent studies showed that needle aspiration alone in the emergency department is at least as safe and effective as a regular chest tube. It also shortened the hospital length of stay.
    For most other pneumothoraces or hemothoraces, a chest tube is generally recommended.

16. **Why avoid rapid pulmonary re-expansion?**
If a lung has been collapsed for a long period of time, rapid re-expansion can lead to re-expansion pulmonary edema, which has a mortality rate as high as 20%. It occurs during rapid evacuation of a chronic pleural effusion or rapid re-expansion of the lung in the case of a chronic pneumothorax. Treatment of re-expansion pulmonary edema is supportive, because the disease is usually self-limited. Supplemental oxygen and, in severe cases, mechanical ventilation may be required. In the case of chronic pneumothorax, asking the patient to breathe deeply and cough to expand the lung before applying suction can prevent rapid re-expansion. In the case of chronic effusion, draining the effusion in serial amounts (no more than 500–1000 cc at a time) using a clamp may also help.

17. **What is the influence of positive-pressure ventilation on chest tube removal?**
A retrospective study showed that PPV does not influence the rate of recurrent pneumothorax or chest tube placements after removal. Consequently, presence of mechanical PPV is not an indication to leave a chest tube in place.

ACKNOWLEDGMENT

The authors wish to acknowledge Drs. Gwendolyn M. van der Wilden, MSc, David R. King, MD, FACS, Madison Macht, MD, and Michael E. Hanley, MD, for the valuable contributions to the previous edition of this chapter.

KEY POINTS; CHEST TUBES AND PNEUMOTHORAX

Chest Tubes

1. All patients in unstable condition with hemothorax or pneumothorax should have a tube thoracostomy.
2. Large tubes are typically chosen for hemothorax, and smaller tubes (placed using Seldinger technique) are selected for pneumothorax or serous effusions.
3. Tube thoracostomy is not required for occult pneumothoraces.
4. Chest tubes placed for a traumatic pneumothorax may safely be removed after 6 hours on water seal.
5. Presence of mechanical PPV is not an indication to leave a chest tube in place.

BIBLIOGRAPHY

1. Ali HA, Lippmann M, Mundathaje U, et al. Spontaneous hemothorax: a comprehensive review. *Chest.* 2008;134:1056.
2. Baumann MH, Strange C, Heffner JE, et al. Management of spontaneous pneumothorax: an American College of Chest Physicians Delphi consensus statement. *Chest.* 2001;119:590.
3. Biffl WL, Narayanan V, Gaudiani JL, et al. The management of pneumothorax in patients with anorexia nervosa: a case report and review of the literature. *Patient Saf Surg.* 2010;4(1):1.
4. Dev SP, Nascimiento B, Jr, Simone C, et al. Videos in clinical medicine. Chest-tube insertion. *N Engl J Med.* 2007;357:e15.
5. Ho KK, Ong ME, Koh MS, et al. A randomized controlled trial comparing minichest tube and needle aspiration in outpatient management of primary spontaneous pneumothorax. *Am J Emerg Med.* 2011;29:1152-1157.
6. Kim YK, Kim H, Lee CC, et al. New classification and clinical characteristics of reexpansion pulmonary edema after treatment of spontaneous pneumothorax. *Am J Emerg Med.* 2009;27:961-967.
7. Martino K, Merrit S, Boyakye K, et al. Prospective randomized trial of thoracostomy removal algorithms. *J Trauma.* 1999;46:369-371 [discussion: 372-373].
8. Maxwell RA, Campbell DJ, Fabian TC, et al. Use of presumptive antibiotics following tube thoracostomy for traumatic hemopneumothorax in the prevention of empyema and pneumonia—a multi-center trial. *J Trauma.* 2004;57:742-748 [discussion: 748-749].
9. Moore FO, Goslar PW, Coimbra R, et al. Blunt traumatic occult pneumothorax: is observation safe? Results of a prospective, AAST multicenter study. *J Trauma.* 2011;70:1019-1025.
10. Schaefer GP, Pender J, Toschlog EA, et al. Endoscopically-assisted tube thoracostomy placement in a super-morbidly obese patient with penetrating thoracoabdominal trauma. *Am Surg.* 2011;77:119-120.
11. Schulman CI, Cohn SM, Blackbourne L, et al. How long should you wait for a chest radiograph after placing a chest tube on water seal? A prospective study. *J Trauma.* 2005;59:92-95.
12. Sethuraman KN, Duong D, Mehta S, et al. Complications of tube thoracostomy placement in the emergency department. *J Emerg Med.* 2011;40:14-20.
13. Tawil I, Gonda JM, King RD, et al. Impact of positive pressure ventilation on thoracostomy tube removal. *J Trauma.* 2010;68:818-821.
14. Zehtabchi S, Rios CL. Management of emergency department patients with primary spontaneous pneumothorax: needle aspiration or tube thoracostomy? *Ann Emerg Med.* 2008;51:91-100.
15. Kwiat M, Tarbox A, Seamon MJ, et al. Thoracostomy tubes: a comprehensive review of complications and related topics. *Int J Crit Illn Inj Sci.* 2014;4:143-155.

CHAPTER 25

BRONCHOSCOPY

Katherine Menson and Garth W. Garrison

1. **What is flexible bronchoscopy?**

   Bronchoscopy is a diagnostic and therapeutic tool used to visualize both the upper airway and lower airways and to perform a number of procedures from within the airway. A flexible bronchoscope, as opposed to a rigid bronchoscope, can be advanced from the upper airway to at least the first or second segmental bronchi. These scopes utilize fiberoptics and/or digital imaging capture to display an image from the distal end in an eyepiece or on a video monitor. Many have working channels that allow for suctioning, instillation of fluid, and placement of specialized tools into the airway. A wide variety of scope sizes exist to allow passage through small neonatal airways as well as larger adult airways.

2. **What are common indications for flexible bronchoscopy?**

   Common indications (Table 25.1) for flexible bronchoscopy include large airway obstruction, foreign body aspiration, hemoptysis, atypical or nonresolving infection, unexplained pulmonary infiltrate, suspected metastatic malignancy, mediastinal mass, or lymphadenopathy. Flexible bronchoscopy can also be used to aid in intubation for patients with difficult airways. Bronchial washings and bronchoalveolar lavage (BAL) can be used for the diagnosis of tuberculosis when noninvasive methods have been exhausted. Bronchoscopy with biopsies can aid in the diagnosis of eosinophilic or granulomatous lung disease but is of limited value in the evaluation of suspected idiopathic interstitial lung diseases.

Table 25-1. Indications for Bronchoscopy

STEP	INDICATION	GOAL
Inspection	Hemoptysis	Localize bleeding
		Search for endobronchial lesion
	Infection	Identify evidence of inflammation or pus
	Aspiration	Look for foreign bodies
	Mass	Look for endobronchial masses
	Chest trauma	Find evidence of airway injury
	Inhalational injury	Find evidence of airway injury
Sample collection	Pulmonary infiltrates (infectious)	Obtain samples for Gram stain, silver stain, bacterial cultures, and viral and fungal studies
	Pulmonary infiltrates (noninfectious)	Identify alveolar hemorrhage
		Check for eosinophilia (analyze cell count and differential)
	Mass or adenopathy	Perform transbronchial biopsy for cytologic or pathologic analysis
Interventions	Hemoptysis	Control bleeding
	Bronchial obstruction	Remove mucus or foreign bodies
		Perform laser removal of masses
		Place stent
	Alveolar proteinosis	Perform lavage
	Intubation	Visualize anatomy for tube placement

3. What types of samples can be obtained during bronchoscopy?
   - Bronchial washings: instillation and aspiration of small fluid volumes from large airways
   - BAL: instillation of sterile saline into a segmental airway followed by aspiration and collection of the lavageate
   - Brushings: using a small brush to collect samples for cytology or culture
   - Needle aspiration: use of a small needle (typically 21–22 g) to collect samples for cytology or culture
   - Forceps biopsy: use of small forceps to collect tissue for histopathology or culture, often done in peripheral locations within the lung (transbronchial biopsies)

4. What are potential complications of bronchoscopy?
   The most common mild complications following bronchoscopy are cough, sore throat, and fever. Sedation can result in hypotension and can reduce respiratory drive, which can lead to respiratory failure. Further complications are typically related to the procedure being performed. Biopsy increases the risk of pneumothorax or bleeding (Table 25.2).

5. What are common contraindications for flexible bronchoscopy?
   Contraindications include conditions that may predispose to cardiopulmonary collapse or hemorrhage during the procedure. Most consider severe hypoxemia and hemodynamic instability to be contraindications. Relative contraindications (those which may increase risk for the procedure) include:
   - Coagulopathy (particularly when performing biopsies)
     - Daily aspirin use is NOT a contraindication to bronchoscopy
   - Inability to provide adequate sedation
   - Severe pulmonary hypertension
   - Severe airflow obstruction (such as asthma exacerbation)
   - Active or recent myocardial ischemia
   - Chronic kidney disease (when performing biopsies)
   - Increased intracranial pressure

Table 25-2. Potential Complications of Bronchoscopy

INTERVENTION	POTENTIAL COMPLICATIONS	PREVENTION
Passing bronchoscope through nose	Epistaxis, nasal discomfort	Topical anesthesia and vasoconstriction
Passing bronchoscope through pharynx	Gagging, emesis, aspiration	Topical anesthesia, benzodiazepines
Passing bronchoscope into trachea	Laryngospasm, cough, laryngeal trauma	Topical anesthesia
	Bronchospasm	Pretreatment with beta agonists
Bronchoalveolar lavage	Postprocedure fever	Minimize lung contamination by oral secretions
	Hypoxemia	Supplemental oxygen; good wedge technique
Cytology brush	Endobronchial hemorrhage	Avoid vascular lesions
Transbronchial biopsy	Hemorrhage	Avoid vascular lesions
	Pneumothorax	Avoid distal biopsies; consider fluoroscopy
Topical lidocaine administration	Arrhythmias, seizures	Use <7 mg/kg (<25 mL) of 2% lidocaine
Conscious sedation	Hypotension	Intravenous access, prehydration in patients with hypovolemia
	Respiratory depression	Avoid oversedation, stimulate patient

6. How is a flexible bronchoscopy performed?

The procedure can be performed on spontaneously breathing patients under conscious sedation or deeply sedated patients on mechanical ventilation. The scope can be introduced via the nose, mouth, or an adequately sized airway device. For nonintubated patients, lidocaine is used first to anesthetize upper airway. A bite block should be placed to prevent scope damage. After adequate sedation and anesthesia are achieved, an airway exam is performed and each segmental bronchus is visualized. Aliquots of lidocaine are instilled topically into the lower airway to provide further anesthesia and reduce cough. Following airway examination, additional testing such as bronchoalveolar lavage and transbronchial biopsy can be performed.

7. Who should be intubated for bronchoscopy?

Intubation should be considered for patients who are at increased risk for respiratory failure from conscious sedation, including those with chronic respiratory failure, altered airway anatomy, severe sleep apnea, impaired mentation, or multiple cardiopulmonary comorbidities. In a patient who can otherwise follow simple commands and does not have uncontrolled coughing at baseline, intubation is not necessary. Given the risk of respiratory depression secondary to sedation, the physician should always be prepared for the need to intubate during and after the procedure. Contraindications are listed in Table 25.2.

8. What additional issues are there for performing a bronchoscopy for mechanically ventilated patients?

The endotracheal tube must be large enough to accommodate the bronchoscope and still allow ventilation during the procedure; typically a 7.5-mm tube or larger is needed for adults. A bite block should still be placed and topical lidocaine should be instilled to limit cough. The ventilator may alarm for increased airway pressures due to obstruction of the lumen by the bronchoscope; therefore limits to peak airway pressures should be increased to allow for adequate ventilation. If air trapping or derecruitment occurs, the bronchoscope might have to be removed temporarily.

9. Are transbronchial biopsies safe in patients on mechanical ventilation?

Transbronchial biopsies in patients on mechanical ventilation may be associated with an increased risk for pneumothorax and are not advised in settings of severe emphysema and high airway pressures. Generally, the alternative diagnostic test after transbronchial biopsy is surgical lung biopsy and therefore this degree of risk should be weighed against those of thoracic surgery.

10. What are the indications for bronchoscopy in the intensive care unit?

Common indications include

- Intubation of patients with difficult airways
- Suctioning of large airway mucous plugs
- Localization of hemoptysis to guide embolization or other therapy
- The need to obtain culture data

11. How is rigid bronchoscopy different from flexible bronchoscopy?

A rigid bronchoscope is essentially a rigid, hollow metal tube that allows for direct visualization of the airways. The procedure is done under general anesthesia. This type of bronchoscope has a side arm that can be attached to a mechanical ventilator. The large working channel allows for a larger area to retrieve foreign bodies, resect endobronchial lesions, place endobronchial stents, perform electrocautery, or if a large degree if suctioning is required. Given the degree of mandibular and cervical spine manipulation, instability of these areas are contraindications to this procedure.

12. What is endobronchial ultrasound?

Ultrasound can be used during bronchoscopic evaluation of the airway either with a radial probe placed into the working channel of the scope (radial ultrasound) or with an integrated ultrasound bronchoscope (linear ultrasound). The term "EBUS" most commonly refers to linear ultrasound. EBUS is helpful in localizing masses or lymph nodes adjacent to airways and can increase the accuracy of sampling with transbronchial needle aspiration. Additionally, Doppler may be utilized to prevent blood vessel puncture. EBUS guided transbronchial needle aspiration (EBUS-TBNA) is useful in diagnosis and staging of malignancy as well as in the diagnosis granulomatous diseases like sarcoidosis.

13. What is navigational bronchoscopy?
    Peripheral lesions are difficult to access in traditional bronchoscopy due to the size limitations of the bronchoscope and traditionally were sampled using percutaneous techniques. Navigational bronchoscopy is an alternate noninvasive technique that employs imaging and a flexible or ultrathin bronchoscope to target peripheral lesions. Specially protocoled noncontrast computed tomography (CT) is used to map a pathway for the bronchoscope, which is followed in real time until the target lesion is reached. Once the bronchoscope reaches the most distal point possible, the navigational system can follow the brush or forceps to the correct location for biopsy. Diagnostic yield is approximately 70%.

14. Does bronchoscopy have a role in the initial evaluation of community-acquired pneumonia?
    Bronchoscopy is of limited benefit in the initial evaluation of community-acquired pneumonia (CAP). However, in patients who have failed appropriate empiric antibiotics, bronchoscopy may aid in the diagnosis or isolation of atypical infectious organisms, which can then tailor therapy.

15. Discuss the role of bronchoscopy in a patient with immunosuppression and pulmonary infiltrates.
    Given the risk of atypical infections, the immunosuppressed patient may be more likely to undergo bronchoscopy to guide therapy. This is particularly helpful if the suspicion for fungal organisms is high, since it is difficult to diagnose without tissue biopsy. Alternatively, immunosuppressed patients are at higher risk for hemorrhage and malignancy, which can also be evaluated with BAL and cytology, respectively.

16. What is the role of bronchoscopy in the diagnosis of ventilator-associated pneumonia?
    Ventilator-associated pneumonia (VAP) is defined as a pneumonia that develops 48 to 72 hours after endotracheal intubation. Studies have shown that bronchoscopic sampling decreases unnecessary antibiotic exposure and length of stay compared with noninvasive sampling. Diagnosis is considered positive if BAL isolates show greater than 10^4 colony forming units (CFUs), or if brushings isolate greater than 10^3 CFUs.

17. What are the alternatives to bronchoscopy for sample collection in the diagnosis of ventilator-associated pneumonia?
    Tracheal aspirates may be suctioned from the endotracheal tube for sampling. Nonbronchoscopic BAL, also known as mini-BAL, is performed by directing a catheter into the airway until resistance is met, at which point saline is irrigated and suctioned back for sampling. Alternatively, the same can be done with a brush biopsy.

18. Can bronchoalveolar lavage be safely performed in patients with acute respiratory distress syndrome?
    Bronchoscopy may cause derecruitment and worsening hypoxia in patients with acute respiratory distress syndrome (ARDS). Due to the risk of hypoxia, a patient should be adequately preoxygenated prior to a BAL examination. The general goal is for the partial pressure of arterial O_2 to be greater than 80 mm Hg when possible. Patients should still be evaluated for other absolute or relative contraindications.

19. How is bronchoscopy used in the evaluation and management of hemoptysis in the intensive care unit?
    Bronchoscopic evaluation of hemoptysis is useful in differentiating diffuse alveolar hemorrhage (DAH) from a focal endobronchial bleed. Additionally, localization of bleeding that cannot be determined on imaging is helpful in directing therapeutic embolization. Certain interventions—such as iced saline lavage, topical vasoconstrictive medications (i.e., epinephrine), or topical coagulants—can be applied to the bleeding. Thermal therapies can be applied via flexible bronchoscopy; however, rigid bronchoscopy allows for better visualization and a greater degree of suction. Last, balloon tamponade using an endobronchial blocker or a Fogarty balloon can stabilize bleeding pending definitive intervention. Most patients expire from hypoxic respiratory failure rather than exsanguination; therefore protecting the unaffected lung is priority.

20. What is the role of bronchoscopy in potential lung donors?
    Most donors are evaluated by bronchoscopy in determination of candidacy. This is to assess the endobronchial anatomy, evaluate for aspiration or trauma, and culture for infection or microbiota. These findings may exclude a patient from donation or alter management after donation.

21. How is bronchoscopy used in performing tracheostomy in the intensive care unit?
    Bronchoscopy is sometimes used to directly visualize the upper airway during placement of routine percutaneous tracheostomy in critically ill patients. This aids in confirming correct placement and

monitoring for complications such a posterior wall puncture. Recent studies have compared guidance with bronchoscopy to ultrasonography and have found outcomes to be noninferior.

ACKNOWLEDGMENT

The authors wish to acknowledge Drs. Amy E. Morris, MD, and Lynn M. Schnapp, MD, for the valuable contributions to the previous edition of this chapter.

KEY POINTS: BRONCHOSCOPY

1. Flexible bronchoscopy is used to examine the airway and collect cytology and/or microbiology samples from the lower respiratory tract.
2. Airway examination and bronchoalveolar lavage are generally safe procedures, whereas risks of bleeding and pneumothorax increase with interventions such as needle aspiration or biopsy.
3. Cardiopulmonary instability and significant coagulopathy increase risks from the procedure.
4. Consider bronchoscopy in patients with hemoptysis, atypical infiltrate on imaging, suspected atypical pneumonia, ventilator-associated pneumonia, suspected malignancy, or large airway occlusion.

BIBLIOGRAPHY

1. Gobatto AL, Besen BA. Comparison between ultrasound- and bronchoscopy-guided percutaneous dilational tracheostomy in critically ill patients: a retrospective cohort study. *J Crit Care.* 2015;30(1):220.e13-220.e17.
2. Guidry CA, Mallicote MU, Petroze RT, et al. Influence of bronchoscopy on the diagnosis of and outcomes from ventilator-associated pneumonia. *Surg Infect.* 2014;15(5):527-532.
3. Jin F, Mu D, Chu D, et al. Severe complications of bronchoscopy. *Respiration.* 2008;76:429-433.
4. Kalil AC, Metersky ML, Klompas M, et al. Management of adults with hospital-acquired and ventilator-associated pneumonia: 2016 Clinical Practice Guidelines by the Infectious Diseases Society of America and the American Thoracic Society. *Clin Infect Dis.* 2016;63:1-51.
5. O'Brien JD, Ettinger NA, Shevlin D, et al. Safety and yield of transbronchial biopsy in mechanically ventilated patients. *Crit Care Med.* 1997;25(3):440-446.
6. Pue CA, Pacht ER. Complications of fiberoptic bronchoscopy at a University Hospital. *Chest.* 1995;107(2):430-432.
7. Steinberg KP, Mitchell DR, Maunder RJ, et al. Safety of bronchoalveolar lavage in patients with adult respiratory distress syndrome. *Am Rev Resp Dis.* 1993;148(3)556-561.
8. Wang MJ, Nietert PJ, Silvestri GA, et al. Meta-analysis of guided bronchoscopy for the evaluation of the pulmonary nodule. *Chest.* 2012;142(2):385-393.

CHAPTER 26

PACEMAKERS AND DEFIBRILLATORS

Scott C. Streckenbach and Kenneth Shelton

1. **What are the general principles of cardiovascular implantable electronic device management according to the Heart Rhythm Society–American Society of Anesthesiologists Consensus Statement published in 2011**
   The recommendation is that the best prescription for the perioperative care of a patient with a cardiovascular implantable electronic device (CIED) will be realized when that patient's CIED team (electrophysiologist or cardiologist) is asked for advice and that advice is effectively communicated to the procedural team. Thus the surgical or procedural team should communicate with the CIED team to identify the type of procedure and the likely risk of electromagnetic interference. The CIED team should then deliver information to the procedure team about the pacer or implantable cardiac defibrillator (ICD) and recommendations for the perioperative management of the patient and the device. Although not published in the consensus statement, we believe that an anesthesiologist well trained in the principles of the perioperative electrophysiology can function as the "CIED team."

2. **What critical information should you obtain related to your patient's pacemaker? List five points.**
   The manufacturer of the device—you must use a manufacturer-specific programmer to interrogate the device, and the effect of a magnet on any device depends on the manufacturer.
   The date of the last interrogation—pacers should be interrogated within 12 months of the procedure and ICDs within 6 months according to the Heart Rhythm Society (HRS) guidelines.
   The pacer mode—this will alert you to the presence of a rate response mode.
   The degree of pacer dependence—this information can be found with a programmer, and it is used to determine the best perioperative management strategy. It may also be on a pacer report.
   The battery life—pacers will change function within 6 months of total battery depletion.

3. **How can one determine if a patient has a pacemaker or an implantable cardioverter defibrillator?**
   Occasionally a patient is seen initially without information about his or her CIED. A critical step is to determine whether the device is a pacemaker or an ICD. The patient may be able to tell you why the device was inserted, and this might provide a clue. However, if the patient's history cannot help, the patient's chest radiograph can. The ICD leads, unlike pacer leads, have one or two radiodense shocking coils. Because of the shocking coils, the ICD leads (Fig. 26.1) are much larger than the pacer leads (Fig. 26.2), and this can be appreciated radiographically.

4. **What is cardiac resynchronization therapy?**
   Cardiac resynchronization therapy (CRT) is the term applied to reestablishing synchronous contraction between the left ventricular (LV) free wall and the ventricular septum in an attempt to improve LV efficiency and subsequently to improve functional class. The LV pacing lead is usually placed in the posterior lateral LV wall via the coronary sinus circulation, and this can be easily appreciated on a chest x-ray (CXR). CRT may be used with a pacemaker (CRT-P) or with an ICD. Indications typically include a low ejection fraction (<35%), a prolonged QRS (>120 ms), and symptoms of class IV heart failure.

5. **Describe the five-letter pacemaker code.**
   - The first position of the code reflects the chamber(s) in which stimulation occurs.
   - The second position refers to the chamber(s) in which sensing occurs.
   - The third position refers to the mode of setting (or how the pacemaker responds to a sensed event).
   - The fourth position reflects rate modulation.
   - The fifth position indicates whether multisite pacing is present (see Table 26.1).

6. **Explain the following pacemaker codes: DOO, VVI, DDD, and DDDRV.**
   - DOO = asynchronous atrial-ventricular pacing with a constant A-V interval. Atrial and ventricular pacing pulses are emitted regardless of the underlying cardiac rhythm.

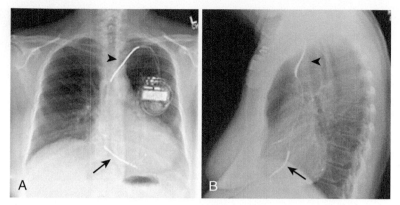

Figure 26-1. Chest radiographs (A and B, posterioranterior and lateral) of an implantable cardioverter defibrillator. (A) The superior vena cava (SVC) shocking coil *(arrowhead)* and the right ventricular shocking coil *(arrow)* are radiopaque and differentiate the implantable cardioverter defibrillator head from a pacemaker head radiographically.

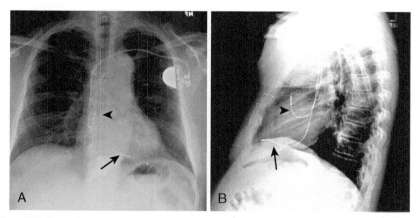

Figure 26-2. Chest radiographs (A and B, posterioranterior and lateral) of a pacemaker. The atrial pacing lead *(arrowhead)* and the ventricular pacing lead *(arrow)* are smaller in diameter and less radiopaque than the leads associated with an implantable cardioverter defibrillator.

Table 26-1. The Generic Pacemaker Code

POSITION 1: CHAMBER(S) PACED	POSITION 2: CHAMBER(S) SENSED	POSITION 3: RESPONSE TO SENSING	POSITION 4: PROGRAMMA-BILITY	POSITION 5: MULTISITE PACING
0 = none	**0** = none	**0** = none	**0** = none	**0** = none
A = atrium	**A** = atrium	**I** = inhibited	**R** = rate modulation	**A** = atrium
V = ventricle	**V** = ventricle	**T** = triggered		**V** = ventricle
D = dual (A + V)	**D** = dual (A + V)	**D** = dual (I + T)		**D** = dual (A + V)

- VVI = ventricular-only antibradycardia pacing. Failure of the ventricle to produce an intrinsic event within the appropriate time window results in ventricular pacing. With no atrial sensing, there can be no atrioventricular (AV) synchrony in a patient with any intrinsic atrial activity.
- DDD = dual-chamber antibradycardia pacing. In the absence of intrinsic activity in the atrium, it will be paced. After any sensed or paced atrial event, an intrinsic ventricular event must occur before the expiration of the AV timer or the ventricle will be paced.
- DDDRV = dual-chamber antibradycardia pacing with rate response mode circuitry (to increase the paced rate in setting of increased metabolic demand) and biventricular pacing capability.

7. What is the effect of placing a magnet on a pacemaker?

Most pacemakers respond to a magnet by converting to an asynchronous pacing mode (e.g., DOO if pacer mode is DDD, or VOO if it is VVI) at a rate dependent on the device manufacturer and the remaining battery life. For adequately charged pacemakers, the following is generally true:
- Medtronic pacemakers pace at 85 beats per minute
- Biotronik pacemakers pace at 90 beats per minute
- St. Jude pacemakers pace at 98 or 100 beats per minute
- Boston Scientific pacemakers pace at 100 beats per minute (see Table 26.2).

   The magnet will also typically inhibit a rate response mode, if present. Finally, no tone is emitted by any pacer in response to magnet application.

8. What is a rate response mode?

The normal heart rate increase with exercise or emotional stress may be compromised in some patients with pacemakers. These "chronotropically incompetent" patients often benefit from that addition of a rate response mode. The three more common types of rate response sensors are based on patient movement (accelerometer), patient ventilation (transthoracic impedance monitor), and ventricular contractility (closed-loop stimulation [CLS]). All of these sensors will increase the patient's paced rate when increased patient activity is detected. The rate at which the heart rate changes is programmable. Typically the heart rate increase is slightly delayed and will return to baseline several minutes after the increased activity subsides. Because these sensors can be falsely activated in a hospital, knowledge of their presence is ideal for optimal patient care.

Table 26-2. Magnet Effect on Pacemakers

MANUFACTURER TONE	BEGINNING OF LIFE	ERI	PROGRAMMABLE	AUDIBLE
Medtronic*	**85** (DOO or VOO)	65 (VOO)	No	No
Biotronik†	—	—	Yes	No
Async	**90** (DOO or VOO)	VOO 80	—	—
Sync	No change	See user manual	—	—
Auto	VOO for 10 beats	See user manual	—	—
ELA/Sorin	**96** (DOO or VOO)	80 (DOO or VOO)	No	No
St. Jude	**98.6** (VOO or DOO) **100** (VOO or DOO)	86.3 <85	Yes‡	No
Boston Scientific (Guidant)	**100**	85 (DOO or VOO)	Yes§	No

Table 26.2 applies only to pacemakers not associated with an ICD. The pacemaker component of an ICD is unresponsive to a magnet.

*Medtronic pacers: The first three beats with magnet application are at 100 beats per minute with a change in pulse width on the third pulse to test threshold safety margin; then the rate is 85 beats per minute.

†Biotronik pacers may be programmed in one of three ways, as noted earlier.

‡Rarely, St. Jude pacers may be programmed to *off*, which will render the pacer unresponsive to a magnet.

§Rarely, Boston Scientific pacers may be programmed to *electrogram*, and magnet application will not result in asynchronous pacing.

ERI, elective replacement indicator.

Modified from Crossley GH, Poole JE, Rozner MA, et al. Heart Rhythm Society/American Society of Anesthesiologists expert consensus statement on the perioperative management of patients with implantable defibrillators, pacemakers and arrhythmia monitors: facilities and patient management. *Heart Rhythm.* 2011;8:1151-1152.

9. How should one manage a patient with a minute ventilation rate response mode?

Minute ventilation sensors should be disabled while the patient is in the hospital. These monitors measure the rate and depth of change in thoracic impedance measured between one of the intracardiac pacing leads and the pulse generator. Increased frequency and depth of change in transthoracic impedance increase the paced rate to match the patient's increased minute ventilation. Electrocautery, ventilators, and patient monitors that measure respiratory rate can all cause significant changes in the paced rate if the minute ventilation rate response mode is not disabled. The rate response mode may be disabled with a device-specific programmer. The minute ventilation sensor is predominantly found in Boston Scientific pacers and ICDs.

10. What is the mode switch function?

The automatic mode switching function describes the capability of a pacemaker both to detect the presence of atrial tachyarrhythmias and to switch automatically from a tracking mode (e.g., DDD) to a nontracking one (e.g., DDI) for the duration of the tachyarrhythmia. In this manner, mode switching prevents the pacemaker-mediated conduction of an atrial tachyarrhythmia to the ventricle. During a mode switch the lower rate limit of the pacer usually increases (to compensate for the loss of the atrial kick) and a rate response mode is often added (e.g., DDIR) to compensate for the loss of atrial tracking capability. These changes may be interpreted as a pacer malfunction if the clinician is not aware of this programmed function.

11. What is the rest or sleep mode?

During sleep the native heart rate decreases to provide a *physiologic rest period* for the heart. Absence of this nightly rest period can decrease overall LV function. Therefore pacemaker manufacturers have created algorithms that allow the lower rate limit to drop during periods of inactivity or at night. For example, the St. Jude rest mode activates whenever perceived patient activity decreases sufficiently for a specified length of time. If the patient takes a nap at noon, the pacer's rate might drop from 60 to 50 approximately 15 minutes into the nap. The Medtronic sleep mode and Biotronik night rate are time based, rather than activity based, and will activate at a preset time, for example, from 9 PM to 5 AM. A programmer is used to turn these modes on or off.

12. What are the options for establishing temporary cardiac pacing?

There are several options available for temporary cardiac pacing in the operating room or the intensive care unit. Epicardial wires are often placed at the end of cardiac surgery and connected to an external pacer. Alternatively, permanent epicardial leads can be placed during surgery and accessed for patients who may require long-term pacing but with a reason not to use a transvenous system (endocarditis, lack of vascular access, etc.), and these leads can be connected to both permanent and temporary pacers. Atrial or ventricular pacing is possible with special pulmonary artery catheters as well, in which a wire is advanced within the right atrial or right ventricular lumen of the pulmonary artery catheter. Temporary transvenous pacing wires can be placed with venous access and connected to an external pacer. Transesophageal atrial pacing is also an option for patients who are intubated whereby a special esophageal probe that can be connected to an external pacemaker is advanced into the esophagus until able to pace the left atrium. Finally, transcutaneous pacing via external defibrillation pads is also always available for emergencies.

13. How does an implantable cardioverter defibrillator work?

ICDs monitor the right ventricular (RV) electrogram (a local QRS signal) of the patient. The time between each QRS signal is measured. If enough intervals are short (e.g., less than 300 ms, which would correspond to a heart rate of 200), the ICD detects ventricular fibrillation (VF). For example, an ICD may require 8 of the next 12 intervals to be short in order to declare an episode of VF. Once VF is detected, the ICD will charge its capacitors to 34 to 40 J. Most devices will reconfirm the presence of the dysrhythmia prior to shocking the patient. If the dysrhythmia has resolved during the reconfirmation period, the charge will be dissipated slowly rather than shocking the patient, but battery life will be diminished. It is worth noting that 2 to 3 seconds of electrocautery can be interpreted as VF.

14. How will a magnet affect an implantable cardioverter defibrillator?

Magnets usually inhibit the antitachycardic functions (defibrillation, cardioversion, antitachy pacing) of an ICD. Because each manufacturer's device has some idiosyncrasies, the clinician must be sure to understand how the magnet will affect the ICD before magnet application. Removal of the magnet usually returns the ICD to the active mode. Boston Scientific devices emit a tone for as long as the magnet is on the ICD. Medtronic devices emit a tone for approximately 15 seconds. The other

Table 26-3. Magnet Effect on Implantable Cardiac Defibrillators

MANUFACTURER	MAGNET EFFECT ON TACHYCARDIA DETECTION OR THERAPY	IS MAGNET PROGRAMMABLE?	MAGNET EFFECT ON PACING	AUDIBLE TONE?
Biotronik	Suspends*	No	No	None
ELA/Sorin	Suspends	No	Rate changes to 96 beats/min	None
Medtronic	Suspends	No	No	Yes†
St. Jude Medical	Suspends‡	Yes	No	None
Boston Scientific	Suspends§	Yes	No	Yes§

*With the Biotronik Lumax series, a magnet placed continuously over the device will disable therapy for a maximum of 8 hours, at which point therapy will be reactivated. To inhibit ICD therapy for longer than 8 hours, the device must be reprogrammed.
†All devices have an audible tone for up to 30 seconds with magnet applied correctly over the device. A steady tone indicates normal magnet placement. Beeping or oscillating tones indicate an *alert* condition; notify ICD care provider.
‡There are two programmable options for St. Jude ICDs: magnet response is nominally programmed to *normal* (ON); response can be programmed to *ignore* (OFF).
§Boston Scientific (formally Guidant and Cardiac Pacemakers Inc. [CPI]) devices, like the St Jude ICDs, can be programmed to ignore a magnet; however, most ICDs will respond to a magnet by inhibiting anti-tachy therapy. In addition, Boston Scientific ICDs will emit an intermittent tone (R-wave synchronous or every second) for as long as the magnet is inhibiting the ICD.
Modified from Crossley GH, Poole JE, Rozner MA, et al. Heart Rhythm Society/American Society of Anesthesiologists expert consensus statement on the perioperative management of patients with implantable defibrillators, pacemakers and arrhythmia monitors: facilities and patient management. *Heart Rhythm.* 2011;8:1153-1154.

ICDs do not emit a tone. A few devices in a specific scenario might not respond to a magnet (see Table 26.3). A magnet does not affect the pacing mode of any ICD except for those made by Sorin.

15. **Why is it important to know when pacemaker or ICD leads were inserted when considering placement of a central line?**
Pacer or ICD leads take time to become secure after implantation. Active fixation leads, which are screwed into the endocardium, usually become secure sooner than passive fixation leads, which rely more on fibrosis for fixation. Coronary sinus leads used for CRT are the least likely to become fixed. Insertion of a central line, and particularly a pulmonary artery (PA) line, may dislodge the newly implanted lead. As a general rule of thumb, the risk for lead dislodgment is highest in the first 3 months after lead implantation. If a central line or PA catheter must be inserted in the first 3 months, it should be done with fluoroscopic guidance, and backup pacing or defibrillation should be immediately available. All pacemakers and ICDs should be evaluated by a qualified specialist after the line has been inserted to ensure proper function.

16. **What are the considerations for placement of a pulmonary artery line in a patient with an active implantable cardioverter defibrillator?**
Caution is required whenever a guidewire is inserted into a heart in the presence of an active ICD. Contact between the guidewire and a sensing electrode (atrial or ventricular) can trigger antitachycardia therapy. If the therapy is a defibrillation, the guidewire can short the proximal coil to the distal coil and cause serious myocardial injury. To prevent this, make sure that the guidewire does not enter the ventricle or temporarily inhibit the ICD during PA line insertion.

17. **What are the considerations for cardioversion or defibrillation in a patient with a cardiovascular implantable electronic device?**
Theoretically, high-voltage cardioversion or defibrillation can damage the pulse generator or the lead-myocardial interface. It appears that application of the defibrillation pads in the anterior-posterior orientation with the anterior pad more than 8 cm away from the pulse generator minimizes this risk. The HRS recommends that if a patient with a CIED undergoes cardioversion or defibrillation, especially in an emergency setting, the patient's device should be interrogated before the patient's discharge from the intensive care unit.

18. **How can electrocautery affect a pacemaker?**
Electrocautery can affect a pacemaker in multiple ways. It can inhibit pacer output if the device is set in a demand mode. This is typically noticed if the electrocautery is sensed by the ventricular lead. The pulse generator presumes that the cautery signal represents native ventricular depolarization and inhibits the ventricular pacing output. Electrocautery may also be sensed by the atrial lead. This can cause rapid atrial tracking (rapid ventricular pacing in response to a sensed high intrinsic atrial rate) to rates up to the upper rate limit of the pacer if the pacemaker is in the DDD mode. Atrial oversensing can also trigger a mode switch if the atrial sensing rate exceeds the mode switch cutoff rate (usually 170–180 beats per minute). Finally, prolonged electrocautery can temporarily convert the pacer to a noise reversion mode or cause permanent pacemaker reset.

19. **How can electrocautery affect an implantable cardioverter defibrillator?**
Electrocautery in close enough proximity to the ICD leads (usually anywhere above the umbilicus) can be detected by the ICD as VF. The device will charge and shock the patient shortly thereafter if the electro-cautery persists during the reconfirmation period (at the end of the charging period). It takes only 2 to 3 seconds of electrocautery to fool the ICD into detecting VF. It takes another 4 to 10 seconds to charge be-fore a shock can be delivered. If, during the reconfirmation period, electrocautery has stopped, the device will abort the charge. The electrocautery will also affect the ICD's pacer function, as described previously.

20. **What should I know about subcutaneous implantable cardioverter defibrillators?**
The Boston Scientific S-ICD consists of a generator placed in anterior axillary line (V6-electrode location) and a single subcutaneous sensing and shocking electrode placed midline above the sternum. Shocks are delivered at higher outputs (80J) than those delivered by conventional ICDs (34–45 J). Only limited postshock pacing (VVI at 50 for 30 seconds) is provided. A magnet can inhibit this ICD; an R-wave synchronous tone will be heard for only 1 minute, but inhibition will persist until the magnet is removed (standard Boston Scientific ICDs emit a tone for as long as the magnet is over the ICD). To reprogram the device, an S-ICD–specific programmer is necessary. The standard Boston Scientific programmer cannot be used. These devices offer a patient freedom from the deleterious effects of intracardiac leads (tricuspid valve injury, endocarditis, lead extraction complications).

21. **Your patient's pacer mode is reported as AAIR<->DDDR. What does this mean?**
There is now evidence that unnecessary ventricular pacing can increase the rate of hospitalization for congestive heart failure (CHF) and increase the rate of atrial fibrillation. Thus companies have devel-oped programs to minimize ventricular pacing whenever possible. Medtronic's Managed Ventricular Pacing (MVP) is one such program, and the mode will appear as AAIR<->DDDR. It basically means that the pacer will pace in the AAIR mode, allowing very long PR intervals. If there is evidence of non-conducted P waves or atrial pacing impulses indicating heart block, the device quickly converts to the DDDR mode. Very long PR intervals (350 ms) may be seen and periodic nonconducted P waves are commonly seen on the ECG and should not be misinterpreted as malfunction.

KEY POINTS: PACEMAKERS AND DEFIBRILLATORS

Regarding Pacemakers and Defibrillators
How will a magnet affect a pacemaker?
1. Magnets convert most pacemakers to an asynchronous pacing mode.
2. The magnet-induced paced rate is manufacturer-specific and dependent on battery life.
3. No audible sound is emitted from a pacemaker when a magnet is applied.
4. Magnets will inhibit any programmed rate response mode in a pacemaker.
5. Magnets do not affect the pacemaker component of an ICD.

WEBSITES

www.biotronik.com
www.bostonscientific.com
www.hrsonline.org (Heart Rhythm Society)
www.medtronic.com
www.PacerICD.com (go to Fundamentals of Pacing, Fundamentals of ICDs, or IBHRE Exam Study Materials for video lectures)
www.sjm.com

BIBLIOGRAPHY

1. American Society of Anesthesiologists. Practice advisory for the perioperative management of patients with cardiac implantable electronic devices: pacemakers and implantable cardioverter-defibrillators: an updated report by the american society of anesthesiologists task force on perioperative management of patients with cardiac implantable electronic devices. *Anesthesiology.* 2011;114:247-261.
2. Crossley GH, Poole JE, Rozner MA, et al. Heart Rhythm Society/American Society of Anesthesiologists expert consensus statement on the perioperative management of patients with implantable defibrillators, pacemakers and arrhythmia monitors: facilities and patient management. *Heart Rhythm.* 2011;8:1114-1152.
3. Lau W, Corcoran S, Mond HG. Pacemaker tachycardia in a minute ventilation rate-adaptive pacemaker induced by electrocardiographic monitoring. *Pacing Clin Electrophysiol.* 2006;29:438-440.
4. Manegold JC, Israel CW, Erlich JR, et al. External cardioversion of atrial fibrillation in patients with implanted pacemaker or cardioverter-defibrillator systems: a randomized comparison of monophasic and biphasic shock energy application. *Eur Heart J.* 2007;28:1731-1738.
5. Maron BJ, Estes M. Medical progress: commotio cordis. *N Engl J Med.* 2010;362:917-927.
6. Smirk FH. R waves interrupting T waves. *Br Heart J.* 1949;11:23-36.

IV
PULMONARY

CHAPTER 27

ACUTE PNEUMONIA

Hui Zhang, Jing Zhao and Lorenzo Berra

1. **What is community-acquired pneumonia and how is it defined?**

   Community-acquired pneumonia (CAP) is defined as an infection of the lung parenchyma that has been acquired outside of a healthcare facility. In order to lower the incidence of mortality, severe CAP (S-CAP) requires intensive care unit (ICU) admission for the purposes of early diagnosis and treatment. Box 27.1 sets forth the criteria defining S-CAP as outlined by the Infectious Diseases Society of America (IDSA)/American Thoracic Society (ATS)

   Infectious Diseases Society of America (IDSA)/American Thoracic Society (ATS) guideline (see Box 27.1). S-CAP is diagnosed when either one of the major criteria or three of the minor criteria have been met.

2. **What is the epidemiology of community-acquired pneumonia?**

   The incidence of CAP is estimated to be between 1.5 and 14 cases per 1000 persons per year. This varies according to the region, season, and population characteristics, specifically age and gender. Children below 5 years of age and adults above age 65 as well as the male population in general have proven to be more susceptible.

   Mortality associated with CAP increases with the severity of presentation. Thirty-day mortality for patients requiring hospital admission ranges between 4% and 18%, while for patients requiring ICU admission it can be as high as 50%. Independent variables associated with increased mortality are age (>65 years), presence of comorbidities, increased frailty, cardiovascular complications, inflammation, and the severity of the initial insult.

3. **What are the criteria for hospital admission for patients with community-acquired pneumonia?**

   Severity-of-illness scores, such as the CURB-65 criteria (confusion, uremia, respiratory rate, low blood pressure, age 65 years or greater) or prognostic models, such as the pneumonia severity index (PSI), can be used to identify patients with CAP who can be treated on an outpatient basis. Outpatient treatment is indicated for those with a CURB-65 score of 0 to 1. Patients should be admitted if their score is equal to 2 and admitted to the ICU if it is equal to or greater than 3. The PSI stratifies patients into five mortality risk classes. It has been suggested that risk class I and II patients should be treated as outpatients, risk class III patients might be admitted to the hospital, and risk class IV and V patients should be treated as inpatients.

4. **How are patients requiring admission to an intensive care unit identified?**

   Patients should be admitted to intensive care when they meet the criteria of septic shock requiring infusion of vasopressor support or develop acute respiratory distress syndrome (the Berlin definition) requiring mechanical ventilation. Direct admission to an ICU or a high-level monitoring unit is recommended for patients with one of the major criteria or three of the minor criteria for severe CAP, as outlined in Box 27.1.

5. **What are the primary pathogens responsible for community-acquired pneumonia?**

   Pneumonia may be caused by a wide variety of pathogens (Table 27.1).
   - *Streptococcus pneumonia* remains the most commonly identified cause of CAP.
   - Other bacteria that cause CAP include *Haemophilus influenzae, Moraxella catarrhalis, Pseudomonas aeruginosa, Staphylococcus aureus*, respiratory viruses, and other gram-negative bacilli.

Box 27-1. Criteria for Severe Community-Acquired Pneumonia

Major Criteria
Invasive mechanical ventilation
Septic shock with need for vasopressors

Minor Criteria
Respiratory rate ≥30 breaths per minute
PaO_2/FiO_2 ratio <250
Multilobar infiltrates

Confusion or disorientation
Uremia (blood urea nitrogen level >20 mg/dL)
Leukopenia (WBCs <4000/mm^3 as a result of infection alone)
Thrombocytopenia (platelets <100,000/mm^3)
Hypothermia (cord temperature <36°C)
Hypotension requiring aggressive fluid resuscitation

Table 27-1. Most Common Etiologies of Community-Acquired Pneumonia

PATIENT TYPE	ETIOLOGY
Outpatient	*Streptococcus pneumoniae* *Mycoplasma pneumoniae* *Haemophilus influenzae* *Chlamydophila pneumoniae* Respiratory viruses*
Inpatient (non-ICU)	*S. pneumoniae* *M. pneumoniae* *C. pneumoniae* *H. influenzae* *Legionella* species Aspiration Respiratory viruses*
Inpatient (ICU)	*S. pneumoniae* *Staphylococcus aureus* *Legionella* species Gram-negative bacilli *H. influenzae*

*Influenza A and B, adenovirus, respiratory syncytial virus, and parainfluenza.
ICU, intensive care unit.

- There is a wide variation in the reported incidence of CAP caused by *Mycoplasma pneumoniae* and *Chlamydophila pneumoniae* due to specific diagnostic techniques that must be used to diagnose "atypical bacterial" pneumonia.
- Another type of bacterial pneumonia caused by *Legionella species* occurs in certain geographic locations and tends to follow specific exposures.
- Mixed microaerophilic and anaerobic bacteria (so-called oral flora) may be responsible for cases in which no cause is found.
- During influenza outbreaks, the circulating influenza virus—including influenza A and B, adenovirus, respiratory syncytial virus, and parainfluenza—becomes the principal cause of CAP that is serious enough to require hospitalization, with secondary bacterial infection as a major contributor.

6. How is community-acquired pneumonia diagnosed?

CAP is diagnosed based on the presence of signs and symptoms as well as radiographic evidence of lung infiltrates. The most common signs and symptoms are dyspnea, cough, fever, sputum production, chills, and pleuritic chest pain, although in some instances clinical presentation can be subtle. An altered state of consciousness, gastrointestinal discomfort, and fever can be absent, particularly in the elderly. For these patients, diagnosis is frequently delayed. Due to the relatively low accuracy of chest radiography for alveolar consolidation and pleural effusion, computed tomography (CT), if available, is considered the gold standard. Although pathogens can be identified in fewer than 50% of cases, microbiologic diagnostic technology is helpful for guidance for antibiotic treatment in ICU patients.

CAP requires early diagnosis and treatment to improve outcome; thus differential diagnosis is a critical step in the management of these patients. The wide differential diagnosis of CAP is summarized in Table 27.2.

7. What techniques are utilized to detect lung infiltrates?

CT is the gold standard technique to identify radiographic evidence for lung infiltrates. However, CT has limitations that include increased cost, radiation exposure, and the inconvenience of performing CT at bedside. For these reasons, CT use is confined to presentations with unclear chest radiographs (e.g., occult pneumonia in chronic obstructive pulmonary disease) or in case of differential diagnosis such as pulmonary embolism, fungal lung infection and detection of complications (e.g., lung abscesses) in nonresponding pneumonia.

Table 27-2. Differential Diagnosis of Community-Acquired Pneumonia

DIAGNOSIS	SYMPTOMS	CHEST X-RAY	KEY POINTS
Acute bronchitis	Mild symptoms, not dyspnea, not lung crackles	No condensation	Limited use of antibiotics (most cases are viral infection)
Acute lung injury secondary to sepsis	Dyspnea, symptoms of another infection	Bilateral alveolar-interstitial pattern	Respiratory symptoms with infection at another site
Congestive heart failure	Dyspnea, tachycardia, chest pain	Bilateral interstitial pattern (>apical), pleural effusion	History of cardiac disease, alteration of echocardiogram, resolution after NIV
Acute exacerbation of COPD	Dyspnea, increased expectoration and cough	No condensation	History of COPD/smoking
Acute exacerbation of asthma	Dyspnea, cough, signs of bronchospasm	No condensation	History of asthma
Pulmonary infarction	DVT, dyspnea, tachycardia, chest pain	Focal condensation, small pleural effusion	Risk factors for thrombosis
Lung cancer or pulmonary metastasis	Dyspnea, constitutional symptoms	Focal or multiple condensation, pleural effusion	History of smoking, nonresolving pneumonia, history of cancer
Acute exacerbation of bronchiectasis	Dyspnea, increased expectoration and cough	No condensation	History of bronchiectasis/repetitive infections
Acute exacerbation of pulmonary fibrosis	Dyspnea, dry cough, fine basal late inspiratory crackles	Interstitial pattern	History of pulmonary fibrosis
Other lung infections (tuberculosis/histoplasmosis)	Constitutional symptoms, prolonged time of symptoms	Focal consolidation, cavitation, Lymphadenopathy	History of specific exposure (contacts)
Autoimmune disease with lung involvement	Dyspnea, extrapulmonary manifestations	Interstitial pattern	History of autoimmune disease Improvement with corticosteroid
Pleural empyema	Dyspnea, constitutional symptoms	Signs of pleural effusion, considered loculated pleural effusion	History of recent respiratory infection
Pulmonary toxicities due to medications	Dyspnea	Prevalent interstitial pattern, condensation and nodules	History of medications

COPD, chronic obstructive pulmonary disease; DVT, deep venous thrombosis; NIV, noninvasive ventilation.
Data from supplementary appendix to Prina E, Ranzani OT, Torres A. Community-acquired pneumonia. *Lancet.* 2015;386:1097–1108.

More recently, the performance of lung ultrasound has acquired popularity in the diagnosis of patients with pneumonia due to its radiation-free technique. As such, it can be delivered at bedside and is safe for use on pregnant women. It also has increased accuracy in the detection of consolidation and pleural effusion compared with chest radiograph. A recent meta-analysis showed a sensitivity of 94% and a specificity of 96%. The use of echo is limited by its learning curve, repeatability, and operator dependency.

8. What techniques are utilized to identify the causative pathogens in patients with severe community-acquired pneumonia?

In S-CAP patients, we favor obtaining Gram staining and cultures of sputum and blood, testing for *Legionella* and pneumococcal urinary antigens, and multiplex polymerase chain reaction (PCR) assays for *M. pneumoniae, C. pneumoniae,* and respiratory viruses as well as other testing as indicated in patients with specific risk factors or exposures.

9. How is select empiric antimicrobial therapy selected and when is it implemented?

Empiric antimicrobial therapy is a broad-spectrum antibiotic treatment that is started upon CAP clinical diagnosis. The choice of the empiric antibiotic depends on the most likely pathogen, individual risk factors, comorbidities, allergies, and cost-effectiveness. The management and antibiotic treatment proposed by CAP guidelines are presented in Table 27.3.

As soon as a clinical diagnosis of pneumonia has been made, antibiotic treatment should be initiated, preferably within 1 to 8 hours of hospital arrival, as a delay in antibiotic therapy increases mortality and a shorter time to the first dose of antibiotic can be a marker of quality of care. In S-CAP patients, antibiotic treatment should start within 1 hour of diagnosis so as to improve mortality.

10. How long should antibiotic treatment last?

The standard duration of uncomplicated pneumonia treatment is 5 to 7 days; 5 days of treatment should be given for low-severity pneumonia and 7 days for severe pneumonia. The duration of antibiotic therapy should be adapted depending on improvements in symptoms and stability. Patients with CAP should not have more than one CAP-associated sign of clinical instability (Box 27.2) before stopping treatment. Patients with extrapulmonary complications or empyema and pneumonia due to a specific pathogens (e.g., *Legionella* spp. and methicillin-resistant *S. aureus* [MRSA]) seem to benefit from prolonged treatment.

A very promising approach in the deescalation of antibiotic treatment has been found with the use of biomarkers. One-time procalcitonin (PCT) values lower than 0.25 μg/mL or a decrease from the peak by 80% to 90% is a strong indication that antibiotics should be discontinued.

11. When should intravenous antibiotic therapy be replaced with oral therapy?

Patients should be switched from intravenous to oral therapy when they are hemodynamically stable, able to ingest medications, and are clinically stable. The criteria for clinical stability are listed in Box 27.2.

12. How is therapy failure identified? What are the patterns and etiologies of failure to respond?

Clinical failure or a lack of response to empiric antimicrobial therapy within 3 days should be considered when patients with CAP present with deterioration. Early failure (<72 h) appears to be related to the severity of the primary infection (e.g., the development of septic shock), whereas the late failures (>72 h) tend to be due to secondary events (e.g., nosocomial superinfection, exacerbation of comorbidities). The possible causes of failure are listed in Box 27.3.

13. When should patients be discharged from the intensive care unit?

Patients should be discharged as soon as they are clinically stable and have a safe environment for continued care. Inpatient observation for those receiving oral therapy is not necessary.

14. What are the risk factors associated with resistant pathogens in community-acquired pneumonia?
   - Comorbidities: chronic lung disease, immunosuppression, cerebrovascular disease, heart failure, diabetes mellitus, chronic renal disease, hemodialysis, previous pneumonia
   - Acquired dysfunction: cognitive impairment, poor functional status, dysphagia
   - Patient status: tube feeding, indwelling catheter
   - Habits: smoking, alcohol abuse
   - Medication: gastric acid suppression, previous antibiotic use
   - Previous infection: MRSA colonization, prior CAP due to resistant pathogen
   - Recent admission to the hospital or living facility

15. What are the primary ways of preventing community-acquired pneumonia?
   - Influenza vaccines are reported to reduce the rate of pneumonia and provide better outcomes. All persons above 50 years of age, others at risk for influenza complications, household contacts of high-risk persons, and healthcare workers should receive inactivated influenza vaccine as recommended by the Advisory Committee on Immunization Practices (ACIP) of the Centers for Disease Control and Prevention (CDC).
   - Smoking and alcohol cessation programs should be encouraged.

Table 27-3. Recommended Empiric Treatment for Community-Acquired Pneumonia

	AMERICA (IDSA/ATS)[1]	CHINA (CTS)[11]	EUROPE[9]
Outpatient without co-morbidities; low severity	Macrolide (azithromycin, clarithromycin/erythromycin) Doxycycline	(1) Amoxicillin, penicillin/lactamase inhibitor (2) First- or second-generation cephalosporin (3) Doxycycline or minocycline (4) Respiratory fluoroquinolone (5) Macrolide	Amoxicillin or tetracycline Macrolide (azithromycin, clarithromycin, erythromycin or roxithromycin)
Outpatient with co-morbidities or high rate bacterial resistance	Lactam* plus macrolide Respiratory[†] fluoroquinolone (moxifloxacin, levofloxacin 750 mg)	(1) Penicillin/lactamase inhibitor (2) Second- or third-generation cephalosporin (oral) (3) Respiratory fluoroquinolone (4) Penicillin/lactamase inhibitor; second-generation cephalosporin, third-generation cephalosporin plus doxycycline, minocycline, or macrolide	Aminopenicillin with or without macrolide Respiratory fluoroquinolone (levofloxacin or moxifloxacin)
Inpatient in ICU; high severity	Lactam[‡] plus respiratory fluoroquinolone Lactam[‡] plus macrolide **If *Pseudomonas* is a consideration:** Antipneumococcal antipseudomonal lactam plus either ciprofloxacin or levofloxacin (750 mg) **OR** Antipneumococcal antipseudomonas lactam plus aminoglycoside and azithromycin **OR** Anitipneumococcal antipseudomonal lactam plus aminoglycoside and antipneumococcal antipseudomonal fluoroquinolone (for penicillin-allergic patients, substitute aztreonam for the lactam)	• Penicillin/lactamase inhibitor, third-generation cephalosporin or plus with lactamase inhibitor, carbapenems plus macrolide • Penicillin/lactamase inhibitor, third- generation cephalosporin or plus with lactamase inhibitor, carbapenems plus respiratory fluoroquinolone **If *Pseudomonas* is a consideration:** (1) Antipseudomonal lactam (2) Antipseudomonal fluoroquinolone (3) Antipseudomonal lactam plus antipseudomonal fluoroquinolone or aminoglycoside (4) Antipseudomonal lactam plus antipseudomonal fluoroquinolone plus aminoglycoside	Third-generation cephalosporin[§] plus macrolide Respiratory fluoroquinolone (moxifloxacin or levofloxacin) with or without a third-generation cephalosporin[§] **If *Pseudomonas* is a consideration:** Antipseudomonal lactam or acylureidopenicillin/lactamase inhibitor or carbapenem (meropenem preferred, up to 6 g possible) **PLUS** Ciprofloxacin **OR PLUS** Macrolide plus aminoglycoside (gentamicin, tobramycin, or amikacin)

*Preferred lactam drugs include cefotaxime, ceftriaxone, and ampicillin.
†Respiratory fluoroquinolone is limited to situations where other options cannot be used or are ineffective (e.g., hepatotoxicity, skin reactions, cardiac arrhythmias, and tendon rupture).
‡Preferred lactam drugs include cefotaxime, ceftriaxone, or ampicillin-sulbactam.
§Third-generation cephalosporin (e.g., cefotaxime, ceftriaxone).
Local or adapted guidelines should be used to adapt for different epidemiology.
ATS, American Thoracic Society; *CTS*, Chinese Thoracic Society; *ICU*, intensive care unit; *IDSA*, Infectious Diseases Society of America; *NICE*, National Institute for Health and Care Excellence.

Box 27-2. Criteria for Clinical Stability

Temperature ≤37.8°C
Heart rate ≤100 beats per minute
Respiratory rate ≤24 beats per minute
Systolic blood pressure ≥90 mm Hg
Arterial oxygen saturation ≥90% or PO_2 ≥60 mm Hg on room air
Ability to maintain oral intake
Normal mental status

Modified from Mandell LA, Wunderink RG, Anzueto A, et al. Infectious Diseases Society of America/American Thoracic Society consensus guidelines on the management of community-acquired pneumonia in adults. *Clin Infect Dis.* 2007;44 (suppl 2):S27–S72.

Box 27-3. Patterns and Etiologies of Types of Failure to Respond

Failure to Improve
Early (<72 h treatment)
Severity of the primary infection (e.g., septic shock)

Delayed (>72 h treatment)
Resistant microorganism
Uncovered pathogen; inappropriate antimicrobial therapy
Parapneumonic effusion/empyema
Nosocomial superinfection
Nosocomial pneumonia; extrapulmonary
Noninfectious
Complication of pneumonia (BOOP)
Misdiagnosis: PE, CHF, vasculitis
Drug fever

Deterioration or Progression
Early (<72 h of treatment)
Severity of illness at presentation
Resistant microorganism

Uncovered pathogen; inappropriate by sensitivity
Metastatic infection
Empyema/parapneumonic
Endocarditis, meningitis, arthritis
Inaccurate diagnosis
PE, aspiration, ARDS, vasculitis (e.g., SLE)

Delayed (>72 h)
Nosocomial superinfection
Nosocomial pneumonia; extrapulmonary
Exacerbation of comorbid illness
Intercurrent noninfectious disease
PE; myocardial infarction; renal failure

ARDS, acute respiratory distress syndrome; *BOOP*, bronchiolitis obliterans organizing pneumonia; *CHF*, congestive heart failure; *PE*, pulmonary embolus; *SLE*, systemic lupus erythematosus.
Modified from Mandell LA, Wunderink RG, Anzueto A, et al. Infectious Diseases Society of America/American Thoracic Society consensus guidelines on the management of community-acquired pneumonia in adults. *Clin Infect Dis.* 2007;44 (suppl 2):S27–S72.

- Respiratory hygiene measures, which include hand and dental hygiene and masks for patients with cough, should be used in outpatient settings and emergency departments (EDs) to reduce the spread of respiratory infections.
- Malnutrition and swallowing disturbance are risk factors for pneumonia. Both need to be corrected as early as possible.

16. What are hospital-acquired pneumonia and ventilator-associated pneumonia?
Hospital-acquired pneumonia (HAP) is defined as a pneumonia not incubating at the time of hospital admission and occurring 48 hours or more after admission. In the 2016 Clinical Practice Guidelines of the IDSA/ATS, HAP denotes an episode of pneumonia without an association with mechanical venti-lation. Ventilator-associated pneumonia (VAP) is defined as a pneumonia occurring at least 48 hours after endotracheal intubation.

17. What criteria should be used to start empiric antibiotic treatment in hospital-acquired or ventilator-associated pneumonia?

Together with clinical criteria and microbiologic cultures, the use of biomarkers (e.g., procalcitonin [PCT], C-reactive protein [CRP], soluble triggering receptor expressed on myeloid cells-1 [sTREM-1]) is recommended, along with clinical pulmonary infection score (CPIS), to decide whether to initiate antibiotic therapy. To guide antibiotic treatment, one should rely on microbiologic samples and/or biomarkers. Microbiologic samples can be collected by noninvasive methods (i.e., endotracheal aspiration, spontaneous expectoration, sputum induction, nasotracheal suctioning in a patient who is unable to cooperate to produce a sputum sample) or invasive methods (i.e., bronchoalveolar lavage [BAL], protected specimen brush [PSB], and blind bronchial sampling [i.e., mini-BAL]). When invasive quantitative culture results are available and below the diagnostic threshold for VAP (PSB with $<10^3$ colony-forming units (CFU)/mL, BAL with $<10^4$ CFU/m), antibiotic treatment is unnecessary. The decision should be based on prudent interpretation of the results when considering the specific clinical situation. PCT levels together with clinical criteria could be also used to guide discontinuation of antibiotic therapy.

18. What is the empiric treatment of ventilator-associated pneumonia?

Selection of broad-spectrum antibiotic treatment for VAP should be based on local antimicrobial susceptibilities if available. Empiric broad-spectrum antibiotic treatment should be quickly narrowed to assure adequate treatment while minimizing side effects and antibiotic resistance.

Empiric antibiotic coverage includes *S. aureus, P. aeruginosa*, and other gram-negative bacilli (Table 27.4).

An antibiotic agent against MRSA is recommended in patients with a risk factor (Box 27.4) for antimicrobial resistance. In the absence of any risk factors, an antibiotic agent against methicillin-sensitive *Staphylococcus aureus* (MSSA) is preferred. In patients with high-risk factors for drug resistance, two antipseudomonal antibiotics from different classes are recommended. In patients without

Table 27-4. Empiric Treatment Regimens for Ventilator-Associated and Hospital-Acquired Pneumonia

	HAP	VAP	ANTIBIOTICS
Empiric therapy	Avoid to use an aminoglycoside as the sole antipseudomonal agent	Avoid aminoglycosides and colistin if alternative agents with adequate gram-negative activity are available	Coverage for *Staphylococcus aureus, Pseudomonas aeruginosa*, and other gram-negative bacilli
Indications for MRSA coverage	• Prior intravenous antibiotic use within 90 days • Hospitalization in an ICU where >20% of *S. aureus* isolates are methicillin-resistant or the prevalence of MRSA is not known • At high risk for mortality (need for ventilatory support due to pneumonia and septic shock)	• Prior intravenous antibiotic use with 90 days • Patients being treated in an ICU where >10%–20% of *S. aureus* isolates are methicillin-resistant or the prevalence of MRSA is not known	Vancomycin 15 mg/kg IV q8–12h (Consider a loading dose of 25–30 mg/kg × 1 for severe illness) **OR** Linezolid 600 mg IV q12h
Indications for MSSA coverage	• Without risk factor for MRSA • Without high risk for mortality	• Without risk factors for antimicrobial resistance • Patients being treated in an ICU where 10%–20% of *S. aureus* isolates are methicillin-resistant	Piperacillin-tazobactam 4.5 g IV q6h **OR** Cefepime 2 g IV q8h **OR** Levofloxacin 750 mg IV q24h **OR** Imipenem 500 mg IV q6h **OR** Meropenem 1g IV q8h

(Continued on following page)

Table 27-4. Empiric Treatment Regimens for Ventilator-Associated and Hospital-Acquired Pneumonia *(Continued)*

	HAP	VAP	ANTIBIOTICS
Suspected *Pseudomonas aeruginosa* victims	• Prior intravenous antibiotic use within 90 days • Patient has structural lung disease, increasing the risk of gram-negative infection (i.e., bronchiectasis or cystic fibrosis)	• Prior intravenous antibiotic use within 90 days • Patients in an ICU where >10% of gram-negative isolates are resistant to an agent being considered for monotherapy • Patients in an ICU where local antimicrobial susceptibility rates are not available	Prescribe two antipseudomonal antibiotics from different classes for empiric treatment
	All patients except the above	Patients without risk factors for antimicrobial resistance who are being treated in ICUs where ≤10% of gram-negative isolates are resistant to the agent	Monotherapy

HAP, hospital-acquired pneumonia; ICU, intensive care unit; MRSA, methicillin-resistant *Staphylococcus aureus*; MSSA, methicillin-sensitive *Staphylococcus aureus*; VAP, ventilator-associated pneumonia.

Box 27-4. Risk Factors for Multidrug-Resistant Pathogens

Risk Factors for MDR VAP
Prior intravenous antibiotic use within 90 days
Septic shock at time of VAP
ARDS preceding VAP
Five or more days of hospitalization prior to the occurrence of VAP
Acute renal replacement therapy prior to VAP onset

Risk Factors for MDR HAP
Prior intravenous antibiotic use within 90 days

Risk Factors for MRSA VAP/HAP
Prior intravenous antibiotic use within 90 days

Risk Factors for MDR *Pseudomonas* VAP/HAP
Prior intravenous antibiotic use within 90 days

HAP, hospital-acquired pneumonia; MDR, multidrug resistant; MRSA, multidrug-resistant S. aureus; VAP, ventilator-associated pneumonia.
Modified from Kalil AC, Metersky ML, Klompas M, et al. Management of adults with hospital-acquired and ventilator-associated pneumonia: 2016 Clinical Practice Guidelines by the Infectious Diseases Society of America and the American Thoracic Society. *Clin Infect Dis.* 2016;63:e61–e11.

high-risk factors for drug resistance, one class of anti *P. aeruginosa* antibiotics is used in the empiric treatment of suspected VAP. Aminoglycoside monotherapy and colistin should be avoided if alternative agents with adequate gram-negative activity are available. Aminoglycosides and colistin are associated with increased adverse events such as nephrotoxicity and ototoxicity. However, due to the increased antibiotic resistance in certain ICUs, colistin is included in the empiric initial antibiotic regimen.

19. **What is the empiric treatment of hospital-acquired (nonventilator-acquired) pneumonia?**
Similarly to VAP, empiric treatment for HAP should be based on local antimicrobial susceptibilities if available. Broad-spectrum antibiotic treatment should be quickly narrowed according to microbiologic cultures to assure adequate treatment while minimizing side effects and antibiotic resistance.

Empiric antibiotic coverage includes *S. aureus, P. aeruginosa*, and other gram-negative bacilli (see Table 27.4).

For patients with HAP who are being treated empirically and have either a risk factor (see Box 27.4) for MRSA infection or are at high risk for mortality, an antibiotic against MRSA is recommended. For patients with HAP who are being treated empirically and have no risk factors for MRSA infection and are not at high risk of mortality, an antibiotic with activity against MSSA is preferred. In patients with high risk factors for *Pseudomonas* or other gram-negative infection or a high risk for mortality, two antipseudomonal antibiotics from different classes are recommended. Meanwhile, an aminoglycoside as the sole antipseudomonal agent is not recommended.

20. How long should antibiotic treatment last in hospital-acquired or ventilator-associated pneumonia?
In most cases, the antibiotic treatment should last 7 days. The duration should depend upon the rate of improvement of clinical, radiologic, and laboratory parameters. Short courses of antibiotics (7 days) compared with long courses (15 days) reduce antibiotic exposure and recurrent pneumonia due to multidrug-resistant (MDR) organisms.

More recently, PCT has been successfully used together with the clinical criteria to guide early discontinuation of antibiotic therapy.

21. What is the role of inhaled antibiotic treatment?
For patients with VAP due to gram-negative bacilli that are susceptible to only aminoglycosides or polymyxins (colistin or polymyxin B), it is suggested to add an inhaled antibiotic to the systemic antibiotic therapy. It is also suggested to consider adjunctive inhaled antibiotic therapy when intravenous antibiotics alone are failing or a high plasma concentration of antibiotic is contraindicated.

22. What is multiple drug resistance?
MDR pathogens are microorganisms that are resistant to one or more classes of antimicrobial agents. Although the term sometimes describes resistance to only one agent (e.g., MRSA, Vancomycin-resistant enterococci [VRE]), these pathogens are frequently resistant to two or more classes of antibiotics.

23. What is the pathogen-specific therapy for hospital-acquired or ventilator-associated pneumonia?
The antibiotic treatment should be definitive therapy based on the results of antimicrobial susceptibility testing and patients-specific conditions. The pathogen-specific therapy for VAP/HAP is listed in Table 27.5.

Table 27-5. Pathogen-Specific Therapies for Ventilator-Associated and Hospital-Acquired Pneumonia

PATHOGENS	ANTIBIOTIC CHOICE
MRSA	Vancomycin or linezolid
Pseudomonas aeruginosa	Based on the results of antimicrobial susceptibility testing aminoglycoside monotherapy is not recommended
ESBL-producing gram-negative bacilli	Based on the results of antimicrobial susceptibility testing
Acinetobacter species	Carbapenem or ampicillin/sulbactam if the isolate is susceptible to these agents; the use of tigecycline is not recommended For species sensitive only to polymyxins, intravenous polymyxin (colistin or polymyxin B) is recommended and adjunctive inhaled colistin is suggested For *Acinetobacter* species sensitive only to colistin, do not use adjunctive rifampicin
Carbapenem-resistant pathogens	In patients with HAP/VAP caused by a carbapenem-resistant pathogen that is sensitive only to polymyxins, intravenous polymyxins (colistin or polymyxin B) is recommended Adjunctive inhaled colistin is suggested

ESBL, extended-spectrum lactamase; *HAP*, hospital-acquired pneumonia; *MRSA*, methicillin-resistant *Staphylococcus aureus*; *VAP*, ventilator-associated pneumonia.

ACKNOWLEDGMENT

The authors wish to acknowledge Drs. Kenneth Shelton, MD, Jeanine P. Wiener-Kronish, MD, and Aranya Bagchi, MBBS, for the valuable contributions to the previous edition of this chapter.

BIBLIOGRAPHY

1. Mandell LA, Wunderink RG, Anzueto A, et al. Infectious Diseases Society of America/American Thoracic Society consensus guidelines on the management of community-acquired pneumonia in adults. *Clin Infect Dis.* 2007; (44 suppl 2):S27-S72.
2. Millett ER, Quint JK, Smeeth L, et al. Incidence of community-acquired lower respiratory tract infections and pneumonia among older adults in the United Kingdom: a population-based study. *PLoS One.* 2013;8:e75131. doi:10.1071/journal.pone.0075131.
3. Ochoa-Gondar O, Vila-Córcoles A, de Diego C, et al. The burden of community-acquired pneumonia in the elderly: the Spanish EVAN-65 study. *BMC Public Health.* 2008;8:222.
4. File Jr TM, Marrie TJ. Burden of community-acquired pneumonia in North American adults. *Postgrad Med.* 2010; 122:130-141.
5. Ranieri VM, Rubenfeld GD, Thompson BT, et al. Acute respiratory distress syndrome: the Berlin Definition. *JAMA.* 2012;307:2526-2533.
6. Chavez MA, Shams N, Ellington LE, et al. Lung ultrasound for the diagnosis of pneumonia in adults: a systematic review and meta-analysis. *Respir Res.* 2014;15:50.
7. Ramirez P, Torres A. Should ultrasound be included in the initial assessment of respiratory patients? *Lancet Respir Med.* 2014;2:599-600.
8. Prina E, Ranzani OT, Torres A. Community-acquired pneumonia. *Lancet.* 2015;386:1097-1108.
9. Woodhead M, Blasi F, Ewig S, et al. Guidelines for the management of adult lower respiratory tract infections–full version. *Clin Microbiol Infect.* 2011;(17 suppl 6):E1-E59.
10. Kalil AC, Metersky ML, Klompas M, et al. Management of Adults With Hospital-acquired and Ventilator-associated Pneumonia: 2016 Clinical Practice Guidelines by the Infectious Diseases Society of America and the American Thoracic Society. *Clin Infect Dis.* 2016;63:e61-e111.
11. Chinese Thoracic Society consensus guidelines on the management of community-acquired pneumonia in adults. *Clin J Tuber Respir Dis.* 2016;39(4):253-279. (Article in Chinese, http://www.medsci.cn/article/show_article.do?id=fcdee2603f3).

CHAPTER 28

ASTHMA

Hill A. Enuh, Gilman B. Allen, and David A. Kaminsky

1. **What are important factors to address in taking the history of a patient with acute severe asthma?**
   Box 28.1 summarizes the important historical points in a patient with acute severe asthma. If the clinician is able to obtain a history from the patient, it is important to first exclude other possible causes of the patient's presentation. A history of heart failure may suggest wheezing and shortness of breath resulting from left ventricular failure and pulmonary edema. A history of bilateral leg swelling or generalized body edema may suggest right ventricular failure or liver or kidney disease. A history of allergies or prior anaphylactic reactions, along with a recent exposure to certain foods, new medications, or other known triggers, could be an important warning of potentially imminent upper airway inflammation and closure. A history of recent-onset cough, wheezing, and hemoptysis with unilateral inspiratory and expiratory wheezes could be clues to an intrabronchial tumor, such as a carcinoid or carcinoma. Pulmonary embolism can also mimic asthma and should especially be considered in the patient with dyspnea, anxiety, and hypoxemia but clear breath sounds. In a patient with dyspnea, anxiety, and inspiratory stridor, vocal cord dysfunction should be considered. Spirometry can be an especially useful tool in the emergency department (ED) when these patients are being evaluated, and flow-volume loops often show the characteristic truncated or flattened inspiratory loops.

2. **List some important indicators of a severe asthma attack.**
   - Use of accessory muscles
   - Inability to speak in full sentences
   - Heart rate greater than 130 beats per minute
   - Pulsus paradoxus greater than 15 mm Hg
   - Respiratory rate greater than 30 breaths per minute
   - Inability to lie down
   - A silent chest
   - Somnolence
   - Worsening fatigue
   - Normal or elevated $PaCO_2$
   - Inability to maintain oxygenation by mask (oxygen saturation <90%)
   - Cyanosis

3. **Which patients are at greatest risk for near-fatal or fatal asthma?**
   A survey of North American adult patients with asthma seen in the ED identified several factors associated with a high number of ED visits, including nonwhite race, Medicaid, other public or no insurance, and markers of chronic asthma severity, such as history of prior hospitalization, intubation, or recent use of inhaled corticosteroids. Also at increased risk for near-fatal asthma are patients with a high degree of bronchial reactivity, those with a history of poor compliance with therapy and follow-up, and those judged to have difficulty perceiving the severity of their own attack, as demonstrated

---

Box 28-1. Important Historical Points in Acute Asthma

- History of asthma (i.e., when diagnosed, type of treatment, common triggers)
- Factors related to asthma control (e.g., frequency of use of medications, nocturnal symptoms, history of hospitalization, intubation, use of oral steroids)
- Timing of onset of symptoms (i.e., gradual vs. sudden)
- Nature of symptoms (e.g., wheezing, chest pain, intermittent versus continuous, associated cough, sputum production, fever)
- Exclusion of other causes of shortness of breath (e.g., heart failure, pulmonary embolus)
- Exclusion of other causes of wheezing (e.g., bronchospasm from allergic reaction, endobronchial tumor)
- Consideration of paradoxical vocal cord closure on inspiration (i.e., vocal cord dysfunction)

by a poor correlation between reported symptoms and peak expiratory flow (PEF) values. These are patients for whom home monitoring of PEF is strongly indicated.

Patients in whom sudden, severe attacks develop or those who have severe, slowly progressive disease are also at increased risk. A history of marked diurnal variation in forced expiratory volume in 1 second (FEV_1) is believed to be a risk factor, but this could simply be related to its being a marker for increased bronchial responsiveness. Historical data indicate that female sex, endotracheal intubation, and prolonged neuromuscular blockade are associated with a more prolonged hospital stay, whereas elevated arterial CO_2 level and lower arterial pH within 24 hours of admission are associated with increased mortality.

Although not widely identified as a true marker of increased risk, the use of inhaled heroin is also frequently associated with near-fatal or fatal attacks of asthma. It is not known whether this is due to a direct effect of the inhaled drug (or its diluents), the degree of airflow limitation, or simply the impaired judgment of the user, which delays arrival at the ED and initiation of appropriate care. However, opioids have long been known to cause bronchoconstriction via mast cell degranulation and histamine release. Although most reports of severe asthma attacks after inhalation of narcotics involve patients with known asthma, they have also been reported in patients without any history of asthma.

4. How should one treat a severe asthma attack?
   - **Oxygen therapy** to achieve an arterial oxygen saturation of 90% or greater.
   - **β-Agonists:** Short-acting beta agonists are the first-line therapy in an acute asthma attack. It is now widely accepted that the inhaled forms of these drugs are superior to the subcutaneous or intravenous (IV) route, with fewer adverse effects, and their administration can be repeated up to three times within the first hour after presentation while monitoring for adverse effects such as tachyarrhythmia and lactic acidosis, the latter of which can be underrecognized. The hyperlactatemia has no clinical significance. Some studies have shown that continuous nebulization significantly reduces hospital admission, with no noticeable increase in side effects when compared with intermittent nebulization. Albuterol is most widely used. Some have suggested using levo-albuterol if the patient has severe tachycardia, but that is more expensive and no randomized trials have found it to be superior to racemic albuterol. The subcutaneous route is still reserved for patients who have such severe dyspnea that they are unable to take deep-enough breaths, but these are usually the patients who later undergo intubation. Metered-dose inhalers are as effective for aerosolized delivery provided that good technique is used with a spacer device. Nebulized or aerosolized delivery is still used frequently in the ED, in part from convention and in part because less instruction and observation are needed to ensure good delivery. Long-acting beta agonists like salmeterol are not recommended as monotherapy during acute asthma. The use of salmeterol as outpatient monotherapy has been shown to increase the risk of hospitalization. However, this increased risk was not seen among patients receiving combined therapy with inhaled corticosteroids and salmeterol (Table 28.1).
   - **Corticosteroids:** These drugs also play a key role in treatment; the typical dosage of methylprednisolone is 60-80 mg IV every 6-12 hours for ICU patients or 40-60 mg every 12-24 hours for hospitalized, non-ICU patients for the first few days of a hospitalization. Then the dose decreases to 40-60 mg orally per day. This must be delivered as soon as possible because peak onset of action can take several hours. Therapy is typically administered every 6 hours until the attack appears to be subsiding and then gradually tapered over days to weeks. A recent Cochrane meta-analysis lacks strong evidence to support high-dose steroid over low-dose or long duration over a short course. This should be individualized. Comparisons between oral prednisone and IV corticosteroids have not demonstrated differences in the rate of improvement of lung function or in the length of the hospital stay. Thus the oral route is preferred for patients with normal mental status and without conditions expected to interfere with gastrointestinal absorption. There is conflicting evidence that an inhaled corticosteroid (ICS) in addition to a systemic steroid reduces risk of admission, but there is insufficient evidence that ICS therapy results in significant changes in pulmonary function or clinical measures when used in addition to systemic steroid during acute asthma.
   - **Anticholinergics:** Many studies have shown a marginal benefit from adding inhaled ipratropium to β-agonist therapy (vs. β-agonists alone) in the treatment of acute asthma.
   - **Aminophylline:** Oral theophylline is a third-line agent in the outpatient management of asthma. This is in part due to the recognition of its intrinsic anti-inflammatory properties, even at serum levels lower than those once thought necessary to achieve significant benefit. However, the use of IV aminophylline in the treatment of acute asthma remains controversial and is generally not recommended, although there is some support for its use in children.
   - **Inhaled epinephrine:** A meta-analysis of using inhaled epinephrine in refractory asthma demonstrated a similar degree of bronchodilation and PEF improvement when compared with albuterol.

Table 28-1. Primary Pharmacologic Treatment of Acute Asthma*

AGENT	DOSE	COMMENTS
β-Agonists	• 4–8 puffs (90 µg/puff) MDI + spacer, every 20 min up to 4 h, then every 1–4 h as needed or • 2.5–5 mg nebulized every 20 min for three doses, then every 1–4 h as needed	• Inhaled better than subcutaneous or IV. • MDI + spacer works as well as nebulized. • Elevated lactate levels seen after high doses.
Corticosteroids	Initial dose for the first few days of a hospitalization is usually 60-80 mg IV every 6-12 hours for ICU patients or 40-60 mg every 12-24 hours for hospitalized, non-ICU patients. Subsequently, the dose typically decreases to 40-60 mg orally per day.	There is no standardized dosing—it depends mainly on clinical context; but less dose is advocated because of side effects. A single 160-mg intramuscular depot injection of methylprednisolone has been found to be as effective as an 8-day tapering course of the same dose of oral methylprednisolone once patients discharged.
Anticholinergics	• 8 puffs (18 µg/puff) MDI + spacer, every 20 min as needed up to 3 h or • 0.5 mg (500 µg) nebulized every 20 min for three doses, then as needed	• Improves lung function and reduces rate of hospitalization when added to standard care. • Combined use with inhaled β-agonists is beneficial.
Oxygen	• Titrate to SaO$_2$ >92%	• Avoid excessive oxygenation, which can result in CO$_2$ retention • Use humidified oxygen

*Per EPR3 Guidelines for treatment of acute asthma in adult patients.
Other agents (magnesium sulfate, heliox, leukotriene antagonists, inhaled anesthetics) discussed in text. IV, intravenous; MDI, metered-dose inhaler; PEF, peak expiratory flow; PO, orally, SaO$_2$, oxygen saturation.

The use of inhaled epinephrine is safer than IV epinephrine, which is associated with a higher risk of acute myocardial infarction and tachyarrhythmias. However, there is no evidence to support the routine use of epinephrine in acute asthma.
• **Inhaled anesthetic agents:** In patients with ongoing severe bronchospasm receiving mechanical ventilation despite aggressive conventional treatment, inhaled anesthetic agents can be used for their intrinsic properties of bronchodilation. Because their delivery requires a special apparatus and conventional therapy is usually more effective, their use is often seen as a rescue therapy only. Isoflurane or enflurane are the agents of choice. There is also some evidence to support the use of ketamine in acute asthma, particularly in children, but further studies will be needed to validate this.
• **Antibiotics:** There is no benefit to the routine use of antibiotics in the management of an acute asthma episode unless findings are suspicious for pneumonia or other bacterial infections.
• **Leukotriene receptor antagonists**: A recent randomized, controlled trial does not show any benefit of adding oral montelukast over conventional treatment in the management of an acute asthma attack. Interestingly, IV montelukast has shown some efficacy in terms of bronchodilation, but it is not recommended clinically for acute asthma.

5. Does magnesium sulfate offer any benefit in the treatment of status asthmaticus?
   Although a small number of controlled trials have yielded mixed results, one controlled study suggests that patients with severe asthma (FEV$_1$ <25% predicted) treated with IV magnesium sulfate in the ED had significantly reduced admission rates compared with those treated with placebo. A more recent meta-analysis did not support these findings. There is no 28-day mortality benefit of using IV magnesium. The 3Mg trial showed no benefit of using nebulized magnesium over placebo. Proposed mechanisms of possible benefit are as follows:
   • Blockage of calcium channels and reduced calcium entry into smooth muscle cells, leading to bronchodilation

- Possible inhibition of mast cell degranulation
- Improved respiratory muscle function due to correction of lower baseline serum levels
    Because the only reported adverse side effects from a single dose of magnesium are flushing, mild fatigue, or burning at the IV site, its use in the treatment of persons with severe asthma may be warranted by its potential for lowering admission rates, but this remains a controversial topic. Magnesium sulfate is generally delivered as 2 g in 50 mL of normal saline solution given IV over a 20-minute period.

6. How can one best decide when to admit a patient and when to discharge a patient from the emergency department?

    Patients who have a poor response to treatment are defined by persistent wheezing, dyspnea, and accessory muscle use at rest despite 3 hours of treatment in the ED. Such patients should be admitted to the hospital. One study suggests that in persons with severe asthma (PEF and FEV_1 <35% of predicted), improvement in PEF measured 30 minutes after initiation of therapy may be an early predictor of response to treatment after 3 hours. Any patient with worsening PEF, rising $PaCO_2$, or advancing fatigue should, at the very least, be monitored in the intensive care unit and possibly undergo intubation. A classification tree for use in risk stratification for hospital admission for acute asthma has been developed. This validated scheme involves three key variables, history of hospitalization, peak flow, and oxygenation, and was entitled the CHOP classification:

- **C**hange in PEF severity category
- History of prior **H**ospitalization for asthma
- **O**xygen saturation with room air
- Initial **P**eak expiratory flow

    Signs of good response to therapy in the ED that would allow a patient to be discharged include a sustained response of at least 1 hour after the last treatment with FEV_1 or PEF equal to or greater than 70% predicted, no distress, and improvement in physical examination results. The Expert Panel Report 3 (EPR3) guidelines emphasize that such patients should be instructed to continue their therapy at home with inhaled short-acting β-agonists; be given a 3- to 10-day course of oral corticosteroids; should be considered for initiation of inhaled corticosteroids; should receive education on medications, inhaler technique, and use of a written action plan and possibly a PEF meter; and should arrange for medical follow-up within the next 1 to 4 weeks.

7. Which patients need to be supported by mechanical ventilation?

    Any patient with progressive lethargy, somnolence, near exhaustion, unresponsiveness, apnea, near apnea, or cardiopulmonary arrest should be intubated and supported by mechanical ventilation. An elevated $PaCO_2$ level on admission, although shown to be associated with increased mortality, may not necessarily warrant immediate endotracheal intubation. Any patient with a progressive rise in $PaCO_2$ despite therapy and increasing fatigue most likely will require intubation. Other potential indicators of the need for intubation would include a silent chest, inability to maintain oxygenation by mask (oxygen saturation <90%), and visible cyanosis. Other relative indications are coexistent medical conditions that can increase minute ventilation requirements or compromise oxygen delivery, such as sepsis, myocardial infarction, metabolic acidosis, or life-threatening arrhythmias.

8. Is normocapnia or hypercapnia an absolute indication for intubation in a person with asthma?

    Most persons with severe asthma are initially seen with hypocapnia because of the hyperventilation associated with dyspnea and hypoxemia. A normal or elevated $PaCO_2$ is usually a sign of fatigue but can also be due to a high dead space–to–tidal volume ratio resulting from air trapping and ineffective ventilation of noncommunicating segments of lung. In either case, it should be taken seriously and can be a sign of impending respiratory failure. Studies indicate, however, that most patients with normal or elevated $PaCO_2$ on blood gas analysis at initial evaluation improve with time in response to conventional therapy and do not require intubation. Analysis of the end-tidal capnography waveform can be used in nonintubated patients to monitor improvement in acute asthma, but the absolute value of the partial pressure of end-tidal CO_2 ($P_{ET}CO_2$) may be inaccurate due to extreme ventilation heterogeneity in asthma. Accordingly, correlation with arterial blood gas is recommended and the monitoring of trends in $P_{ET}CO_2$ is more important than the absolute value. Because mechanical ventilation in severe asthma can be complicated by increased air trapping and barotrauma, it is advisable not to perform intubation and mechanical ventilation in a patient with acute asthma merely on the basis of an elevated $PaCO_2$ unless concomitant somnolence, progressive fatigue, or worsening acidosis exists.

9. Can noninvasive mechanical ventilation be used safely to avoid intubation in a person with asthma?

Noninvasive positive-pressure ventilation (NIPPV) via face mask has been shown to be safe and effective when applied to a patient with severe asthma and hypercapnia whose condition fails to improve with conventional therapy. It can be effective in unloading respiratory muscles, improving dyspnea, lowering respiratory rate, and improving gas exchange. NIPPV has been shown to be an effective potential means of avoiding endotracheal intubation and may also help avoid the need for reintubation after extubation. However, it is also critical to determine early in a patient's course whether he or she is responding appropriately to NIPPV, because delays in endotracheal intubation may be associated with worse outcomes. NIPPV should not be used in persons with asthma who have life-threatening hypoxemia, somnolence, or hemodynamic instability; it should be aborted in patients whose condition fails to improve or who cannot tolerate the mask.

10. What about using high-flow oxygen via nasal cannula in acute asthma?

High-flow oxygen allows the delivery of a very high oxygen concentration and flow and is playing an increasingly important role in treating patients with acute hypoxemic respiratory failure. The typical patient with acute asthma has respiratory failure mainly on the basis of hypercarbia and not hypoxemia; thus noninvasive ventilation may be a more rational first choice for ventilatory support. However, there is some evidence that the high flow of gas provided by high-flow nasal cannula may provide a small degree of CPAP and therefore offload some of the work of breathing and provide dead space washout, so it may be worth trying if hypercarbic respiratory failure is not a prominent feature of acute asthma.

11. Are helium admixtures of any proven benefit in treating severe asthma?

When helium (He) is blended with oxygen (in a 20% O_2, 80% He or 30% O_2, 70% He mixture), the gas density becomes approximately one-third that of room air and viscosity is increased, leading to increased laminar flow and a reduction in airway resistance in areas of greatest turbulent flow. This can result in a reduction in the work of breathing required to meet the same minute ventilation requirement when breathing room air. Because work of breathing is reduced, it would seem likely that respiratory fatigue might be delayed until conventional therapy has had time to take effect. Despite numerous trials and two meta-analyses, no evidence yet exists that helium-oxygen (heliox) admixtures can prevent the need for endotracheal intubation. However, heliox has been shown to improve PEF and reduce the degree of pulsus paradoxus in acute asthma attacks. This is presumably due to the decrease in airway resistance and lower generated negative pleural pressures but also possibly due to improved expiratory flow and less dynamic hyperinflation (DHI). The improved laminar flow afforded by heliox may also allow deeper lung deposition of inhaled aerosols. Because heliox mixtures typically include only 20% to 30% oxygen, hypoxemia is a barrier to the use of heliox. However, when the patient does not have hypoxemia, it is safe and worthwhile to use, particularly in those with fatigue and hypercapnia who are at risk for progressing to the point of requiring mechanical ventilation. A recent meta-analysis has shown that heliox-driven nebulization of albuterol significantly decreased the risk of hospitalization and improved PEF over oxygen-driven nebulization.

12. What is the best approach when a patient requires intubation?

Intubation: Blind nasoendotracheal intubation is often better tolerated by an awake patient, but oral endotracheal intubation is the preferred method of intubation because it permits the use of an endotracheal tube (ETT) with a larger internal diameter. This will lead to lower resistance within the respiratory circuit and allow easier deep suctioning of secretions and mucous plugs. It is important to remember that the resistance of a tube is indirectly proportional to its internal radius (to the fourth power), and the resistance of an 8-mm ETT is roughly one-half that of a 7-mm ETT. Oral intubation is indicated for patients with apnea and cyanosis.

Intubation in a person with asthma is often difficult and may induce laryngospasm or lead to increased bronchospasm, so it should be performed by the most experienced person available and rapid-sequence technique should be used. Because of its intrinsic sympathomimetic and bronchodilating properties, ketamine has been advocated by many as the induction agent of choice to avoid the possible loss of sympathetic tone and drug-induced vasodilation, thus helping to prevent cardiovascular collapse. The usual dose of ketamine for intubation is 1 to 2 mg/kg given IV over a 2-minute period. Sedation is usually necessary, and although sometimes warranted, paralysis should be avoided if possible. Barbiturates such as thiopental should not be used because of their association with histamine release and potential worsening of bronchoconstriction. Although the narcotic fentanyl is often

useful because it inhibits airway reflexes and causes less histamine release than morphine, one should be aware of its potential to trigger bronchoconstriction and laryngospasm.
- **Avoiding potential complications:** Some authors advocate using a hand bag to ventilate patients with asthma immediately after intubation to assess the severity of bronchospasm and avoid DHI by slowly delivering a rate of 4 to 5 breaths per minute as a bridge to mechanical ventilation. Ensuring adequate humidification of inspired gas is particularly important to prevent thickening of secretions and drying of airway mucosa, which can promote mucous plugging and further bronchospasm.

13. What ventilator settings should be used?
- The best mode of ventilation is one that minimizes minute ventilation and allows for sufficient exhalation time to minimize DHI while also trying to maintain oxygen saturation above 92% (use 100% oxygen initially) (Box 28.2). This can generally be achieved with low tidal volumes of 6 to 8 mL/kg, a respiratory rate of 8 to 10 breaths per minute, minimal added positive end-expiratory pressure (PEEP), and moderate inspiratory flow rates of 80 to 90 L/min. Decelerating flow waveforms may improve overall flow distribution and hence optimize gas exchange. Higher inspiratory flow rates with square waveforms allow for a shorter inspiratory time and hence, at the same respiratory rate, a longer expiratory time. It is the longer expiratory time, and not just the inspiratory-to-expiratory ratio, that is critical to limiting DHI. Lowering total minute ventilation is the most crucial goal, because a longer expiratory time and smaller burden of volume to be exhaled minimize DHI. Intentional hypoventilation with low minute volumes can significantly reduce the risk of DHI and barotrauma. Thus allowing for a maximum $PaCO_2$ of 80 mm Hg or a minimum pH of 7.20 is a safe and acceptable practice when performing ventilation in patients with severe airflow limitation. However, because an elevated $PaCO_2$ can increase cerebral perfusion, such use of "permissive hypercapnia" should be avoided in patients with intracranial bleeding, edema, or space-occupying brain lesions.

14. What are the complications of mechanical ventilation in these patients?
- **DHI:** When airflow limitation is severe, the next ventilated breath can be initiated before the lungs can fully empty to a normal functional residual capacity, resulting in progressive air trapping. This leads to DHI and elevated end-expiratory alveolar pressures, referred to as *intrinsic positive end-expiratory pressure* (PEEP$_i$). The measurement of PEEP$_i$ can be problematic, and it is often underestimated by the brief end-expiratory pause used to estimate it on the ventilator. This is due to the heterogeneous distribution of early airway closure, which can prevent many hyperinflated segments from communicating their alveolar pressures to the transducer at the airway opening. Ideally, PEEP$_i$ should be kept below 15 cm H_2O. The key determinants of DHI are minute ventilation, tidal volume, exhalation time, and severity of airflow limitation. DHI can often be predicted by elevated plateau pressures and failure to achieve zero expiratory flow before the next delivered breath. DHI can lead to less effective respiratory muscle contraction and added work because of less optimal curvature of the diaphragm, which in turn can lead to less effective triggering of the ventilator. DHI can also lead to decreased venous return and right ventricular preload, increased right ventricular afterload (via extrinsic compression of the pulmonary vasculature), and decreased left ventricular compliance, which can all lead to diminished cardiac output and hypotension. When DHI is strongly suspected, the best immediate solution (and test) is to briefly disconnect the ETT from the ventilator circuit to allow for more complete exhalation. The other concern with DHI is that the high degree of associated PEEP$_i$ can ultimately lead to barotrauma.

Box 28-2. Principles of Management of Mechanical Ventilation in Acute Asthma

The goal is to minimize DHI through the use of the following:
- Minimal minute ventilation (low tidal volumes [e.g., 6–8 mL/kg]), low respiratory rate (8–10 beats per minute)
- Minimal (or zero) PEEP
- Relatively high inspiratory flow rate (80–100 L/min), to reduce inspiratory time
- Maintenance of plateau pressures ≤35 cm H_2O, and PEEP$_i$ ≤15 cm H_2O
- Permissive hypercapnia up to 80 mm Hg (contraindicated in patients with intracranial bleeding, cerebral edema, or a space-occupying lesion), while trying to maintain pH ≥ 7.20

DHI, dynamic hyperinflation; *PEEP*, positive end-expiratory pressure.

- **Barotrauma:** High airway pressures can potentially lead to pulmonary interstitial emphysema, subcutaneous emphysema, pneumomediastinum, pneumothorax, and even pneumoperitoneum. Barotrauma correlates directly with the degree of DHI. Plateau pressures are traditionally thought to be a good indicator of the degree of DHI, and a level below 35 cm H_2O is still a widely recommended upper limit of plateau pressure for minimizing barotrauma. However, one study has shown that elevated end-inspiratory lung volume (the exhaled volume measured from end inspiration to the relaxation volume during a period of apnea) may be a more reliable predictor of barotrauma than are airway pressures. The most feared consequence of barotrauma is tension pneumothorax, typically characterized by a precipitous rise in airway pressures (peak and plateau), a drop in oxygen saturation, hypotension, tachycardia, unilaterally absent breath sounds and chest excursions, and possibly tracheal deviation. Tension pneumothorax is a clinical diagnosis and, if strongly suspected in a patient in unstable condition, should be treated immediately with needle thoracotomy followed by chest tube placement. Bedside ultrasound of the lung is being more commonly used to quickly diagnose pneumothorax without the need to wait for a chest x-ray. Bedside ultrasound is more sensitive than chest x-ray in diagnosing pneumothorax. Fatal air embolism may also occur because of barotrauma.

15. What is the role of sedation?
    - **Sedation:** Agitation and inadequate sedation can lead to hyperventilation and asynchrony with the mechanical ventilator and hence DHI and unacceptably high airway pressures with increased risk of barotrauma. Deep anesthesia with benzodiazepines or propofol is often necessary to achieve optimal control and prevent dyssynchrony between patient and ventilator, especially in using intentional hypoventilation and permissive hypercapnia. Paralytics should and often can be avoided if sufficient levels of sedatives are used.

16. Can added positive end-expiratory pressure help reduce air trapping in patients with asthma who are receiving mechanical ventilation?
    Some argue that added PEEP can help minimize air trapping by *stenting* open peripheral airways. Although this may be true to some extent in patients with emphysema and easily collapsible central airways, it is unlikely to be of much benefit in persons with severe asthma. In the classic model of airflow limitation, airway collapse occurs when the extraluminal pressure overcomes intraluminal pressures (and any architectural properties of the airway itself). In patients who already have significant $PEEP_i$, and in whom distal alveolar pressures already exceed extraluminal pressures at end-expiration, added PEEP will likely only increase distal alveolar pressures and worsen hyperinflation. It is important to remember that, because DHI can occur even in the absence of airflow limitation if the respiratory rate is high enough, the previously mentioned strategies are still best for minimizing DHI. However, once patients begin to recover and breathe spontaneously while using the ventilator, it is important to add sufficient PEEP to reduce the work of breathing necessary to trigger the next breath.

ACKNOWLEDGMENT

The authors wish to acknowledge Dr. Ali Al-Alwan, MD, for the valuable contributions to the previous edition of this chapter.

KEY POINTS: ASTHMA

Assessment and Treatment of Acute Asthma

1. Risk factors for acute asthma include poor perception of symptoms, poor compliance with therapy, lack of medical insurance, and previous hospitalization or intubation.
2. Examination findings suggesting impending respiratory failure in acute asthma include use of accessory muscles, inability to speak full sentences, inability to lie down, and a silent chest.
3. Patients with acute asthma should be admitted to the hospital when they have failed to respond to treatment in the ED within 3 hours or when they have a rising PCO_2.
4. Ventilator settings that minimize DHI and its complications include low minute ventilation (preferably via both reduced tidal volume and respiratory rate), high inspiratory flow rate to minimize inspiratory time, and no external PEEP.

BIBLIOGRAPHY

1. Camargo Jr CA, Gurner DM, Smithline HA, et al. A randomized placebo- controlled study of intravenous montelukast for the treatment of acute asthma. *J Allergy Clin Immunol.* 2010;125:374-380.
2. Dennis RJ, Solarte I, Rodrigo G. Advances in acute asthma. [Review]. *Curr Opin Pulm Med.* 2015;21(1):22-26.
3. Edmonds ML, Camargo Jr CA, Pollack Jr CV, et al. Early use of inhaled corticosteroids in the emergency department treatment of acute asthma (Cochrane review). *Cochrane Database Syst Rev.* 2001;(1):CD002308. doi:10.1002/14651858. CD002308.pub2.
4. Gallegos-Solórzano MC, Perez-Padilla R, Hernandez-Zenteno RJ. Usefulness of inhaled magnesium sulfate in the coadjuvant management of severe asthma crisis in an emergency department. *Pulm Pharmacol Ther.* 2010;23:432-437.
5. Goodacre S, Cohen J, Bradburn M, et al. The 3Mg trial: a randomised controlled trial of intravenous or nebulised magnesium sulphate versus placebo in adults with acute severe asthma. *Health Technol Assess.* 2014;18(22):1-168.
6. Griswold SK, Nordstrom CR, Clark S, et al. Asthma exacerbations in North American adults: Who are the "frequent fliers" in the emergency department? *Chest.* 2005;127:1579-1586.
7. Hodder R, Lougheed MD, FitzGerald JM, et al. Management of acute asthma in adults in the emergency department: assisted ventilation. *CMAJ.* 2010;182:265-272.
8. Hodder R, Lougheed MD, Rowe BH, et al. Management of acute asthma in adults in the emergency department: nonventilatory management. *CMAJ.* 2010;182:E55-E67.
9. Holley AD, Boots RJ. Review article: management of acute severe and near-fatal asthma. *Emerg Med Australas.* 2009;21:259-268.
10. Howe TA, Jaalam K, Ahmed R. et al. The use of end-tidal capnography to monitor non-intubated patients presenting with acute exacerbation of asthma in the emergency department. *J Emerg Med.* 2011;41(6):581-589.
11. Lazarus SC. Emergency treatment of asthma. *N Engl J Med.* 2010;363:755-764.
12. Lugogo NL, MacIntyre NR. Life-threatening asthma: pathophysiology and management. *Respir Care.* 2008;53:726-735.
13. National Heart, Lung, and Blood Institute. *Expert Panel Report 3 (EPR3): Guidelines for the Diagnosis and Management of Asthma. Section 5: Managing exacerbations of asthma.* Bethesda, MD: National Heart, Lung, and Blood Institute; 2007.
14. Normansell R, Kew KM, Mansour G. Different oral corticosteroid regimens for acute asthma. (Cochrane Review). *Cochrane Database Syst Rev.* 2016;(5):CD011801. doi:10.1002/14651858.CD011801.pub2.
15. Ram FS, Wellington S, Rowe BH, et al. Non-invasive positive pressure ventilation for treatment of respiratory failure due to severe acute exacerbations of asthma. *Cochrane Database Syst Rev.* 2005;(3):CD004360. doi:10.1002/14651858.CD004360.pub4.
16. Rodrigo GJ, Castro-Rodriguez JA. Heliox-driven beta2-agonists nebulization for children and adults with acute asthma: a systematic review with meta-analysis (Review). *Ann Allergy Asthma Immunol.* 2014;112(1):29-34.
17. Rodrigo GJ. Comparison of inhaled fluticasone with intravenous hydrocortisone in the treatment of adult acute asthma. *Am J Respir Crit Care Med.* 2005;171:1231-1236.
18. Rodrigo GJ, Nannini LJ. Comparison between nebulized adrenaline and beta2 agonists for the treatment of acute asthma. A meta-analysis of randomized trials. *Am J Emerg Med.* 2006;24:217-222.
19. Rodrigo G, Rodrigo C, Pollack CV, et al. Use of helium-oxygen mixtures in the treatment of acute asthma: a systematic review. *Chest.* 2003;123:891-896.
20. Sarwar Zubairi AB, Salahuddin N, Khawaja A, et al. A randomized, double-blind, placebo-controlled trial of oral montelukast in acute asthma exacerbation. *BMC Pulm Med.* 2013;13:20.
21. Traver AH, Milan SJ, Camargo Jr CA, et al. Addition of intravenous beta(2)-agonists to inhaled beta(2)-agonists for acute asthma (Cochrane review). *Cochrane Database Syst Rev.* 2012;12:CD010179. doi:10.1002/14651858. CD010179.
22. Tsai CL, Clark S, Camargo Jr CA. Risk stratification for hospitalization in acute asthma: the CHOP classification tree. *Am J Emerg Med.* 2010;28:803-808.

CHAPTER 29

CHRONIC OBSTRUCTIVE PULMONARY DISEASE

Charlotte C. Teneback and Timothy Leclair

1. **What is chronic obstructive pulmonary disease?**
   Chronic obstructive pulmonary disease (COPD) is a systemic disease characterized by airflow limitation that is not fully reversible; thus spirometry is required to make the diagnosis. This should be done when the patient is clinically stable and not acutely ill. Chronic airflow limitation results from a combination of small airways disease and parenchymal destruction due to inflammatory processes. In addition to pulmonary disease, COPD patients often have significant muscle weakness, balance problems, and other systemic disease manifestations.

2. **How many people are affected by chronic obstructive pulmonary disease?**
   COPD is the third-ranked cause of death in the United States, killing more than 120,000 individuals each year. The number of people affected by COPD worldwide continues to increase because of exposure to tobacco smoke and aging of the population. Historically the prevalence of disease was higher in men, but, with changing patterns of exposure to tobacco, women are now affected as frequently as men. Worldwide, exposure to indoor pollution from heating and cooking fuels substantially contributes to COPD in women.

3. **What processes are involved in the pathogenesis of chronic obstructive pulmonary disease?**
   COPD is characterized by chronic inflammation throughout the lung, with increased neutrophils, macrophages, and CD8+ T lymphocytes. An imbalance between proteinase-antiproteinase activity and oxidative stress contributes to the pathogenesis, but the primary injury is thought to be caused by human leukocyte elastase in combination with proteinase-3 and macrophage-derived matrix metalloproteinases (MMPs), cysteine proteinases, and a plasminogen activator. These, together with free radicals produced by chemicals found in cigarette smoke and other environmental exposures, cause apoptosis and cell death.

4. **How is severity graded in chronic obstructive pulmonary disease?**
   Once airflow obstruction is determined by forced expiratory volume in 1 second (FEV1)/forced vital capacity (FVC) ratio less than 0.70 or less than the lower limit of normal (both are used and there is some controversy regarding the best cutoff), severity can be assessed using one of several grading systems. One used commonly is the Global Initiative for Chronic Obstructive Lung Disease (GOLD) guidelines which stages severity based on airflow limitation (Table 29.1) as well as symptoms and frequency of exacerbations.

5. **What are the benefits of smoking cessation for a patient with chronic obstructive pulmonary disease?**
   Smoking cessation is the most effective intervention to attenuate the progression of COPD, as well as improve survival and reduce morbidity. Ideally smoking cessation should utilize a support program in combination with two forms of nicotine replacement therapy and varenicline or bupropion sustained release for 3 months. If successful, the rate of decline in the FEV_1 may be reduced. In some cases the rate of decline may be reduced to the rate found in healthy nonsmokers (± 30 mL/year).

6. **Why are bronchodilators used in the treatment of chronic obstructive pulmonary disease?**
   Bronchodilators treat airway obstruction in patients with COPD. By reducing bronchomotor tone, they decrease airway resistance, which can improve airflow. This will improve emptying of the lungs and reduce hyperinflation. Acutely ill patients are often unable to use metered-dose inhalers, and other similar delivery devices, and may require nebulized bronchodilators in order to achieve maximum benefit, though data on this is inconclusive. Both anticholinergic and β_2-adrenergic medications can and should be used during acute exacerbations. Short-acting preparations are preferred in this setting.

Table 29-1. Staging of Severity of Airflow Limitation in Chronic Obstructive Pulmonary Disease

STAGE/SEVERITY	SPIROMETRIC RESULTS IN PATIENT WITH FEV_1/FVC <70% OR <LLN
0. At risk	Normal spirometry Chronic symptoms (e.g., cough, sputum production) and exposure to known risk factors
I. Mild COPD	$FEV_1 \geq 80\%$ predicted
II. Moderate COPD	$50\% \leq FEV_1 <80\%$ predicted
III. Severe COPD	$30\% \leq FEV_1 <50\%$ predicted
IV. Very severe COPD	$FEV_1 <30\%$ predicted or $FEV_1 <50\%$ predicted plus chronic respiratory failure

FEV_1, forced expiratory volume in 1 second; FVC, forced vital capacity; LLN, lower limit of normal.

7. **Why are anticholinergic agents used in the treatment of chronic obstructive pulmonary disease?**
   These medications inhibit cholinergically mediated bronchomotor tone and also block vagally mediated reflex arcs that cause bronchoconstriction. Ipratropium is short-acting and has a duration of action of 6 to 8 hours. Alcinidium bromide and tiotropium bromide are more potent and have a longer duration of action, allowing twice and once-daily administration, respectively. Both have been shown to significantly reduce the frequency of COPD exacerbations and to improve quality of life. Caution should be used in prescribing these drugs to older males with COPD as they can increase the risk of urinary retention.

8. **Why are β_2-Adrenergic adrenergic agonists used in the treatment of chronic obstructive pulmonary disease?**
   β_2-adrenergic agents act on the surface of airway smooth muscle. These drugs increase intracellular cyclic adenosine monophosphate and cause relaxation. Inhaled, short-acting β_2-adrenergic agents are readily absorbed systemically and can lead to numerous systemic adverse effects, such as tachycardia, tremor, and arrhythmias. Long-acting inhaled β_2-adrenergic agents are more effective and convenient but more expensive.

9. **Can patients with chronic obstructive pulmonary disease benefit from monotherapy with combined β_2-adrenergic agonist and anticholinergic medications?**
   The SPARK trial showed that patients with severe COPD who took a once-daily fixed-dose combination of indacaterol (a β_2-agonist) and glycopyrronium (a muscarinic antagonist) had very modest improvement in lung function (FEV_1 improved by 100 mL) and a reduction in exacerbation rate compared with monotherapy with glycopyrronium or tiotropium. Although other studies have been published revealing favorable results, concern remains about the potential increased risk of acute coronary syndrome or heart failure associated with combination therapy. If used, such agents should be considered in patients without significant cardiac disease (Wedzicha JA, et al, 2013).

10. **What role do phosphodiesterase inhibitors play in the treatment of chronic obstructive pulmonary disease?**
    Phosphodiesterase (PDE) inhibitors increase cyclic adenosine monophosphate (cAMP) and cause airway dilation. Theophylline is a nonspecific PDE inhibitor. Owing to its narrow therapeutic window, weak beta agonist activity, and adverse event profile—which includes cardiac arrhythmia and stroke—it is primarily used for patients with severe disease or those who cannot tolerate inhaled medication. Roflumilast and cilomaslast specifically target PDE-4, reducing inflammation by inhibiting the breakdown of intracellular cAMP; they appear to reduce the risk of exacerbations in patients with severe COPD and chronic bronchitis.

11. **Can methylxanthines be used to treat chronic obstructive pulmonary disease?**
    Methylxanthines are weak bronchodilators but have multiple other effects that might be important: an inotropic effect on diaphragmatic muscle, reduced muscle fatigue, increased mucociliary clearance

and central respiratory drive, and some anti-inflammatory effects. Because of the potential for toxicity, other bronchodilators are preferred when available. Methylxanthines are contraindicated in the setting of PDE use and should not be used in the acute setting.

12. **When are inhaled corticosteroids beneficial in chronic obstructive pulmonary disease?**
Inhaled corticosteroids in combination with long-acting bronchodilators have been recommended for patients with severe disease (FEV$_1$ <50% predicted) and recurrent exacerbations. Recent data, however, suggests that inhaled corticosteroids are overprescribed and often used for patients with less severe disease. Several studies have suggested that it is likely safe to withdraw inhaled corticosteroids in most low-risk COPD patients. They are not beneficial during acute illness.

13. **What other pharmacologic treatments may benefit patients with chronic obstructive pulmonary disease?**
    - **α1-Antitrypsin replacement:** This is recommended for patients with emphysema related to deficiency of α_1-antitrypsin, with low levels of residual activity, who are nonsmokers.
    - **Vaccines:** Patients with COPD are at risk for increased morbidity and mortality from respiratory tract infections. Pneumococcal and influenza vaccinations, both alone and in combination, have been shown to reduce hospitalizations and mortality rates.
    - **Opiates:** Patients with severe COPD who have a constant sensation of breathlessness will benefit from this drug class. However, caution should be used when prescribing and monitoring patients taking opiates as they may have an increased risk of death.

14. **Are chronic antibiotics useful in treating patients with stable chronic obstructive pulmonary disease?**
Macrolide therapy has been shown decrease airway inflammation and exacerbation frequency in patients with COPD. Careful selection should be made when considering who should be prescribed these drugs due to an increased risk for cardiac arrhythmia, qTc prolongation, and hearing loss. Moreover, evidence suggests that patients who continue to smoke will not likely benefit from these medications. It is important to note that macrolide therapy is used as an anti-inflammatory therapy rather than a strictly antimicrobial one.

15. **What is an exacerbation of chronic obstructive pulmonary disease?**
The GOLD report defines an exacerbation as an acute worsening of respiratory symptoms beyond normal day-to-day variations that leads to medication change. Symptoms typically include increased cough frequency, increased dyspnea, and/or increased sputum production or color.

16. **What organisms cause chronic obstructive pulmonary disease exacerbations?**
Bacteria and viruses cause COPD exacerbations. In mild exacerbations *Streptococcus pneumoniae* is common. As severity of COPD increases, *Haemophilus influenzae* and *Moraxella catarrhalis* become more common, and, in severe COPD, *Pseudomonas aeruginosa* may occur.

17. **Should patients with chronic obstructive pulmonary disease exacerbations receive empiric antibiotics?**
Antibiotics are indicated when patients have increased sputum purulence associated with increased sputum volume and/or dyspnea. Antibiotics are also administered to patients receiving mechanical ventilation for COPD exacerbation because studies have shown that withholding antibiotics in these patients may increase the risk of hospital-acquired pneumonia or death.

18. **What is the role of steroids in the treatment of chronic obstructive pulmonary disease exacerbations?**
Systemic glucocorticoids shorten the duration of the exacerbation and lead to faster improvements in lung function. Additionally, they may reduce the risk of relapse and require fewer hospital days. Modest doses, not exceeding 1 mg/kg of prednisone or equivalent, are likely sufficient even in intensive care unit (ICU) patients.

19. **What are the causes of acute respiratory failure in patients with chronic obstructive pulmonary disease?**
Causes include bronchial infection, pulmonary emboli, cardiac failure, pneumonia, pneumothorax, respiratory depression (usually by the injudicious use of sedatives or narcotic analgesic drugs), surgery (especially of the chest and upper abdomen), stopping of medications, or occasionally malnutrition.

20. **What defines acute respiratory failure in patients with chronic obstructive pulmonary disease?**
    - Hypoxemia (PaO$_2$ <60 mm Hg)
    - Hypercapnia (PaCO$_2$ >50–70 mm Hg)

- Respiratory acidosis (pH <7.35) associated with worsening of the patient's respiratory symptoms compared with baseline

21. **What are indications for admission to an intensive care unit for a patient with a chronic obstructive pulmonary disease exacerbation?**
    - Continued severe dyspnea despite initial emergency therapy including nebulized bronchodilators and systemic corticosteroids
    - Ongoing hypoxemia (PaO_2 <40 mm Hg) and/or severe respiratory acidosis (pH 7.25) despite oxygen therapy and noninvasive ventilation (NIV)
    - Hemodynamic instability and the need for vasopressors.

22. **What is the role of noninvasive ventilation in the treatment of chronic obstructive pulmonary disease exacerbations?**
    NIV has been used for patients with moderate to severe dyspnea and moderate to severe acidosis from a COPD exacerbation. A number of trials report improvements in acid-base balance, reduced $PaCO_2$, and decreased length of stay. Intubation rates are also reduced by NIV. Table 29.2 summarizes the indications and contraindications for NIV in COPD exacerbations. Somnolence alone is not a contraindication to noninvasive support as it may improve rapidly as ventilation improves. Invasive ventilation is indicated when noninvasive therapy fails or is contraindicated.

23. **Does high-flow oxygen by nasal cannula play a role in treating patients suffering from a chronic obstructive pulmonary disease exacerbation?**
    A high-flow nasal cannula (HFNC) is a device that provides oxygen at high flow rates. The high flow rates can produce low levels of positive pressure and may decrease physiologic dead space, which could decrease the work of breathing. Although this device may be used in COPD patients with hypoxemia and potentially reduce the likelihood of intubation, it should not be used in patients who have acute or acute on chronic hypercapnia as is provides little support of ventilation.

24. **Where should a central venous catheter ideally be placed in a patient with chronic obstructive pulmonary disease?**
    The optimal location is in the internal jugular vein. Placement of subclavian lines in patients with COPD is associated with a higher risk of pneumothorax due to significant hyperinflation of the lungs, especially in intubated patients. Although femoral access is an option, it is inferior to the internal jugular site due to infection and other risk factors.

25. **What is the prognosis for a patient requiring mechanical ventilation?**
    Many studies report reasonable short-term mortality rates (25%–30%) for patients requiring mechanical ventilation for a COPD exacerbation. Mortality is lower than that among patients with COPD requiring mechanical ventilation for non-COPD causes. High mortality rates in the long term occur in patients with poor lung function (FEV_1 <30%) before intubation and those with significant other comorbidities.

26. **What are the objectives of mechanical ventilation in patients with chronic obstructive pulmonary disease?**
    - Supporting oxygenation
    - Supporting ventilation
    - Minimizing the work of breathing
    - Avoiding dynamic hyperinflation

27. **What is the preferred mode of invasive mechanical ventilation in a chronic obstructive pulmonary disease exacerbation?**
    No mode of mechanical ventilation has been shown to be superior to another during a COPD exacerbation. In general, the principles of ventilation are to minimize hyperinflation by allowing adequate

Table 29-2. Indications and Contraindications for Noninvasive Ventilation in Chronic Exacerbations of Obstructive Pulmonary Disease

INDICATIONS	CONTRAINDICATIONS
Moderate to severe dyspnea	Altered mental status or inability to protect airway
Moderate to severe acidosis and hypercapnia	Craniofacial abnormalities making mask fit difficult
Moderate to severe tachypnea	High aspiration risk

expiratory time and avoiding high tidal volumes. Oxygen should be titrated to maintain an arterial partial pressure of approximately 60 mm Hg. Overventilation should be avoided: these patients frequently have hypercapnia and a compensatory metabolic alkalosis at baseline.

28. What modalities can be used to provide exercise therapy to critically ill patients in respiratory failure?
Early physical activity is important to decrease physical deconditioning, muscle weakness, and long-term deficits following an acute respiratory exacerbation. Passive leg cycle ergometers can be used even in unconscious patients for early mobility training. Joint mobilization, muscle stretching, and neuromuscular stimulation have also been successfully used. In conscious but intubated patients, specialized teams can train the patient in activities ranging from transferring from bed to chair to ambulating with or without support.

29. Who should get pulmonary rehabilitation?
Patients with a recent admission for a COPD exacerbation should be referred to pulmonary rehabilitation following discharge. Pulmonary rehabilitation has been shown to improve functional status, decrease dyspnea, and reduce healthcare use. It does not improve pulmonary function. Additional indications include
- Stable outpatients with moderate, severe, and very severe COPD
- Patients with advanced disease seeking lung transplantation

30. What are the indications for *chronic* noninvasive ventilatory support (biphasic positive airway pressure) in patients with chronic obstructive pulmonary disease?
Patients with advanced disease may benefit from chronic nocturnal noninvasive support, which can be initiated on an inpatient or outpatient basis. The current guidelines support therapy for those who meet the following criteria:
- Obstructive sleep apnea considered and ruled out
- Arterial blood gas with PCO_2 equal to or greater than 52 mm Hg
- Nocturnal desaturation to 88% or below for a minimum of 5 minutes on 2 L supplemental oxygen or the patient's current prescribed oxygen, whichever is higher.

ACKNOWLEDGMENT

The authors wish to acknowledge Dr. Anne E. Dixon, MA, BM, BCh, for the valuable contributions to the previous edition of this chapter.

KEY POINTS: CHRONIC OBSTRUCTIVE PULMONARY DISEASE

1. There is no single preferred mode of mechanical ventilation in COPD. The best mode is the one that achieves the ventilator goals of the individual patient.
2. Bronchodilators play a key role in the treatment of both acute exacerbations of COPD as well as in management of chronic symptoms.
3. Chronic macrolide therapy may have a benefit in select patients but is not without risk.

BIBLIOGRAPHY
1. Celli BR, MacNee W, ATS/ERS Taskforce. Standards for the diagnosis and treatment of patients with COPD: a summary of the ATS/ERS position paper. *Eur Respir J.* 2004;23:932-946.
2. Davidson AC, Banham S, Elliott M, et al. BTS/ICS Guidelines for the ventilator management of acute hypercapneic respiratory failure in adults. *Thorax.* 2016;(71 suppl 2):ii1-ii35.
3. *Global strategy for the diagnosis, management, and prevention of chronic obstructive pulmonary disease. Global initiative for Chronic Obstructive Lung Disease (GOLD) 2016.* Available at https://goldcopd.org. Accessed October 21, 2016.
4. Spruit MA, Singh SJ, Garvey C, et al. An Official American Thoracic Society/European Respiratory Society Statement: key concepts and advances in pulmonary rehabilitation. *Am J Respir Crit Care Med.* 2013;188(8):e13-e64.
5. Tunis S, Whyte J, Spencer F, et al. *Decision memo for non-invasive positive pressure RADs for COPD (CAG-00052).* Available at http://www.cms.gov. Accessed October 13, 2016.
6. Wedzicha JA, Decramer M, Ficker JH, et al. Analysis of chronic obstructive pulmonary disease exacerbations with the dual bronchodilator QVA149 compared with glycopyrronium and tiotropium [SPARK]: a randomised, double-blind, parallel-group study. *Lancet Resp Med.* 2013;1(3):199–209.
7. Yawn BP, Suissa S, Rossi A. Appropriate use of inhaled corticosteroids in COPD: the candidates for safe withdrawal. *NPJ Prim Care Respir Med.* 2016;26:16068.

CHAPTER 30

ACUTE RESPIRATORY FAILURE/ ACUTE RESPIRATORY DISTRESS SYNDROME

Timothy Leclair and Gilman D. Allen

1. **What is acute respiratory failure?**

   Acute respiratory failure (ARF) is a syndrome in which the respiratory system fails in gas exchange in either oxygenation, carbon dioxide elimination, or both. ARF can occur within minutes or over hours.

2. **What are the types of acute respiratory failure and how are they diagnosed?**

   ARF can involve either hypoxemia, hypercapnia, or a combination of both. The gold standard for the diagnosis of either of these causes is done using arterial blood gas analysis. An arterial partial pressure of oxygen (PaO_2) of less than 50 mm Hg while breathing ambient air defines hypoxemia, whereas partial pressure of carbon dioxide ($PaCO_2$) of greater than 50 mm Hg defines hypercapnia.

3. **What are the mechanisms and causes of hypoxemic respiratory failure?**

   Mechanisms of hypoxemia are as follows:
   - Ventilation/perfusion (V/Q) mismatch
   - Alveolar hypoventilation
   - Shunt: physiologic (alveolar level) and anatomic (proximal to lung)
   - Diffusion limitation
   - Low inspired oxygen fraction

   Common causes of hypoxemia and their respective primary mechanisms are as follows:
   - Chronic obstructive pulmonary disease (COPD): V/Q mismatch, diffusion limitation
   - Pneumonia, pulmonary edema, and acute respiratory distress syndrome (ARDS): V/Q mismatch and intrapulmonary shunt
   - Pulmonary fibrosis: diffusion limitation
   - Obesity: alveolar hypoventilation (and intrapulmonary shunt if atelectasis is present)
   - Pulmonary embolism: V/Q mismatch early in the disease process

4. **What are the mechanisms and causes of hypercapnic respiratory failure?**

   Mechanisms (all related to alveolar hypoventilation) are as follows:
   - Decreased central respiratory drive
   - Abnormalities of the chest wall, leading to excessive restriction
   - Airway abnormalities leading to excessive dead space or increased work of breathing and fatigue
   - Neuromuscular diseases (peripheral nervous system)

   Causes are as follows:
   - Severe asthma
   - Drug overdose
   - Myasthenia gravis
   - Cervical cord injuries
   - Brain stem injuries
   - Obesity and hypoventilation
   - Kyphoscoliosis

5. **What are the most important immediate goals of therapy for acute respiratory failure?**

   Hypoxemia is the major immediate threat to organ function; therefore initial goals should be directed toward oxygen supplementation and reversal or prevention of tissue hypoxia. Hypercapnia is generally better tolerated unless in the setting of sudden onset or associated severe acidosis, which can lead to cardiac arrest and death if not treated. Immediate goals for therapy are to enhance carbon dioxide

removal or buffer the blood if immediate removal is not attainable. Supplemental oxygen should be delivered to achieve a PaO_2 greater than 55 mm Hg. This can be achieved through several modalities including:
- Nasal prongs or face mask
- Biphasic positive-pressure noninvasive ventilation
- High-flow nasal cannula
- Mechanical ventilation

6. **What are the main indications for endotracheal intubation and mechanical ventilation?**
   Bradypnea, apnea, or respiratory arrest; ARDS; respiratory muscle fatigue; obtundation or coma; PaO_2 less than 55 mm Hg despite supplemental oxygen; $PaCO_2$ greater than 50 mm Hg with arterial pH less than 7.2 despite noninvasive ventilation modalities.

7. **What is the definition of acute respiratory distress syndrome?**
   ARDS is an acute, diffuse, inflammatory lung injury that leads to increased pulmonary vascular permeability, increased lung weight, and a loss of aerated tissue. Diagnostic evaluation is done using The Berlin definition of ARDS, published in 2012. This definition replaces the American-European Consensus Conference's definition of ARDS published in 1994. The Berlin definition requires all of the following:
   - Respiratory symptoms within 1 week of a known clinical insult or worsening symptoms during the previous week.
   - Bilateral opacities consistent with pulmonary edema on chest radiography or computed tomography (CT) scan that are not fully explained by pleural effusions, lobar/lung collapse, or pulmonary nodules.
   - Not fully explained by heart failure or fluid overload.
   - Moderate to severe impairment of oxygenation defined by the ratio of arterial oxygen tension to fraction of inspired oxygen (PaO_2/FiO_2). Severity of hypoxemia defines severity of ARDS.
   - Mild: PaO_2/FiO_2 greater than 200 mm Hg, but equal to or less than 300 mm Hg on positive end-expiratory pressure (PEEP) or continuous positive airway pressure (CPAP) equal to or greater than 5 cm H_2O.
   - Moderate: PaO_2/FiO_2 greater than 100 mm Hg but equal to or less than 200 mm Hg on PEEP equal to or greater than 5 cm H_2O.
   - Severe: PaO_2/FiO_2 is equal to or less than 100 mmHg on PEEP equal to or greater than 5 cm H_2O.

8. **What is the pathogenesis of acute respiratory distress syndrome?**
   The early phase of ARDS is characterized by injury and increased permeability of the endothelial and epithelial barriers of the lung, which leads to an accumulation of protein-rich edema fluid in the interstitium and alveolar air space. The fluid contains plasma protein, inflammatory cells (mostly neutrophils), and necrotic debris that can pack down into dense eosin-staining hyaline membranes—collectively termed *diffuse alveolar damage*—which are pathognomonic for the histopathology of ARDS. Patients usually begin to recover in the first 5 to 14 days of disease. During the later phase, the epithelium regenerates and heals or can progress to fibrosis. This latter *fibroproliferative phase* can cause worse morbidity and mortality or can be self-limited and resolve entirely.

9. **What are risk factors for the development of acute respiratory distress syndrome?**
   Several conditions can lead to the development of ARDS, including aspiration of gastric contents, pneumonia, sepsis (most common cause), trauma, transfusion of blood products (particularly plasma-rich products), pancreatitis, fat emboli, and near drowning. Alcoholism and sepsis both greatly increase the likelihood of developing ARDS in patients at risk, whereas diabetes (for yet unclear reasons) reduces the likelihood of ARDS in at-risk patients. Comorbid conditions can also be predictive of outcome (see Question 11).

10. **What is multiple organ dysfunction syndrome?**
    Multiple organ dysfunction syndrome (MODS) is characterized by incremental physiologic derangement in major organs, such as the liver, gut, kidney, brain, or cardiovascular and hematologic systems. MODS can vary widely from a mild to irreversible organ failure. MODS is the single most important predictor of death in ARDS and a much more common cause of death compared with refractory hypoxemia caused by the lung damage alone.

11. **What is the mortality associated with acute respiratory distress syndrome?**
    When ARDS was first described in 1967, the mortality rate was approximately 58%. The overall mortality rate of patients with ARDS over the past several decades has been approximately 43%.

The mortality rate of ARDS has progressively declined over the last decade to approximately 30% but is still 41% to 45% in those between 65 and 84 years of age and approximately 60% in patients over the age of 85 years. Numerous clinical factors have been shown to predict a higher mortality rate in ARDS patients. These include male sex, African American race, advanced age (>70 years), alcohol abuse, malignancy, liver disease, chronic steroid use, infection with human immunodeficiency virus, and ARDS secondary to sepsis or aspiration.

12. **How do patients with acute respiratory distress syndrome die?**
The leading cause of death in patients with ARDS is sepsis syndrome with MODS. Unsupportable respiratory failure is a much less common cause of death.

13. **What medical therapy is available for the treatment of acute respiratory distress syndrome?**
Currently no specific pharmacologic therapy has been proven effective in reducing ARDS mortality. Recombinant surfactant protein C has been effective in improving lung function but has not demonstrated a reduction in mortality. The only interventions thus far shown to reduce ARDS mortality are the use of low-tidal-volume ventilation (LTV), neuromuscular blockade (NMB) for the first 48 hours, and more recently prone positioning, which is discussed in greater detail further on. Although LTV has been adopted as best practice, the data on NMB are limited, and controversy remains over early NMB. For this reason, early NMB is currently being restudied by the Prevention and Early Treatment of Acute Lung Injury (PETAL) study group.

14. **How should respiratory failure associated with acute respiratory distress syndrome be managed?**
Most patients with ARDS require intubation and mechanical ventilation. The use of high-flow nasal cannula in patients with severe hypoxemia may prevent intubation; however, data on its use in patients with hypoxemia secondary to ARDS alone is lacking. Several clinical studies have shown a benefit from using LTV in patients with ARDS. The most influential of these studies, conducted by the ARDS Network, showed a nearly 9% absolute reduction in the risk of death in patients with ARDS receiving ventilation with LTVs (6 mL/kg predicted body weight) and targeted plateau pressures of equal to or less than 30 cm H_2O.

15. **Are there modes of ventilation for patients with acute respiratory distress syndrome that decrease mortality?**
Ventilation using higher PEEP, alveolar recruitment maneuvers, and modes of ventilation such as high-frequency oscillatory ventilation (HFOV) and airway pressure release ventilation have yet to demonstrate a mortality benefit in ARDS. HFOV was recently discredited as first-line therapy for ARDS in two large multicenter randomized controlled trials (RCTs). Pressure-targeted and esophageal pressure–targeted PEEP has shown some benefits in lung function and ventilator-free days, but no benefits in reducing mortality have been demonstrated to date with any of the modes or maneuvers mentioned here.

16. **What is the role of prone positioning for patients with acute respiratory distress syndrome who require mechanical ventilation?**
Prone positioning was initially shown to improve oxygenation for patients with hypoxemic respiratory failure in the mid-1970s, yet a reduction in mortality was not demonstrated. Since then, the Proning Severe ARDS Patients study group concluded a multicenter RCT demonstrating a significant reduction in 28- and 90-day mortality in patients with "severe" ARDS (PaO_2/FiO_2 <150 mm Hg) using prone positioning for at least 16 hours a day, LTV, and targeted plateau pressures of equal to or less than 30 mm H_2O. Unfortunately complication rates are high; thus proning should be limited to patients with severe hypoxemia and undertaken in centers with experience in safe technique.

17. **What are the sequelae in survivors of acute respiratory distress syndrome?**
The spectrum of impairments in survivors of ARDS is broad. Surprisingly, limitations in lung function are typically minimal based on mean values of pulmonary function after 5 years. However, the range of values for forced vital capacity and diffusing capacity among survivors suggests a wide spectrum from moderate to no impairment at all. The majority of the physical impairment is related to decreased exercise capacity and musculoskeletal weakness. Quality of life among survivors is also negatively impacted by a large prevalence of cognitive deficits, depression, and anxiety as far as 2 years out from discharge as well as a reduced rate of return to work or prior line of work (~50%) by 5 years from discharge.

18. **What is acute chest syndrome?**
Acute chest syndrome (ACS) is a frequent complication of sickle cell disease. It is defined as a combination of acute-onset fever, chest pain, new pulmonary infiltrates, and signs and symptoms of pulmonary

disease (i.e., tachypnea, dyspnea, and cough). ACS resembles bacterial pneumonia clinically but is entirely different in its pathology. It can be brought on by various physiologic insults or stressors, including infection, vaso-occlusive crisis, embolization of marrow fat from infarcted bone, and lung infarction, but it uniformly involves an acute occlusion of the pulmonary vascular bed by sickled erythrocytes.

19. **What are the treatment options for acute chest syndrome?**
    Blood transfusion, hydration, pain control, and antibiotics are the current mainstays of therapy. Red cell transfusion has no proven benefit over standard supportive care, but it can improve oxygenation and thus is still recommended. The role of corticosteroids is unclear. Studies examining the use of glucocorticoids have generated variable results. Some experts recommend the use of dexamethasone, primarily in patients with asthma and ACS. However, the risk for increased pain and subsequent readmission remains a limitation. Incentive spirometry has proven beneficial in preventing ACS in patients with chest or rib pain and should be considered for all patients with ACS.

20. **Is there a role for exchange transfusion in sickle cell disease?**
    Simple or exchange transfusion successfully and rapidly increases oxygenation in patients with ACS. In patients requiring mechanical ventilation with multilobar processes who have already received simple transfusions, the current expert recommendation is to proceed with red cell exchange transfusions, but no RCTs have been done to date that demonstrate proven benefit from exchange transfusion in ACS.

21. **Is pulse oximetry reliable in patients with sickle cell disease?**
    Pulse oximetry measurements may overestimate the oxygen saturation by including methemoglobin and carboxyhemoglobin, which are both slightly increased in hemoglobin (Hgb) S disorders. Automated blood gas analyzers may also overestimate the saturation because they calculate O_2 saturation on the basis of standard HgbA. Co-oximetry is the most accurate method for analyzing oxygen saturation in HgbS disorders.

22. **What is the mortality for acute chest syndrome?**
    The overall mortality for ACS is 3%. However, adult patients have a higher overall mortality rate of 9%. The leading causes of death are respiratory failure and bronchopneumonia, but sepsis, pulmonary hemorrhage, hypovolemic shock, and intracranial hemorrhage are additional common causes of death in ACS.

ACKNOWLEDGMENT

The authors wish to acknowledge Dr. Prema R. Menon, MD, for the valuable contributions to the previous edition of this chapter.

KEY POINTS: ACUTE RESPIRATORY FAILURE/ACUTE RESPIRATORY DISTRESS SYNDROME

1. Definition of ARF
   - Hypoxemic respiratory failure: PaO_2 less than 50 mm Hg
   - Hypercapnic respiratory failure: PCO_2 greater than 50 mmHg
2. Berlin criteria for ARDS
   - Within 1 week of insult or worsening symptoms
   - Bilateral infiltrates not fully explained by other lung pathology
   - Respiratory failure not fully explained by heart failure or volume overload
     - Need objective assessment for this, that is, echocardiography
   - Severity: dictated by oxygenation with PEEP or CPAP equal to or greater than 5 H_2O
     - Mild: PaO_2/FiO_2 less than or equal to 300 mm Hg and greater than 200 mm Hg
     - Moderate: PaO_2/FiO_2 less than or equal to 200 mm Hg and greater than 100 mm Hg
     - Severe: PaO_2/FiO_2 less than or equal to 100 mm Hg
3. Treatment of ACS
   - Blood transfusion/exchange transfusion
   - Hydration
   - Incentive spirometry
   - Pain control
   - Antibiotics

BIBLIOGRAPHY

1. Allen GB, Parsons PE. Acute respiratory failure due to acute respiratory distress syndrome and pulmonary edema. In: Irwin RS, Rippe JM, eds. *Intensive Care Medicine*. 8th ed. Philadelphia: Lippincott Williams & Wilkins; 2016.
2. The Acute Respiratory Distress Syndrome Network. Ventilation with lower tidal volumes as compared with traditional tidal volumes for acute lung injury and the acute respiratory distress syndrome. *N Engl J Med*. 2000;342:1301-1308.
3. Graham Jr LM. The effect of sickle cell disease on the lung. *Clin Pulm Med*. 2004;11:369.
4. Guérin C, Reignier J, Richard JC, et al. Prone positioning in severe acute respiratory distress syndrome. *N Engl J Med*. 2013;368:2159-2168.
5. Herridge MS, Tansey CM, Matté A, et al. Functional disability 5 years after acute respiratory distress syndrome. *N Engl J Med*. 2011;304:1293-1304.
6. Papazian L, Forel JM, Gacouin A, et al. Neuromuscular blockers in early acute respiratory distress syndrome. *N Engl J Med*. 2010;363:1107-1116.
7. Rubenfeld GD, Caldwell E, Peabody E, et al. Incidence and outcomes of acute lung injury. *N Engl J Med*. 2005;353: 1685-1693.
8. Turner JM, Kaplan JB, Cohen HW, et al. Exchange versus simple transfusion for acute chest syndrome in sickle cell anemia adults. *Transfusion*. 2009;49:863-868.
9. Vichinsky EP, Neumayr LD, Earles AN, et al. Causes and outcomes of the acute chest syndrome in sickle cell disease. National Acute Chest Syndrome Study Group. *N Engl J Med*. 2000;342:1855-1865.
10. Ware LB, Matthay MA. The acute respiratory distress syndrome. *N Engl J Med*. 2000;342:1334-1349.

CHAPTER 31

HEMOPTYSIS

Mark T. Kearns and Michael E. Hanley

1. **What is hemoptysis?**

   Hemoptysis is the expectoration of blood originating from the lower respiratory tract. It is classified on the basis of the volume of expectorated blood or the rate of bleeding.
   - *Scant hemoptysis* refers to expectoration of sputa with streaks or specks of blood or that is blood-tinged.
   - *Frank hemoptysis* is characterized by sputa that are grossly bloody but of a low volume (<100–200 mL in 24 hours).
   - *Massive hemoptysis* refers to bleeding that is potentially acutely life threatening because it involves expectoration of a large volume of blood and/or a rapid rate of bleeding. The exact volume of blood that constitutes massive hemoptysis is controversial; various studies have defined it from as high as a minimum of 1000 mL per 24 hours to as low as 100 mL if there is coexistent hemodynamic instability or abnormal gas exchange. Most authors limit the definition of massive hemoptysis to expectoration of more than 500 to 600 mL of blood in 24 hours or bleeding at a rate greater or equal to 100 mL/hour.

2. **How are hemoptysis and pseudohemoptysis different?**

   Pseudohemoptysis is expectoration of blood originating from a source other than the lower respiratory tract. It results from expectoration of blood either aspirated from the gastrointestinal tract or draining into the larynx and trachea from bleeding sites in the oral cavity, nasopharynx, or larynx.

3. **Describe the differential diagnosis of hemoptysis.**

   The differential diagnosis of hemoptysis is based on the site of bleeding. Hemoptysis in general results from either a focal or diffuse airway or pulmonary parenchymal process (Table 31.1). Occasionally nonpulmonary processes, in particular cardiac, vascular, or hematologic disorders, may result in bleeding in the lungs. The frequency with which hemoptysis is associated with these conditions is determined by the age of the patient, the population being studied (e.g., surgical vs. medical, veterans hospital vs. city or county indigent hospital), and the amount of expectorated blood. Approximately 30% of cases are cryptogenic, and no explanation for hemoptysis is determined despite extensive evaluation.

4. **What are the common causes of massive hemoptysis?**

   Although there are no recent large studies describing the frequency of the causes of massive hemoptysis, historically 90% of cases were due to either chronic bronchiectasis, active or inactive tuberculosis, necrotizing pneumonia (including lung abscess), or fungal infections. The latter included both mycetoma (aspergilloma) and, less commonly, chronic necrotizing pulmonary aspergillosis. The relative frequency of these etiologies has changed in the past few decades and depends on both the institution and country from which the data are reported. Pulmonary neoplasm, arteriovenous malformation, pulmonary vasculitis, valvular heart disease (especially mitral stenosis), and bleeding diathesis are also potential causes of massive hemoptysis but occur less frequently.

5. **Name iatrogenic causes of hemoptysis that occur in critically ill patients.**

   When hemoptysis begins after endotracheal intubation, upper airway trauma caused by the intubation procedure, endotracheal tube, or endotracheal suction catheters should be considered. If hemoptysis begins after a latent period of 1 or more weeks postintubation, a tracheoarterial fistula may be the source of hemorrhage. This possibility is increased if a tracheostomy tube is present and has been placed in a low position in the neck. Pulmonary artery rupture and pulmonary infarction should be considered when hemoptysis occurs in a patient with a pulmonary artery catheter. Pulmonary infarction should be suspected if a wedge-shaped infiltrate develops distal to the catheter on the chest radiograph. Finally, hemoptysis can occur following pulmonary vein isolation during cryoballoon ablation for atrial fibrillation.

Table 31-1. Causes of Hemoptysis

AIRWAY DISORDERS	LOCALIZED PARENCHYMAL DISEASES	VASCULAR DISORDERS	DIFFUSE PARENCHYMAL DISEASES
Acute tracheobronchitis	Nontuberculous pneumonia	Aortic aneurysm	Disseminated angiosarcoma
Amyloidosis	Actinomycosis	Congenital heart disease	Farmer's lung
Gastric aspiration	Amebiasis	Congestive heart failure	Goodpasture syndrome
Bronchial adenoma	Ascariasis	Fat embolism	Idiopathic pulmonary hemosiderosis
Bronchial endometriosis	Aspergilloma	Mitral stenosis	Mixed IgA nephropathy
Bronchial telangiectasia	Bronchopulmonary sequestration	Postmyocardial infarction syndrome	Legionnaires disease
Bronchogenic carcinoma	Coccidioidomycosis	Pulmonary arteriovenous malformation	Mixed connective tissue disease
Broncholithiasis	Congenital and acquired cyst	Pulmonary artery aneurysm	Mixed cryoglobulinemia
Chronic bronchiectasis	Cryptococcosis	Pulmonary embolus	Polyarteritis nodosa
Chronic bronchitis	Histoplasmosis	Pulmonary venous varix	Scleroderma
Cystic fibrosis	Hydatid mole	Schistosomiasis	Systemic lupus erythematosus
Endobronchial metastasis	Lung abscess	Superior vena cava syndrome	Wegener granulomatosis
Endobronchial tuberculosis	Lipoid pneumonia	Tumor embolization	**OTHER**
Foreign body aspiration	Lung contusion	**HEMATOLOGIC DISORDERS**	Idiopathic
Bronchial mucoid impaction	Metastatic cancer	Anticoagulant therapy	Iatrogenic
Tracheobronchial trauma	Mucormycosis	Disseminated intravascular coagulation	Drug- and toxin-induced (cocaine, bevacizumab, nitrogen dioxide)
Tracheoesophageal fistula	Nocardiosis	Leukemia	
	Paragonimiasis	Thrombocytopenia	
	Pulmonary endometriosis		
	Pulmonary tuberculosis		
	Sporotrichosis		

IgA, Immunoglobulin A.
Modified from Irwin RS, Hubmayr R. Hemoptysis. In: Rippe JM, Irwin RS, Alpert JS, et al., eds. *Intensive Care Medicine*. Boston: Little, Brown; 1985.

6. Explain the significance of massive hemoptysis.
   Ninety percent of cases of massive hemoptysis are due to hemorrhaging from the bronchial artery circulation as opposed to the pulmonary artery circuit. The bronchial artery circulation is characterized by high pressure and provides the blood supply to the airways and airway lesions; bleeding from this system can rapidly deliver a large amount of blood to the airways and produce life-threatening hemorrhage. Mortality from untreated massive hemoptysis in some studies is 75% to 100%.

7. List the tests that should be included in a routine evaluation of patients with hemoptysis.
   History, physical examination, complete blood cell counts including platelet count, coagulation studies, urinalysis, oxygenation by either pulse oximetry or arterial blood gas analysis, creatinine, and chest radiograph. Additional testing is directed towards specific diagnoses as suggested by this initial evaluation.

8. What is the initial approach to the evaluation of a patient admitted to the intensive care unit with hemoptysis?
   Evaluation should begin with the routine tests previously described. After the patient has been hemodynamically stabilized, the site, etiology, and extent of bleeding should be determined. Identifying the site of bleeding requires visualization of the airways of both the upper and lower respiratory tract and examination of the chest radiograph.
   If the radiograph is normal or does not localize the site of bleeding a computed tomography (CT) scan of the chest may be helpful, as it is more sensitive at detecting subtle parenchymal lesions (such as bronchiectasis) that may not be apparent on the radiograph.
   Pernasal fiberoptic laryngoscopy and bronchoscopy allow examination of the nasopharynx, larynx, and major airways and may reveal whether hemorrhaging is focal or diffuse. The presence of an endotracheal tube may compromise this examination. In this instance, upper airway bleeding may be detected by clearing the trachea of blood with a bronchoscope while the endotracheal cuff is inflated and then observing fresh blood flow down from above the cuff when it is decompressed. Rigid bronchoscopy may be required if hemorrhaging is massive, such that blood cannot be adequately removed with a flexible bronchoscope.
   Bronchoscopy and CT scanning are complementary in the evaluation of hemoptysis as each has advantages for different clinical situations. Bronchoscopy is better at detecting airway lesions (especially subtle mucosal abnormalities), while CT scanning is superior for parenchymal disease. The timing of these modalities depends on the stability of the patient and whether active hemoptysis is continuing.

9. How does the chest radiograph assist in the evaluation of hemoptysis?
   Examination of the radiograph gives clues to both the site and etiology of hemoptysis but with some caveats. The presence of an infiltrate suggests a pulmonary parenchymal process. However, occasionally an infiltrate may occur after aspiration of blood that is actually originating from an airway source. Similarly, the presence of diffuse infiltrates suggests diffuse parenchymal disease, although this radiographic pattern can also occur with localized bleeding associated with severe coughing, which disperses blood throughout the lungs.

10. Do all patients with hemoptysis require bronchoscopy?
    No. Bronchoscopy may not be indicated if the initial evaluation strongly suggests that hemoptysis is due to a cardiovascular etiology, a lower respiratory tract infection, or a single episode of frank hemoptysis caused by acute or chronic bronchitis. However, bronchoscopy should be reconsidered in these clinical settings if the patient's hemoptysis does not improve or resolve after 24 hours of empiric therapy. Bronchoscopy is not indicated to make the specific diagnosis of a tracheoarterial fistula.

11. Describe the immediate management of massive hemoptysis.
    The goals of immediate management of patients with massive hemoptysis are as follows:
    1. Establish which side is bleeding.
    2. Maintain airway patency.
    3. Ensure adequate gas exchange.
    4. Establish hemodynamic stability.
    5. Stop ongoing hemorrhage.
       These goals should be pursued simultaneously as opposed to in a sequential manner. Identifying which side is bleeding is important because it facilitates establishing a patent airway. Old as well as current chest radiographs may be helpful in demonstrating pre-existing focal disease which now may be the source of hemorrhage. The history may also be helpful in this regard as patients may report an abnormal sensation on the side of the chest that is bleeding. Maintenance of airway patency is of

paramount importance because death from massive hemoptysis more commonly results from asphyxiation due to major airway obstruction than from exsanguination. The first step in maintaining airway patency involves properly positioning the patient. If hemorrhage is occurring from a focal site and the site of hemorrhage is known, the patient should be positioned with the bleeding side dependent to prevent contamination of noninvolved airways. If the site of hemorrhage is unknown or diffuse, the patient should be placed in the Trendelenburg position. Other approaches to protect uninvolved airways include bronchoscopically guided selective intubation of the nonbleeding main stem bronchus or placement of a double-lumen endotracheal tube. The utility of double-lumen tubes is limited by the need for specialized training in their insertion and the tendency for double-lumen tubes to become dislodged. Patients may need to be paralyzed to prevent the latter.

12. What specific therapies may be useful to stop ongoing hemorrhage?

If the etiology of hemorrhage is known, specific therapy directed at the cause (such as antibiotics for bronchiectasis or corticosteroids for pulmonary vasculitis) should be started to stop ongoing hemorrhage. Coagulopathies should be corrected with administration of appropriate blood products. If the patient is receiving anticoagulant therapy it should be discontinued.

Life-threatening hemorrhage from a focal site requires a more aggressive strategy. The most common of these is bronchial artery embolization (see Question 14). Surgical resection may be considered in patients with adequate underlying lung function; however, because of the higher mortality associated with this approach when used emergently and the safety and efficacy of bronchial artery embolization, it is usually reserved for those patients who have persistent bleeding despite other interventions. A number of bronchoscopic techniques are also available to control bleeding. These include the following:

- Balloon tamponade with an airway blocker (such as a Fogarty catheter or an Arndt endobronchial blocker) placed under bronchoscopic guidance
- Bronchoscopy-guided topical hemostatic tamponade therapy with use of either oxidized regenerated cellulose mesh or infusions of thrombin alone or fibrinogen with thrombin
- Iced normal saline lavage of hemorrhaging lung segments
- Regional instillation of vasoconstrictor agents such as epinephrine or vasopressin
- Electrocautery, laser photocoagulation, or cryotherapy of focal airway lesions that are bleeding

The efficacies of these bronchoscopic techniques have not been studied in a rigorous manner and in general they are felt to be inferior to embolization as a means to stop hemorrhaging.

13. Describe the management of a tracheoarterial fistula.

Tracheoarterial fistulas are rare complications of tracheostomy, occurring in 0.7% of tracheostomies. However, they are life-threatening with survival of only 14% and require immediate surgical intervention. The goals of immediate management are to control bleeding and to maintain a patent airway while preparing the patient for prompt surgical correction. Diagnostic procedures including bronchoscopy and angiography should be avoided as they may delay emergent intervention.

Bleeding from a tracheoarterial fistula usually occurs at one of three sites: the tracheostomy tube stoma, the tracheostomy tube balloon, or the intratracheal cannula tip. Temporizing maneuvers to control bleeding while the patient is transported to the operating room include the following:

1. Bleeding at the tracheostomy stoma can sometimes be tamponaded by applying forward and downward pressure on the top of the tracheostomy tube. Bleeding at the site of the balloon can be tamponaded by overinflating the balloon. Both of these maneuvers should be performed immediately; however, they will not be helpful if bleeding is occurring at the cannula tip.
2. If bleeding stops or slows either spontaneously or subsequent to these efforts, an endotracheal tube should be placed distal to the bleeding site. However, the initial tracheostomy tube should not be removed without a surgeon present because a sudden increase in the rate of hemorrhage may necessitate blunt dissection down the anterior tracheal wall posterior to the sternum to attempt direct digital tamponade of the bleeding site.
3. If bleeding still persists, a finger may be placed through the tracheostomy stoma and lifted anteriorly to compress the artery against the sternum. Enough force must be applied to lift the sternum. Compression must be continued and bag valve ventilation provided until surgery can be performed.

14. What is the role of bronchial artery embolization in the management of massive hemoptysis?

Bronchial artery embolization is important in the management of both surgical and nonsurgical causes of massive hemoptysis. It is a temporary measure for surgical lesions, facilitating the stabilization of patients while they undergo evaluation and preparation for surgery. It allows surgery to be performed in a more controlled setting. Bronchial artery embolization has become the primary mode of therapy for patients whose conditions are considered inoperable because of either diffuse lung disease or poor pulmonary function. Such patients may undergo multiple episodes of embolization over many years if hemoptysis recurs.

15. What is the success rate of bronchial artery embolization?
Various studies have reported success rates in the initial 24-hour period after embolization from 73% to 98%. However, 16% to 30% of patients rebleed in the first year after embolization. Rebleeding tends to be bimodal in occurrence, with peaks in the first month (generally because of inadequate initial embolization) and at 1 to 2 years (because of progression of underlying disease).

16. What complications are associated with bronchial artery embolization?
Bronchial artery embolization is associated with low morbidity rates. The most common complications include pleuritic chest pain, fever, leukocytosis, and dysphagia. These symptoms may last for 5 to 7 days. Other complications are quite rare and are related to the vascular compromise of organs supplied from vessels that arise downstream from the site of catheter insertion. Examples include spinal cord infarction, transverse myelitis, bronchial stenosis, bronchial-esophageal fistula, transient cortical blindness, and cerebrovascular accidents.

17. When should surgery be considered in the management of massive hemoptysis?
Bronchial artery embolization has largely replaced surgical resection as the initial therapy in massive hemoptysis. Embolization is associated with much lower morbidity and early mortality rates than emergent surgery. However, because of high rates of recurrence after embolization, surgery should be considered for patients who have been stabilized with embolization and have hemoptysis due to focal lung lesions and good pulmonary reserve. Surgery is contraindicated in patients with advanced lung disease associated with limited pulmonary reserve, significant comorbidities (especially advanced heart disease), or lung malignancies invading the trachea, mediastinum, heart, great vessels, and parietal pleura. It remains the treatment of choice for patients with hemoptysis related to trauma, aortic aneurysm, and bronchial adenomas.

CONTROVERSY

18. Should fiberoptic bronchoscopy always be performed before bronchial artery embolization in patients with massive hemoptysis?

FOR:

Fiberoptic bronchoscopy:
- Is important in guiding bronchial artery embolization by identifying the site of bleeding.
- Is complementary to chest computed tomography in identifying the cause of hemoptysis, allowing the institution of specific therapy aimed at the underlying lung pathologic condition.
- Facilitates the use of a number of techniques that can control bleeding.

AGAINST:

- A retrospective review of 29 patients who underwent bronchial artery embolization to control massive hemoptysis revealed that the site of bleeding could be identified in 80% of patients by chest radiograph alone. Bronchoscopy was essential to localizing the site of hemorrhage in only 10% of patients.
- The site of embolization is generally identified by angiography at the time of bronchial catheterization.
- Emergent bronchoscopy results in unnecessary delays before performance of bronchial artery embolization.
- Endobronchial tamponade is inferior to embolization as a temporary measure to control hemorrhage before the institution of more specific therapy and should be reserved for patients with contraindications to embolization.

KEY POINTS: HEMOPTYSIS

Management Goals in Massive Hemoptysis
1. Identify which side is bleeding.
2. Maintain airway patency.
3. Ensure adequate gas exchange.
4. Establish hemodynamic stability.
5. Stop hemorrhage.
6. Prevent repeated hemorrhage.

BIBLIOGRAPHY

1. Bussières JS. Iatrogenic pulmonary artery rupture. *Curr Opin Anaesthesiol.* 2007;20:48-52.
2. de Gracia J, de la Rosa D, Catalán E, et al. Use of endoscopic fibrinogen-thrombin in the treatment of severe hemoptysis. *Respir Med.* 2003;97:790-795.
3. Fartoukh M, Khoshnood B, Parrot A, et al. Early prediction of in-hospital mortality of patients with hemoptysis: an approach to defining severe hemoptysis. *Respiration.* 2012;83:106-114.
4. Hsiao EI, Kirsch CM, Kagawa FT, et al. Utility of fiberoptic bronchoscopy before bronchial artery embolization for massive hemoptysis. *Am J Roentgenol.* 2001;177:861-867.
5. Ibrahim WH. Massive haemoptysis: the definition should be revised. *Eur Respir J.* 2008;32:1131-1132.
6. Jean Baptiste E. Clinical assessment and management of massive hemoptysis. *Crit Care Med.* 2000;28:1642-1647.
7. Jougon J, Ballester M, Delcambre F, et al. Massive hemoptysis: what place for medical and surgical treatment. *Eur J Cardiothorac Surg.* 2002;22:345-351.
8. Komatsu T, Sowa T, Fujinaga T, et al. Tracheo-innominate artery fistula: two case reports and a clinical review. *Ann Thorac Cardiovasc Surg.* 2013;19:60-62.
9. Martí-Almor J, Jauregui-Abularach ME, Benito B, et al. Pulmonary hemorrhage after cryoballoon ablation for pulmonary vein isolation in the treatment of atrial fibrillation. *Chest.* 2014;145:156-157.
10. Menchini L, Remy-Jardin M, Faivre JB, et al. Cryptogenic haemoptysis in smokers: angiography and results of embolisation in 35 patients. *Eur Respir J.* 2009;34:1031-1039.
11. Razazi K, Parrot A, Khalil A, et al. Severe haemoptysis in patients with nonsmall cell lung carcinoma. *Eur Respir J.* 2015;45:756-764.
12. Sakr L, Dutau H. Massive hemoptysis: an update on the role of bronchoscopy in diagnosis and management. *Respiration.* 2010;80:38-58.
13. Savale L, Parrot A, Khalil A, et al. Cryptogenic hemoptysis: from a benign to a life-threatening pathologic vascular condition. *Am J Respir Crit Care Med.* 2007;175:1181-1185.
14. Sopko DR, Smith TP. Bronchial artery embolization for hemoptysis. *Semin Intervent Radiol.* 2011;28:48-62.
15. Shigemura N, Wan IY, Yu SC, et al. Multidisciplinary management of life-threatening massive hemoptysis: a 10-year experience. *Ann Thorac Surg.* 2009;87:849-853.
16. Valipour A, Kreuzer A, Koller H, et al. Bronchoscopy-guided topical hemostatic tamponade therapy for the management of life-threatening hemoptysis. *Chest.* 2005;127:2113-2118.
17. Woo S, Yoon CJ, Chung JW, et al. Bronchial artery embolization to control hemoptysis: comparison of N-butyl-2-cyanoacrylate and polyvinyl alcohol particles. *Radiology.* 2013;269:594-602.
18. Yoon W, Kim JK, Kim YH, et al. Bronchial and nonbronchial systemic artery embolization for life threatening hemoptysis: a comprehensive review. *Radiographics.* 2002;22:1395-1409.

CHAPTER 32

VENOUS THROMBOEMBOLISM AND FAT EMBOLISM

Peter D. Sottile and Marc Moss

1. **What are the sources of pulmonary embolism?**
   The majority of pulmonary embolisms (PEs) arise from thromboses in the deep veins of the legs, particularly the iliac, femoral, and popliteal veins. Thromboses can also originate on central venous catheters and from the pelvic veins in women with a history of obstetric difficulties or recent gynecologic surgery. Nonhematologic sources of PE include fat particles, amniotic fluid, air introduced through central venous catheters, and foreign bodies such as talc and cotton fibers in intravenous drug users.

2. **What are some of the risk factors for pulmonary embolism and deep venous thrombosis?**
   In general, three broad conditions that increase the risk of venous thrombosis are called *Virchow's triad:* venous stasis, thrombophilia, and injury to the endothelium of vessel walls. A list of specific risk factors is listed in Table 32.1.

3. **How common is venous thromboembolism in critically ill patients?**
   Deep venous thrombosis (DVT) and PE are common and often underdiagnosed in critically ill patients. In prospective studies, 33% of medical patients in the intensive care unit (ICU) had DVTs on routine clinical screening, and 18% of trauma patients had proximal DVTs. In a retrospective series of respiratory ICU patients, 27% had PE on autopsy.

4. **What are the signs and symptoms of an acute pulmonary embolism?**
   The symptoms of an acute PE depend on the thromboembolic burden, the degree of underlying pulmonary parenchymal disease, and the ability of the right ventricle to accommodate acute pressure changes. Patients can present with syncope, shock, tachycardia, acute right ventricular failure, increased dead space, or refractory hypoxemia. However, patients may also be relatively asymptomatic. In patients with underlying cardiac or pulmonary disease, significant hemodynamic compromise may occur with less occlusion of the pulmonary vasculature.

5. **Are any laboratory test result abnormalities helpful in diagnosing pulmonary embolism?**
   No arterial blood gas values have adequate operating characteristics to exclude PE. Elevated serum D-dimer levels are highly sensitive but have low specificity. The serum D-dimer was validated in outpatients, when clinical suspicion for PE was low. In the setting of moderate to high pre-test probability of acute PE, the ability of even a low D-dimer to exclude PE is limited. Troponin and brain naturetic

Table 32-1. Risk Factors for Venous Thromboembolism

VENOUS STASIS	THROMBOPHILIA	ENDOTHELIAL INJURY
Prolonged bed rest	Malignancy	Major surgical procedures
Prolonged air travel (>8 h)	Heparin-induced thrombocytopenia	Trauma
Heart failure	Antiphospholipid antibodies	Prior venous thrombosis
	Nephrotic syndrome	
	Inflammatory bowel disease	
	Pregnancy	
	Hormone replacement therapy	
	Oral contraceptives	
	Specific chemotherapy agents	

peptide (BNP) are neither sensitive nor specific to diagnose acute PE but assist in risk stratification when PE is present.

6. **What are the electrocardiographic findings associated with pulmonary embolism?**
   Electrocardiographic (ECG) findings are also variable and relatively nonspecific. Sinus tachycardia and nonspecific ST-segment and T-wave changes occur most commonly. The classic ECG findings of S_1, Q_3, T_3, or right bundle branch block occur in fewer than 15% of patients. The development of ECG findings of acute right ventricular strain (i.e., rightward shift of the QRS axis or peaked P waves in the inferior leads) in a critically ill patient should raise concern about potential PE.

7. **What are some findings of pulmonary embolism visible on chest radiography?**
   Chest radiography can be used neither to make nor to exclude the diagnosis of PE. However, the chest radiograph does assist in ruling out alternative diagnoses. Small to moderate unilateral, exudative pleural effusions occur in approximately one-third of patients with PE. Although not specific for the diagnosis, patients with a pulmonary infarct may occasionally have a wedge-shaped opacity that abuts the pleura (Hampton hump). In addition, focal oligemia may be visible (Westermark sign) and when present should prompt further evaluation for PE.

8. **When should a ventilation-perfusion scan be ordered in the diagnostic work-up of acute pulmonary embolism?**
   Ventilation-perfusion (V/Q) scans can be particularly useful in patients for whom computed tomography angiography (CTA) is contraindicated (renal failure or radiocontrast allergy). Eighty-seven percent of patients with a high-probability V/Q scan have a PE, whereas the diagnosis can essentially be excluded in patients with a normal V/Q scan. Unfortunately, more than 50% of V/Q scans are nondiagnostic (i.e., intermediate), and further testing is needed. Importantly, V/Q scans are more difficult to interpret in patients with pre-existing concurrent lung disease and are logistically difficult to organize in a patient with critical illness. Performing a V/Q scan on an intubated patient is often impossible.

9. **What about computed tomography angiography for the diagnosis of pulmonary embolism?**
   The sensitivity and specificity of CTA exceed 90%. Higher imaging resolution and more experienced radiologists have contributed to this increase in CTA sensitivity and specificity. The sensitivity of CTA for small, subsegmental emboli is lower, although the clinical significance of subsegmental PE is unclear and may not warrant treatment. Several studies have demonstrated that subsequent DVT will develop in fewer than 1% of patients with a negative CTA for the diagnosis of PE over the next 3 months. Additionally, CTA will assist with the evaluation for alternative diagnoses in the thoracic cavity. Utility of CTA in the ICU is limited in patients with impaired renal function, the inability to lie flat, or illnesses that prohibit transportation.

10. **What is the role of echocardiography in the evaluation of pulmonary embolism?**
    Echocardiography is useful for risk stratification, and for those patients whose condition is too unstable for them to be transported for further imaging procedures. As many as 25% of patients with PE exhibit abnormalities of the right ventricle (RV). Findings of RV volume and pressure overload include abnormal motion of the intraventricular septum, RV dilation, and RV hypokinesis. Echocardiography also may diagnose conditions that simulate PE, such as aortic aneurysm, myocardial infarction, and pericardial tamponade.

11. **How is the severity of pulmonary embolism classified?**
    PE is generally classified as massive, submassive, and low-risk. *Massive PE* or *high-risk* is characterized by hemodynamic instability, generally defined as a systolic blood pressure less than 90 mm Hg over 15 minutes despite adequate fluid resuscitation. *Submassive PE* or *intermediate-risk* is characterized by evidence of RV strain or dysfunction. This has been broadly defined by EKG changes (right bundle branch block or RV strain pattern), RV dilation and dysfunction on echocardiogram, an enlarged RV on CTA, or an elevated troponin or BNP. *Low-risk PE* include patients with hemodynamic stability and no evidence of RV dysfunction.

12. **What is the recommended algorithm for the diagnosis of pulmonary embolism in the intensive care unit for a patient who is hemodynamically stable?**
    In hemodynamically stable patients in whom PE is suspected, the initial diagnostic test should be a CTA. V/Q scan should be considered if a CTA is contraindicated. If these tests are nondiagnostic, a Doppler ultrasound and scan of the legs and echocardiogram should be performed. If the diagnosis is still not confirmed and the clinical suspicion for PE is high, pulmonary angiography may be performed, although many centers lack experience interpreting traditional angiography.

13. **What is the recommended algorithm for the diagnosis of pulmonary embolism in the intensive care unit for a patient who is hemodynamically unstable?**
Anticoagulation should be started (if not contraindicated) as soon as PE is suspected. Because moving an unstable patient is difficult and potentially unsafe, the initial tests should be a Doppler ultrasound scan of the legs and cardiac echocardiography to look for signs of right ventricular dilatation or dysfunction. Occasionally, clot can be seen in transit in the RV. If patient anatomy allows, the main, left, and right pulmonary arteries can be imaged with echocardiography to evaluate for clot. A portable chest radiograph should be obtained to evaluate for alternative diagnoses. Evidence of DVT with new RV dysfunction on echocardiogram without another alternative diagnosis is often sufficient to make a presumed diagnosis of PE.

14. **What are the goals of treatment for submassive or low-risk pulmonary embolism, and how are they achieved?**
The major goals of submassive and low-risk PE therapy are to prevent further thrombotic and embolic complications and to promote resolution of the existing thrombosis. In the short term, unfractionated (UF) or low-molecular-weight (LMW) heparin should be administered. Oral anticoagulation therapy can be started when the patient's condition is stable and no invasive procedures are planned. The role of systemic thrombolytic therapy or catheter direct thrombolysis is still debated and without clear guidelines in the literature. A recent randomized control trial of systemic thrombolytic therapy for submassive PE showed no difference in mortality with systemic thrombolytics.

15. **What are the goals of therapy for massive pulmonary embolism and how are they achieved?**
The major goal of therapy in massive PE is to reverse the obstructive shock caused by acute RV failure. Fluid resuscitation to ensure adequate RV preload and inotropic infusions are often used. On the basis of limited clinical evidence, systemic thrombolytic therapy is recommended for patients with PE associated with massive PE who lack contraindications related to bleeding risk (Table 32.2). If successful, this can reverse the obstructive shock. However, the risk of significant bleeding is not inconsequential, with a risk of intracranial hemorrhage approaching 6% in a recent randomized control trial.

16. **What is the role for newer oral anticoagulant agents in the treatment of deep venous thrombosis or pulmonary embolism?**
In several clinical trials, patients taking warfarin have an international normalized ratio (INR) within a therapeutic range only 60% of the time. Two new classes of oral anticoagulants, direct thrombin inhibitors and factor Xa inhibitors, are currently being studied in this disease. In the recent 2016 American College of Chest Physicians Anticoagulation guidelines, these agents were recommended as first-line therapy for venus thromboembolism (VTE) and PE over warfarin.

17. **When should low-molecular-weight heparin be used?**
LMW heparin is preferred to warfarin or the novel oral anticoagulation agents in the setting of active malignancy. In the 2003 CLOT Trial, patients with active malignancy were randomized to either receive

Table 32-2. Contraindications to Thrombolytic Therapy

ABSOLUTE	RELATIVE
History of intracranial hemorrhage	Recent internal bleeding
Intracranial neoplasm, arteriovenous malformation, or aneurysm	Recent surgery or organ biopsy
Significant head trauma	Recent trauma, including cardiopulmonary resuscitation
Active internal bleeding (intracranial, retroperitoneal, gastrointestinal, genitourinary, respiratory)	Venipuncture at a noncompressible site
Known bleeding diathesis	Acute pericarditis
Intracranial or intraspinal surgery within 3 months	Subacute bacterial endocarditis or septic thrombophlebitis
Cerebrovascular accident within 2 months	Pregnancy
	Age >75 years

either 6 months of LMW heparin or warfarin. Patients in the LMW heparin group had nearly an 8% absolute risk reduction in recurrent VTE with a detectible difference in bleeding risk.

18. How long should a patient with pulmonary embolism or deep venous thrombosis be treated with anticoagulation?
   - Patients with their first episode of PE or DVT due to a transient (reversible) risk factor (e.g., surgery, trauma, immobilization, pregnancy, venous catheter, hip fracture) should receive anticoagulation for 3 months.
   - Patients with their first episode of an unprovoked PE or DVT should be treated for *at least* 3 months, with a recommendation for life-long anticoagulation with an annual assessment and a discussion of the risks and benefits of long-term treatment.

19. When should the placement of an inferior vena cava filter be considered?
   The most common and agreed-on indications for inferior vena cava (IVC) filter placement are as follows: (1) an acute PE or proximal DVT with contraindication to anticoagulation, (2) recurrent acute PE despite therapeutic anticoagulation. Patients with a large acute PE and poor cardiopulmonary reserve are often considered for IVC filter placement—IVC filter may reduce the risk of recurrent PE in the first 7 days by 4%, but does not change the rate of recurrence long term and may cause additional complications without anticoagulation. Given the greatly increased risk for subsequent DVT (21%) and IVC thrombosis (2%–10%) in patients with IVC filters, resumption of anticoagulants is recommended when bleeding risk decreases and to remove the filter when safely indicated.

20. Are there important long-term sequelae of a pulmonary embolism?
   Pulmonary hypertension occurs in approximately 4% of patients within 2 years after their first episode of PE, which is called chronic thromboembolic pulmonary hypertension (CTEPH). It is unknown if thrombolytic therapy reduces the risk of CTEPH development. Patients suspected of having CTEPH should be evaluated with V/Q scan, CTA chest, and right heart catheterization with pulmonary arteriogram. Surgical thromboembolectomy remains first-line therapy. Riociguat is a pharmacologic therapy approved in the United States for CTEPH and is often used in patients without surgical options.

21. What is the recommended prophylactic therapy for patients at risk for the development of deep venous thrombosis or pulmonary embolism?
   Pharmacologic prophylaxis is recommended in all high-risk patients who lack contraindications and has been reported to decrease the incidence of DVT by 67%. Multiple risk stratification scores exist. Although mechanical methods of thromboprophylaxis (intermittent pneumatic compression devices) are generally less efficacious, they are recommended in patients for whom anticoagulants are contraindicated. The most common recommended medications for DVT or PE prophylaxis are as follows:
   - UF heparin (5000 units subcutaneously every 8–12 hours).
   - LMW heparin (dose depends on the specific drug and the patient's renal function).

22. What is the fat embolism syndrome? Who is at risk for development of it?
   Embolism of fat occurs in nearly all patients with traumatic bone fractures and during orthopedic procedures. It can also occur in patients with pancreatitis or sickle cell crises and during liposuction. Most cases are asymptomatic. Fat embolism syndrome (FES) occurs in the minority of these patients who have signs and symptoms, usually affecting the respiratory, neurologic, and hematologic systems and the skin. Symptoms typically occur 12 to 72 hours after the initial injury. The presentation may be catastrophic with RV failure and cardiovascular collapse.

23. How is fat embolism syndrome diagnosed?
   Fat embolism is a clinical diagnosis. The use of bronchoscopy or pulmonary artery catheterization to detect fat particles in alveolar macrophages or blood from the pulmonary artery lacks both sensitivity and specificity for the diagnosis of FES. The Gurd criteria are the most widely used method of diagnosis (Box 32.1).

24. What is the recommended treatment for fat embolism syndrome?
   Treatment of FES is primarily supportive. Although it has been studied extensively, no compelling evidence exists that the use of corticosteroids is indicated for FES. Some studies have suggested that early stabilization of long bone fractures can minimize bone marrow embolization into the venous system.

Box 32-1. Gurd Diagnostic Criteria for Fat Embolism Syndrome

Major Criteria (One Necessary for Diagnosis)
Petechial rash
Respiratory failure
Cerebral involvement

Minor Criteria (Four Necessary for Diagnosis)
Tachycardia (heart rate >120 beats per minute)
Fever (temperature >39°C)
Retinal involvement
Jaundice
Renal insufficiency

Additional Laboratory Criteria (One Necessary for Diagnosis)
Thrombocytopenia
Anemia
Elevated erythrocyte sedimentation rate
Fat macroglobulinemia

ACKNOWLEDGMENT

The authors wish to acknowledge Dr. Madison Macht, MD, for the valuable contributions to the previous edition of this chapter.

KEY POINTS: VENOUS THROMBOEMBOLISM AND FAT EMBOLISM

1. Critically ill patients have high rates (up to 33%) of VTE.
2. Clinical findings, including laboratory and EKG results, are neither sensitive nor specific for the diagnosis of PE. CT chest angiography or V/Q scan is necessary to confirm the diagnosis.
3. PE severity is graded as: (1) massive PE (with evidence of shock), (2) submassive PE (with evidence of RV strain), or (3) low-risk PE (no evidence of shock or RV strain).
4. The novel oral anticoagulants, rivaroxaban or apixaban, are now first-line therapy for the treatment of VTE once the patient is stable.

BIBLIOGRAPHY

1. Tapson VF. Acute pulmonary embolism. *N Engl J Med.* 2008;358:1037-1052.
2. Anderson Jr FA, Spencer FA. Risk factors for venous thromboembolism. *Circulation.* 2003;107(23 suppl 1):I9-I16.
3. Chunilal SD, Fikelboom JW, Attia J, et al. Does this patient have pulmonary embolism? *JAMA.* 2003;290:2849-2858.
4. Moores LK, King CS, Holley AB. Current approach to the diagnosis of acute nonmassive pulmonary embolism. *Chest.* 2011;140:509-518.
5. Kearon C, Akl EA, Ornelas J, et al. Antithrombotic therapy for VTE disease: CHEST guideline and expert panel report. *Chest.* 2016;149:315-352.
6. Yoo HH, Queluz TH, El Dib R. Anticoagulant treatment for subsegmental pulmonary embolism. *Cochrane Database Syst Rev.* 2014;(4):CD010222. doi:10.1002/14651858.CD010222.pub2.
7. Moores LK, Holley AB. Computed tomography pulmonary angiography and venography: diagnostic and prognostic properties. *Semin Respir Crit Care Med.* 2008;29:3-14.
8. Klok FA, Meyer G, Konstantinides S. Management of intermediate-risk pulmonary embolism: uncertainties and challenges. *Eur J Haematol.* 2015;95:489-497.
9. van der Hulle T, Dronkers CE, Klok FA, et al. Recent developments in the diagnosis and treatment of pulmonary embolism. *J Intern Med.* 2016;279:16-29.
10. Konstantinides S, Torbicki A. Management of venous thrombo-embolism: an update. *Eur Heart J.* 2014;35:2855-2863.
11. Meyer G, Vicaut E, Danays T, et al. Fibrinolysis for patients with intermediate-risk pulmonary embolism. *N Engl J Med.* 2014;370:1402-1411.
12. Konstantinides S, Geibel A, Heusel G, et al. Heparin plus alteplase compared with heparin alone in patients with submassive pulmonary embolism (MAPPET-3). *N Engl J Med.* 2002;347:1143-1150.
13. Snow V, Qaseem A, Barry P, et al. Management of venous thromboembolism: a clinical practice guideline from the American College of Physicians and the American Academy of Family Physicians. *Ann Intern Med.* 2007;146:204-210.

14. Cohen AT, Dobromirski M. The use of rivaroxaban for short- and long-term treatment of venous thromboembolism. *Thromb Haemost.* 2012;107(6):1035-1043.
15. Büller HR, Prins MH, Lensin AW, et al. Oral rivaroxaban for the treatment of symptomatic pulmonary embolism. *N Engl J Med.* 2012;366:1287-1297.
16. Lee AY, Levine MN, Baker RI, et al. Low-molecular-weight heparin versus a coumarin for the prevention of recurrent venous thromboembolism in patients with cancer. *N Engl J Med.* 2003;349:146-153.
17. Agnelli G, Prandoni P, Becattini C, et al, Warfarin Optimal Duration Italian Trial Investigators. Extended oral anticoagulant therapy after a first episode of pulmonary embolism. *Ann Intern Med.* 2003;139:19-25.
18. Decousus H, Leizorovicz A, Parent F, et al. A clinical trial of vena caval filters in the prevention of pulmonary embolism in patients with proximal deep-vein thrombosis. Prévention du Risque d'Embolie Pulmonaire par Interruption Cave Study Group. *N Engl J Med.* 1998;338:409-415.
19. PREPIC Study Group. Eight-year follow-up of patients with permanent vena cava filters in the prevention of pulmonary embolism: The PREPIC (Prévention du Risque d'Embolie Pulmonaire par Interruption Cave) randomized study. *Circulation.* 2005;112:416-422.
20. Mismetti P, Laporte S, Pellerin O, et al. Effect of a retrievable inferior vena cava filter plus anticoagulation vs anticoagulation alone on risk of recurrent pulmonary embolism: a randomized clinical trial. *JAMA.* 2015;313:1627-1635.
21. Mayer E, Jenkins D, Lindner J, et al. Surgical management and outcome of patients with chronic thromboembolic pulmonary hypertension: results from an international prospective registry. *J Thorac Cardiovasc Surg.* 2011;141:702-710.
22. Kakkos SK, Caprini JA, Geroulakos G, et al. Combined intermittent pneumatic leg compression and pharmacological prophylaxis for prevention of venous thromboembolism in high-risk patients. *Cochrane Database Syst Rev.* 2008;(4):CD005258. doi:10.1002/14651858.CD005258.pub2.
23. Guyatt GH, Akl EA, Crowther M, et al. Executive summary: antithrombotic therapy and prevention of thrombosis, 9th ed: American College of Chest Physicians evidence-based clinical practice guidelines. *Chest.* 2012;141(suppl 2):S7-S47.

V

CARDIOLOGY

CHAPTER 33

HEART FAILURE AND VALVULAR HEART DISEASE

Amir Azarbal and Martin M. LeWinter

HEART FAILURE

1. What are the types of cardiomyopathy resulting in the syndrome of heart failure?
   - **Reduced ejection fraction** (HFrEF; also referred to as systolic heart failure [HF], dilated cardiomyopathy): impaired contraction, often with loss of cardiomyocytes. Multiple causes but approximately 65% ischemic.
   - **Normal or preserved ejection fraction** (HFpEF; also referred to as diastolic HF): a prominent component of abnormal relaxation and/or increased stiffness of the left ventricle (LV), commonly associated with hypertension and increased arterial stiffness, concentric LV remodeling, type 2 diabetes mellitus and insulin resistance, obesity, chronic kidney disease, and aging. Comorbidities (e.g., atrial fibrillation, chronic obstructive pulmonary disease, obstructive sleep apnea) are very common.
   - **Infiltrative cardiomyopathy:** markedly decreased biventricular compliance leading to impaired diastolic filling and elevated right- and left-sided filling pressures. The most common cause is amyloidosis.
   - **Hypertrophic cardiomyopathy (HCM):** LV hypertrophy usually with asymmetric septal thickening and often dynamic outflow tract systolic pressure gradient. In most patients, HCM is an inherited disease caused by sarcomeric protein mutations. The mechanisms of HF in HCM are complex.
   - **Right ventricular (RV) failure:** Common causes are LV failure with type 2 pulmonary hypertension, obstructive sleep apnea, type 1 pulmonary hypertension, pulmonary embolus, and RV myocardial infarction (MI).

2. What are some other causes of heart failure with reduced ejection fraction besides ischemic heart disease or myocardial infarction?
   See Table 33.1.

3. How do we classify heart failure by functional status or stage?
   See Table 33.2.

4. What is the role of brain natriuretic peptide in the diagnosis of heart failure?
   - Not required to diagnose HF
   - Helpful when diagnostic uncertainty exists and for prognosis
   - Lower in HFpEF than in HFrEF
   - Lower in obese patients

Table 33-1. Causes of Heart Failure with Reduced Ejection Fraction

TYPE	CAUSE
Myocarditis	Infectious (viral) or inflammatory (e.g., systemic lupus erythematosus), giant cell (often requires transplantation)
Toxins	EtOH, cocaine, cancer chemotherapy
Stress-induced cardiomyopathy	Catecholamine surge during stress, most common pattern is apical ballooning (Takotsubo syndrome)
Genetic	Idiopathic, familial (multiple mutations)
End stage of chronic valvular disease	Aortic, mitral (see valvular disease section)
Other	Peripartum, sustained tachycardia, HTN, DM, endocrine or nutritional, acidosis, sepsis

DM, Diabetes mellitus; *EtOH*, ethyl alcohol; *HTN*, hypertension.

Table 33-2. Classifying Heart Failure by Functional Status/Stage

NYHA Functional Classification	
Class I	No limitation of physical activity
Class II (mild)	Slight limitation of physical activity
Class III (moderate)	Marked limitation of physical activity
Class IV (severe)	Unable to carry out any physical activity without discomfort, symptoms at rest
ACC-AHA Staging System	
Stage A	Patients at high risk for development of HF in the future but no functional or structural heart disease
Stage B	Structural heart disease but no symptoms
Stage C	Previous or current symptoms of HF in the context of underlying structural heart disease, adequately managed with medical treatment
Stage D	Advanced disease requiring hospital-based support, heart transplantation or mechanical support, or palliative care

ACC, American College of Cardiology; AHA, American Heart Association; HF, heart failure; NYHA, New York Heart Association.

5. How is acute decompensated heart failure treated?
   Patients can be categorized and treatment based on the presence or absence of signs and symptoms of congestion ("wet" versus "dry") and impaired perfusion ("cold" versus "warm"). **Congestion:** dyspnea, orthopnea, crackles, elevated venous pressure, ascites, peripheral edema.
   Impaired perfusion: reduced pulse pressure, cold extremities, altered mentation.
   - Dry and warm: Normal, requires no intervention.
   - Dry and cold: Pump failure without marked pulmonary congestion. Usually found in end-stage HF. Patients require inotropic support: dobutamine (β_1-adrenergic agonist), milrinone (phosphodiesterase inhibitor), mechanical support (LV assist devices); consider cardiac transplantation evaluation.
   - Wet and warm: Adequate perfusion with volume overload and increased filling pressures. The treatment focus is intravenous (IV) loop diuretics (furosemide). In the presence of hypertension, reduction of preload and afterload with IV vasodilators (morphine sulfate, nitroglycerin or nitroprusside, hydralazine, angiotensin-converting enzyme inhibitors [ACEIs]) should be a primary treatment focus.
   - Wet and cold: Volume overload with pump failure. These patients require diuretics, inotropes, vasodilators, and consideration of mechanical support and transplantation.
   Worsening renal function (cardiorenal syndrome): very common in acute decompensated heart failure (ADHF) and may require modification of treatment. In oliguric patients, dialysis may be the only effective way to achieve decongestion.

6. How is diastolic dysfunction diagnosed?
   An elevated LV end-diastolic or pulmonary capillary wedge pressure in a patient with a normal or preserved LV ejection fraction (EF) and normal or reduced end-diastolic volume by echocardiography establishes the presence of diastolic dysfunction. Various two-dimensional echocardiographic-Doppler parameters are also used, including increased ratio of early transmitral flow velocity to early diastolic velocity of the mitral valve annulus (E/e′), left atrial enlargement, and concentric LV remodeling.

VALVULAR HEART DISEASE

AORTIC STENOSIS

7. What are the causes of aortic stenosis?
   - Supravalvular, subvalvular (discrete, tunnel), extremely rare in adults
   - Valvular: congenital, degenerative

Congenital:

- Age 1 to 30 years, unicuspid (very rare)
- Age 40 to 60 years, usually bicuspid with secondary calcification

Degenerative:

- Age more than 70 years (most common form in developed countries)
- Rheumatic (incidence now markedly reduced in developed countries, usually associated with mitral valve disease)

8. What is the pathophysiology of aortic stenosis?
   1. Increase in afterload
   2. Impaired subendocardial blood flow regulation
   3. Progressive hypertrophy with diastolic dysfunction

   An increase in afterload caused by LV outflow obstruction causes concentric hypertrophy and increased wall thickness. By Laplace's law, the increased wall thickness normalizes systolic wall stress and maintains shortening (EF). These structural changes are associated with diastolic dysfunction (impaired relaxation, reduced chamber compliance), which increases LV filling pressures and, in turn, increases pressures in the pulmonary circulation. In a minority of patients, the ability to hypertrophy is exhausted, EF decreases, and the LV dilates.

9. What are the classic symptoms of aortic stenosis?

   Aortic stenosis (AS) results in a triad of symptoms: dyspnea (HF), angina, and dizziness or syncope. The appearance of these symptoms directly correlates with mortality. Fifty percent of patients are deceased 5 years after presentation with angina, 3 years after presentation with syncope, and 2 years after presentation with HF. The rate of progression of disease by valve gradient and area is another important predictor of mortality.

10. How is the severity of aortic stenosis graded using echocardiographic-Doppler methods?

    See Table 33.3.

11. How is aortic stenosis managed in the critically ill patient?

    The only definitive treatment for AS is valve replacement, either surgical or, increasingly, transcutaneous. For patients with circulatory congestion, IV furosemide should be used as in any patient with decompensated HF, but care must be taken to avoid over-diuresis. As a temporizing measure, critically ill patients with adequate blood pressure can sometimes be managed with vasodilators, in particular, nitroprusside. In carefully selected patients, nitroprusside increases cardiac index and stroke volume (SV) and reduces mean and diastolic arterial pressure and systemic vascular resistance. Vasodilator therapy should not be used without hemodynamic monitoring with a systemic arterial and flow-directed pulmonary artery catheter. Excessive vasodilation can cause severe deterioration by decreasing coronary perfusion. In some patients with reduced EF, dobutamine can be considered as a temporary alternative.

12. When should aortic valvuloplasty be considered?

    In carefully selected patients, balloon valvuloplasty can be used as a bridge to valve replacement for patients who are hemodynamically unstable. Balloon valvuloplasty has a high rate of early restenosis and poor long-term survival, and is therefore not a definitive treatment.

MITRAL STENOSIS

13. What are the causes of mitral stenosis?
    - Rheumatic disease
    - Congenital

Table 33-3. Grading Aortic Stenosis Using Echocardiographic-Doppler Methods

SEVERITY	FLOW VELOCITY (m/sec)	MEAN GRADIENT (mm Hg)	VALVE AREA (cm²)
Mild	2–2.9	<25	>1.5
Moderate	3–3.9	25–40	1.0–1.5
Severe	≥4	≥40	≤1.0

- Other: calcification related to aging and/or end-stage renal disease, obstructive left atrial myxoma, carcinoid heart disease

14. **How does mitral stenosis affect cardiac function and hemodynamics?**
    As the mitral valve orifice narrows, the left atrial pressure rises and a diastolic pressure gradient develops between the left atrium (LA) and the LV. The latter is required to maintain forward flow. The increased LA pressure is transmitted backward, in turn increasing pressure in the pulmonary veins, capillaries, pulmonary artery, and RV. In the lungs, this results in congestion and symptoms of HF. Over time, the increased LA pressure and secondary increases in pulmonary artery pressure may result in RV pressure overload and failure. The transmitral gradient is directly proportional to heart rate. Atrial fibrillation is extremely common in mitral stenosis (MS) and often leads to decompensation because of a rapid ventricular response.

15. **How is mitral stenosis graded with use of echocardiographic-Doppler methods?**
    See Table 33.4.

16. **How are critically ill patients with mitral stenosis managed?**
    As discussed above, the most common cause of decompensation in patients with MS is a rapid heart rate associated with atrial fibrillation. If tachycardia is present, this should be the focus of treatment through the use of β-blockers or calcium channel antagonists such as diltiazem. Direct current cardioversion for atrial fibrillation often has a role, but may be contraindicated in the acute setting in patients who have not been receiving prior anticoagulant therapy. Diuretics should also be used if necessary to reduce circulatory congestion. Vasodilators and positive inotropic agents generally have no role. Some patients with MS, even if critically ill, are candidates for percutaneous mitral balloon valvotomy, which is currently available in a limited number of centers.

17. **What are the indications for percutaneous mitral balloon valvotomy for mitral stenosis?**
    In centers performing the procedure, this is the preferred treatment for patients with moderate to severe MS who continue to have significant symptoms on medical management and who have pliable, noncalcified mitral valve leaflets, and who do not have moderate or worse mitral regurgitation (MR). Contraindications to valvotomy include left atrial thrombus and more than moderate MR.

AORTIC REGURGITATION

18. **What are the causes of aortic regurgitation?**
    The causes of aortic regurgitation (AR) can be divided into those related to disease of the valve itself or diseases of the aorta resulting in root dilatation (see Table 33.5).

Table 33-4. Grading Mitral Stenosis with Use of Echocardiographic Doppler Methods

SEVERITY	DIASTOLIC PRESSURE HALF-TIME (msec)	MITRAL VALVE AREA (cm²)
Progressive MS	≤150	>1.5
Asymptomatic Severe	≥150	1.0–1.5
Symptomatic Severe	≥150	<1.0

MS, Mitral stenosis.

Table 33-5. Causes of Aortic Regurgitation

VALVULAR DISEASE	AORTIC DISEASE
Rheumatic	Aortopathy: • Associated with bicuspid aortic valve • Marfan, Ehlers Danlos
Bicuspid	Type A aortic dissection
Endocarditis (bacterial or marantic)	Inflammatory (syphilis, Reiter syndrome)
Degenerative or calcified	
Vasculitis	

19. What is the pathophysiology of aortic regurgitation?

AR represents combined volume and pressure overload. Regurgitant flow in diastole increases the end-diastolic pressure and volume. This initiates LV hypertrophy with both increased wall thickness and further increases in diastolic volume. This combination initially helps to maintain SV. Approximately 50% of patients in whom severe AR is diagnosed progress to HF. Tachycardia reduces diastolic filling time and decreases the regurgitant fraction. In contrast, bradycardia does the opposite and is often poorly tolerated in patients with AR.

20. What is the management of acute, severe aortic regurgitation in the critical care setting?

Most acute, severe AR will require surgical intervention, depending on the cause (e.g., endocarditis, valvular vs. aortic disease). The first line of hemodynamic medical management in patients with normal blood pressure is diuretics and/or nitroprusside or another arteriolar dilator to reduce LV filling pressure, decrease the regurgitant fraction, and improve forward flow. Care must be taken not to cause excessive hypotension. The LV is typically hyperdynamic and does not require inotropic support. Vasopressors in general are contraindicated because they increase arterial load and promote a higher regurgitant fraction. When AR is stabilized, medical treatment consists of vasodilators such as hydralazine, nifedipine, and angiotensin-converting enzyme inhibitors.

21. What are the indications for surgery in aortic regurgitation?

Patients with prosthetic valve failure, aortic dissection, and most forms of acute, severe AR should be considered for urgent or emergent surgical intervention. Patients with HF, symptoms provoked by stress testing, EF less than 55%, or end-systolic dimension by echocardiography greater than 55 mm should in general have surgical intervention. A decreased EF and elevated end-systolic volume reduces 10-year survival after surgery. In the setting of endocarditis, surgical intervention should be balanced with antibiotic sterilization. Active infection is not a contraindication for valve replacement in critically ill patients.

MITRAL REGURGITATION

22. What are the causes of mitral regurgitation?
- Degenerative (mitral prolapse and/or chordal rupture): most common
- Functional (dilated cardiomyopathy, LV annular dilatation)
- Ischemia or infarction of the posterior LV wall or papillary muscle
- Rheumatic: rare in developed countries
- Other (e.g., endocarditis)

23. What is the pathophysiology of mitral regurgitation?

The mitral apparatus (leaflets, chordae tendineae, papillary muscles, and underlying LV wall) works in a coordinated fashion to maintain valve competence. In acute, severe MR, LV filling increases and afterload is decreased, which increases EF and total SV, although forward SV is often reduced. This combination results in pulmonary vascular congestion. Over time, the LV and LA chambers enlarge and become more compliant via rearrangement of myocardial fibers (eccentric remodeling). This allows maintenance of total and forward SV. Eventually, the LV cannot meet the demands of worsening MR and volume overload. Further dilation occurs, which is associated with an increased end-systolic volume and eventually a decrease in EF.

24. How is acute, severe mitral regurgitation managed?

A major goal of medical management is to pharmacologically reduce MR. This can be done by reducing systemic vascular resistance with arterial dilators such as nitroprusside. Diuretics should be used to relieve circulatory congestion. Acute MR often responds well to vasodilators alone. In patients whose condition is unstable or who have hypotension, nitroprusside should be used. In patients with reduced EF, an inotrope such as dobutamine can be used cautiously. Almost all patients with severe MR will eventually require surgical treatment.

25. What are the indications for surgery in mitral regurgitation?
- Symptoms of HF, even if mild
- LV dysfunction (EF <60%, end-systolic dimension >40 mm)
  Note: EF less than 30% is usually prohibitive for surgery because of high operative mortality.

ACKNOWLEDGMENT

The authors wish to acknowledge Dr. Neil Agrawal, MD, for the valuable contributions to the previous edition of this chapter.

KEY POINTS: HEART FAILURE AND VALVULAR HEART DISEASE

1. Classifications and Definitions:
   - Types of cardiomyopathy
   - HFrEF (systolic failure)
   - HFpEF (diastolic failure)
   - Infiltrative cardiomyopathy
   - HCM
   - RV failure
2. Treatment of ADHF
   - Dry-cold → inotropes
   - Wet-warm → diuretics, vasodilators
   - Wet-cold → inotropes, vasodilators, diuretics
3. AS and mortality
   - Syncope → 50% mortality after 5 years
   - Angina → 50% mortality after 3 years
   - Congestive HF → 50% mortality after 2 years
4. Treatment of AS in the critically ill
   - Valve replacement, balloon valvuloplasty
   - Nitroprusside
5. The pathophysiology of AR
   - Volume and pressure overload
6. Management of severe AR in the critically ill
   - Valve replacement in acute, severe AR
   - Nitroprusside, hydralazine, nifedipine, and ACEIs
   - Vasopressors contraindicated
7. Main causes of MS:
   - Rheumatic, congenital, calcific
8. The pathophysiology of MS
   - Elevated diastolic pressure gradient between LA and LV
   - Elevated pulmonary pressures and RV failure
   - Exacerbated by atrial fibrillation and rapid heart rates
9. Major causes of MR
   - Degenerative, functional, ischemia, rheumatic
10. Management of acute severe MR
    - Diuresis
    - Hypotension → Nitroprusside
    - Low EF → inotropes
    - Surgery if HF symptoms, EF less than 60% (preferably >30 percent), LV ESD greater than 40 mm
    - If technically feasible, mitral valve repair is preferred over replacement

BIBLIOGRAPHY

1. Yancy CW, Jessup M, Bozkurt B, et al. 2013 ACCF/AHA Guideline for the Management of Heart Failure: A Report of the American College of Cardiology Foundation/American Heart Association Task Force on Practice Guidelines. *J Am Coll Cardiol.* 2013;62:e147-e239. doi:10.1016/j.jacc.2013.05.019.
2. Felker GM, Thompson RE, Hare JM, et al. Underlying causes and long-term survival in patients with initially undiagnosed cardiomyopathy. *N Engl J Med.* 2000;342:1077.
3. Nohria A, Mielniczuk LM, Stevenson LW. Evaluation and monitoring of patients with acute heart failure syndromes. *Am J Cardiol.* 2005;96:32G.
4. Lindenfeld J, Albert NM, Boehmer JP, et al. HFSA 2010 Comprehensive Heart Failure Practice Guideline. *J Card Fail.* 2010;16:e1-e194.
5. Nishimura RA, Otto CM, Bonow RO, et al. 2014 AHA/ACC Guideline for the Management of Patients With Valvular Heart Disease: Executive Summary: A Report of the American College of Cardiology/American Heart Association Task Force on Practice Guidelines. *J Am Coll Cardiol.* 2014;63:2438-2488.

CHAPTER 34

ACUTE MYOCARDIAL INFARCTION

Sreedivya Chava and Harold L. Dauerman

1. Who is at risk for acute myocardial infarction?
   - **Nonmodifiable:** older age, noncardiac atherosclerotic disease, first-degree relative with early atherosclerosis (male age <55 years, female age <65 years).
   - **Modifiable:** diabetes mellitus; hypertension; smoking; elevated low-density lipoprotein (LDL), high-density lipoprotein (HDL), and triglycerides; C-reactive protein; lipoprotein (a); low HDL; hypertriglyceridemia; metabolic syndrome; sedentary lifestyle; atherogenic diet.
   - **Unclear:** In more than 10% of patients, no obvious risk factor is seen for coronary artery disease (CAD).

2. What causes an acute myocardial infarction?
   Coronary arterial atherosclerotic plaque with a thin fibrous cap is the ideal substrate for myocardial infarction (MI). Shear stress created by turbulent flow through an irregular, diseased segment of coronary artery can result in sudden rupture of this thin-capped vulnerable plaque. Procoagulants from the plaque's lipid core are extruded into the bloodstream, forming an occlusive thrombus at the site of insult. Plaque rupture accounts for roughly three-quarters of fatal acute myocardial infarctions (AMIs). The remaining 25% are due to erosion of the endothelial monolayer, uncovering a nidus for clot formation and extension into the arterial lumen.

3. How are patients typically seen initially with an acute myocardial infarction?
   - Severe retrosternal pressure with radiation to arms, neck, or jaw. Usually greater than or equal to 30 minutes in duration and associated with dyspnea, weakness, or diaphoresis. May be provoked by exertion, emotional stress, or extreme temperatures.
   - Rales, diaphoresis, hypotension, bradycardia or tachycardia, and transient murmur of mitral regurgitation are potential physical findings, though the examination results are most often unremarkable.
   - The key considerations in differential diagnosis are aortic dissection, pulmonary embolism, and pericarditis.

4. Which biomarkers diagnose acute myocardial infarction?
   The recently adopted universal definition of AMI includes elevation in cardiac biomarkers above the 99th percentile of the upper reference limit. See Table 34.1.

5. How do you diagnose an ST-elevation myocardial infarction (STEMI)?
   - New left bundle branch block or greater than or equal to 1-mm ST elevations in two or more contiguous leads. Absence of these electrocardiogram (ECG) changes leads to the alternative diagnosis: non–ST-elevation myocardial infarction (NSTEMI). Both types of MI demonstrate positive cardiac biomarkers.
   - Formation of a fibrin-rich *red clot*, which adheres to activated platelets, causing total occlusion of the affected artery and probable transmural infarction.
   - This syndrome was formerly termed Q-wave MI, but this terminology has been abandoned in favor of the more specific ST-elevation myocardial infarction (STEMI) term.

6. In whom does cardiogenic shock develop?
   - Shock complicating MI is most common among elderly patients.
   - Criteria for cardiogenic shock include persistent hypotension with a systolic blood pressure less than 90 mm Hg, cardiac index less than 1.8 $L/min^1/m^2$, left ventricular end-diastolic pressure greater than 18 mm Hg, or need for pressors or hemodynamic support.
   - Causes of cardiogenic shock include ventricular septal rupture, free wall or papillary muscle rupture, large MI, and nonischemic causes (myocarditis, Takotsubo cardiomyopathy, valvular heart disease).

Table 34-1. Biomarkers to Diagnose Acute Myocardial Infarction

BIOMARKER	ONSET/PEAK	DURATION	SENSITIVITY	SPECIFICITY
Myoglobin	1–4 h/6–12 h	24–36 h	Very high	Low
CK-MB	2–4 h/5–9 h	18–30 h	High	High
Troponin T or I	4–6 h/12–24 h	7–10 days	Very high	Very high

CK-MB, Creatine kinase MB.

7. What is the prognosis of a patient with acute myocardial infarction and out-of-hospital cardiac arrest?
   - The cause of cardiac arrest is AMI in greater than or equal to 50% of patients. Other causes include arrhythmias due to nonischemic etiologies (i.e., nonischemic cardiomyopathy).
   - Less than 40% of patients with cardiac arrest may survive to hospital discharge. Predictors of discharge from hospital include witnessed arrest, initial ventricular tachycardia or ventricular fibrillation, bystander cardiopulmonary resuscitation, cooling or hypothermia, younger age, male sex, acute myocardial ischemia or heart failure, early invasive management of CAD, and absence of comorbidities.

8. You diagnose a ST-elevation myocardial infarction at a rural clinic without a catheterization laboratory; what do you do?
   Reperfusion via percutaneous coronary intervention *(primary PCI)* is the preferred treatment for STEMI. A clear mortality benefit exists if this is done within 90 minutes of first contact with the medical system. In this case, door to balloon time is expected to exceed 120 minutes, and reperfusion should be achieved with fibrinolytics (with half dose lytic given to elderly patients to limit risk of intracranial bleeding). In addition to fibrinolysis, adjunctive therapy with heparin, aspirin, and clopidogrel (300 mg) is warranted. A pharmacoinvasive approach leads to decreased risk of recurrent ischemia and infarction compared to fibrinolysis alone; thus all patients in the postlytic period should be transferred for cardiac catheterization and possible revascularization.

9. Which antithrombotic therapy should be administered to the patient in Question 8?
   After receiving fibrinolytics, choices of anticoagulant include weight-based dosing of unfractionated heparin, enoxaparin, or fondaparinux. The most common regimen in patients being referred for early catheterization is unfractionated heparin, along with aspirin and clopidogrel. Bivalirudin is an alternative to unfractionated heparin use during primary PCI, but there is limited data on its use with pharmacoinvasive approaches.

10. Which antiplatelet therapies are indicated for the patient in Question 8?
    Aspirin (162–325 mg followed by 81 mg daily) and clopidogrel (300 mg loading dose followed by 75 mg daily) are the mainstays of antiplatelet therapy in STEMI and are indicated in patients who received full-dose fibrinolytic therapy. In the primary PCI population only, treatment with ticagrelor (180 mg loading dose followed by 90 mg BID) as compared with clopidogrel significantly reduced the rate of death from cardiovascular causes, via reductions in MI, stent thrombosis, and stroke. Similarly, prasugrel (60 mg loading dose followed by 10 mg daily) reduces stent thrombosis compared with clopidogrel in patients with AMI, but is contraindicated in patients with prior stroke or transient ischemic attack. Addition of glycoprotein inhibition of platelets to unfractionated heparin as bailout (for slow flow in the culprit artery) is also possible.

11. Which patients with unstable angina or non–ST-elevation myocardial infarction have the highest mortality?
    Thrombolysis in Myocardial Infarction (TIMI), Global Registry of Acute Coronary Events (GRACE), and Platelet Glycoprotein IIb/IIIa in Unstable Angina: Receptor Suppression Using Integrilin (PURSUIT) are risk stratification schemes that aid in patient selection for early invasive versus conservative therapies. The TIMI risk score is composed of seven variables: age 65 years or older, three or more CAD risk factors, aspirin use within a week, two or more episodes of severe angina in the past day, elevated cardiac biomarkers, ST deviation greater than or equal to 0.5 mm, and known greater than or equal to 50% coronary stenosis. The presence of three variables indicates intermediate risk (13% chance of death, MI, or need for urgent revascularization within 14 days), and five or more predicts a doubling of this risk.

Table 34-2. Risk Factors Associated with Referral for Invasive Management Strategy

SYMPTOMS	TESTING	HISTORY	PHYSICAL EXAMINATION	OTHER
Refractory symptoms	New ST depressions	Prior PCI	Hemodynamic instability	Sustained ventricular tachycardia
—	Elevated biomarkers	Prior CABG	Heart failure	High risk score (i.e., TIMI)
—	EF <40%	—	New mitral regurgitation	High-risk noninvasive testing

CABG, coronary artery bypass grafting; *EF,* Ejection fraction; *TIMI,* thrombolysis in myocardial infarction.
Modified from O'Connor RE, Brady W, Brooks SC, et al. Part 10: acute coronary syndromes, 2010 American
 Heart Association Guidelines for Cardiopulmonary Resuscitation and Emergency Cardiovascular Care.
 Circulation. 2010;122(18 suppl 3):S787–S817.

12. You are evaluating a patient with unstable angina. What patient characteristics would lead to early
    referral to the catheterization laboratory and possible revascularization?
    See Table 34.2.

13. What medications do you start in a patient initially seen with a non–ST-elevation myocardial
    infarction?
    Aspirin (162–325 mg) should be administered to every patient. Intermediate- or high-risk patients
    should receive ticagrelor (180 mg) or clopidogrel (300 or 600 mg) plus weight-adjusted unfractionated
    heparin or renal function–adjusted enoxaparin. Upstream use of glycoprotein inhibitors prior to
    angiography is no longer recommended. For the early invasive strategy, pretreatment with a statin
    may decrease periprocedural infarction. Prasugrel (60 mg) could be loaded after coronary angiography
    and may be given in place of ticagrelor or clopidogrel as long as the patient is not at high risk for
    bleeding (defined as age ≥75 years, previous stroke, or weight ≤60 kg). Relief of chest pain may be
    achieved with nitrates and morphine but should alert the care team to a high-risk situation. Ongoing
    chest pain should warrant consideration for emergent catheterization because it may represent
    coronary occlusion and progression to STEMI.

14. Your acute myocardial infarction patient is ready to go home. What prescriptions do you consider
    at discharge?
    Dual antiplatelet therapy should be continued in patients after AMI, including a P2Y12 inhibitor and aspi-
    rin. Potent P2Y12 inhibitors (ticagrelor or prasugrel) have shown a decreased risk of recurrent ischemic
    events in patients with acute MI, as compared with the clopidogrel, but with an increased risk of bleed-
    ing. P2Y12 inhibitors should be continued at least 1 year after the percutaneous intervention in all AMI
    patients (and 81 mg of aspirin is continued indefinitely). In patients with AMI treated with coronary stent
    implantation who have tolerated dual antiplatelet therapy (DAPT) without a bleeding complication and
    who are not at high bleeding risk, continuation of DAPT for longer than 12 months may be reasonable.
    β-Blockers, statins (goal LDL <70 mg/dL), and angiotensin-converting enzyme (ACE) inhibitors reduce
    cardiovascular morbidity and mortality and should be initiated in hospital.

15. Your acute myocardial infarction patient has cardiogenic shock. What is the only therapy that can
    improve mortality?
    Early revascularization is recommended in all patients with AMI complicated by shock. Previous
    studies have shown early revascularization with PCI or coronary artery bypass grafting (CABG)
    improves mortality and quality of life significantly compared to initial medical stabilization and
    intra-aortic balloon pump (IABP) placement alone. The IABP—SHOCK—II trial randomly assigned
    patients with AMI and cardiogenic shock who were planned to undergo early revascularization to
    IABP or no IABP. The 30-day all-cause mortality is similar in both groups (39.7% vs 41.3%:
    $P = .69$). Though there are several mechanical circulatory support devices (percutaneous left
    ventricular assist devices, extracorporeal membrane oxygenation), available for management
    of acute cardiogenic shock patients, there is a lack of randomized trial data evaluating the
    effectiveness of these new devices.

16. Name the most appropriate first and second choice of vasopressor in cardiogenic shock.

After PCI or early revascularization with CABG, vasopressors may be required for a period of time to allow hemodynamic stabilization. Dopamine and norepinephrine are the medications most often used for hypotension in cardiogenic shock. Both agents have α- and β-adrenergic properties, though in different degrees, resulting in disparate effects on renal and splanchnic perfusion. A recent multicenter randomized trial established norepinephrine as the first-line vasopressor in cardiogenic shock, with dopamine resulting in more arrhythmic events and a lower survival at 28 days. In patients with refractory hemodynamic instability, referral for left ventricular assist support devices and cardiac transplantation may be warranted.

17. What are the indications for cooling or hypothermia after acute myocardial infarction and cardiac arrest?

- Adult successfully resuscitated from a witnessed out-of-hospital or in-hospital cardiac arrest and now hemodynamically stable
- Patient with a presenting rhythm of ventricular fibrillation or nonperfusing ventricular tachycardia who remains comatose after restoration of spontaneous circulation

After cooling, patients should be monitored for electrolyte abnormalities, coagulation disturbances, pancreatitis, and leukopenia or thrombocytopenia.

ACKNOWLEDGMENT

The authors wish to acknowledge Dr. Cameron Donaldson, MD, for the valuable contributions to the previous edition of this chapter.

KEY POINTS: ACUTE MYOCARDIAL INFARCTION

1. Distinguish between unstable angina (UA)-NSTEMI and STEMI: STEMI is an occluded artery and requires immediate reperfusion with PCI or fibrinolysis; UA-NSTEMI requires medical therapy and invasive approach (within 4–48 hours of presentation) for all patients at increased risk.
2. Oral antiplatelet therapy should be initiated including aspirin and early clopidogrel or ticagrelor, or prasugrel at the time of angiography.
3. Antithrombotics (heparin, enoxaparin, fondaparinux, or bivalirudin) should be administered with weight- and glomerular filtration rate–adjusted dosing to avoid bleeding risks.
4. Statin, β-blocker, and ACE inhibitors should be considered in all patients with AMI regardless of baseline LDL level, blood pressure, and heart rate.
5. Revascularization (PCI, CABG) is warranted immediately (STEMI–primary PCI), urgently (STEMI–pharmacoinvasive approach) or within 4 to 48 hours of presentation (high-risk UA-NSTEMI).

BIBLIOGRAPHY

1. Antman EM, Cohen M, Bernink PJ, et al. The TIMI risk score for unstable angina/non-ST elevation MI: a method for prognostication and therapeutic decision making. *JAMA.* 2000;284:835-842.
2. Stone GW, Maehara A, Lansky AJ, et al. A prospective natural-history study of coronary atherosclerosis. *N Engl J Med.* 2011;364:226-235.
3. Tian J, Dauerman H, Toma C, et al. Prevalence and characteristics of TCFA and degree of coronary artery stenosis: an OCT, IVUS, and angiographic study. *J Am Coll Cardiol.* 2014;64(7):672-680.
4. Thygesen K, Alpert JS, White HD. Universal definition of myocardial infarction. *J Am Coll Cardiol.* 2007;50: 2173-2195.
5. White HD, Chew DP. Acute myocardial infarction. *Lancet.* 2008;372:570-584.
6. Dauerman HL, Sobel BE. Synergistic treatment of ST-segment elevation myocardial infarction with pharmacoinvasive recanalization. *J Am Coll Cardiol.* 2003;42:646-651.
7. Armstrong PW, Gershlick AH, Goldstein P, et al, for the STREAM Investigators. Fibrinolysis or primary PCI in ST-segment elevation myocardial infarction. *N Engl J Med.* 2013;368:1379-1383.
8. Dauerman HL, Bates ER, Kontos MC, et al. A Nationwide Perspective on the STEMI Transfer Process: Findings from the AHA Mission Lifeline Program. *Circ Cardiovasc Interv.* 2015;8(5):e002450. doi:10.1161/CIRCINTERVENTIONS. 114.002450.
9. Chava S, Raza S, El-Haddad MA, et al. A regional pharmacoinvasive therapy strategy incorporating selected bleeding avoidance strategies. *Coron Artery Dis.* 2014;26(1):30-36.
10. De Backer D, Biston P, Devriendt J, et al. Comparison of dopamine and norepinephrine in the treatment of shock. *N Engl J Med.* 2010;362:779-789.
11. Holzer M. Targeted temperature management for comatose survivors of cardiac arrest. *N Engl J Med.* 2010;363: 1256-1264.

12. Reynolds HR, Hochman JS. Cardiogenic shock: current concepts and improving outcomes. *Circulation.* 2008;117:
     686-697.
13. Thiele H, Zeymer U, Neumann FJ, et al., for the IABP-SHOCK II Trial Investigators. Intraaortic balloon support for
     myocardial infarction with cardiogenic shock. *N Engl J Med.* 2012;367:1287-1296.
14. Wiviott SD, Braunwald E, McCabe CH, et al. Prasugrel versus clopidogrel in patients with a acute coronary
     syndromes. *N Engl J Med.* 2007;357:2001-2015.
15. Dauerman HL. Anticoagulation strategies for primary PCI: current controversies and recommendations. *Circ
     Cardiovasc Interv.* 2015;8(5):e001947. doi.org/10.1161/CIRCINTERVENTIONS.115.001947.
16. Wallentin L, Becker RC, Budaj A, et al. Ticagrelor versus clopidogrel in patients with acute coronary syndromes.
     N Engl J Med. 2009;361:1045-1057.

CHAPTER 35

CARDIAC ARRHYTHMIA

Pierre Znojkiewicz and Peter S. Spector

1. How do you treat tachycardia in the intensive care unit?
   The first step in treating an arrhythmia in the intensive care unit (ICU) is determination of the urgency with which it must be resolved; hemodynamically unstable rhythms require immediate treatment at times not affording the clinician the luxury of full diagnostic assessment. Even in the patient whose condition is unstable, a very quick look at a telemetry recording allows one to answer several key questions: Is this a wide (QRS >120 ms) or narrow complex rhythm? Is the rhythm irregular or regular? **Unstable rhythms can be electrically cardioverted or defibrillated.** With better-tolerated rhythms it is important to gather some diagnostic information that may be required for both short- and long-term arrhythmia management.

2. How do you determine the cause of wide complex tachycardias?
   Whenever possible, a 12-lead electrocardiogram (ECG) should be obtained. The first distinction to make is between supraventricular and ventricular arrhythmias. A detailed description of how to make this distinction is beyond the scope of this chapter, but a few rules of thumb can be helpful. Narrow complexes indicate that the ventricles are being depolarized via the conduction system (His-Purkinje [HP]). A wide QRS complex indicates that ventricular activation is *not* entirely via an intact conduction system. This can occur with ventricular tachycardia (VT), ventricular pacing, bundle branch block (BBB), accessory pathway (AP) conduction, or rarely with ventricular conduction delay (e.g., hyperkalemia).

3. How do you differentiate a ventricular tachycardia from an aberrantly conducted supraventricular tachycardia?
   In wide complex tachycardias, one must distinguish supraventricular tachycardia (SVT) with aberrancy from VT. Step 1 is to identify P waves and assess the relationship between atrial and ventricular activation. A 1:1 relationship can occur with conduction from atria to ventricles (or vice versa and therefore does not distinguish SVT from VT). Atrioventricular (AV) dissociation, on the other hand, can identify VT (V faster than A) or SVT with aberrancy (A faster than V). Other indicators that suggest VT (though not definitively) are a very wide QRS (>160 ms), precordial concordance (leads V1–V6 all positive or all negative), and fusion beats (indicating intermittent conduction via the HP system during VT). Finally, inspection of an old ECG can help identify the prior presence of BBB or pre-excitation. Irregularly irregular rhythms are likely to be atrial fibrillation (AF) .

4. What rhythms produce a wide complex tachycardia that can be mistaken for ventricular tachycardia?
   SVTs that are conducted with BBB (pre-existing or rate related) are referred to as SVT with aberrancy. In patients with an AP conduction from atria to ventricles over the AP will produce a wide complex. This will occur whether the AP is part of the arrhythmia circuit (antidromic AV reentrant tachycardia [AVRT]; conduction antegrade over the AP and retrograde over the AV node) or a *bystander* that simply conducts activation resulting from some other arrhythmia (e.g., atrial flutter).

5. What should you think of when you see a very wide QRS (and no P waves)?
   Hyperkalemia leads to baseline depolarization of cardiac cell membranes. This in turn results in an increased proportion of inactivated sodium channels. The global consequence of increased inactivation is decreased conduction velocity. In the atria this creates long low-amplitude P waves (which can be difficult to see), and in the ventricle it creates a very wide QRS. With sufficient hyperkalemia a sine wave–appearing rhythm can result. If the underlying rhythm is fast (e.g., sinus tachycardia) the wide QRS and apparent lack of P waves can be mistaken for VT. It is critical **not** to give sodium channel blocking antiarrhythmics (e.g., lidocaine) in this setting because they further increase sodium channel inactivation and can result in asystole and death. Treatment should be aimed at stabilizing the cell membrane (calcium) and reducing potassium (insulin, glucose, Kayexalate, and/or dialysis). See Fig. 35.1.

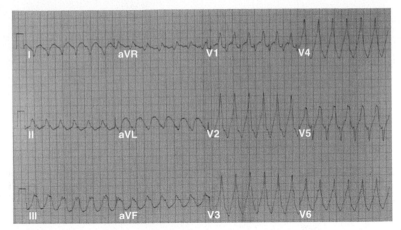

Figure 35-1. Example of a wide complex tachycardia in a patient with hyperkalemia; note how this could be mistaken for ventricular tachycardia.

6. What is *torsades de pointes*, and what predisposes a patient to it?

Torsades de pointes, French for *twisting of the points*, is a specific polymorphic VT that is frequently self-limiting but can degenerate into ventricular fibrillation (VF). It must be distinguished from polymorphic VT due to ischemia. Torsades is defined by the following:
- Constellation of one long QT interval (QTc >440 ms in men and >460 ms in women)
- Initiation with a *long-short* interval (tachycardia begins after a pause [long cycle])
- Premature ventricular contraction that begins during the T wave (short cycle)

Long QT (and torsade) can result from a congenital ion channel abnormality or be acquired from ion channel blocking medication (Fig. 35.2) and can be exacerbated by hypomagnesemia, hypokalemia, and hypocalcemia.

7. What drugs commonly used in the intensive care unit can cause QT prolongation?

See Table 35.1. See also www.torsades.org.

8. What is the Wolff-Parkinson-White syndrome?

Wolff-Parkinson-White (WPW) syndrome occurs in patients who have an abnormal extra connection between the atria and the ventricles: an AP. This can result in evidence of pre-excitation on surface ECG. The atrial wave front travels down the AP and begins depolarizing ventricular tissue before ventricular activation through the HP system, resulting in a short PR interval and initial slurring of the QRS (delta wave). This is followed by rapid activation of the remaining ventricular tissue through the HP system. A patient with preexcitation and documented AVRT is said to have WPW syndrome. Note that a subset of APs will only conduct retrograde and will not produce evident preexcitation; these are so-called concealed APs.

9. Why are patients with Wolff-Parkinson-White syndrome at increased risk for sudden cardiac death?

Patients who have an AP lack the protection offered by AV node refractoriness. If their AP can conduct antegrade (from the atria to the ventricles) at high frequency, they are at risk for very rapid ventricular

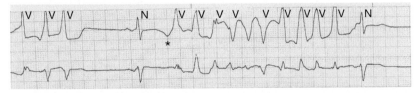

Figure 35-2. Example of torsade de pointes. Notice the long QT, long-short interval *(asterisk)*, and self-limiting polymorphic ventricular tachycardia with twisting of the points.

Table 35-1. Common Drugs That Cause QT Prolongation	
Amiodarone	Quinidine
Clarithromycin	Sotalol
Haloperidol	Dofetilide
Amitriptyline	Lithium
Methadone	Fluconazole

rates should atrial fibrillation develop. Such rapid rates can lead to VT or VF. Any patient who is initially seen with an irregularly irregular wide complex tachycardia should raise the suspicion of pre-excited AF. AV nodal blocking agents should be avoided in such patients because they can increase conduction down the AP, leading to increased risk for VF or VT. Drugs that slow conduction of the pathway such as procainamide or amiodarone should be considered.

10. What is the main effect of adenosine on cardiac conduction?
Adenosine's main clinically relevant effect on cardiac conduction is transient AV nodal block. As such, it can be used in the diagnosis of various narrow complex tachycardias where the P waves are difficult to discern on the surface ECG. A bolus of adenosine produces rapid-onset, short-duration AV block. This can result in *unmasking* of P waves previously obscured by the QRST complex. In AV node–dependent rhythms (such as AVRT and AVNRT [described later]), adenosine will cause termination of tachycardia. Thus adenosine injection can be a diagnostic and therapeutic maneuver. Termination of a narrow complex tachycardia by adenosine strongly suggests an AV node–dependent rhythm, but rarely can indicate adenosine-sensitive focal atrial tachycardias. It is important always to have a 12-lead ECG running when giving adenosine. See Fig. 35.3.

11. How do you treat hemodynamically stable tachycardias?
There are two issues to consider when identifying arrhythmias:
1. Is the rhythm symptomatic (and hence treatment is aimed at relief from symptoms)? and/or
2. Does the rhythm identify an underlying risk (e.g., an increased risk for sudden cardiac death or stroke)?

Atrial fibrillation and rapid atrial tachycardias (e.g., atrial flutter) are associated with increased risk for stroke, and measures must be taken to reduce this risk *independent of* whether the rhythm is

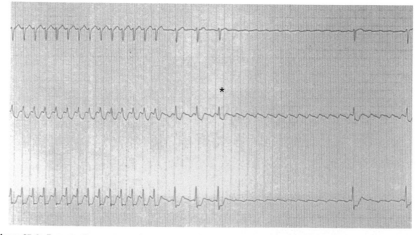

Figure 35-3. Example of a narrow complex tachycardia proven to be atrial flutter by unmasking of the flutter waves once transient atrioventricular block is achieved by adenosine, the asterisk shows the onset of AV block.

controlled. In some patients (e.g., those with decreased ventricular function), VT can indicate an increased risk for sudden cardiac death. Finally, pre-excitation (antegrade conduction via an AP) *may* indicate an increased risk for sudden death depending on the refractory properties of the AP. Such patients may require an electrophysiologic study to assess the pathway's refractory period.

12. **What drugs can be used to control ventricular response rate in a patient with hypotension and atrial fibrillation?**
An unfortunate side effect of most rate-controlling medications such as β-blockers and calcium channel blockers is that they are vasodilators and negative inotropes and hence can lead to lowered systemic blood pressure. For this reason, physicians are often hesitant to give these medications to a patient with AF and rapid ventricular response rate who have low pressure. In the vast majority of cases, repeated small doses of intravenous (IV) medication (e.g., 5 mg of diltiazem) will reduce heart rate without decreasing blood pressure (the increased diastolic filling time offsets the vasodilatory and negative inotropic effects). Direct current cardioversion (DCCV) is the treatment of choice for hemodynamically unstable rapid AF.

13. **How should you treat AF in a hemodynamically stable patient?**
A patient with highly symptomatic atrial fibrillation should have attempts made at restoring and maintaining sinus rhythm. Cardioversion (chemical or electrical) is the usual first step in any patient who has new-onset atrial fibrillation of less than 48 hours. After 48 hours of AF without adequate anticoagulation, the risk for thromboembolic events increases. Under these circumstances, the patient should have rate control and adequate anticoagulation for at least 3 weeks and then cardioversion. If the patient cannot tolerate AF for that period of time and if transesophageal echocardiography reveals no thrombus, cardioversion may be performed and anticoagulation started. Antiarrhythmic agents can be used for patients with symptoms either in whom DCCV has failed or who are going in and out of AF (in which case DCCV is not appropriate). In patients without symptoms, it is reasonable to allow AF to continue and control ventricular response rates. Management of anticoagulation *is independent of rhythm control.*

14. **Who needs anticoagulation?**
In patients with new-onset AF of less than 48 hours duration, the need for anticoagulation before and after cardioversion may be based on the patient's long-term risk for thromboembolism (see Table 35.2). For patients with AF of more than 48 hours duration, anticoagulation should be initiated before cardioversion (for at least 3 weeks if possible, or IV heparin if requiring immediate cardioversion for hemodynamic instability) and continued for 4 weeks after cardioversion. The decision for long-term anticoagulation is based on the CHA_2DS_2-VASc score. Patients with a score of 1 can receive no therapy, therapy with aspirin, or full anticoagulation; patients with a score of 2 or more should receive long-term anticoagulation.

Table 35-2. CHA2DS2-VASc Score

RISK FACTOR	SCORE
Congestive heart failure/LV dysfunction	1
Hypertension	1
Age >75	2
Diabetes Mellitus	1
Stroke/TIA	2
Vascular disease (PAD, MI)	1
Age 65–74	1
Sex category (i.e., female gender)	1

LV, left ventricular; TIA, transient ischemic attack; PAD, peripheral artery disease; MI, myocardial infarction.

Lip GY, Nieuwlaat R, Pisters R, et al. Refining clinical risk stratification for predicting stroke and thromboembolism in atrial fibrillation using a novel risk factor based approach—The Euro Heart Survey on Atrial Fibrillation. *Chest.* 2010;137:263–272.

15. **Are there nonpharmacologic approaches to acute rate control with atrial tachycardias?**

In patients with atrial tachycardia who have a pacemaker with atrial pacing leads in place, a nonpharmacologic alternative to AV node–blocking drugs exists for controlling ventricular response rate. In an atrial tachycardia that cannot be otherwise rate-controlled, efforts can be made to pace the atria *faster* than the rate of the atrial tachycardia; this can lead to a higher degree of block in the AV node (i.e., 3:1 vs. 2:1) and therefore paradoxically lower the ventricular rate.

16. **How do you treat rapid regular narrow-complex tachycardias?**

Adenosine can be a helpful diagnostic maneuver (see earlier). Typical atrial flutter can be recognized by its characteristic appearance: "sawtooth" P waves in the inferior leads and a narrow upright P wave in V_1. This ECG pattern reliably indicates counterclockwise re-entry around the tricuspid annulus, a rhythm with a very high rate of cure with catheter ablation. Other atrial tachycardia can be treated with antiarrhythmic medication or ablation. Ablation of SVT has a high success rate and low complication rate. AV nodal–blocking agents can also be used for long-term suppression of SVT.

17. **How do you decide which antiarrhythmic medication to use?**

The choice of antiarrhythmic medication can be complex, but one should know major contraindications to the various antiarrhythmic agents. Amiodarone is contraindicated in patients with chronic lung disease and baseline thyroid dysfunction; patients taking amiodarone should have annual chest radiographs and biannual liver and thyroid function tests. Dronedarone is contraindicated in patients with congestive heart failure. Flecainide is contraindicated in patients with coronary artery or structural heart disease. Dofetilide and sotalol should be avoided in patients with renal insufficiency; with preserved renal function, therapy with these agents should be started in the hospital where the QTc can be monitored until steady states have been achieved.

18. **How are bradycardias described?**

Bradycardia can result from abnormalities of impulse formation (e.g., sinus bradycardia, sinus arrest) or from failure of impulse conduction (i.e., AV node or HP system disease).

19. **How do you describe the different degrees of AV block?**

- **First-degree** heart block: conduction delay with PR interval greater than 200 ms. First-degree AV *block* is therefore a misnomer; all p waves are conducted through the AV node, and electrophysiology purists will use the term first-degree AV *delay*.
- **Second-degree** heart block: periodic interruptions of AV conduction, leading to nonconducted beats. Second-degree heart block is divided into Mobitz type I (Wenckebach: progressive PR prolongation followed by a nonconducted beat) and Mobitz type II (intermittent nonconducted beats with a fixed PR interval that is typically not prolonged).
- **Third-degree** heart block: complete interruption of AV conduction, with AV dissociation (if there are ventricular escape beats) or ventricular asystole.

20. **Which type of second-degree heart block is worrisome and why?**

Second-degree AV block is rarely symptomatic and by itself is not dangerous. The question is whether second-degree block indicates increased risk for complete AV block, and if so, whether asystole is likely to occur. AV node block rarely progresses to third-degree block and often has a reliable escape rhythm if it does. HP block is more likely to progress to complete block and is more likely to result in asystole. AV node suppression typically results in Mobitz I block, whereas HP block leads to Mobitz II block. Therefore Mobitz II block is an indication for permanent pacemaker placement. In the presence of 2:1 AV block, Mobitz I and II cannot be distinguished; widened QRS and normal PR interval suggest that block is at the HP level. Atropine improves AV node conduction. It has no direct effect on HP conduction, but by causing increased sinus rate, can *paradoxically* increase HP block and therefore should be avoided in this setting.

21. **How would you know whether transcutaneous pacing pads are capturing?**

Transcutaneous pacing is a temporary solution for hemodynamically unstable bradycardia. Electric current is delivered between the pacing/defibrillation pads on the patient's chest. It can be difficult to assess whether myocardial capture has been achieved; the surface electrogram and telemetry are frequently obscured by a large-amplitude pacing artifact, and palpation of the pulse can be misleading because of contraction of the skeletal muscles mimicking cardiac pulsation. One can look for T waves on the cardiogram, monitor arterial blood pressure, or palpate the femoral pulse. **Note:** the default setting on most external pacing machines is to start pacing at the machine's **minimum** output current.

22. What are some common causes of out-of-hospital cardiac arrest?

The most common causes of out-of-hospital cardiac arrest are coronary artery disease and acute coronary syndrome. Another common cause is underlying structural heart disease (i.e., systolic dysfunction, prior myocardial infarction (MI), and cardiac scarring facilitating VT). In younger, otherwise healthy patients with no evidence of structural heart disease, congenital cardiac channelopathies should be suspected.

23. How do you determine the etiology of cardiac arrest?

A focused history, either from the patient or anyone witnessing the event, should be obtained. Unfortunately this is not always immediately possible, but can be extremely valuable in trying to ascertain whether cardiac arrhythmia is the primary culprit or is secondary to a preceding event (acute coronary syndrome, respiratory arrest, intentional overdose of cardiac medications). In patients requiring defibrillation in the field, attempts should be made to recover the rhythm strips from the defibrillator which is usually possible, even in the case of automated devices. Determination of the underlying rhythm (Monomorphic VT, Polymorphic VT, *Torsades* or VF) can help narrow down possible etiologies. An ECG and assessment of left ventricular (LV) function are paramount and ischemic evaluation should be performed in the vast majority of patients.

24. What intervention has been shown to dramatically increase neurologic recovery and survival after out-of-hospital cardiac arrest?

Therapeutic hypothermia (TH) should be initiated in all patients who have had recovery of a perfusing rhythm after out-of-hospital arrest but exhibit neurologic symptoms (not following commands or showing purposeful movements). Although there remains some debate about the optimal temperature goal, there is no doubt that lowering core temperature to 33 to 36°C has been shown in multiple trials to dramatically improve neurologic recovery and even long term survival. There are different commercially available devices and systems to achieve this strategy and it is usually implemented by a multidisciplinary team combining intensive care, neurology, and cardiology.

25. Name possible complications or adverse events secondary to therapeutic hypothermia.

Shivering is a natural reaction to hypothermia and is the body's way of trying to increase its temperature. It must be controlled with the use of sedatives; otherwise, achieving hypothermia might be difficult. Hypothermia also slows cardiac conduction and impulse generation and can lead to bradycardia, most commonly sinus bradycardia, which is usually not an issue if the mean blood pressure remains within acceptable range. Lastly, hypothermia induces a mild coagulopathy and this should be monitored closely if there is any suspicion of bleeding as can be the case if there was significant trauma with the initial cardiac arrest.

26. Name conditions that can cause cardiac arrest in patients without apparent underlying heart disease.

In patients without underlying structural heart disease and cardiac arrest, especially in younger patients, one should suspect inherited channelopathies. Examples of such conditions are: arrhythmogenic right ventricular cardiomyopathy, congenital long-QT syndrome, Brugada syndrome, and catecholaminergic polymorphic ventricular tachycardia (CPVT). A detailed family history is very important in patients suspected of any of these conditions. Particular scrutiny should be directed towards any relatives having possible syncopal events or cardiac arrest. The astute clinician should be careful when laymen describe someone as having a "heart attack": was it an acute coronary syndrome with preceding angina or was it sudden cardiac arrest due to arrhythmia?

27. What is Arrhytmogenic right ventricular cardiomyopathy (ARVC)?

Previously referred to as arrhythmogenic right ventricular dysplasia (ARVD), this condition is characterized by fibrofatty infiltration of cardiac tissue predominantly in the right ventricle, although it is now known to frequently affect both ventricles and rarely, only the left ventricle. Clinically ARVC manifests as frequent premature ventricular contractions (PVCs), palpitations, syncope, and possible sudden cardiac arrest. It is thought to be secondary to mutations to genes responsible for desmosomal proteins and a variety of these mutations have been described, the majority being transmitted in autosomal dominant fashion. It is likely this is an under-recognized cause of sudden cardiac death/cardiac arrest.

28. How is ARVC diagnosed?

As with most conditions where a single gold standard test for diagnosis does not exist, ARVC is diagnosed by a combination of criteria. A complete listing of the criteria is beyond the scope of this chapter, but some notable major criteria are: RV akinesis, dyskinesia or aneurysm and enlarged RV outflow tract on echo, MRI or RV angiography, presence of less than 60% myocytes on RV free wall biopsy,

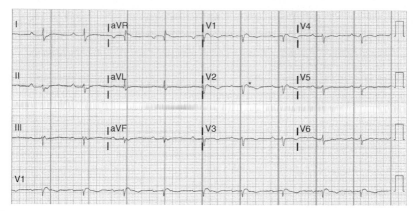

Figure 35-4. Epsilon wave electrocardiogram. Note the epsilon wave visible after the QRS in V2 *(asterisk)*. This is caused by delayed activation of portions of the right ventricule due the slow conduction through tissue affected by fibrofatty infiltration.

inverted T waves in right precordial lead (V1, V2 and V3), Epsilon wave on surface ECG (Fig. 35.4), nonsustained or sustained VT of left bundle-branch morphology with superior axis (negative in II, III or aVF), or a first-degree relative with confirmed ARVC.

29. **What is congenital long-QT syndrome?**
    Long-QT syndrome (LQTS) can be acquired (most likely secondary to medications that prolong QT, see Question 7) or congenital. A large number of mutations have been described that results in congenital LQTS and the phenotypic constellation of prolonged QTc and increased risk of characteristic polymorphic VT *(Torsades des pointes)*. Clinically, this disorder is characterized by syncopal episodes and possible cardiac arrest related to the sudden onset of this arrhythmia, frequently with preceding triggers such as exercise; in some forms of the disorder, loud sounds; or in other cases, facial immersion into water (swimming).

30. **How is congenital long-QT syndrome diagnosed?**
    No single gold standard test exists to diagnose a patient with congenital LQTS. As mentioned previously, many mutations are known to cause this condition, but a fair number of patients with clinically proven congenital LQTS do not have any of the mutations discovered to date. Genetic testing is certainly not first-line evaluation and should be approached with caution. Diagnosis is usually made by criteria from the LQTS score, which includes points for various factors including: QTc length (with more points if >480 ms), QTc at fourth minute of exercise recovery >480 ms, clinical *Torsade* in the absence of QT prolonging drugs, syncope (with more points if with stress or exercise), and family members with proven LQTS. Lastly, keep in mind that a patient with definite LQTS might very well have a QTc within normal range, depending on his physiological state when the ECG is taken.

31. **What is Brugada syndrome and how is it diagnosed?**
    Brugada syndrome is defined by a combination of a specific pattern on surface ECG (Fig. 35.5), called Brugada ECG, and clinical symptoms related to sustained ventricular tachyarrhythmia (suspicious syncope or sudden cardiac arrest). It is an autosomal dominant disorder that is in most cases due to mutations in cardiac cell sodium channels. It is more common in males. Note that the ECG pattern can be transient and vary over time; it can also be elicited by fevers or various medications and drugs including cocaine. Patients with a suspect ECG that does not completely meet criteria can undergo a challenge with drugs (commonly procainamide) to try to elicit a more typical Brugada pattern.

32. **How to treat a patient who is receiving repeated implantable cardioverter defibrillator (ICD) shocks?**
    The first order of business is to determine whether the patient is having recurrent ventricular arrhythmias and receiving appropriate ICD shocks, or if the device is somehow getting fooled when there is no malignant arrhythmia present. If the patient is having recurrent ventricular arrhythmia, then treatment of the underlying condition is in order. If the patient is not having ventricular arrhythmias, placement of a magnet over the ICD should disable all therapies and prevent further inappropriate shocks. If the distinction cannot be made, it is not unreasonable to place defibrillator pads on the patient and place a magnet over the device, with the ICU team effectively becoming the patient's defibrillator were he to need any more shocks.

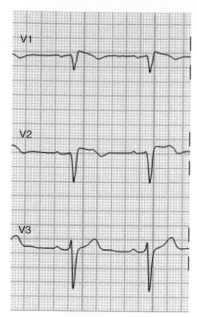

Figure 35-5. Brugada electrocardiogram. Note the cove pattern in V1.

KEY POINTS: CARDIAC ARRHYTHMIA

1. Characteristics of a wide complex tachycardia that point towards it being VT:
   - AV dissociation
   - Very wide QRS complex
   - Precordial lead concordance
   - Fusion beats
2. Risk factors for stroke in patients with atrial fibrillation or atrial flutter:
   - Congestive heart failure (LV dysfunction)
   - Hypertension
   - Age, with greater risk over 75
   - Diabetes mellitus
   - History of prior stroke or transient ischemic attack (TIA)
   - Vascular disease
   - Female sex

BIBLIOGRAPHY

1. Jalife J, Delmar M, Davidenko J, et al. *Basic Cardiac Electrophysiology for the Clinician.* New York: Futura/Wiley-Blackwell; 1999.
2. Lip GY, Nieuwlaat R, Pisters R, et al. Refining clinical risk stratification for predicting stroke and thromboembolism in atrial fibrillation using a novel risk factor based approach—The Euro Heart Survey on Atrial Fibrillation. *Chest.* 2010;137: 263–272.
3. Marcus FI, McKenna WJ, Sherill D, et al. Diagnosis of arrhythmogenic right ventricular cardiomyopathy/dysplasia: proposed modification of the task force criteria. *Circulation.* 2010;121(13):1533.
4. Schwartz PJ, Crotti L. QTc Behavior during exercise and genetic testing for the long-QT syndrome. *Circulation.* 2011;124(20): 2181–2184.
5. Vargas M, Servillo G, Sutherasan Y, et al. Effects of in-hospital low targeted temperature after out of hospital cardiac arrest: a systematic review with meta-analysis of randomized clinical trials. *Resuscitation.* 2015;91:8–18.
6. Zipes DP, Jalife J. *Cardiac Electrophysiology: From Cell to Bedside.* Philadelphia: Saunders; 2009.

CHAPTER 36

AORTIC DISSECTION

Lydia Miller and Sheri Berg

1. Define acute aortic syndrome and aortic dissection

The term acute aortic syndrome (AAS) refers to several life-threatening conditions characterized by separation of the walls of the aorta, including aortic dissection (AD), intramural hematoma, and penetrating aortic ulcer. The different types of AAS are distinguished based on the mechanism of separation of the aortic wall. AD is caused by a tear in the intima. An intramural hematoma does not have an intimal entry tear and is believed to be caused by rupture of vasa vasorum. A penetrating aortic ulcer is caused by atherosclerotic plaque eroding through the intimal layer.

In all these conditions, blood enters the media layer, creating a false lumen that propagates in an anterograde and/or retrograde direction. This false lumen compromises blood flow to branch vessels, causing myocardial, cerebral, mesenteric, renal, or limb ischemia. The three types of AAS are indistinguishable based on clinical signs and symptoms and carry high morbidity and mortality if not identified and treated immediately. Diagnosis and treatment of the three types of AAS are similar. AD is the most common AAS (accounting for 90%) and will be the focus of this chapter.

2. Describe the DeBakey and Stanford classifications of aortic dissection

Identifying the location of AD is crucial in determining immediate management. AD involving the ascending aorta carries very high mortality if untreated and is a surgical emergency. The ascending aorta is defined as the segment proximal to the brachiocephalic artery, and the descending aorta begins at the left subclavian artery. Fig. 36.1 depicts the Stanford and DeBakey classifications.

The **Stanford** classification describes **two** types of dissection and is more commonly used:
- *Type A*: involves the ascending aorta
- *Type B*: does not involve the ascending aorta

   The **DeBakey** classification describes **three** types of dissection:
- *Type I*: involves the ascending aorta, arch, and usually descending aorta
- *Type II*: involves only the ascending aorta
- *Type III*: involves only the descending aorta and has two subtypes:
- *Type IIIA*: limited to the thoracic aorta
- *Type IIIB*: extends below the diaphragm

3. What is the mortality of aortic dissections?

Type A dissections have a higher mortality than Type B. The overall in-hospital mortality of Type A is 22% and Type B is 14%. Medically managed Type A dissections have a mortality of about 50%.

4. Which is more common: Type A or B dissection?

Two-thirds of dissections are Type A; one-third are Type B. This is because the ascending aorta has greater wall stress.

5. What factors determine aortic wall stress?

Aortic wall stress is determined by heart rate, blood pressure, and the rate of change of pressure with time. Wall stress is directly proportional to radius and inversely proportional to thickness, meaning aneurysms or areas of dissection are subject to especially high wall stress (Law of Laplace).

6. What are the risk factors for aortic dissection?

Risk factors for AD include factors that increase aortic wall stress and acquired or inherited aortic pathology. Some risk factors are less well understood (e.g., male sex).
- Hypertension: the most common risk factor, in 77% of patients
- Older age: the average age of patients presenting with AD is early 60s
- Male sex: about two-thirds of patients are male. Women presenting with AD are typically older, have more atypical symptoms, delayed diagnosis, and higher mortality
- Smoking
- Hyperlipidemia
- Atherosclerosis

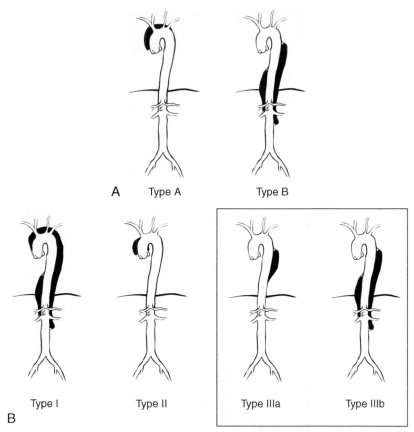

Figure 36-1. Stanford (A) and DeBakey (B) classifications of aortic dissection. (Illustration by Samuel Rodriguez, MD.)

- Aortic aneurysm
- Stimulant drugs including cocaine, amphetamines
- Connective tissue diseases, namely Marfan, Loeys-Dietz, Ehlers-Danlos, Turner syndromes, and bicuspid aortic valve. Genetic disorders account for about 20% of AD and should be suspected in patients under 40 presenting with AD
- Family history of dissection or thoracic aortic aneurysm without an identified syndrome
- Aortic inflammation or infection: large-vessel arteritis including Giant-cell, Takayasu, Behçet; syphilis
- Deceleration trauma
- Pregnancy
- Chronic steroid use
- Iatrogenic: AD is an uncommon complication of instrumentation of the aorta in cardiac or vascular surgery

7. What are the clinical signs and symptoms of aortic dissection?
   - Severe, acute onset chest, back, or abdominal pain is the most common symptom, reported in over 90% of patients. Pain is most commonly described as sharp or stabbing; the classic description of tearing or ripping pain is reported in only about 25% of patients.
   - Hypertension, more common in Type B (66%) vs. A (28%)
   - Weak pulse, more common in Type A (31%) vs. B (19%)

- Syncope, more common in Type A (19%) vs. B (3%). Syncope is concerning for involvement of cerebral branch vessels or cardiac dysfunction (acute aortic insufficiency, ischemia, or tamponade)
- Systolic BP differential in limbs greater than 20 mmHg
- Focal neurologic deficits, concerning for ischemic stroke, spinal cord ischemia, or ischemic peripheral neuropathy
- New murmur concerning for aortic regurgitation
- Hypotension/shock is concerning for acute cardiac dysfunction (tamponade, acute aortic insufficiency, myocardial ischemia), rupture, or compression of true lumen

8. How is aortic dissection diagnosed?

Diagnosis of AD requires imaging. Computed tomography angiography (CTA) is the most commonly used initial imaging modality in diagnosis of AD. CTA is fast, noninvasive, and can identify the site of intimal tear, extent of dissection, rupture, true and false lumen dimensions, involvement of branch vessels, and pleural and pericardial effusion. CTA has 100% sensitivity and specificity for AD. Transesophageal echocardiography (TEE) has comparable sensitivity (86%–100%) and specificity (90%–100%) and may be preferred in unstable patients. Fig. 36.2 shows TEE images of a Type A dissection flap extending from the ascending aorta to descending aorta. Transthoracic echocardiography provides limited views of the aorta but could be useful in rapid bedside evaluation for acute aortic regurgitation, pericardial effusion/tamponade, and heart failure. Chest x-ray may show widened mediastinum, but this is not a consistent finding, reported in only 52% in Type A and 39% in Type B. Magnetic resonance imaging also has high sensitivity and specificity for AD, but is rarely used in the acute setting and is better suited for long-term surveillance of aortic remodeling after AD.

9. What other potentially fatal conditions should be in your differential diagnosis in a patient with acute chest or back pain?

Acute coronary syndrome, pulmonary embolism, pneumothorax, and esophageal perforation should be considered. A "triple rule-out" CT protocol has been proposed for simultaneous evaluation for AD, coronary artery disease, and pulmonary embolism in a patient presenting with acute chest or back pain.

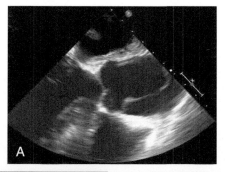

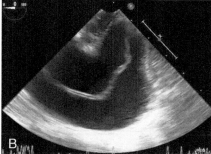
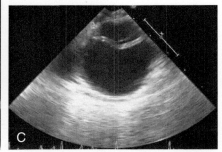

Figure 36-2. Transesophageal echocardiography images of a Type A aortic dissection. The dissection flap extends from the ascending aorta (A) through the arch (B) to the descending aorta (C). (Images courtesy of Genevieve Staudt, M.D.)

10. How is the chronicity of aortic dissection defined?

Guidelines define acute AD as the two-week period following the onset of symptoms, subacute between 2 to 6 weeks, and chronic as greater than 6 weeks.

11. What are the short- and long-term complications of aortic dissection?

- End-organ ischemia results when the dissection flap obstructs blood flow to branch vessels. This can result in stroke, paraplegia, coronary, limb, renal, and mesenteric ischemia. Mesenteric ischemia is the leading cause of death in patients with Type B dissections.
- Cardiac complications occur when dissection involves the aortic root, valve, coronary arteries, and pericardium, resulting in acute aortic insufficiency (most common cardiac complication), myocardial ischemia, pericardial effusion/tamponade, and heart failure.
- Pleural effusion
- Aortic rupture
- Aneurysm

12. What are the indications for surgery in aortic dissection?

All patients presenting with AD should be immediately evaluated by a cardiac surgeon.

1. **Type A.** Any dissection involving the ascending aorta requires emergent open surgical repair under cardiopulmonary bypass. The mortality for medically managed Type A dissections is around 50%. Open aortic replacement with or without aortic valve replacement is the gold standard; endovascular repair of Type A dissections is currently being investigated.
2. **Complicated Type B.** Immediate surgery is indicated for Type B dissections if there are signs of end-organ ischemia, aortic rupture, rapidly expanding dissection or aneurysm, or refractory pain or hypertension. Endovascular repair is recommended over open repair when possible.
3. **Hypotension/shock.** Hypotension or shock in a patient with AD is very concerning for an acute cardiac complication (tamponade, severe aortic insufficiency, or coronary ischemia), true lumen obstruction, or rupture, and should prompt immediate surgical re-evaluation.

    While the standard of care for uncomplicated Type B dissections has traditionally been medical management, two recent randomized controlled trials have shown benefit of early endovascular repair in uncomplicated Type B dissections in aorta-specific mortality and aortic remodeling. This has led some authors to propose that early endovascular repair should be considered in management of uncomplicated Type B dissections.

13. Describe the initial medical management of a patient with acute aortic dissection.

If immediate surgery is not indicated, the patient should be admitted to an ICU for close monitoring of hemodynamics and end-organ perfusion. The goal of medical management in AD is to reduce aortic wall stress by tight control of heart rate and blood pressure. Decreasing wall stress reduces the risk of dissection propagation and rupture. All patients should have an arterial line placed for continuous blood pressure monitoring, and tight heart rate and blood pressure control achieved with intravenous agents. Bilateral upper extremity arterial lines should be considered, particularly for Type A dissections. If there is a blood pressure differential between arms, medications should be titrated to the higher reading. Intravenous beta-blockers are the first-line therapy and should be titrated to goal heart rate less than 60 and systolic blood pressure of 100 to 120 mm Hg. Nondihydropyridine calcium channel blockers (namely verapamil or diltiazem) should be used in patients with contraindications to beta-blockers. Patients with acute aortic insufficiency may not tolerate lower heart rate.

If systolic blood pressure goals are not met with heart rate control, intravenous vasodilators should be added; options include nitroprusside, nitroglycerin, and nicardipine. Vasodilators should only be initiated after heart rate control is achieved; otherwise, reflex tachycardia could result. Good pain control, which usually requires IV opioids, will also help achieve hemodynamic goals.

In all cases, large-bore IVs should be placed and blood products made available in case of emergency surgery or rupture.

14. Besides hemodynamics, what other parameters should be monitored closely in the intensive care unit?

Evidence of end-organ ischemia or worsening pain could indicate progression of dissection or rupture and warrants urgent re-imaging or surgical intervention. Rising creatinine and lactate is concerning for renal and mesenteric ischemia, respectively. Of note, the rise in lactate often lags in mesenteric ischemia, making it important to monitor closely for abdominal pain. A Foley catheter should be placed for close monitoring of urine output. Pulses should be checked in all extremities to monitor limb perfusion. Altered mental status or focal neurologic deficits are concerning for cerebral or spinal cord ischemia or ischemic peripheral neuropathy.

15. Describe the long-term management of patients with aortic dissection.

Once patients have been transitioned to oral heart rate and blood pressure control agents and have been monitored for several days in the ICU without signs of end-organ ischemia, patients can be discharged with close follow-up with a cardiac or vascular surgeon. Long-term medical management includes aggressive heart rate and blood pressure control, lipid-lowering therapy, smoking cessation, and surveillance imaging for aortic remodeling. Many patients with Type B dissections initially managed medically will require endovascular or open aneurysm repair in the future.

ACKNOWLEDGMENT

The authors wish to acknowledge Drs. Asheesh Kumar, MD, and Rae M. Allain, MD, for the valuable contributions to the previous edition of this chapter.

KEY POINTS: AORTIC DISSECTION

1. AD carries high morbidity and mortality if untreated and should be suspected in any patient presenting with acute-onset severe chest, back, or abdominal pain. CT angiography has very high sensitivity and specificity for diagnosis of AD and is the most commonly used imaging modality to diagnose AD.
2. The major risk factors for AD are hypertension, male sex, smoking, and older age. Inherited connective tissue diseases should be suspected in patients under age 40 presenting with AD.
3. All patients presenting with AD should be immediately evaluated by a surgeon. Type A dissections require emergent open repair. Type B dissections complicated by end-organ ischemia, rupture, rapidly expanding dissection or aneurysm, or intractable pain or hypertension require surgery; endovascular repair is preferable if possible.
4. The goal of medical management in AD is to reduce aortic wall stress by tight control of heart rate and blood pressure. Intravenous beta-blockers are first-line therapy, followed by the addition of vasodilators if needed once heart rate goal is achieved.
5. Complications of AD include aortic rupture, obstruction of flow to branch vessels causing end-organ ischemia, cardiac complications of acute aortic insufficiency, tamponade, myocardial ischemia and heart failure, and aneurysm formation.

BIBLIOGRAPHY

1. Brunkwall J, Kasprzak P, Verhoeven E, et al. Endovascular repair of acute uncomplicated aortic type B dissection promotes aortic remodeling: 1 year results of the ADSORB trial. *Eur J Vasc Endovasc Surg*. 2014;48:285–291.
2. Clough RE, Nienaber CA. Management of acute aortic syndrome. *Nat Rev Cardiol*. 2015;12:103–114.
3. Hiratzka LF, Bakris GL, Beckman JA, et al. 2010 ACCF/AHA/AATS/ACR/ASA/SCA/SCAI/SIR/STS/SVM Guidelines for the diagnosis and management of patients with thoracic aortic disease. *J Am Coll Cardiol*. 2010;55:e27–e129.
4. Mussa FF, Horton JD, Moridzadeh R, et al. Acute aortic dissection and intramural hematoma: a systematic review. *JAMA*. 2016;316:754–763.
5. Nienaber CA, Clough RE. Management of acute aortic dissection. *Lancet*. 2015;385:800–811.
6. Nienaber CA, Fattori R, Mehta RH, et al. Gender-related differences in acute aortic dissection. *Circulation*. 2004;109: 3014–3021.
7. Nienaber CA, Kische S, Rousseau H, et al. Endovascular repair of type B aortic dissection: Long-term results of the randomized investigation of stent grafts in aortic dissection trial. *Circ Cardiovasc Interv*. 2013;6:407–416.
8. Pape LA, Awais M, Woznicki EM, et al. Presentation, diagnosis, and outcomes of acute aortic dissection: 17-Year trends from the International Registry of Acute Aortic Dissection. *J Am Coll Cardiol*. 2015;66:350–358.
9. Rogers IS, Banerji D, Siegel EL, et al. Usefulness of comprehensive cardiothoracic computed tomography in the evaluation of acute undifferentiated chest discomfort in the emergency department (CAPTURE). *Am J Cardiol*. 2011;107:643–650.

PERICARDIAL DISEASE (PERICARDIAL TAMPONADE AND PERICARDITIS)

Elliott L. Woodward and Alexander S. Kuo

CHAPTER 37

PERICARDIAL DISEASE

1. Describe the basic structure of the pericardium.

   The pericardium is a sac composed of two distinct layers known as the visceral and the parietal pericardium. The visceral pericardium is continuous with the epicardium of the myocardium and consists of a single layer of mesothelial cells. The parietal pericardium is the fibrous, outer layer and is composed of collagen and elastic fibrils with a single layer of mesothelium lining its inner surface.

2. What is normally found between the visceral and parietal layers of the pericardium?

   A potential space exists between the visceral and parietal pericardium which forms a small pericardial reserve volume. This is typically filled with 15 to 50 mL of a serous plasma ultrafiltrate known as pericardial fluid. Pericardial fluid volumes in excess of this are designated as pericardial effusions.

3. Describe the function of the pericardium.
   - Restraint: The pericardium helps to limit cardiac dilation and enhance mechanical interaction between cardiac chambers.
   - Protection: The pericardium reduces friction, thereby allowing for rotation and translation of the heart during the normal cardiac cycle. It is also an important barrier that helps to prevent the spread of infection and malignancy from other intrathoracic structures.
   - Secretory: The pericardium secretes a number of important biochemical substances that regulate local processes ranging from fibrinolysis to control of coronary tone.

4. What electrocardiogram (ECG) changes are often seen with pericardial effusions?
   - Electrical alternans: Oscillations in the axis and/or QRS amplitude between beats due to swinging of the heart in the fluid filled pericardium.
   - Low-voltage QRS: Limb lead amplitude less than 0.5 mV.

5. What is cardiac tamponade?

   Cardiac tamponade is a *clinical* diagnosis and a medical emergency. It occurs when fluid accumulation in the pericardial space exceeds the ability of the pericardium to distend, ultimately resulting in compression of the cardiac chambers and hemodynamic compromise. The compression usually occurs first in the lower pressure right heart during diastole. However, fluid and pressure accumulation within the pericardium does not always occur uniformly (such as in the setting of a loculated effusion) and regional tamponade may localize to other cardiac chambers.

6. How much pericardial fluid is required in order to produce tamponade?

   The absolute volume of pericardial fluid is less important than the rate of accumulation. The visceral pericardium can distend over time to accommodate slowly developing effusions. This explains why a chronic effusion of greater than 500 mL may not result in tamponade, while an acute effusion of much smaller volume might.

7. What are the signs and symptoms of tamponade?

   Beck's Triad: Low blood pressure, elevated jugular venous pressure (JVP), and muted/distant heart sounds
   - Chest pain/fullness: Caused by acute pericardial irritation
   - Tachycardia: A physiologic response important in maintaining cardiac output
   - Shock: Low cardiac output with peripheral venous congestion
   - Pulsus paradoxus (see below): May be absent if there is a localized effusion

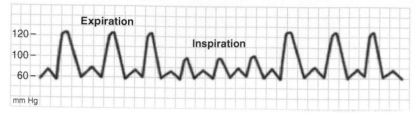

Figure 37-1. Arterial blood pressure tracing of *pulsus paradoxus*: exaggerated respirophasic variation in systolic blood pressure greater than 10 mm Hg.

8. What is pulsus paradoxus?
   Pulsus paradoxus is an exaggeration of the normal respirophasic variation in systolic blood pressure. It is defined as a decrease in systolic blood pressure of greater than 10 mm Hg with inspiration. See Fig. 37-1.

9. Describe how *inspiratory* changes in intrathoracic pressure affect ventricular preload in the normovolemic, spontaneously breathing patient.
   Intrathoracic pressure becomes more *negative* during *inspiration* in *spontaneously breathing* patients. This negative intrathoracic pressure draws blood into the chest, augmenting right heart filling. Due to *ventricular interdependence*, this inspiratory increase in right heart volume can result in a reduction in left ventricular volume and filling. Inspiratory decreases in intrathoracic pressure also dilate the pulmonary vasculature, resulting in pulmonary venous pooling and a further decrease in venous return to the left heart.

10. Describe the respirophasic variation in *cardiac output* and *blood pressure* that is typically seen in the normovolemic, spontaneously breathing patient.
    Left ventricular preload is decreased during *inspiration* as a result of the phenomenon described above. This *inspiratory* decrease in left ventricular filling/preload results in decreased stroke volume and cardiac output. This effect on cardiac output and blood pressure is enhanced by increased left ventricular afterload that occurs during inspiration (think of the negative intrathoracic pressure resisting the left ventricle ejection of blood). During expiration, these changes in preload, blood pressure, and cardiac output are reversed.

11. Why is pulsus paradoxus frequently seen in cardiac tamponade?
    - Tamponade limits right heart filling: As a result, the heart becomes more preload-sensitive and the effects of respiration on preload are exaggerated.
    - Tamponade limits total cardiac volume: This enhances *ventricular interdependence* and exaggerates the respirophasic swings in cardiac output associated with it.

12. Why is initiation of positive pressure ventilation/intubation so dangerous in patients with pericardial tamponade?
    Positive pressure ventilation *increases* intrathoracic pressure, reducing venous return and impeding right heart diastolic filling. In cardiac tamponade, right ventricular filling is already restricted, and further reduction may lead to complete cardiovascular collapse.

13. Is there a role for echocardiography in pericardial tamponade?
    It is a Class 1 indication (ACC/AHA/ASE) for the use of echocardiography in cardiac tamponade (Cheitlin et al., 2003).

14. What are the important echocardiographic findings associated with pericardial tamponade?
    - Presence of a pericardial effusion. See Fig. 37.2.
    - Right atrial and/or ventricular collapse. See Fig. 37.2.
    - Inspiratory septal bounce: Abnormal movement of the intraventricular septum as a result of exaggerated ventricular interdependence. *See pulsus paradoxus explanation above.
    - Exaggerated and reciprocal changes in transmitral and transtricuspid diastolic flow velocities with respiration (inspiratory reduction in mitral peak E-wave velocity >30%).
    - Inferior vena cava (IVC) distention greater than 20 mm with less than 50% reduction in size with spontaneous inspiration.
    - Hepatic vein diastolic flow blunting or reversal on pulse-wave Doppler.

15. Does the absence of a pericardial effusion on transthoracic echocardiography rule out the possibility of tamponade? Why or why not?
    No, the absence of a pericardial effusion on transthoracic echocardiography does *not* completely rule out the possibility of tamponade because localized/loculated effusions may be poorly visualized.

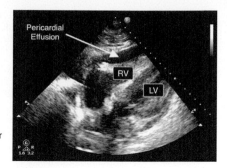

Figure 37-2. An echocardiographic subcostal four-chamber view demonstrating *pericardial effusion* with *right ventricular collapse.*

Transesophageal echocardiography and cardiac computer tomography (CT) imaging can help to identify these pathologies.

16. What is the definitive treatment for pericardial tamponade?
    Pericardial drainage is the treatment for tamponade. Notably, in tamponade resulting from ascending aortic dissection, pericardiocentesis is relatively contraindicated and immediate cardiac surgical evaluation should be obtained.

17. What is the temporizing hemodynamic strategy for patients with pericardial tamponade until definitive treatment can be accessed?
    - *Fast:* Tachycardia can be an important factor in maintaining cardiac output in the setting of a fixed or falling stroke volume (no β-blockers!).
    - *Full:* Maintain/increase preload (fluids wide open).
    - *Tight:* Avoid vasodilation/vasodilating agents.

18. What is pericarditis?
    Pericarditis is inflammation of the pericardium which can occur as a result of either a primary pericardial process or as a manifestation of systemic disease.

19. What are the most common causes of acute pericarditis?
    Acute pericarditis is most commonly attributed to idiopathic or viral causes. The list of other causes is extensive, including but not limited to bacterial infection (e.g., tuberculosis), collagen vascular disease, uremia, postmyocardial infarction (Dressler syndrome), postcardiac surgery, post-traumatic, post radiation, neoplasm, toxins, drugs, etc.

20. What diagnostic triad is often present in patients presenting with acute pericarditis?
    - Chest pain: Typically sudden in onset, retrosternal with or without radiation to the neck, arms, shoulder, and/or trapezius. It is worsened during inspiration and when supine and improved when the patient is sitting forward.
    - Pericardial friction rub: High pitched, scratchy, and heard best at the left sternal boarder.
    - ST changes on ECG: Initially, diffuse, upward-concave ST-segment elevation and PR-segment depression with reciprocal changes in aVR and/or V1 leads are seen. Later, the ST and T waves normalize prior to the development of widespread T-wave inversion. In some, the T waves ultimately normalize again with time and in others, T-wave inversions persist indefinitely.

21. Are there elevations in troponin and creatine kinase (CK) levels in patients with acute pericarditis?
    Acute pericarditis is frequently associated with a mild elevation in troponin T without a concomitant increase in total blood creatine kinase levels. It is postulated that this mild troponin elevation is the result of epicardial inflammation and its presence in patients with acute pericarditis is usually not associated with abnormalities on coronary angiogram.

22. How can echocardiography be useful in differentiating patients with pericarditis versus those with coronary disease?
    Echocardiographic findings consistent with the diagnosis of pericarditis include new or worsening pericardial effusion with or without tamponade and increased pericardial brightness. Segmental wall motion abnormalities may be seen in cases of pericarditis that are complicated by significant myocardial involvement (myopericarditis). However, demonstration of normal left ventricular regional contractility in patients whose presentation is otherwise consistent with pericarditis may help avoid unnecessary coronary angiography.

23. List some other high-risk features associated with acute pericarditis.
High-risk features associated with acute pericarditis include: fever, leukocytosis, a large pericardial effusion, cardiac tamponade, a history of acute trauma, immunosuppression, anticoagulation, troponin elevation, recurrent pericarditis, and/or failure of non-steroidal anti-inflammatory drug (NSAID) therapy.

24. Describe the basic treatment strategy for acute pericarditis without tamponade.
   • Acute pericarditis without high-risk features can frequently be treated as an outpatient.
   • For viral or idiopathic acute pericarditis: NSAIDs (with a proton pump inhibitor or other form of gastric protection), colchicine ± corticosteroids.
   • For secondary acute pericarditis: treatment of the underlying primary disease.

25. What is constrictive pericarditis?
Constrictive pericarditis is an uncommon disease characterized by impairment in cardiac filling and limitation in total cardiac volume by a thickened and inelastic pericardium. Frequently, it is the result of chronic pericarditis, infiltrative, or connective tissue disorder.

26. What is Kussmaul's sign and why is it frequently seen in constrictive pericarditis?
Kussmaul's sign describes the *absence* of the inspiratory *drop* in JVP that normally occurs during spontaneous inspiration. In constrictive pericarditis, the stiff pericardium isolates the cardiac chambers from changes in intrathoracic pressure (in contrast to pericardial tamponade where changes in intrathoracic pressure are transmitted to the cardiac chambers).

27. What role does echocardiography have in the diagnosis of constrictive pericarditis?
Echocardiography plays an important role in diagnosing constrictive pericarditis and differentiating constrictive pericarditis from restrictive cardiomyopathy.

28. How is constrictive pericarditis treated?
In cases of acute pericardial constriction caused by pericardial inflammation, medical therapy alone with anti-inflammatory agents, colchicine ± steroids may suffice. In cases of chronic pericardial constriction, surgical pericardiectomy is the definitive treatment.

ACKNOWLEDGMENT

The authors wish to acknowledge Drs. Stuart F. Sidlow, MD, and C. William Hanson, III, MD, for the valuable contributions to the previous edition of this chapter.

KEY POINTS: PERICARDIAL DISEASE (PERICARDIAL TAMPONADE AND PERICARDITIS)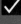

1. Cardiac tamponade is a medical emergency that may lead to cardiac arrest if untreated.
2. Tamponade is a clinical diagnosis, based on physiology, not size of effusion.
3. In cardiac tamponade, positive pressure ventilation, may cause hemodynamic collapse.
4. Pericarditis can result in diffuse ST changes on ECG, and mild troponin elevation.
5. Echocardiography is a primary tool in the diagnosis and assessment of pericardial disease.

BIBLIOGRAPHY

1. Busch C, Penov K, Amorim PA, et al. Risk factors for mortality after pericardiectomy for chronic constrictive pericarditis in a large single-centre cohort. *Eur J Cardiothorac Surg.* 2015;48(6):e110-e116.
2. Cheitlin MD, Armstrong WF, Aurigemma GP, et al. ACC/AHA/ASE 2003 guideline update for the clinical application of echocardiography: summary article: a report of the American College of Cardiology/American Heart Association Task Force on Practice Guidelines (ACC/AHA/ASE Committee to Update the 1997 Guidelines for the Clinical Application of Echocardiography). *Circulation.* 2003;108(9):1146-1162.
3. Dal-Bianco JP, Sengupta PP, Mookadam F, et al. Role of echocardiography in the diagnosis of constrictive pericarditis. *J Am Soc Echocardiogr.* 2009;22(1):24-33.
4. Khandaker MH, Espinosa RE, Nishimura RA, et al. Pericardial disease: diagnosis and management. *Mayo Clin Proc.* 2010; 85(6):572-593.
5. Klein AL, Abbara S, Agler DA, et al. American Society of Echocardiography clinical recommendations for multimodality cardiovascular imaging of patients with pericardial disease: endorsed by the Society for Cardiovascular Magnetic Resonance and Society of Cardiovascular Computed Tomography. *J Am Soc Echocardiogr.* 2013;26(9):965-1012.e15.
6. Lachman N, Syed FF, Habib A, et al. Correlative anatomy for the electrophysiologist, part II: Cardiac ganglia, phrenic nerve, coronary venous system. *J Cardiovasc Electrophysiol.* 2011;22(1):104-110.
7. Little WC, Freeman GL. Pericardial disease. *Circulation.* 2006;113(12):1622-1632.

VI
INFECTIOUS DISEASE

CHAPTER 38

SEPSIS AND SEPTIC SHOCK

Jimmy L. Moss and Aranya Bagchi

1. What is sepsis?

Sepsis has recently been redefined (the Sepsis 3 definition) as a **life-threatening organ dysfunction caused by a deregulated host response to infection**. This new definition emphasizes the importance of differentiating between previously accepted nonspecific "sepsis" criteria (systemic inflammatory response syndrome [SIRS] plus infection), which may simply represent adaptive host responses, and the pathobiology underlying nonhomeostatic host responses to infection.

2. Explain the historical nomenclature for disorders related to sepsis.

Sepsis is derived from the Greek word "F073hFO6Ahh (sipsi)," that means to make rotten. Hippocrates first introduced the term sepsis. Another physician from antiquity, Ibn Sina documented the coincidence of "blood putrefaction" and fever. The next development in our understanding of sepsis took place more than two millennia later, when Ignaz Semmelweis identified the link between hand hygiene and transmission of puerperal fever. The concept of sepsis as an uncontrolled inflammatory response to inflammation was popularized by Lewis Thomas, and formalized in 1991 by the American College of Chest Physicians and the Society of Critical Care Medicine (SCCM) consensus conference. The following terms were implemented to describe the progression of signs and symptoms regarding this complex syndrome and came to be known as Sepsis-1. They are included here as it is not uncommon for physicians to continue to use this terminology:

- **Sepsis:** a suspected or documented source of infection plus two or more SIRS criteria.
- **SIRS:** characterized by:
  - Temperature greater than 38°C or less than 36°C
  - Heart rate greater than 90 beats per minute
  - Respiratory rate greater than 20 breaths per minute or the need for mechanical ventilation
  - White blood cell count greater than 12,000 cells/mm^3 or less than 4000 cells/mm^3
- **Severe sepsis:** sepsis with acute sepsis-induced organ dysfunction of one or more organ systems.
- **Septic shock:** severe sepsis with cardiovascular dysfunction. Specifically, sepsis-induced hypotension (mean arterial pressure [MAP] <65 mm Hg) that persists despite adequate and aggressive volume resuscitation.
- **Multiple organ dysfunction syndrome (MODS):** Failure in more than one organ system that requires acute intervention. Once the patient reaches this degree of illness, the chances of making a meaningful recovery can often be quite low.

In 2001, the International Sepsis Definitions Conference convened to once again address the difficulties in defining sepsis. In our opinion, this definition added complexity without improving understanding, and it was largely ignored by practicing clinicians.

In 2014, aiming to better categorize septic patients, the European Society of Intensive Care Medicine (ESICM) and the SCCM created a task force and redefined sepsis as a process more complicated than inflammation and infection. This definition, noted above (Answer 1), was created to eliminate misleading terminologies that often lead to clinical discrepancies in both treatment and evaluation. Septic shock, defined as patients with evidence of hypoperfusion (serum lactate >2 mmol/L) or requirement of vasopressor to maintain MAP greater than or equal to 65 mm Hg after appropriate volume resuscitation, was noted as a subset of sepsis that signifies a higher mortality risk than sepsis alone and should be quickly identified. Additionally, the task force suggested using a modified sequential organ failure (SOFA) score (qSOFA), in lieu of traditional SIRS criteria, to identify patients with higher mortality risks. A patient with a suspected infection and qSOFA score (which assesses a point to patients with RR ≥22, altered mental status [GCS <15], and systolic blood pressure ≤100 mm Hg,) greater than or equal to 2 is the proposed cutoff point that should prompt clinicians to implement hospital-based sepsis-driven treatment and monitoring protocols. Although reported to be superior to previous sepsis defining guidelines, this new approach (Sepsis-3) has not been uniformly endorsed by all Critical Care organizations and societies. The fear is that using a mortality-screening tool (SOFA, qSOFA) alone could possibly eliminate other useful/validated clinical markers/tools (e.g., CURB-65) that are traditionally followed and also "miss" a large cohort of patients (newborns, pediatrics, elderly) who may have other signs and symptoms of sepsis.

3. **What is the incidence of sepsis?**

Sepsis and septic shock are relatively common and associated with substantial mortality and consumption of healthcare resources. In 2013, an estimated 1.6 million cases of severe sepsis occurred in the United States alone, with more than 258,000 deaths. The incidence of sepsis is substantially higher in elderly than in younger people, and the projected growth of the aforementioned population is expected to continue increasing. However, even when adjusting for population size, the incidence of sepsis is reported to increase 8% each year—notably higher in the elderly and nonwhites. Importantly, earlier clinical recognition, increased awareness, escalating invasive procedures, expansion in immunosuppressive and chemotherapy drug usages, as well as rising antimicrobial resistance are thought to contribute to these increases. The annual healthcare cost of treating patients with sepsis-related illnesses is approximately $25 billion; however, 50% of patients who survive (postsepsis syndrome) still have an annual economic impact of nearly $2 billion.

4. **How does the nomenclature relate to outcome?**

Previous studies have shown that as the disorder progresses from SIRS to septic shock, the mortality rate increases. Of interest, some data support the concept that, although the degree of illness at presentation may have some correlation with outcomes, it is the change in clinical status from baseline that may have the closest correlation with outcomes. The mortality rate for patients with acute renal failure in the setting of sepsis ranges from 50% to 80%. For most patients with sepsis syndrome, the failure of three or more organ systems results in a mortality rate greater than 90%. It is important to note, however, that the actual cause of death in patients with sepsis is often ill-defined. Frailty, major comorbidity, and unsurvivable injuries are often important contributors to the death of patients with sepsis. Many patients with sepsis die as a result of discontinuation of care deemed to be futile. More work is needed to parse the difference between patients who die "with sepsis" versus those that die "of sepsis."

5. **Discuss current understanding of the pathogenesis of sepsis and septic shock.**

The pathophysiology of sepsis is extraordinarily complicated and not truly well understood. A number of factors influence the nature of the host response.
- **Host-pathogen-environment interactions**: Humans harbor an enormous quantity of microbial fauna that is collectively referred to as the "microbiome." In addition to the traditional host factors (age, comorbidities, medications), the structure and function of the microbiome can be acutely altered in critical illness, with important consequences for the host immune response.
- **Initiation of the acute inflammatory response**: The initial host response is determined by the interaction between the factors described above. The innate immune system of the host responds to the presence of "Pathogen Associated Molecular Patterns" (PAMPs) or "Damage Associated Molecular Patterns" (DAMPs) in a preprogrammed immune response. Microbe-associated PAMPs and host-associated DAMPs can evoke similar responses, partly accounting for the similar initial presentation among patients with severe infectious and noninfectious insults. Severe sepsis sets off a "genomic storm" with large-scale activation of the leukocyte transcriptome. Recent work has shown that, rather than a sequence of a hyperinflammatory responses followed by immune suppression, both pro- and anti-inflammatory pathways are altered simultaneously (see Chapter 84).
- **End Organ Damage**: The pathophysiologic "triad" of septic shock includes epithelial dysfunction, endothelial dysfunction, and mitochondrial dysfunction. It is intriguing that there is a discrepancy between the severity of organ dysfunction and the relatively modest structural damage to the organs. This has led some investigators to propose that sepsis-induced organ dysfunction is a "hibernation" phenotype, with cells reverting to a minimally functional state until the initial insult has passed.

6. **Which microorganisms are most commonly associated with sepsis?**

A recent study of nosocomial bloodstream infections found the following infecting organisms in the intensive care unit (ICU):
- **Gram positive (65%):** coagulase-negative staphylococci (36% of isolates), *Staphylococcus aureus* (17%), enterococci (10%).
- **Gram negative (25%):** *Escherichia coli* (4%), *Klebsiella* sp. (4%), *Pseudomonas aeruginosa* (5%), *Enterobacter* sp. (5%), *Serratia* sp. (2%), *Acinetobacter* sp. (2%). Clinically, however, the problem of resistant gram-negative organisms in the ICU is rapidly becoming a serious one nationwide.
- **Fungi (9%):** primarily *Candida* species (*albicans* 54%, *glabrata* 19%, *parapsilosis* 11%, *tropicalis* 11%).
- Coagulase-negative staphylococci, *Pseudomonas* species, *Enterobacter* species, *Serratia* species, and *Acinetobacter* species were more likely to cause infections in patients in ICUs. The proportion of *S. aureus* isolates with methicillin resistance increased from 22% in 1995 to 57% in 2001.

7. **What are the most common primary sources of infection?**
   The order of incidence varies throughout regions throughout the United States and the rest of the world; however, the most common causes are: pneumonia (half of all cases in the United States), intra-abdominal, urinary tract, skin, and hematologic infections.

8. **What clinical signs and symptoms should raise suspicion of sepsis, and septic shock?**
   Most available data suggest that the rapid identification of patients with sepsis and the rapid administration of appropriate antibiotics are associated with lower mortality in patients with sepsis. The focus of the clinical care should therefore be to identify patients at high risk of developing sepsis and initiating appropriate treatment promptly. Multiple studies suggest that delays in recognition and care for patients with sepsis are common and contribute to poor outcomes. The following guidelines may be used to identify patients with sepsis:
   - The presence of an infection (documented or suspected) AND greater than or equal to 2 qSOFA points (see Answer 2)
   - The Centers for Medicare and Medicaid SEP-1 criteria:
     - All 3 of the following occurring within a 6-hour period:
       - Suspected/documented infection
       - greater than or equal to 2 SIRS criteria (see Answer 2)
       - Acute organ dysfunction attributable to infection (any ONE of the following):
         - Systolic blood pressure (SBP) less than 90 mm Hg, mean arterial pressure less than 65 mm Hg, or SBP drop from baseline greater than 40 mm Hg
         - Lactate greater than 2.0 mmol/L
         - Respiratory failure (need for noninvasive or invasive ventilation)
         - Creatinine greater than 2.0 mg/dL or urine output less than 0.5 cc/kg/h X 2 h
         - Bilirubin greater than 2.0 mg/dL
         - Platelets less than 100 k
         - International normalized ratio (INR) greater than 1.5 or partial thromboplastin time (PTT) greater than 60

   The criteria for septic shock include sepsis as defined by the above criteria, in addition to persisting hypotension requiring vasopressors to maintain MAP greater than 65 mm Hg AND a lactate greater than 2.0. Of note, the Centers for Medicare and Medicaid Services (CMS) definition for septic shock differs slightly. The CMS defines septic shock as sepsis and EITHER hypotension in spite of adequate fluid resuscitation OR a lactate greater than 4 mmol/L. It is useful to keep in mind that not all patients may be captured by these definitions and a high index of suspicion is required to identify some patients.

9. **What are the Surviving Sepsis Campaign Guidelines? What are some of the high points?**
   The Surviving Sepsis Guidelines were originally published in 2004 and were codified by 11 international critical care organizations. They were updated in 2008, 2012, and more recently in 2016. Many of the guideline's merits are founded on the principles originally outlined in the Rivers trial on early goal-directed therapy in 2001. Aimed at providing a state-of-the-art evidence-based approach to the management of severe sepsis and septic shock, many of their recommendations have spearheaded numerous Early Warning Systems for institutional sepsis management. Each campaign update attempts to address limitations of the previous one in the face of evolving recognition that having rigid approaches towards sepsis can indeed lead to worse outcomes. Although there are reasonable disagreements with regards to some of their suggestions (lactate as a "sole" marker for tissue perfusion, synergistic double-coverage for gram negative microbes, initial resuscitation fluid dosages, etc.), it is uniformly accepted that "appropriate clinical assessment" should be at the forefront of providing care for septic patients. Some of the highlights of this important document (modified by our institutional practice patterns) are in Box 38.1.

10. **What is the evidence base for the use of the pulmonary artery catheter?**
    Since its initial description in the *New England Journal of Medicine* in 1970, the pulmonary artery catheter (PAC) has been an important tool for the critical care clinician. Its major roles have been to:
    - Distinguish cardiogenic from noncardiogenic pulmonary edema
    - Determine which particular shock state (cardiogenic, distributive, hypovolemic) a patient may be in
    - Serve as a guide for therapeutic interventions for patients in shock
    - Guide the titration of medications for the acute management of pulmonary hypertension

    Recent data from large randomized trials have been unable to document a particular subgroup of patients in which the use of the PAC has been associated with improved outcomes. It should be remembered that it is extraordinarily difficult for a monitor to be linked to improved outcomes, particularly a monitor that is often misinterpreted, like the PAC tracing. Nevertheless, it can be stated with some certainty that the placement of a PAC is no longer considered essential for the successful diagnosis and management of a patient with sepsis.

Box 38-1. Highlights of the Surviving Sepsis Campaign Guidelines (Modified According to Our Institutional Practice)

Initial Resuscitation

Resuscitation guidelines of the surviving sepsis campaign are derived from the landmark Early Goal Directed Therapy (EGDT) trial, that have been further modified based in recent evidence. The ARISE, ProCESS and ProMISE trials have demonstrated that "usual care" or non-protocolized care is equivalent to EGDT derived protocols. Thus, targeting CVP and central venous oxygen saturation targets is no longer emphasized, although targeting lactate clearance is still recommended. The initial resuscitation phase of a patient with severe sepsis or in septic shock should be completed within 3 h of identification, based on the most recent data available. The mode of intravenous access (central vs. peripheral catheter) is less important than establishing adequate access. It is reasonable to individualize resuscitation goals rather than dogmatically following specific volume recommendations. At our institution, we typically use a combination of focused bedside ultrasonography, lactate, and the base deficit on the arterial blood gas while addressing the adequacy of fluid resuscitation.

Cultures and Broad Spectrum Antibiotics:

The use of effective intravenous antimicrobial treatment within **3 h (ideally within 1 h)** of the recognition of septic shock remains one of the cornerstones in the management of these patients. Typical empiric therapy often begins using a combination of antibiotics that can be expected to be active against all likely pathogens in a specific clinical situation. Adequate dosing is as important as prompt initiation of antibiotics, particularly for frequently underdosed antibiotics such as Vancomycin. A number of studies have shown that every hour of delay in the appropriate initiation of antibiotics increases the risk of death in patients with septic shock. Blood and other relevant cultures form the bedrock of the diagnosis of sepsis. Cultures should be drawn prior to starting antibiotics whenever possible but should not delay initiation of antibiotic therapy.

Source control: If a *nidus* of infection is identified, surgical or percutaneous intervention should be considered as soon as possible. The choice of intervention is based on patient stability, resources available, and the source of the infection, and should target the least invasive option that will provide adequate source control (for example, choosing percutaneous drainage for intra-abdominal abscess when possible rather than open surgery).

Hemodynamic Support:

Type of Fluid: Crystalloids are the initial fluids of choice in most patients. Of note, **chloride** containing fluids (such as **normal saline**) may be associated with worse renal function. Large volume resuscitations with normal saline also causes a hyperchloremic acidosis that makes it, paradoxically, an inferior choice compared to Ringer's lactate in patients with impaired renal function. **Hydroxyethyl starch solutions** should **not be used** in patients with septic shock as multiple trials (VISEP, 6S and CHEST) have shown worse renal function and mortality with their use in patients with septic shock. **Albumin** has been proven to be safe (and perhaps beneficial) in patients with septic shock. The ALBIOS trial showed that using 20% albumin to keep serum albumin levels >3 gm% in patients with septic shock had a mortality benefit (albeit in a *post hoc* analysis). It is reasonable to use albumin in hypoalbuminemic patients with septic shock, although the relatively high cost of albumin should temper its indiscriminate use.

Vasopressors and Ionotropes: Norepinephrine is the initial vasopressor agent of choice in septic shock. **Vasopressin** is often added to norepinephrine in an effort to limit norepinephrine dosage although the vasopressin and septic shock (VASST) study shown no survival benefit. **Epinephrine** can be used if additional hemodynamic support is required, especially chronotropy. Norepinephrine has been shown to be superior to dopamine as a primary agent in cardiogenic shock as well as septic shock (SOAP II trial), particularly in the presence of hypotension. **Dobutamine** can be added to increase cardiac output, provided there is no significant hypotension, and the cardiac output is low. Recent studies have shown that there is no benefit to raising cardiac output to supranormal levels.

Adjunctive Therapy Within the First 24 H
Bicarbonate Therapy

It has been common practice to give bicarbonate therapy for vasopressor-dependent patients to improve hemodynamics. However, it is important to state that—to the extent that it has been studied—no data support this intervention. Current recommendations are not to give bicarbonate for hypoperfusion-induced lactic acidosis unless the serum pH is <7.15.

Blood Product Administration

Red blood cell transfusions should only occur when the hemoglobin level has fallen to <7.0 g/dL, with a target hemoglobin level of 7.0–9.0 g/dL. However, it may need to be higher in special circumstances (i.e., ongoing or recent myocardial ischemia, acute hemorrhage). Fresh frozen plasma should not be administered to correct coagulation abnormalities unless the patient is bleeding. Recent studies do not suggest any advantage of fresh blood over moderately old blood.

Glucose

"Tight glycemic control" that is, maintaining blood glucose between 80 and 110 mg/dL is no longer recommended. Current recommendations for critically ill patients, including those with severe sepsis, include some form of a glucose control protocol

Box 38-1. Highlights of the Surviving Sepsis Campaign Guidelines (Modified According to Our Institutional Practice)—cont'd

using low-dose insulin infusion. Though the precise glucose target for the critically ill patient remains controversial, ≤180 mg/dL is the current recommendation in the Surviving Sepsis Guidelines. Some populations of patients, such as those with global or focal cerebral damage, may benefit from more close glucose monitoring, although strong recommendations are not available.

Mechanical Ventilation of Sepsis-Induced Acute Lung Injury or Acute Respiratory Distress Syndrome

The lungs are the most common organ system to fail in patients with sepsis, many of whom eventually require mechanical ventilation. The lungs are the most likely source of initial infection as well, and patients are at great risk for nosocomial and ventilator-associated pneumonias. For details on management of ARDS please see chapter 30.

Steroids

The use of intravenous steroids in patients with persistent vasopressor-dependent septic shock is controversial but may be considered for refractory shock. At this time, laboratory testing of serum cortisol levels is not recommended.

Consideration for Limitation of Support

Severe sepsis and septic shock are serious diseases with significant mortality. It is important for the multidisciplinary critical care team to be in frequent communication with the family with appropriate updates regarding the status and prognosis of their loved one so that the family can set realistic expectations. It is paramount that the team be aware of any previous wishes the patient may have had regarding resuscitation, heroic measures, and artificial life support.

ACKNOWLEDGMENT

The authors wish to acknowledge Drs. David Shimabukuro, MDCM, Richard H. Savel, MD, FCCM, and Michael A. Gropper, MD, PhD, for the valuable contributions to the previous edition of this chapter.

KEY POINTS: SEPSIS AND SEPTIC SHOCK

1. Sepsis is a syndrome of life-threatening organ dysfunction caused by the dysregulated host immune response to an infection.
2. Early diagnosis and initiation of treatment for sepsis is associated with a reduction in mortality.
3. The pathophysiology of sepsis is complex, involving host-pathogen-microbiome interactions that lead to the activation of the innate immune system and defects in epithelial, endothelial, and mitochondrial function.
4. The Surviving Sepsis Campaign Guidelines provide a reasonable evidence-based approach to the current management of sepsis and septic shock.

BIBLIOGRAPHY

1. ARISE Investigators. Goal-directed resuscitation for patients with early septic shock. *N Engl J Med.* 2014;371:1496.
2. Gotts JE, Matthay MA. Sepsis: pathophysiology and clinical management. *BMJ.* 2016;353:i1585.
3. Kumar A, Roberts D, Wood KE, et al. Duration of hypotension before initiation of effective antimicrobial therapy is the critical determinant of survival in human septic shock. *Crit Care Med.* 2006;34:1589.
4. Liu V, Escobar GJ, Greene JD, et al. Hospital deaths in patients with sepsis from two independent cohorts. *JAMA.* 2014;312:90.
5. Perner A, Haase N, Guttormsen AB, et al. Hydroxyethyl Starch 130/0.42 versus Ringer's Acetate in severe sepsis. *N Engl J Med.* 2012;367:124.
6. Rhodes A, Evans LE, Alhazzani W, et al. Surviving Sepsis Campaign: International Guidelines for the management of Sepsis and Septic Shock: 2016. *Crit Care Med.* 2017;45:486.
7. Seymour CW, Gesten F, Prescott HC, et al. Time to treatment and mortality during mandated emergency care for sepsis. *N Engl J Med.* 2017;376:2235.
8. Singer M, Deutschman CS, Seymour CW, et al. The third international consensus definitions for sepsis and septic shock (sepsis-3). *JAMA.* 2016;315:801.

CHAPTER 39

ENDOCARDITIS

Lindsay M. Smith and Louis B. Polish

1. What are the important clinical manifestations of endocarditis?

   The clinical presentation of a patient with infective endocarditis can be quite variable. Fever, occurring in up to 80% of patients, is the most common complaint. Patients can also report symptoms of chills, rigors, or drenching night sweats. Other nonspecific symptoms such as anorexia, weight loss, malaise, fatigue, nausea, vomiting, and weakness are common. Many patients have joint complaints, which can range from relatively innocuous low back pain, myalgias, or arthralgias, or more severe complaints consistent with septic arthritis or severe low back pain, concerning for epidural abscess with neurologic compromise. Physical exam may reveal abnormal vital signs (fever, tachycardia, tachypnea, or hypotension). Although heart murmurs are common, the so-called changing murmur is relatively uncommon. There may be evidence of septic emboli, such as splenomegaly with left upper quadrant tenderness, or costovertebral angle tenderness from emboli to the kidney, or evidence of necrotic fingers or toes. If there are coronary emboli, the patient may present with symptoms of myocardial infarction. Patients may complain of headache or have neurologic signs or symptoms consistent with stroke, which are worrisome for cerebral septic emboli or mycotic aneurysm. Cutaneous and mucosal membrane manifestations of infective endocarditis include petechiae, Oser nodes, Janeway lesions, and splinter hemorrhages. New, worsening, or unexplained heart failure should prompt an investigation for infectious endocarditis.

2. Are there differences in the manifestations of endocarditis in elderly patients?

   There does appear to be an increased incidence of endocarditis in elderly patients that may be related to an increased life span in patients with rheumatic and other cardiovascular diseases, with a commensurate increase among patients with calcific and degenerative heart disease. In addition, the increase in prolonged catheter use, implantable devices, and dialysis catheters increases the incidence of nosocomial endocarditis. Endocarditis in elderly persons is more likely to occur in men, with a ratio of approximately 2 to 8:1 in patients older than 60 years of age. Staphylococci and streptococci account for approximately 80% of the cases in elderly persons, and *Streptococcus bovis* may be noted more frequently in elderly patients associated with underlying colonic malignancy. The clinical presentation of endocarditis may be nonspecific, including lethargy, fatigue, malaise, anorexia, failure to thrive, and weight loss (which may be attributed to aging or other medical illnesses common in the elderly). In addition, fever, which occurs in roughly 80% of patients with endocarditis, is more likely to be absent in elderly patients. Worsening heart failure and murmurs may be attributed to underlying disease and therefore erroneously neglected. Consequently, a high index of suspicion is necessary.

3. What are the Duke criteria for the diagnosis of endocarditis? How have they been modified?

   The original Duke criteria for the diagnosis of infective endocarditis stratified patients into three categories:

   - **Definite**—Identified by using clinical or pathologic criteria (Box 39.1).
   - **Possible**—Findings consistent with infective endocarditis that fall short of definite, but the diagnosis cannot be rejected.
   - **Rejected**—Firm alternative diagnosis for manifestations of endocarditis *or* resolution of manifestations of endocarditis, with antibiotic therapy for 4 days or less, *or* no pathologic evidence of infective endocarditis at surgery or autopsy, after antibiotic therapy for 4 days or less

     Since the original Duke criteria were published in 1994, several refinements have been made based on studies evaluating the sensitivity and specificity of the criteria:

   - Bacteremia with *Staphylococcus aureus* was originally included as a major criterion only if it was community acquired. Subsequent research has shown that a significant proportion of patients with nosocomially acquired staphylococcal bacteremia will have documented infective endocarditis. Consequently, *S. aureus* bacteremia is now included as a major criterion regardless of whether the infection is nosocomial or community acquired.
   - An additional major criterion was added as follows: single blood culture result positive for *Coxiella burnetii* or anti–phase 1 immunoglobulin G antibody titer ≥1:800.

Box 39-1. Original Duke Pathologic and Clinical Criteria for Diagnosis of Endocarditis

Pathologic Criteria

Pathologic criteria include microorganisms demonstrated by culture *or* histology in a vegetation *or* in a vegetation that has embolized *or* in an intracardiac abscess *or* pathologic lesions, including vegetation or intracardiac abscess, confirmed by histologic analysis showing active endocarditis.

Clinical Criteria

Clinical criteria include either two major criteria *or* one major and three minor criteria *or* five minor criteria from the following list:

Major criteria are the following:

- Positive blood culture results with a typical microorganism for infective endocarditis from two separate blood cultures (viridans streptococci, including nutritionally variant strains; *Streptococcus bovis*, HACEK group, or community-acquired *Staphylococcus aureus* or enterococci in absence of a primary focus)
- Persistently positive blood culture result, defined as recovery of a microorganism consistent with infective endocarditis from blood cultures drawn more than 12 h apart *or* all of three or a majority of four or more separated blood cultures with first and last drawn at least 1 h apart
- Echocardiogram result positive for infective endocarditis, including one of the following:
  - Oscillating intracardiac mass on valve or supporting structures, in the path of regurgitant jets, or on implanted material in the absence of an alternative anatomic explanation
  - Abscess
  - New partial dehiscence of prosthetic valve
  - New valvular regurgitation (increase or change in preexisting murmur not sufficient)

Minor criteria are the following:

- **Predisposition**—Predisposing heart condition or IV drug use
- **Fever**—Body temperature >38°C (100.4°F)
- **Vascular phenomena**—Major arterial emboli, septic pulmonary infarcts, mycotic aneurysm, intracranial hemorrhage, conjunctival hemorrhages, Janeway lesions
- **Immunologic phenomena**—Glomerulonephritis, Osler nodes, Roth spots, rheumatoid factor
- **Microbiologic evidence**—Positive blood culture result but not meeting major criterion as noted previously *or* serologic evidence of active infection with organism consistent with infective endocarditis
- **Echocardiogram**—Consistent with infective endocarditis but not meeting major criterion as noted previously

- An additional statement was added to the major criteria regarding endocardial involvement and an echocardiogram positive for infective endocarditis. The statement now includes the following: Transesophageal echocardiography (TEE) is recommended for patients with prosthetic valves, diagnoses rated at least "possible infective endocarditis" by clinical criteria, or complicated infective endocarditis (paravalvular abscess); transthoracic echocardiography (TTE) should be the first test in other patients.
- The echocardiogram minor criterion was eliminated.
- The category of "possible endocarditis" was adjusted to include the following criteria: one major and one minor criterion or three minor criteria. This so-called floor was designated to reduce the proportion of patients assigned to the "possible" category.

4. What is the optimal timing, volume, and number of blood cultures for a patient in whom infective endocarditis is suspected?

Multiple blood cultures are necessary to increase the yield, help distinguish between contamination and true bacteremia, and prove continuous bacteremia characteristic of infective endocarditis. Two to three blood cultures obtained over several minutes with adequate volumes of blood (20 mL for each two-bottle set) will identify approximately 99% of patients with culture-positive bacteremia. If the patient has a clinical course suggestive of subacute endocarditis, obtaining two to three sets of blood cultures over several hours, prior to antibiotic administration, to document continuous bacteremia would be prudent. It should also be stressed that each blood culture set requires a separate venipuncture site.

Patients with fungal endocarditis, or organisms that are difficult to culture, may have negative blood cultures (though Candida spp grow readily in blood culture bottles). If the first set of blood culture results is negative, it is important to realize that repeating blood cultures may be important if the pretest probability of endocarditis remains high. If the clinical situation evolves and endocarditis appears less likely, repeating blood cultures may be counterproductive. If blood cultures grow an organism, cultures should be repeated to ensure clearance of the bacteremia.

5. What are the organisms that most often cause endocarditis?
The etiologic agents of infective endocarditis include the following:
- Streptococci: 60% to 80%
- Viridans streptococci: 30% to 40%
- Enterococci: 5% to 18%
- Other streptococci: 15% to 25%
- Staphylococci: 20% to 35%
- Coagulase-positive organisms: 10% to 27%
- Coagulase-negative organisms: 1% to 3%
- Gram-negative aerobic bacilli: 1% to 13%
- Fungi: 2% to 4%

S. aureus tends to be the most common etiologic agent of infective endocarditis in intravenous (IV) drug users. *Pseudomonas aeruginosa* is also more commonly seen in patients using IV drugs. In patients with prosthetic valves, the microbiology is somewhat dependent on whether they have early (<2 months after valve replacement) versus late (>12 months) endocarditis. Staphylococci account for 40% to 60% of the cases of early onset prosthetic valve endocarditis. Coagulase-negative staphylococci account for approximately 30% to 35% of cases, and *S. aureus* accounts for approximately 20% to 25%. Patients who have late-onset prosthetic valve endocarditis are more likely to have the organisms most commonly seen in patients with native valve endocarditis, with one exception: coagulase-negative staphylococci are seen more frequently (approximately 10%–12%) in patients with prosthetic valves. Patients who have fungal endocarditis are often IV drug users, have recently undergone cardiovascular surgery, or have received prolonged IV antibiotic therapy.

6. How do you distinguish a case of *Staphylococcus aureus* endocarditis from uncomplicated *Staphylococcus aureus* bacteremia?
In a classic 1976 study, Nolan and Beaty suggested that, among 105 patients with *S. aureus* bacteremia retrospectively identified, most of the 26 patients with endocarditis could be identified on the basis of three characteristics: community-acquired infection, the absence of a primary focus of infection, and the presence of metastatic foci of infection. However, in prospectively identified patients with *S. aureus* bacteremia who undergo early echocardiography, approximately 25% will have evidence of endocarditis by TEE. Clinical findings and predisposing heart disease did not distinguish those with or without endocarditis. In addition, a substantial portion of these patients had hospital-acquired *S. aureus* bacteremia.

7. What are the HACEK organisms? How often do they cause endocarditis?
HACEK is an acronym for a group of fastidious, slow-growing, gram-negative bacteria:
- **H**—*Haemophilus influenza, Haemophilus parainfluenzae, Haemophilus aphrophilus, Haemophilus paraphrophilus* (subsequently called *Aggregatibacter aphrophilus* and *Aggregatibacter paraphrophilus*)
- **A**—*Actinobacillus actinomycetemcomitans* (subsequently called *Aggregatibacter actinomycetemcomitans*)
- **C**—*Cardiobacterium hominis*
- **E**—*Eikenella corrodens*
- **K**—*Kingella kingae, Kingella denitrificans*

These organisms account for approximately 5% to 10% of cases of community-acquired endocarditis. Because an increasing number of these organisms produce β-lactamase, they should be considered resistant to ampicillin. The treatment of choice is ceftriaxone or other third- or fourth-generation cephalosporins. Gentamicin is no longer recommended.

8. What are the causes of culture-negative endocarditis?
Approximately 2% to 30% of patients with infective endocarditis will have sterile blood culture specimens; however, it is more likely to be 5% with use of strict diagnosis criteria. Potential causes of culture-negative endocarditis include the following:
- Prior antibiotic usage
- Nonbacterial thrombotic endocarditis (NBTE) or an incorrect diagnosis
- Slow growth of fastidious organisms, including anaerobes, HACEK organisms, nutritionally variant streptococci, or *Brucella* species

- Obligate intracellular organisms, including rickettsia, chlamydiae, *Tropheryma whippelii*, or viruses
- Other organisms, including *C. burnetii* (the etiologic agent of Q fever) and *Legionella*, *Bartonella*, or *Mycoplasma* species
- Subacute right-sided endocarditis
- Fungal endocarditis
- Mural endocarditis, as in patients with ventricular septal defects, postmyocardial infarction thrombi, or infection related to implanted cardiac devices
- Culture specimens taken at the end of a long course, usually more than 3 months

9. **What is the prevalence of healthcare–associated endocarditis?**
   Data from the International Collaboration on Endocarditis–Prospective Cohort Study (ICE-PCS) suggested that healthcare–associated native valve endocarditis was present in 34% of non–IV drug–using patients (557 of 1622 patients). Of these 557 patients, 54% had nosocomial and 46% had nonnosocomial infections (infections developing outside the hospital but with extensive healthcare contact [i.e., dialysis centers, outpatient antibiotic programs, nursing homes]). Patients with healthcare–associated native valve endocarditis and without a history of injection drug use were more likely to have *S. aureus* (including methicillin-resistant *S. aureus* [MRSA]) and had a higher mortality rate than those with community-acquired infections.

10. **What is the appropriate empirical therapy (cultures pending) for patients with presumptive infective endocarditis?**
    Infectious diseases consultation for aid in antibiotic therapy is strongly recommended. Several regimens considered by authorities to be appropriate while awaiting results of blood cultures would include the following, based on native or prosthetic valve and symptom duration:
    - **Acute native valve**—Therapy should target *S. aureus*, β hemolytic streptococci, and aerobic gram-negative bacilli. Possible antibiotics would include vancomycin 15-20 mg/kg IV every 12 hours (dosing interval based on creatinine clearance) plus cefepime 2 g IV every 8 hours (dosing interval based on creatinine clearance). Some experts would add ampicillin, 2 g IV every 4 hours, to cover the possibility of enterococci.
    - **Subacute native valve**—Organisms to consider would include *S. aureus*, viridans group streptococci, the HACEK organism, and enterococcal species. Empiric therapy could include ampicillin and sulbactam, 3 g IV every 4 to 6 hours, plus vancomycin, 15-20 mg/kg every 12 hours IV (dosing interval based on creatinine clearance).
    - **Prosthetic valve within 1 year from surgery**—Organisms of concern are staphylococci, enterococci, and gram-negative bacilli. Empiric treatment could include vancomycin, 15-20 mg/kg IV every 12 hours (dosing interval based on creatinine clearance), plus gentamicin, 1 mg/kg every 8 hours IV, plus rifampin, 300 mg orally every 8 hours, plus cefepime 2 g IV every 8 hours (dosing interval based on creatinine clearance).
    - **Prosthetic valve beyond 1 year from surgery**—Staphylococci, viridans group streptococci, and enterococci should be considered for these infections, and empiric therapy could include vancomycin 15-20 mg/kg IV every 12 hours (dosing interval based on creatinine clearance) plus ceftriaxone.

11. **What valves are most commonly affected in patients with endocarditis?**
    This depends on the etiology of the endocarditis. In patients with native valve endocarditis, the mitral valve alone is involved in 28% to 45% of cases, 5% to 36% for the aortic valve alone, and 0% to 35% for both valves combined. The tricuspid valve is involved alone 0% to 6% of the time, and the pulmonic valve is involved in less than 1% of the cases of endocarditis. Endocarditis occurs in approximately 5% to 15% of injection drug users admitted to the hospital for acute infection. In these patients, the frequency of valvular involvement is as follows: tricuspid valve alone or in combination, 50%; aortic valve alone, 19%; mitral valve alone, 11%; and aortic plus mitral, 12%. In patients with prosthetic valve endocarditis, a difference does not seem to exist in the incidence of endocarditis at the aortic compared with the mitral location. The overall risk of endocarditis is similar with a mechanical valve compared with a bioprosthetic valve; however, slight differences exist in the risk on the basis of the length of time after surgery. Within the first 6 postoperative months, mechanical valves have a slightly increased risk of infection; however, no significant increased risk was seen within the first 5 years after surgery with mechanical valves compared with bioprosthetic valves. After 5 years, the risk for endocarditis for bioprosthetic valves is slightly greater than that for mechanical valves. In patients with fungal endocarditis, the aortic valve was involved 44% of the time either alone or in combination with other valves; the mitral valve, 26% alone or in combination; and the tricuspid valve, 7%; other locations were documented in 18% of patients.

12. What are the clinical differences between right-sided and left-sided endocarditis?

In patients with right-sided endocarditis (either the tricuspid or pulmonic valve), particularly injection drug users with tricuspid valve endocarditis, only 35% will have an audible murmur. In general, symptoms and complications arise from involvement of the pulmonary vasculature and are characterized by multiple pulmonary septic emboli that may cause pulmonary infarction, abscesses, pneumothoraces, pleural effusions, or empyema. In addition, multiple pulmonary emboli may result in right-sided heart failure with chamber dilatation and worsening tricuspid regurgitation. Clinical symptoms associated with these complications may include chest pain, dyspnea, cough, and hemoptysis. Peripheral embolic phenomena and neurologic involvement are generally absent in patients with right-sided endocarditis, and when they do occur in the setting of right-sided endocarditis, involvement of the left side or paradoxical embolization should be considered. Patients with left-sided endocarditis (aortic or mitral) generally have greater hemodynamic consequences and are more likely to have congestive heart failure. Systemic embolization (brain, kidney, spleen) is more common with left-sided lesions.

13. What is the appropriate role of echocardiography in the diagnosis and management of endocarditis?

Echocardiography is an essential tool in the diagnostic workup of a patient with suspected endocarditis. The primary objective is to identify, localize, and characterize valvular vegetations. However, echocardiography is also potentially important in the management of endocarditis. Identification of an abscess may indicate the need for surgical intervention. Patients may also benefit from repeating the echocardiography once a definitive diagnosis has been established to assess complications, including congestive heart failure and atrioventricular block, which suggest worsening valvular and myocardial function. It is important to emphasize that echocardiographic findings should always be interpreted in coordination with clinical information.

The TEE is more sensitive than a TTE for the diagnosis of endocarditis. Sensitivities of the different modalities have ranged from 48% to 100% for TEE and from 18% to 63% for TTE. This is in part related to the fact that the transesophageal approach allows closer proximity to the heart and therefore can be performed at higher frequencies, providing greater spatial resolution. It can identify structures as small as 1 mm. TEE is the preferred modality in patients with prosthetic valves. The spatial resolution of the TTE may be limited by overlying fat in obese patients or hyperinflated lungs from chronic obstructive pulmonary disease or mechanical ventilation. The TTE may only be able to identify structures as small as 5 mm. Both modalities, however, are highly specific, in the range of 95%.

A cost-effectiveness analysis study conducted by Heidenreich and colleagues suggested that the prior probability of endocarditis was the most important factor in choosing the appropriate modality. Because echocardiography is an essential component to the diagnosis of infective endocarditis, TTE should be performed in all cases of suspected infective endocarditis. If the TTE is negative, but clinical suspicion for infective endocarditis remains high, then a TEE should be performed. TEE is the preferred modality in patients with a higher pretest probability of disease, particularly in patients with *S. aureus* bacteremia, or in patients in whom the TTE would be less sensitive—that is, with obesity, lung hyperinflation, prosthetic valve, or new atrioventricular block. Echocardiography can identify patients at high risk for complications or with a need for surgery. These features include:

- Large vegetations (>10 mm in diameter)
- Severe valvular insufficiency
- Abscess cavities
- Pseudoaneurysm
- Valvular perforation or dehiscence
- Decompensated heart failure

Although echocardiography has become an essential diagnostic tool in patients with suspected endocarditis, no definitive echocardiographic features can reliably distinguish infection from those lesions that are noninfective. Cardiac computed tomography (CT) and magnetic resonance imaging have been used in diagnosing complications of infective endocarditis, and in at least one study cardiac multislice CT was shown to be as effective as TEE. However, at this time, they are not part of the current standard of care in diagnosing infective endocarditis.

14. What conduction abnormalities can be associated with endocarditis?

Right and left bundle branch blocks, second-degree atrioventricular block, and complete heart block can be found with infective endocarditis. Heart block generally is the result of extension of infection to the atrioventricular node or the bundle of His. Most patients with heart block have involvement of the aortic valve. Mitral valve endocarditis may cause first- or second-degree heart block, but third-degree heart block would be unusual. Aortic valve endocarditis can cause first- or second-degree heart block as well as bundle branch blocks, hemiblocks, and complete heart blocks. It should be remembered that the electrocardiogram (ECG) is specific but not sensitive for involvement of the conduction system. Consequently, one could have a valve ring abscess but not have conduction abnormalities on the ECG. Complete heart block may be preceded by prolongation of the PR interval or a left bundle branch block. Conduction abnormalities in the setting of endocarditis may occur for other reasons as well, including myocardial infarction (rarely), myocarditis, or pericarditis. ECG findings may also have prognostic implications, because patients with persistent conduction abnormalities have an increased 1-year mortality compared with patients who have normal ECG findings.

15. **What are the neurologic manifestations of endocarditis?**
Overall, the incidence of central nervous system involvement during the course of infective endocarditis ranges between 20% and 40%. Neurologic symptoms are the presenting manifestations in endocarditis approximately 16% to 23% of the time; however, there are generally other clues to the diagnosis. The most common neurologic manifestation is stroke, and this accounts for approximately 50% to 60% of all neurologic complications. Stroke generally occurs from cerebral emboli with infarction, but hemorrhage or abscess may occur as well. When hemorrhage is suspected, either a CT angiogram or magnetic resonance angiography (MRA) should be obtained. Recent studies have shown that CT angiography and MRA have similar results in the detection of noninfectious intracranial aneurysms, and it is likely that the same would be true for infectious intracranial aneurysms. If hemorrhage has been confirmed and surgery is considered, conventional angiography is still the most appropriate diagnostic procedure to pinpoint location and anatomic relationships.

Other neurologic manifestations with their associated main clinical presentations include encephalopathy (decreased level of consciousness), seizures, severe or localized headache, psychiatric syndromes from minor personality changes to more severe psychiatric syndromes (generally in elderly patients), various dyskinesias, visual disturbances, spinal cord involvement (paraplegia or tetraplegia), peripheral nerve involvement (mononeuropathy), and meningitis, which is more common with *S. aureus* and *Streptococcus pneumoniae* (with or without focal signs). Ocular complications include acute embolic occlusion of the central retinal artery, which may result in sudden vision loss. Other complications that have been well documented include involvement of cranial nerves III, IV, and VI, which can lead to diplopia, deviation of the eyes, nystagmus or unequal pupils, retinal hemorrhages, and endophthalmitis.

16. **How often do intracranial mycotic aneurysms occur?**
Intracranial mycotic aneurysms (ICMAs) are uncommon, and although they constitute only 2% to 6% of all intracranial aneurysms, 80% of these are identified in the setting of infective endocarditis. Among patients with endocarditis, only 1% to 5% will have a recognized ICMA. The mortality rate is approximately 60%, and many patients are seen initially with a sudden subarachnoid or intracerebral hemorrhage. Rupture of an ICMA may occur while the patient is being treated for endocarditis or after completion of therapy.

17. **What are the indications for surgical therapy?**
Clinical situations that warrant surgical intervention include moderate and severe (i.e., New York Heart Association class III or IV) or progressive and refractory congestive heart failure (CHF), valve dehiscence, rupture, or fistula. Although CHF has a worse prognosis with medical therapy alone, an increased surgical risk also exists. Delay in surgery may also lead to worsening cardiac decompensation or perivalvular extension, which will increase operative mortality as well as secondary complications. Several studies have shown benefits in mortality statistics with surgical intervention. Progressive heart failure in the presence of aortic or mitral valve regurgitation requires surgery. Other indications for surgery include perivalvular extension of infection, persistent bacteremia without evidence of an extracardiac source of bacteremia, mechanical valve obstruction, prosthetic valve endocarditis, and difficult-to-treat organisms, including *Pseudomonas* species, *C. burnetii*, *Brucella* species, and *Staphylococcus lugdunensis*. Surgery may also be indicated to avoid embolizations or further embolization, particularly if the vegetation is greater than 10 mm after an embolization event. Conventional wisdom has been that indications for surgery to avoid embolization have been two or more major embolic events during therapy. However, determining the number and timing of embolic events may be difficult, given that the detection of damage may occur well after the actual embolism. The risk of embolization also decreases significantly during the first 1 to 2 weeks of antibiotic therapy.

Right-sided endocarditis with tricuspid regurgitation is reasonably well tolerated if the pulmonary vascular resistance is not increased, and surgery is often not required. Surgery could be indicated if there is a poor response to medical therapy. Valve repair is preferred over replacement. The decision to proceed with valvular surgery in the presence of an intracranial hemorrhage or cerebral mycotic aneurysm is complicated, and there are ongoing studies to determine optimal timing of surgery.

18. Is there a relationship between duration of antibiotic therapy before surgery and operative mortality?

Although it is important to have adequate antibiotic coverage during surgery, the duration of antibiotic therapy does not generally influence operative mortality. The incidence of reinfection of newly implanted valves is approximately 3% and may be as high as 10%.

19. What is nonbacterial thrombotic endocarditis?

NBTE refers to small, sterile vegetations on cardiac valves from platelet-fibrin deposits. The cardiac lesions most commonly resulting in NBTE include mitral regurgitation, aortic stenosis, aortic regurgitation, ventricular septal defect, and complex congenital heart disease. NBTE may also result from a hypercoagulable state, and sterile vegetations can be seen in systemic lupus erythematosus (i.e., Libman-Sacks endocarditis), antiphospholipid antibody syndrome, and collagen vascular diseases. Noninfectious vegetations can also be seen in patients with malignancy (e.g., renal cell carcinoma or melanoma), burns, or even acute septicemia. Other lesions that may be somewhat misleading include myxomatous valves, benign cardiac tumors, and degenerative thickening of the valves. Lambl excrescences, which are multiple small tags on heart valves seen in a large number of adults at autopsy, can also be confused with infectious vegetations; however, these tend to be much more filamentous in appearance.

KEY POINTS: ENDOCARDITIS

1. The Duke criteria for the diagnosis of endocarditis include two major criteria, one major and three minor criteria, or five minor criteria (Box 39-1).
2. The HACEK organisms are fastidious, slow-growing, gram-negative bacteria and include *Haemophilus*, *Aggregatibacter*, *Cardiobacterium*, *Eikenella*, and *Kingella* species.
3. *S. aureus* endocarditis cannot be distinguished from bacteremia on the basis of community-acquired infection, lack of a primary focus, and presence of metastatic foci of infection.
4. Symptoms and complications of right-sided endocarditis generally result from involvement of the pulmonary vasculature, whereas complications of left-sided endocarditis are generally characterized by greater hemodynamic consequences, congestive heart failure, and systemic embolization.
5. Nervous system involvement occurs in 20% to 40% of patients and may be the presenting symptom in approximately 20% of the cases of infective endocarditis.

BIBLIOGRAPHY

1. Baddour LM, Wilson WR, Bayer AS, et al. Infective endocarditis in adults: diagnosis, antimicrobial therapy and management of complications. A statement for healthcare professionals for healthcare professionals from the American Heart Association. *Circulation*. 2015;132:1435-1486.
2. Barton TL, Mottram PM, Stuart RL, Cameron JD, Moir S. Transthoracic echocardiography is still useful in the initial evaluation of patients with suspected infective endocarditis: evaluation of a large cohort at a tertiary referral center. *Mayo Clin Proc*. 2014;89:799-805.
3. Cavassini M, Meuli R, Francioli P. Complications of infective endocarditis. In: Scheld WM, Whitley RJ, Marra CM, eds. *Infections of the Central Nervous System*. 3rd ed. Philadelphia: Lippincott Williams & Wilkins; 2004:537-568.
4. Chu VH, Park LP, Athan E, et al. Association between surgical indications, operative risk, and clinical outcome in infective endocarditis: a prospective study from the International Collaboration on Endocarditis. *Circulation*. 2015;131:131-140.
5. Chun JY, Smith W, Halbach VV, Higashida RT, Wilson CB, Lawton MT. Current multimodality management of infectious intracranial aneurysms. *Neurosurgery*. 2001;48:1203-1213. [discussion: 1213-1214].
6. Dhawan VK. Infective endocarditis in the elderly patients. *Clin Infect Dis*. 2002;34:806-812.
7. Di Salvo G, Habib G, Pergola V, et al. Echocardiography predicts embolic events in infective endocarditis. *J Am Coll Cardiol*. 2001;37:1069-1076.
8. Ellis ME, Al-Abdely H, Sandridge A, Greer W, Ventura W. Fungal endocarditis: evidence in the world literature, 1965-1995. *Clin Infect Dis*. 2001;32:50-62.
9. Fowler VG, Scheld WM, Bayer AS. Endocarditis and intravascular infections. In: Mandell GL, Bennett JE, Dolin R, eds. *Principles and Practice of Infectious Diseases*. 8th ed. New York: Churchill Livingstone; 2015:990-1028.

10. González-Juanatey C, González-Gay MA, Llorca J, et al. Rheumatic manifestations of infective endocarditis in non-addicts: a 12 year study. *Medicine (Baltimore)*. 2001;80:9-19.
11. Heidenreich PA, Masoudi FA, Maini B, et al. Echocardiography in patients with suspected endocarditis: a cost-effectiveness analysis. *Am J Med*. 1999;107:198-208.
12. Li JS, Sexton DJ, Mick N, et al. Proposed modifications to the Duke Criteria for the Diagnosis of Infective Endocarditis. *Clin Infect Dis*. 2000;30(4):633-638.
13. Mehta NJ, Nehra A. A 66 year old man with fever, hypotension and complete heart block. *Chest*. 2001;120:2053-2056.
14. Benito N, Miró JM, de Lazzari E, et al. Health care–associated native valve endocarditis: importance of non-nosocomial acquisition. *Ann Intern Med*. 2009;150:586-594.
15. Nolan CM, Beaty HN. Staphylococcus aureus bacteremia—current clinical patterns. *Am J Med*. 1976;60:495-500.
16. Olaison L, Pettersson G. Current best practices and guidelines indications for surgical intervention in infective endocarditis. *Infect Dis Clin North Am*. 2002;16:453-475.
17. Petti CA, Fowler VG Jr. Staphylococcus aureus bacteremia and endocarditis. *Infect Dis Clin North Am*. 2002;16:413-435.
18. Rosen AB, Fowler VG Jr, Corey GR, et al. Cost-effectiveness of transesophageal echocardiography to determine the duration of therapy for intravascular catheter–associated Staphylococcus aureus bacteremia. *Ann Intern Med*. 1999;130:810-820.
19. Sachdev M, Peterson GE, Jollis JG. Imaging techniques for diagnosis of infective endocarditis. *Infect Dis Clin North Am*. 2002;16:319-337.
20. Towns ML, Reller LB. Diagnostic methods: current best practices and guidelines for isolation of bacteria and fungi in infective endocarditis. *Infect Dis Clin North Am*. 2002;16:363-376.
21. Yoshioka D, Toda K, Sakaguchi T, et al. Valve surgery in active endocarditis patients complicated by intracranial haemorrhage: the influence of the timing of surgery on neurological outcomes. *Eur J Cardiothorac Surg*. 2014; 45(6):1082-1088.

MENINGITIS AND ENCEPHALITIS IN THE INTENSIVE CARE UNIT

Cindy Noyes

MENINGITIS

1. **Describe the most common signs and symptoms of acute meningitis syndrome.**
   Fever, neck stiffness, and altered mental status are the classic triad, but they occur together only approximately 45% of the time. In a systematic review, 95% of patients had two of the three classic signs. The onset is hours to days, although historical detail may be limited if the patient's sensorium is altered.

2. **What is the pathophysiology of meningitis?**
   The pathogen gains entry via attachment on epithelial mucosal cells, endocytosis by dendritic cells, or direct vascular access. In the setting of bacterial meningitis, infection causes cytokine production and influx of inflammatory cells. The blood-brain barrier may have changes in permeability, allowing for protein entry in addition to inflammatory cells and fluid. Vasculature initially vasodilates but then becomes stenotic with infiltration of inflammatory cells. This vasculitis can result in ischemia and/or infarction. Glucose metabolism is increased, and transport across the blood-brain barrier is possibly decreased.

3. **What is the distinction between acute versus chronic meningitis?**
   Acute meningitis syndrome consists of fever, neck stiffness, and altered mental status, with an onset of hours to days. Patients with acute bacterial meningitis may have rapid progression of signs and symptoms. This is in contrast to chronic meningitis, which is defined by the presence of symptoms and abnormal cerebrospinal fluid (CSF) that persists for 4 weeks or more. The two syndromes have very distinct causes.

4. **What host factors are important to consider regarding risk and cause for acute bacterial meningitis?**
   Factors such as age, immune deficiency or suppression, recent central nervous system (CNS) instrumentation, and possible exposures should be considered and will influence empiric therapy. See Table 40.1.

5. **What are the most common causes of community-acquired acute bacterial meningitis in adults?**
   Table 40.2 includes the most common organisms in descending order based on case series with preferred antimicrobial therapy and suggested duration of treatment.

6. **What is adequate empirical therapy while awaiting culture results?**
   Empiric therapy should reflect suspected pathogens on the basis of host factors as well as local antibiotic susceptibility patterns. For example, *Streptococcus pneumoniae* is commonly known to have resistance to penicillin. Some strains are also resistant to third-generation cephalosporins. As a result, empiric therapy for *S. pneumoniae* should include high-dose third-generation cephalosporin as well as vancomycin. Empiric therapy with third-generation cephalosporin is also suggested for *Neisseria meningitidis*. For *Listeria monocytogenes*, preferred treatment is ampicillin, although trimethoprim-sulfamethoxazole is another option if the patient is penicillin allergic. Thus in an adult older than 50 years, an initial empiric regimen including vancomycin, high-dose ceftriaxone, and ampicillin would be suggested to treat the most likely community-acquired pathogens.

   In the event that a patient has undergone recent neurosurgical instrumentation and has risk for nosocomial pathogens, one would also want to include therapy directed at methicillin-resistant *Staphylococcus aureus* (MRSA) and resistant nosocomial gram-negative bacilli, such as *Pseudomonas aeruginosa*.

   Risk factors that may additionally influence empiricism must be identified with each patient. Prompt and detailed history should be explored. Factors including exposures, such as contaminated

Table 40-1. Important Considerations Regarding Risk and Cause for Acute Bacterial Meningitis

HOST FACTORS	COMMON PATHOGENS					EMPIRIC THERAPY
Age						
<1 month	Streptococcus agalactiae	—	Escherichia coli	Listeria monocytogenes	Klebsiella species	—	—	Ampicillin + third-generation cephalosporin
1–23 months	S. agalactiae	E. coli	Haemophilus influenzae	Streptococcus pneumoniae	—	Vancomycin + third-generation cephalosporin
2–50 years	S. pneumoniae	N. meningitidis	—	—	Neisseria meningitidis	Vancomycin + third-generation cephalosporin
>50 years	S. pneumoniae	N. meningitidis	L. monocytogenes	Aerobic gram-negative bacilli	—	Vancomycin + third-generation cephalosporin + ampicillin
Immune Suppression	S. pneumoniae	N. meningitidis	L. monocytogenes	Aerobic gram-negative bacilli, including nosocomial organisms	—	Vancomycin + carbapenem or fourth-generation cephalosporin + ampicillin
Post Neurosurgery	S. aureus (including methicillin resistant)	Coagulase-negative staphylococci	Aerobic gram-negative bacilli	—	—	Vancomycin + carbapenem or fourth-generation cephalosporin or ceftazidime

Table 40-2. Most Common Causes of Community-Acquired Bacterial Meningitis in Adults

PATHOGENS	PREFERRED ANTIMICROBIAL	SUGGESTED DURATION OF THERAPY
Streptococcus Pneumoniae PCN MIC <0.1 mcg/mL PCN MIC 0.1–1 mcg/mL PCN MIC ≥1 mcg/ml	PCN or ampicillin Third-generation cephalosporin Vancomycin + third-generation cephalosporin	10–14 days
Neisseria Meningitidis PCN MIC <0.1 mcg/mL PCN MIC >0.1 mcg/mL	PCN or ampicillin Third-generation cephalosporin	7 days
Listeria Monocytogenes	Ampicillin or PCN	≥21 days
Streptococcus Agalactiae, Pyogenes	Ampicillin or PCN	21 days
Staphylococcus Aureus	MSSA → nafcillin, oxacillin MRSA → vancomycin	14 days
Haemophilus Influenzae β-Lactamase negative β-Lactamase positive	Ampicillin Third-generation cephalosporin	7 days

MIC, Minimum inhibitory concentration; *MSSA*, methicillin-sensitive *Staphylococcus aureus*; *PCN*, penicillin.

food consumption, travel, and sick contacts should be identified. The presence of immune suppression should also be elicited. The type and degree of immune suppression, including medications, absence of spleen, advanced HIV, and administration of chemotherapy should be sought. Risk factors for nosocomial pathogens, including recent neurosurgical procedures, epidural injection, presence of a foreign body within the CNS (such as a ventricular drain), and trauma are also important to determine.

7. When and to whom should steroids be administered?
Adults suspected of having bacterial meningitis should receive steroids before or with the administration of antibiotics. On the basis of a prospective, randomized, placebo-controlled trial, dexamethasone was shown to reduce morbidity and mortality in adults who received corticosteroid therapy before or at the same time as administration of antibiotics. This had the greatest benefit in patients with pneumococcal meningitis. The dose used in the study was 10 mg of dexamethasone every 6 hours for 4 days. Shorter durations and alternative dosing regimens have not been evaluated in adults.

8. What are the contraindications to lumbar puncture?
Lumbar puncture (LP) is critical to diagnostic evaluation. If clinical suspicion for meningitis exists, one should perform an LP. Conditions such as elevated intracranial pressure, mass lesion, uncorrected coagulopathy, and skin infection overlying intended puncture site are to be considered before LP.

9. When would one consider imaging before lumbar puncture?
Most patients do not require imaging before LP. Computed tomography (CT) of the head should occur before LP if the patient has any signs or symptoms that suggest elevated intracranial pressure. These include new-onset neurologic deficits, new-onset seizure, and papilledema. Consideration should also be given to imaging in patients with moderate to severe cognitive impairment and immune compromise.

10. Is there harm in awaiting computed tomography and lumbar puncture results before initiating therapy?
Yes. Delay in initiating antimicrobial therapy has been associated with increase in mortality. If imaging is needed before LP:
• Obtain blood cultures.
• Initiate antibiotic therapy and steroids.
• Obtain CT of head, and perform LP if safe. CSF cultures may be affected by pretreatment with antibiotics before LP, but CSF findings including cell counts, chemical analyses, and Gram stain

Table 40-3. Typical Cerebrospinal Fluid Findings in Bacterial and Aseptic Meningitis

	BACTERIAL DISEASE LIKELY	EARLY BACTERIAL/ VIRAL/SYPHILIS	MENINGITIS UNLIKELY
White blood cell count	>1000 cells/mcL	100–1000 cells/mcL	<5 cells/mcL
White blood cell differential	Neutrophil predominance (although 10% have 50% lymphocytes)	Lymphocyte predominance	—
Glucose	<34 mg/dL	>45 mg/dL	Normal
Protein	>250 mg/dL	50–250 mg/dL	Normal

should remain helpful. Van de Beek, in his review, noted that yield of Gram stain was similar in patients who had been treated with antibiotics before LP as compared with those who had not.

11. **What cerebrospinal fluid studies are important?**
A number of studies help determine likelihood for bacterial meningitis based on various CSF markers, although it is important to know that none are absolute. See Table 40.3 for specific indicators.

A positive Gram stain confirms bacterial meningitis. However, culture data remain important for speciation (especially if morphology is not characteristic) and antimicrobial sensitivities. Low glucose level can be very helpful in indicating acute bacterial meningitis, but it is important to remember that other factors can contribute to a low glucose finding. For example, *Mycobacterium tuberculosis* meningitis, which is typically chronic, is commonly associated with low CSF glucose level. Malignancies are also associated with low CSF glucose level.

In addition, other tests have been studied to improve performance when trying to distinguish bacterial versus nonbacterial causes of meningitis. One such marker, CSF lactate, was shown to add predictive value when trying to distinguish between bacterial meningitis and nonbacterial meningitis shortly after neurosurgery. In a study of patients after neurosurgery by Lieb and colleagues, a value of greater than 4 mmol/L CSF lactate was 88% sensitive and 98% specific for diagnosis of bacterial meningitis. Of interest, CSF lactate levels did not vary with the presence or absence of red blood cells (RBCs), nor was there a correlation with days after surgery.

12. **How does one correct for a suspected traumatic lumbar puncture?**
In the event of traumatic LP, one general guideline is subtraction of one white blood cell (WBC) for every 500 to 1500 RBCs. More precise calculation would be to tabulate the adjusted WBC count per microliter according to the following formulas:
a) Adjusted CSF WBC count/mcL = Observed WBC count/mcL minus Predicted CSF WBC count/mcL, where
b) Predicted WBC count/mcL = CSF RBC count/mcL × (peripheral blood WBC/peripheral blood RBC)
Per Mayefski and colleague, the ratio of observed CSF WBC over predicted CSF WBC, especially if the multiple exceeded 10, was a sensitive and specific indicator of bacterial meningitis in setting of traumatic LP.

13. **In the setting of documented bacterial meningitis, who gets postexposure prophylaxis?**
The goal of postexposure prophylaxis is to eradicate nasopharyngeal carriage. There are two pathogens for which one would consider postexposure prophylaxis, with specific indications listed as follows.

N. meningitidis
1. Extended period of contact (>8 hours) in close proximity (within 3 feet)
2. Contact with oral secretions, with such activities as kissing, mouth-to-mouth resuscitation, intubation
3. Household contacts, including communal living (military recruits, college dormitory residents)
4. Exposure 1 week before symptom onset until after 24 hours of effective antibiotic therapy is considered significant. Postexposure prophylaxis should occur despite history of vaccination, because not all people respond to vaccination.
Suggested regimens:
- Ciprofloxacin 500 mg orally (PO) × 1
- Rifampin 10 mg/kg PO every 12 hours for 2 days (or 600 mg every 12 hours in adults)
- Ceftriaxone 250 mg intramuscularly (IM) × 1 in adults; 125 mg IM × 1 in children

> **Box 40-1.** Determining Possible Etiologic Viral Pathogens for Aseptic Meningitis
>
> Time of year or season
> Exposures
>   Animal
>   Insect (tick, mosquito)
>   Travel
>   Water
>   Sick contacts
>
> Environmental (day care, college dormitory, military recruit)
>   Sexual history
>   Skin rash
>   Genital lesions
>   HIV status
>   As primary cause
>   As a risk for secondary cause

Haemophilus influenzae: If there is a partially vaccinated child or child younger than 4 years of age, prophylaxis is suggested for all household contacts, including adults. Prophylaxis of day-care contacts can be considered if applicable. The highest risk is in children under the age of 2 years.

Suggested regimen: Rifampin 20 mg/kg per day (maximum dose of 600 mg daily) for 4 days

14. **What is aseptic meningitis?**
    Aseptic meningitis is defined by a syndrome of meningeal symptoms accompanied by abnormal CSF, usually with lymphocytic pleocytosis, in the setting of negative routine stains and cultures. Symptoms can be severe. Differential diagnosis includes infectious as well as noninfectious causes. This syndrome is usually associated with viral pathogens but can be caused by bacteria such as *M. tuberculosis*, *Treponema pallidum*, and *Borrelia burgdorferi*, or fungi. This constellation of findings could also reflect a partially treated bacterial meningitis or a parameningeal focus. Medications, connective tissue disorders, and malignancy can also cause aseptic meningitis. It is imperative that the common bacterial causes be excluded.

15. **What are important historical data to obtain to help determine possible etiologic viral pathogens?**
    The list of possible causes is extensive. Various factors can help narrow the possibilities. See Box 40.1.

16. **What are the most common viral causes of meningitis?**
    The most common viruses associated with meningitis are nonpolio enteroviruses. These include various coxsackievirus, echovirus, and enterovirus strains. Diagnosis was historically made by viral culture, although polymerase chain reaction (PCR) evaluation of CSF is now readily available in many laboratories. Treatment is supportive in nature, and the illness is usually self-limited with complete recovery. Exceptions to this are neonates less than 2 weeks of age and persons with immune deficiencies, such as agammaglobulinemia, in whom severe disease can develop. Other common viruses include flaviviruses, such as St. Louis encephalitis (SLE) and West Nile virus (WNV), and herpes family viruses, such as herpes simplex virus 2 (HSV-2) and varicella-zoster virus (VZV). These too can be confirmed by PCR. It is important to note that other viral illnesses can cause meningitis. These include acute HIV infection and various respiratory viruses such as influenza and parainfluenza. It is important to remember that to diagnose acute HIV, viral load RNA quantification of serum is necessary because antibody testing is usually negative during acute seroconversion.

ENCEPHALITIS

17. **What symptoms and signs are commonly associated with encephalitis?**
    Encephalitis is defined by inflammation of brain parenchyma. Most causal pathogens are viral and gain access to the CNS via the bloodstream, although some viruses such as HSV-1 and rabies directly invade via neuronal transport. Acute encephalitis usually occurs over a brief period of time (days) as compared with chronic encephalitis, which can progress over weeks to months. Many patients will present with a prodromal illness with symptoms of fever, myalgias, and anorexia, which corresponds to viremia. Neurologic manifestations that follow can range from headache, focal neurologic defect, and behavioral changes to seizure and coma. Meningeal inflammation can also occur resulting in symptoms suggestive of meningitis. Various viruses may have slightly different neural tropism, which can suggest a cause based on presentation. For example, HSV-1 has a predilection for the temporal lobe. Encephalitis is associated with high morbidity and mortality.

18. **What are the most common causes of acute encephalitis?**
    Despite often aggressive diagnostics, the cause of encephalitis in the majority of patients remains unknown. Any epidemiologic clues should be identified to guide diagnostic workup as well as to initiate prompt empiric therapy. In the United States, when a cause is identified, the most common pathogens are HSV-1, WNV, and enteroviruses.
    Possible infectious causes include but are not limited to the following:
    - Viral: HSV-1, enterovirus, WNV, VZV, SLE, influenza, HIV, Epstein-Barr virus, measles, rabies, cytomegalovirus (CMV)
    - Bacterial: *Bartonella henselae*, *L. monocytogenes*
    - Rickettsial: *Ehrlichia*, *Rickettsia rickettsii*, *Anaplasma*
    - Parasitic: *Toxoplasma gondii*, *Naegleria fowleri*
    - Fungal: *Histoplasma capsulatum*, *Cryptococcus neoformans*, *Coccidioides immitis*

    Up to 5% to 10% of sporadic cases of encephalitis, when diagnosis is available, are attributable to HSV-1. Postinfectious, postimmunization, and noninfectious causes, such as connective tissue disease and paraneoplastic phenomena, must also be explored if diagnosis is elusive. Acute disseminated encephalomyelitis may follow a viral illness or vaccine and is important to differentiate from an infectious cause.

19. **What should the initial diagnostic workup include?**
    After careful history and physical examination, neuroimaging is recommended. This can suggest possible causes, dependent on regions of involvement, and may also exclude other possible causes, such as brain abscess. The most sensitive neurologic imaging is magnetic resonance imaging (MRI). If MRI cannot be performed, CT with contrast is the next preferred method. CSF evaluation is also suggested, unless contraindicated. CSF studies should include the usual cell count with differential, protein, and glucose markers. CSF should be sent for PCR evaluation for HSV and enteroviruses. A positive test is helpful, but a negative first test does not exclude infection if the clinical suspicion is high. Repeated testing within 3 to 7 days is suggested. Of note, the presence of hemoglobin can interfere with HSV PCR and cause a false negative result. PCR can also be performed to evaluate for VZV, EBV, and CMV. If acute HIV is considered, one would need to obtain serum quantification of HIV RNA levels, because initial antibody testing may be negative. CSF cultures have not been helpful in elucidating viral causes but should be obtained if concern exists for nonviral causes, including bacteria and fungal organisms. Brain biopsy is usually reserved for those cases in which initial evaluation has been unrevealing and the patient continues to have clinical decline.
    Additional studies should be obtained in the context of a patient's epidemiologic risks. For example, travel to endemic areas could heighten concern for rickettsial disease or flaviviruses. An animal bite, particularly in a developing nation, could increase suspicion for rabies.

20. **What empiric therapy is suggested?**
    In any person with suspected encephalitis, acyclovir should be initiated at 10 mg/kg every 8 hours. If a patient has had travel to regions where rickettsial disease is endemic, doxycycline should also be administered. Given the overlap of encephalitis and meningitis syndromes, in the appropriate clinical context, empiric therapy for bacterial meningitis can be considered. However, the combination of tetracyclines and β-lactam antibiotics should be used cautiously because historical data suggest this combination to have static-cidal inhibition and an increase in mortality when used in patients with pneumococcal meningitis.

ACKNOWLEDGMENT

The authors wish to acknowledge Dr. Christopher D. Huston, MD, for the valuable contributions to the previous edition of this chapter.

KEY POINTS: MENINGITIS AND ENCEPHALITIS IN THE INTENSIVE CARE UNIT

Delayed Lumbar Puncture
When LP is delayed during evaluation for acute bacterial meningitis, the following diagnostic and management actions are suggested:
1. Obtain blood cultures.
2. Initiate antibiotic and steroid therapy.
3. Obtain head CT.
4. Perform LP if safe.

BIBLIOGRAPHY

1. Attia J, Hatala R, Cook DJ, et al. Does this adult patient have acute meningitis? *JAMA.* 1999;282:175-181.
2. Bijlsma MW, Brouwer MC, Kasanmoentalib ES, et al. Community-acquired bacterial meningitis in adults in the Netherlands, 2006-14: a prospective cohort study. *Lancet Infect Dis.* 2016;16:339-347.
3. Durand ML, Calderwood SB, Weber DJ, et al. Acute bacterial meningitis in adults: a review of 493 episodes. *N Engl J Med.* 1993;328:21-28.
4. de Gans J, van de Beek D, European Dexamethasone in Adulthood Bacterial Meningitis Study Investigators. Dexamethasone in adults with bacterial meningitis. *N Engl J Med.* 2002;347:1549-1556.
5. Glimåker M, Johansson B, Grindborg Ö, et al. Adult bacterial meningitis: earlier treatment and improved outcome following guideline revision promoting prompt lumbar puncture. *Clin Infect Dis.* 2015;60:1162-1169.
6. Hasbun R, Abrahams J, Jekel J, et al. Computed tomography of the head before lumbar puncture in adults with suspected meningitis. *N Engl J Med.* 2001;345:1727-1733.
7. Leib SL, Boscacci R, Gratzl O, et al. Predictive value of cerebrospinal fluid (CSF) lactate levels versus CSF/blood glucose ratio for the diagnosis of bacterial meningitis following neurosurgery. *Clin Infect Dis.* 1999;29:69-74.
8. Lepper MH, Dowling HF. Treatment of pneumococcic meningitis with penicillin compared with penicillin plus aureomycin; studies including observations on an apparent antagonism between penicillin and aureomycin. *AMA Arch Intern Med.* 1951;88:489-494.
9. Mayefsky JH, Roghmann KJ. Determination of leukocytosis in traumatic spinal tap specimens. *Am J Med.* 1987;82:1175-1181.
10. McCarthy M, Rosengart A, Schuetz AN, et al. Mold infections of the central nervous system. *N Engl J Med.* 2014;371:150-160.
11. Sawyer MH, Rotbart HA. Viral meningitis and aseptic meningitis syndrome. In: Scheld WM, Whitley RJ, Marra CM, eds. *Infections of the Central Nervous System.* 3rd ed. Philadelphia: Lippincott Williams & Wilkins; 2004:75-93.
12. Tunkel AR, Glaser CA, Bloch KC, et al. Computed tomography of encephalitis: clinical practice guidelines by the Infectious Diseases Society of America. *Clin Infect Dis.* 2008;47:303-327.
13. Tunkel AR, Hartman BJ, Kaplan SL, et al. Practice guidelines for the management of bacterial meningitis. *Clin Infect Dis.* 2004;39:1267-1284.
14. Tunkel AR, Van de Beek D, Scheld WM. Acute meningitis. In: Mandell G, Bennett J, Dolin R, et al., eds. *Mandell, Douglas, and Bennett's Principles and Practice of Infectious Diseases.* 8th ed. Philadelphia: Churchill Livingstone; 2015;1097-1137.
15. van de Beek D, Drake JM, Tunkel AR. Nosocomial bacterial meningitis. *N Engl J Med.* 2010;362:146-154.

CHAPTER 41

DISSEMINATED FUNGAL INFECTIONS

Maged Muhammed, Themistoklis Kourkoumpetis, and Eleftherios Mylonakis

1. **What is the definition of disseminated fungal infection?**
   Disseminated infection is defined as the presence of the same infectious agent in two noncontagious sites. We define disseminated fungal infection as the presence of a fungal pathogen in the blood (fungemia) and/or any other sterile deep-seated structure attributed to hematogenous seeding. This distinguishes disseminated infection from superficial infection, which mostly involves the mucocutaneous structures (i.e., dermatitis, onychitis, stomatitis, esophagitis, and keratitis), as well as from simple colonization, which is the isolation of a fungal pathogen from a nonsterile site without any sign of infection attributable to the specific pathogen. Invasive fungal infection is a different term. Invasive fungal infection is defined in detail according to the European Organization for Research and Treatment of Cancer/Invasive Fungal Infections Cooperative Group and the National Institute of Allergy and Infectious Diseases Mycoses Study Group (EORTC/IFICG and NIAID/MSG).

2. **What are the most clinically important fungal pathogens?**
   Candida spp., *Aspergillus* spp., and *Cryptococcus* spp. are by far the most common fungal pathogens encountered in the hospital setting. Other important fungal infections that are less frequently encountered in the hospital setting are fusariosis, mucormycosis, blastomycosis, coccidioidomycosis, and histoplasmosis.

3. **What is the epidemiology of fungal infections in hospitalized patients?**
   Candida spp. are the leading cause of fungal infection. *Candida* spp. are the fourth most commonly recovered blood culture isolates in the United States. The incidence of candidemia in US hospitals increased from 3.65 cases per 100,000 in 2000 to 5.56 cases per 100,000 in 2005. *Aspergillus* spp., as a cause of fungal infection, have been steadily increasing, specifically in the intensive care unit (ICU) setting as well as among specific populations, such as immunocompromised patients.

4. **Why has the incidence of fungal infection increased so dramatically?**
   With the numbers of immunosuppressed patients increasing through cancer and chemotherapy, transplantation, and HIV infection, as well as with the increased use of vascular and urinary catheters and broad-spectrum antibacterial agents, an alarming increase of deep-seated fungal infections has been seen in clinical practice.

5. **What fungi are responsible for invasive infection in humans?**
   Candida spp. account for the majority of invasive fungal infections (up to 73.4% of all invasive fungal infections in one nationwide study in the United States), followed by *Aspergillus* spp. (13.3 % in the same study), other yeasts (6.2%; mainly *Cryptococcus* spp.), other molds, endemic fungi, and zygomycetes. Interestingly, in some centers, non–*albicans Candida* spp., such as *Candida tropicalis, Candida glabrata,* and *Candida krusei,* account for most *Candida* infections (52.2%).

6. **What are the most important risk factors for disseminated *Candida* infection?**
   - Neutropenia
   - Immunosuppression (hematological malignancy, hematopoietic stem cell transplantation, HIV infection, and immunosuppressive therapy such as steroids and chemotherapeutic regimens)
   - ICU stay
   - Total parenteral nutrition
   - Comorbidities and a high APACHE (Acute Physiology, Age, and Chronic Health Evaluation) score
   - Broad-spectrum antimicrobial agents
   - *Candida* colonization in multiple sites
   - Acute renal failure
   - Hemodialysis

- Central venous catheter (CVC), arterial catheter, or urinary catheters
- General and especially abdominal surgery

7. List the diagnostic criteria for disseminated fungal infection.
   Definitive:
   - Positive blood culture (never mistake a positive fungal blood culture as a contaminant)
   - Fungus cultured from biopsy specimen
   - Histopathology. Burn wound invasion
   - Endophthalmitis
   - Fungus cultured from peritoneal or cerebrospinal fluid

8. How reliable are these diagnostic criteria?
   Blood culture is positive in only 30% to 50% of patients with disseminated fungal infection. Therefore a high index of suspicion must be maintained.
   Clinical manifestation of invasive candidiasis typically ranges from fever not responding to antibiotics to severe sepsis and shock. Presence of skin lesions and eye involvement is highly suggestive of fungal infection.

9. Should asymptomatic candiduria be treated?
   Among most low-risk individuals, no treatment is recommended.
   Among high-risk patients, with high probability of dissemination (such as patients with neutropenia or with urologic manipulations, and low birth weight infants), treatment is similar to the one used for invasive candidiasis.

10. Should a central venous catheter be removed once candidemia is confirmed?
    Clinical practice guidelines for the management of candidiasis indicate that in nonneutropenic patients, CVC removal is strongly recommended (when it is safe) once candidemia is confirmed, and CVC is presumed to be source the of candidemia (Table 41.1). In the neutropenic patient, CVC removal is individualized.

11. When should you suspect disseminated candidiasis?
    Unfortunately, disseminated candidiasis has a wide spectrum of manifestations, from a mild fever to a sepsis syndrome with multiorgan failure and shock. On certain occasions the hematogenous spread of Candida produces visible changes throughout the body, including muscle, skin, and eyes, making a bloodstream process clinically apparent. However, this is not always the case, and that is why there must be a low threshold for the disease, especially in patients with multiple risk factors for candidiasis. As mentioned previously, refractory fever despite broad-spectrum antibiotics with the presence of skin lesion and eye involvement is highly suggestive of fungal infection (*Candida* spp.).

12. If disseminated candidiasis is suspected, where should you look for it?
    The first consideration is to perform blood cultures. Also, Candida detection in the blood can be facilitated with the recently FDA-approved T2MR technology that can definitely help in establishing the diagnosis in a few hours and should be considered, when available, for high-risk patients. Also, ophthalmological exam/dilated funduscopic examinations are important in candidemia to evaluate for eye involvement. Keep in mind that patients with neutropenia may have no symptoms until they regain their normal counts. You can also look for endocarditis; the osteomyelitis; and the liver, spleen, and renal abscesses and candiduria (remember that hepatosplenic candidiasis can present during

Table 41-1. Recommendation on Central Venous Catheter Removal in Patients with Candidemia

VENOUS ACCESS	RECOMMENDATION
Normal venous access	*Remove* CVC, and send tip for culture.
Limited venous access (not safe to remove catheter)	*Exchange* CVC over a guidewire, and perform catheter tip cultures. If catheter is colonized with the same *Candida* sp. that is found in the blood, then it is prudent to remove catheter.

CVC, Central venous catheter.
Modified from www.guidelines.gov and Mermel LA, Allon M, Bouza E, et al. Clinical practice guidelines for the diagnosis and management of intravascular catheter-related infection: 2009 update by the Infectious Diseases Society of America. *Clin Infect Dis.* 2009;49:1-45.

the resolution of neutropenia, can have negative blood cultures, and imaging is needed for diagnosis). Also make sure to perform a biopsy of skin lesions to add extra yield to the diagnosis along with blood cultures.

13. **What is the overall mortality associated with candidemia?**
The overall mortality associated with candidemia is 40% to 68%, with an attributable mortality of 25% to 40%. However, the earlier the initiation of antifungal agents, the better the prognosis. Early targeted antifungal therapy is difficult to accomplish because cultures take at least 24 to 48 hours to yield the species and antifungal resistance profiles. That is why empirical therapy should take into account risk factors for antifungal resistance—that is, prolonged exposure to antifungal agents or long length of hospital stays—and also risk factors for non-*albicans* species intrinsically resistant to fluconazole.

14. **Should antifungal therapy be delayed until blood cultures are positive for fungus?**
Absolutely not! Early therapy means lower mortality. Blood cultures have been found to be only 30% to 50% sensitive. Systemic antifungal therapy should be strongly considered, especially in a patient who is at high risk for disseminated fungal infection, if:
- Fever persists despite antibiotics and negative blood cultures.
- High risk patients presenting with high grade funguria.
- Fungus is cultured from at least two body sites.
- Visceral fungal lesions are confirmed.

15. **What are the major classes of antifungal drugs in use today?**
Antifungal drugs in clinical use today fall into three broad categories: polyene antifungals (amphotericin B), antifungal azoles, and the echinocandins.

16. **So, how do we treat?**
According to recent guidelines, echinocandins are first-line agents for invasive candidiasis. Other agents include azoles, amphotericin B preparations, or combination of amphotericin B with flucytosine. The therapeutic strategy should take into account any previous use of antifungal agents (due to resistant species issues), the epidemiology of fluconazole-resistant or non-*albicans* strains in the community, and any comorbid conditions (which could influence drug pharmacokinetics or worsen coexisting conditions such as renal failure). As noted previously, in general, echinocandins (or amphotericin B preparations) should be preferred over fluconazole, especially among patients with neutropenia and critically ill patients, as well as those known to be exposed to fluconazole-resistant strains. Of course the physician can always switch to fluconazole whenever an antifungal resistance profile becomes available.
Other alternatives are voriconazole, isavuconazole, amphotericin B preparations, posaconazole, and itraconazole, especially in invasive aspergillosis (voriconazole) or when broad coverage (amphotericin B product or isavuconazole, posaconazole) is needed.
Regarding less common infections, for cryptococcosis, amphotericin B preparations in combination with flucytosine are part of the induction therapy. Alternatives are amphotericin B preparations in combination with fluconazole (inferior treatment). High doses of fluconazole alone or in combination with flucytosine can be used if amphotericin B preparations are not available. For mucormycosis, amphotericin B preparations are first-line treatment, while posaconazole or isavuconazole can be used as salvage therapy. For fusariosis, amphotericin B preparations alone or in combination with voriconazole are first-line agents (while posaconazole can be used as salvage therapy). For blastomycosis and most cases of histoplasmosis in the ICU, amphotericin B preparations are first-line agents. Finally, for coccidioidomycosis the first-line agents are itraconazole or fluconazole.

17. **How do amphotericin B and flucytosine work?**
Amphotericin B, a polyene, is fungicidal. It binds irreversibly to ergosterol (but not to cholesterol, the major sterol in mammalian cell membranes), creating a membrane channel that allows leakage of cytosol leading to cell death. Flucytosine is sometimes used in conjunction with amphotericin B and is synergistic against *Cryptococcus* spp. Flucytosine acts on fungal organisms by inhibition of nucleic acid and protein synthesis.

18. **What antifungal azoles are available, and how do they work?**
Fluconazole, itraconazole, voriconazole, and posaconazole, which are triazoles, are fungistatic against *Candida* spp. They inhibit C-14 α-demethylase, a cytochrome P-450–dependent fungal enzyme required for synthesis of ergosterol, the major sterol in the fungal cell membrane. This alters cell membrane fluidity, decreasing nutrient transport, increasing membrane permeability, and inhibiting cell growth and proliferation.

19. **How do echinocandins work, and are they being used?**
The target for echinocandins is the complex of proteins (β [1-3] glucan synthetase) responsible for synthesis of cell wall polysaccharides. Caspofungin, anidulafungin, and micafungin are used in the treatment of candidemia and other forms of disseminated Candida infections.

20. **What advantages does fluconazole offer over amphotericin B in the treatment or prevention of disseminated fungal infections?**
- Fluconazole is available in both intravenous (IV) and oral (PO) forms; patients have been successfully treated with 7 days of IV fluconazole followed by PO if the patient is able. Administration by mouth is both easier and less costly than IV administration.
- Fluconazole is not nephrotoxic and has fewer overall adverse effects than amphotericin B, which can cause renal failure, hypokalemia, fever, and chills.

21. **Are there any limitations to the use of fluconazole?**
Yes. Fluconazole is not active against *Aspergillus* spp. or *C. krusei* and other resistant *Candida* spp. Also, remember that fluconazole may inhibit the P-450 detoxification system and cause hepatotoxicity, increasing phenytoin and cyclosporin levels and potentiating warfarin's anticoagulant effects. But, in general, fluconazole is well tolerated and has fewer overall adverse effects compared to amphotericin B.

22. **What should be done when a Candida infection fails to respond to fluconazole?**
An echinocandin agent or an amphotericin B preparation should be considered. Make sure that the diagnosis is confirmed, the dosage is appropriate, and drug-drug interactions are ruled out (e.g., rifampin decreases fluconazole levels). Keep in mind that resistance can happen to all antifungal agents. For example, *C. krusei* and *C. glabrata* can be resistant azoles, *C. lusitaniae* can be resistant to amphotericin B, and *C. parapsilosis* can have higher minimum inhibitory concentration to echinocandins.

23. **Are there less toxic forms of amphotericin B available?**
Yes. To reduce the toxicity associated with amphotericin B, lipid formulations have been produced. The earliest and most widely studied of these is AmBisome, which in randomized trials has been shown to be safer than amphotericin B, with many fewer side effects. Other lipid-associated, nonliposomal products are amphotericin B lipid complex (Abelcet) and amphotericin B colloidal dispersion (Amphocil). The disadvantage of these alternative forms of amphotericin B is their currently high cost.

24. **Can healthcare providers help prevent the spread of fungal colonization in the intensive care unit?**
Basic prevention measures can be helpful, such as washing hands and wearing gloves when working directly with patients. *Candida* spp. were found on the hands of 33% to 75% of ICU staff in one study.

CONTROVERSY

25. **Does the strategy of presumptive or preemptive treatment of high-risk patients prevent severe candidiasis in critically ill surgical patients?**
The effectiveness of fluconazole in treating overt candidiasis has unfortunately provoked its widespread, unjustified use in patients without neutropenia in the ICU setting. This practice has likely led to an increase in non-*albicans* species, which are resistant to fluconazole. Several studies have shown decreased incidence of colonization and the risk of candidiasis with such empirical treatment but have failed to show decreased mortality in any group other than high-risk patients who have received a transplant. Recent reviews have suggested that targeted preemptive strategy may be of benefit in preventing candidiasis in the ICU. This concept requires further study before continued practice.

ACKNOWLEDGMENT

Dr. Mylonakis wish to acknowledge the research support provided by Astellas Pharma US and T2 Biosystems.

KEY POINTS: DISSEMINATED FUNGAL INFECTIONS

1. Fungal infections are an increasing source of morbidity and mortality in ICUs.
2. Simple colonization does not require treatment.
3. Candida and Aspergillus account for more than 90% of disseminated fungal infections.
4. Do not wait for confirmation by culture to treat, because up to 50% of lethal infections may be culture negative before death.
5. The earlier the administration of antifungal treatment, the lower the mortality.

BIBLIOGRAPHY

1. Azie N, Neofytos D, Pfaller M, et al. The PATH (Prospective Antifungal Therapy) Alliance® registry and invasive fungal infections: update 2012. *Diagn Microbiol Infect Dis.* 2012;73:293-300.
2. Horn DL, Neofytos D, Anaissie EJ, et al. Epidemiology and outcomes of candidemia in 2019 patients: data from the prospective antifungal therapy alliance registry. *Clin Infect Dis.* 2009;48:1695-1703.
3. Kourkoumpetis TK, Velmahos GC, Ziakas PD, et al. The effect of cumulative length of hospital stay on the antifungal resistance of Candida strains isolated from critically ill surgical patients. *Mycopathologia.* 2011;171:85-91.
4. Piarroux R, Grenouillet F, Balvay P, et al. Assessment of preemptive treatment to prevent severe candidiasis in critically ill surgical patients. *Crit Care Med.* 2004;32:2443-2449.
5. Rex JH, Bennett JE, Sugar AM, et al. A randomized trial comparing fluconazole with amphotericin B for the treatment of candidemia in patients without neutropenia. *N Engl J Med.* 1994;331:1325-1330.
6. Richardson MD. Changing patterns and trends in systemic fungal infections. *J Antimicrob Chemother.* 2005;(56 suppl 1):i5-i11.
7. Sipsas NV, Kontoyiannis DP. Invasive fungal infections in patients with cancer in the Intensive Care Unit. *Int J Antimicrob Agents.* 2012;39:464-471.
8. Spanakis EK, Aperis G, Mylonakis E. New agents for the treatment of fungal infections: clinical efficacy and gaps in coverage. *Clin Infect Dis.* 2006;43:1060-1068.
9. Yapar N. Epidemiology and risk factors for invasive candidiasis. *Ther Clin Risk Manag.* 2014;10:95-105.
10. Zilberberg MD, Shorr AF, Kollef MH. Secular trends in candidemia-related hospitalization in the United States, 2000-2005. *Infect Control Hosp Epidemiol.* 2008;29:978-980.

CHAPTER 42

MULTIDRUG-RESISTANT BACTERIA

Krystine Spiess and Christopher Grace

1. What is antibiotic resistance?

   Antibiotic resistance is an increasing threat to patients in the intensive care unit (ICU). If bacteria no longer respond to antibiotics designed to treat them, they are resistant. This happens through various mechanisms detailed as follows. Bacteria have the ability to express more than one mechanism of resistance leading to multidrug resistance (MDR). The generally accepted definition for MDR is bacteria showing resistance to antibiotics in three or more classes. An increasing number of bacteria are now considered extensively drug-resistant (XDR) to most standard regimens. Pandrug-resistant (PDR) species are resistant to all available antibiotic agents. Although there is now a large array of agents with activity against resistant gram-positive organisms, including *Staphylococcus* spp. and *Enterococcus* spp., there are very few options for patients infected with MDR-gram-negative rods. It is feared these options will only become more limited as times goes on. Newer agents to fill the breech are not on the horizon. For the foreseeable future, our best defense against this growing menace will be the judicious use of our current limited resources.

2. How common is multidrug-resistant bacterial resistance?

   Gram-positive pathogens make up about 41% of healthcare-associated infections (HAI), but only about 25% of ventilator-acquired pneumonia (VAP). Aerobic GNRs make up about 41% of HAI, but 54% of VAP. The most common VAP pathogens have been *Staphylococcus aureus, Pseudomonas aeruginosa*, and *Klebsiella* spp. Nearly half of *S. aureus* have been methicillin resistant (methicillin-resistant *S. aureus* [MRSA]), and more than 80% of *Enterococci* have been vancomycin resistant *Enterococci* (VRE). *P. aeruginosa, Klebsiella* spp., *Escherichia coli*, and *Acinetobacter* spp. are often MDR species.

3. Why is antibiotic resistance important?

   The associated morbidity and mortality and costs are high. Centers for Disease Control and Prevention (CDC) data indicate that in the United States alone more than 2 million infections and 23,000 deaths are caused every year by resistant bacteria. Bacteria that are resistant to antibiotics are difficult to treat and oftentimes require utilization of more costly or more toxic treatment options, if any treatment is available at all. In most cases, antibiotic resistant infections require extended hospitalizations, resulting in a significant economic burden. The total costs are difficult to calculate, but estimates range as high as $20 billion in excess direct costs per year, with additional cost to society for lost productivity as high as $35 billion per year. Additional costs of $16,450 per patient and 9.7 days of hospitalization have been demonstrated in patients with resistant *E. coli* and *Klebsiella* spp.

4. How does resistance begin and spread among bacteria?

   Over many millennia, bacteria have evolved chemical defenses (antibiotics) to fight off other bacteria in their environment. In turn, bacteria have developed antibiotic resistance mechanisms to block or neutralize these antibiotics, thus rendering them intrinsically resistant to attack. Bacteria develop resistance to antibiotics by point mutations in the bacterial genome. Bacteria may also acquire resistance genes from other bacteria via transfer of plasmids (small circular extrachromosomal DNA) or transposons (small DNA segments inserted into the bacterial genome) or from bacteriophages (viruses carrying resistance genes that infect bacteria). Often this genetic transfer may carry genes causing resistance to multiple classes of antibiotics. Antibacterial resistance gives the bacteria a survival advantage, thus allowing it to replicate and pass on the resistance gene(s). Antibiotics help select out those resistant bacteria, thus driving the evolution of antibiotic resistance in ICU patients.

5. How do antibiotics work?

   See Fig. 42.1. For antibiotics (shown in italics) to work, they must first pass through the outer membrane porin channel (in gram-negative bacteria only). They must then interact with the bacterial

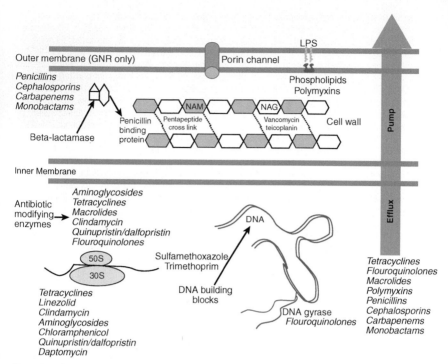

Figure 42-1. Bacterial structure and sites of activity of antibiotics. The diagram shows the inner and outer cell membrane and cytoplasm of a gram-negative bacteria. The cell wall is made up of repeating carbohydrate units of N-acetylmuraminc acid (NAM) and N-acetyl glucosamine (NAG). These are cross-linked by pentapeptide side chains by enzymatic penicillin binding proteins. Cell membranes are composed of phospholipids and lipopolysaccharides (LPS). Bacterial protein synthesis is accomplished at the 50S and 30S ribosomal units. The prokaryotic DNA is not enclosed in a nucleus. Efflux pumps can remove antibiotics from the bacterial cytoplasm. Antibiotics are shown in italics. Sites of bacterial resistance are shown in bold. *GNR*, Gram-negative rod.

target. Beta-lactam antibiotics (penicillins, cephalosporins, carbapenems, monobactams) bind to the bacterial penicillin binding proteins (PBP), which enzymatically cross-link the pentapeptide side chain, stabilizing the cell wall. In the case of vancomycin and teicoplanin, they bind to and inactivate the pentapeptide side chain. Polymyxins such as colistin interfere with outer membrane phospholipids, disrupting the membrane. The antibiotic target may also be in the cytoplasm of the bacteria. Tetracyclines, linezolid, clindamycin, aminoglycosides, chloramphenicol, and quinupristin/dalfopristin interfere with protein synthesis at the 50S or 30S ribosomal level. Sulfonamides and trimethoprim block DNA synthesis by blocking folate metabolism. DNA synthesis can also be blocked by fluoroquinolones, which interfere with the DNA gyrase coiling and uncoiling of the DNA.

6. What are the mechanisms for the development of antibiotic-resistant bacteria?
Please see Fig. 42.1. Bacteria have evolved multiple resistance mechanisms that diminish or eliminate the activity of the antibiotic.
- Porin channel—Reduction in the number or size of porin channels by *Pseudomonas, Acinetobacter,* and *Enterobacteriaceae* can reduce entry of antibiotics such as the carbapenems, cephalosporins, aminoglycosides, and fluoroquinolones.
- Alteration of the outer membrane—Mutations in the lipid outer membrane will stop the binding of polymyxins to the outer membrane, rendering the organism resistant.
- Beta-lactamase—Beta-lactamases are enzymes that open the amide bond of the beta-lactam antibiotic, rendering it inactive. There are currently more than 1000 unique beta-lactamase enzymes. The genes for these enzymes may be on the bacterial chromosome or transferable plasmids, allowing this resistance to be spread among bacterial species. Initially beta-lactamases had activity limited to penicillins. Extended spectrum beta-lactamases (ESBL) have emerged that have the

ability to inactivate many generations of cephalosporins and penicillins. AmpC an inducible beta-lactamase, can be found in Enterobacter, indole-positive Proteus, Morganella, Serratia, Providencia, Acinetobacter, Citrobacter, and rarely Pseudomonas. It is capable of inactivating almost all of the current cephalosporins. AmpC cephalosporinases are beta-lactamases that confer resistance to cephalosporin antibiotics by *Enterobacter, Nitrobacteria, Morganella, Serratia,* and *P. aeruginosa.* In contrast to ESBL enzymes, they are most often chromosomally encoded and not transferable. Paradoxically, they are inducible by third-generation cephalosporins (although they may look susceptible to third-generation cephalosporins on susceptibility testing, giving a patient one of these drugs may actually induce resistance while on therapy). Carbapenem-resistant Enterobacteriaceae (CRE) are particularly alarming. They are primarily transmitted in health care settings with mortality rates of 40% to 50%. Resistance is mediated through the production of carbapenemase. Carbapenemases, such as the *Klebsiella pneumoniae* carbapenemase (KPC) inactivate carbapenem antibiotics such as imipenem, meropenem, and ertapenem. These enzymes can inactivate all classes of beta-lactam antibiotics and are resistant to beta-lactamase inhibitors. Organisms found to carry these MDR genes include *P. aeruginosa, Acinetobacter, Stenotrophomonas, Klebsiella spp., Serratia, Enterobacter, E. coli,* and *Citrobacter.* Metallo-β-lactamase-1 (NDM-1), first isolated in 2009 in New Delhi, India, are able to cause resistance to all beta-lactam antibiotics except aztreonam. Now spreading worldwide, the genes for these enzymes are often part of larger gene cassettes that house resistance to other antibiotic classes. They are carried on plasmids, thus allowing transfer among bacteria. These beta-lactamases are rendering many *Pseudomonas, Acinetobacter,* and *Enterobacteriaceae* species increasingly resistant.

- Efflux pumps—Removal of the antibiotic from the bacterial cytoplasm by efflux pumps is a widespread and common mechanism of MDR. Beta-lactams, tetracyclines, macrolides, fluoroquinolones, and polymyxins can be removed by *Pseudomonas, Stenotrophomonas, Enterobacteriaceae, Staphylococci,* and *Streptococci.* The efflux pump genes can be carried by chromosomes or plasmids.
- Overproduction of antibiotic target—Sulfonamides and trimethoprim interfere with DNA synthesis by blocking folate metabolism. Bacteria can overcome this interference by overproducing dihydropteroate synthetase (DHPS) and dihydrofolate reductase (DHFR), key enzymes needed for folate synthesis.
- Enzymatic inactivation of the antibiotic—Aminoglycosides, tetracyclines, macrolides, clindamycin, fluoroquinolones, and quinupristin/dalfopristin can be inactivated by bacterial enzymes.
- Alteration of antibiotic target:
  - Ribosomes—Altered ribosomal binding sites can render aminoglycosides, macrolides, tetracyclines, clindamycin, linezolid, chloramphenicol, and quinupristin/dalfopristin inactive. These altered genes have been found in both gram-negative and gram-positive bacteria.
  - Cell wall—Bacteria can alter the terminal amino acids of the pentapeptide cross-link between layers of peptidoglycan cell wall. This can cause resistance by *Enterococci* to vancomycin and teicoplanin, leading to the emergence of VRE. *Staphylococci* have also acquired some of these genes (Van A, B, C), leading to vancomycin-intermediate *S. aureus* (VISA) and rarely, so far, vancomycin-resistant *S. aureus* (VRSA).
  - PBP—Beta-lactam antibiotics work by binding to PBP, thus blocking cell wall synthesis. Mutations in the Staphylococcal *mec* gene produce an altered PBP. Although referred to as MRSA, these bacteria are resistant to all the beta-lactam antibiotics, except the newer cephalosporin, ceftaroline fosamil.
  - DNA gyrase—Theses enzymes are needed during bacterial DNA uncoiling involved in bacterial cell division and DNA repair. Flouroquinolones interfere with DNA gyrase interfering with these vital processes. DNA gyrase mutations in *S. aureus, Enterobacteriaceae,* and *Pseudomonas,* along with bacterial proteins that bind to the DNA, block fluoroquinolone activity.
- Auxotrophs—Bacteria can develop mutant growth requirements (e.g., folate from the environment) that allow it to bypass the target of the antibiotic.
- Multiple mechanisms—Bacteria may acquire numerous resistance mechanisms that render it resistant to multiple classes of antibiotics (MDR). This can occur by accumulation of point mutations or acquisition of resistance genes from plasmids and transposons from other bacteria or bacteriophages that are able house multiple resistance genes.

7. What puts people at risk for multidrug-resistance infection?
Risk factors for acquiring resistant bacteria include prior and recent antibiotic use, hospitalization, admission to an ICU, residence in a long-term acute care facility or nursing home, presence of an indwelling medical device, chronic wounds, poor functional status, advanced age, transplant or other immune suppression, and travel to or receipt of healthcare in an endemic area.

8. What are the most common multidrug-resistant pathogens seen in the intensive care unit?
   - Gram-positive organisms—MRSA and VRE. MRSA is resistant to all penicillins and cephalosporins (except ceftaroline fosamil). MRSA has been recognized as a nosocomial pathogen for years but is now frequently acquired in the community as well. The scope of infection is wide and includes skin and soft tissue infections, blood-stream/endovascular and line infections, osteomyelitis, and pneumonia. Without the presence of foreign material (Foley catheter, recurrent I/O catheter, nephrostomy tubes), *S. aureus* should not be seen in the urine. The presence of this organism in the urine should always raise suspicion for bacteremia with hematogenous seeding of the urinary tract. VRE have become increasingly common in recent years. They are frequently found as part of the bowel flora and often colonize the urine. They can cause serious infections with a spectrum similar to those seen with *S. aureus*. Other concerning resistant gram-positive organisms seen in the ICU include penicillin and fluoroquinolone-resistant *S. pneumoniae,* erythromycin-resistant Group A Streptococcus, and clindamycin-resistant Group B Streptococcus.
   - Gram-negative organisms—A great number of resistant gram-negative infections are encountered in the ICU, including MDR-*Enterobacteriaceae* (*E. coli, Klebsiella* spp., *Enterobacter, Serratia, Proteus* spp.), *Acinetobacter* spp., *Stenotrophomonas maltophilia* and resistant *Pseudomonas* species. These pathogens can cause urinary tract infections, pneumonia, wound infections, osteomyelitis, and bloodstream/line infections. *Enterobacteriaceae* have developed extensive resistance, including ESBL and carbapenemases. *Acinetobacter* spp. have multiple beta-lactamases, loss of outer membrane porin channels, and efflux pumps, resulting in resistance to most beta-lactams, quinolones and aminoglycosides. *S. maltophilia* is another inherently highly resistant organism seen in patients with extensive broad-spectrum antibiotic exposure.

9. What antibiotic regimens are available to treat multidrug-resistance infections in the intensive care unit?
   Antibiotics with activities against resistant gram-positive and gram-negative bacteria are summarized in Table 42.1.

10. Why have new antibiotics not been developed for multidrug-resistant GNR?
   Antibiotic development is time-consuming and expensive. It can take 12 to 15 years and cost $5 billion to bring a drug from bench to market. Only about 10% to 20% of drugs in development make it to market. Further blocking the pipeline of new agents are high failure rates and toxicities discovered during clinical trials and regulatory complexity. Even if an antibiotic makes it to market, its usage may be discouraged or restricted and the duration of use is limited. Because of these barriers, many pharmaceutical companies are no longer developing new antibiotics. Over the past several decades, the number of new antibiotics making it to market has dropped precipitously, especially those for MDR gram negatives.

11. How can one control and reduce the emergence of multidrug-resistant bacteria?
   Since the emergence of MDR bacteria is related to selective antibiotic pressure, the best means of reducing or controlling MDR bacteria is by limiting antimicrobial exposure through hospital-based antimicrobial stewardship programs. Although challenging in the ICU setting because of the critical nature of illness, antibiotic usage can be curtailed by careful differentiation of colonization from true infection and narrowing of "broad spectrum" empiricism once cultures are available. Minimizing the duration of antimicrobial use will also decrease exposure. Guidance developed by the Infectious Diseases Society of America (IDSA) and the American Thoracic Society (ATS) suggests 5 days of an active antibiotic for community-acquired pneumonia and 7 days for uncomplicated hospital or VAP is adequate. Limitation of excess culturing can also avoid repeated sampling of universally positive cultures from endotracheal tubes and urinary catheters. Strict use of infection control measures can also limit healthcare worker transfer of resistant bacteria from one patient to another. This is especially true for hand-washing prior to and after each patient contact. Patients with MDR bacteria (gram-positive cocci [GPC] and gram-negative rod [GNR]) should be placed in a private room and contact precautions (gown and gloves) practiced by all those entering the room. On a societal level, removing antibiotics from animal feed products will also lessen antibiotic pressure and selection of resistant strains.

Table 42-1. Antibiotic Options for Resistant Gram-Positive and Gram-Negative Bacteria

MRSA*	VRE†	ESBL	CRE	ACINETOBACTER Spp.	PSEUDOMONAS	STENOTROPHOMONAS MALTOPHILA
Vancomycin	Daptomycin‡	Cefoxitin Cefotetan	Combination Therapy: Polymyxin B or E (Colistin) AND Meropenem Tigecycline Ceftazidime-avibactam Aztreonam††	Cefepime	Ceftazidime Cefepime	Trimethoprim-Sulfamethoxazole
Daptomycin‡	Linezolid Tidezolid	Clavulanate Tazobactam	Double carbapenem: high dose with extended infusion	Sulbactam	Piperacillin-tazobactam	Piperacillin-tazobactam
Linezolid Tidezolid	Tetracyclines	Imipenem Meropenem Doripenem Ertapenem	Complicated UTI or intra-abdominal infection: Ceftolozane-tazobactam	Imipenem Meropenem Doripenem	Ciprofloxacin Levofloxacin	Moxifloxacin
Trimethoprim-Sulfamethoxazole	Quinupristin/Dalfopristin§	Complicated UTI or intra-abdominal infection: Ceftazidime-avibactam Ceftolozane-tazobactam	Uncomplicated UTI: Fosfomycin‡‡	Polymyxin B Polymyxin E (Colistin)	Imipenem Meropenem Doripenem	Tigecycline Minocycline
Clindamycin	Ciprofloxacin**	—	—	Minocycline Tigecycline	Aztreonam	Polymyxin B Polymyxin E (Colistin)
Tetracyclines	Uncomplicated UTI: Fosfomycin Nitrofurantoin	—	—	—	Tobramycin Gentamicin Amikacin	—
Quinupristin/dalfopristin	—	—	—	—	Polymyxin B Polymyxin E (Colistin)	—

Ceftaroline fosamil	—	—	—	—	Complicated UTI or intra-abdominal infection: Ceftazidime-Avibactam Ceftolozane-tazobactam
Oritavancin Dalbavancin Telavancin	—	—	—	—	—

*MRSA: MRSA isolates with a vancomycin MIC greater than or equal to 2 ug/mL are increasingly frequent. Although an MIC of two is considered susceptible by established breakpoints, if seen, it should encourage providers to treat serious infection with an alternative to vancomycin.

†VRE: Occasionally susceptibility to ampicillin is retained and it can be used at high doses.

‡Daptomycin: Should not be used for pulmonary infections.

††Aztreonam should not be used to treat carbapenem-resistant enterobacteriaceae (CRE) infections due to Class A carbapenemase (KPCs) but is often an acceptable component of combination therapy in disease due to class B (metallo-beta-lactamases) and class D carbapenemases.

§Quinupristin/Dalfopristin for treatment of VRE—only active against *Enterococcus faecium*.

‡‡Monotherapy with fosfomycin should never be attempted in critically ill patients. Even in the case of uncomplicated UTI, combination therapy may be warranted due to potential for emerging resistance.

**Ciprofloxacin for treatment of VRE—not acceptable for treatment of systemic infection.

ESBL, Extended spectrum beta-lactamases; *MRSA*, methicillin-resistant *Staphylococcus aureus*; *UTI*, urinary tract infection; *VRE*, vancomycin resistant *Enterococci*.

KEY POINTS: MULTIDRUG-RESISTANT BACTERIA

1. GNR and GPC MDR bacteria are becoming an increasingly greater problem.
2. Increasing bacterial resistance is caused by excessive antibiotic use both by physicians and in animal feeds.
3. Before initiating antibiotic therapy, it is vital to differentiate between colonization and infection.
4. Due to the lack of new agents with activity against MDR-GNRs, older drugs such as colistin will be required more often.
5. The key to reducing the emergence of MDR is to use fewer antibiotics through antimicrobial stewardship programs.

BIBLIOGRAPHY

1. Sievert DM, Ricks P, Edwards JR, et al. Antimicrobial-resistant pathogens associated with healthcare-associated infections: Summary of Data Reported to the National Healthcare Safety Network at the Centers for Disease Control and Prevention, 2009–2010. *Infect Control Hosp Epidemiol.* 2013;34(1):1-14.
2. Sader HS, Farrell DJ, Flamm RK, et al. Antimicrobial susceptibility of Gram-negative organisms isolated from patients hospitalized in intensive care units in United States and European Hospitals (2009–2011). *Diagn Microbiol Infect Dis.* 2014;78:443-448.
3. Blair JM, Webber MA, Baylay AJ, et al. Molecular mechanisms of antibiotic resistance. *Nat Rev Microbiol.* 2015;13: 42-51.
4. Vasoo S, Barreto JN, Tosh PK. Emerging issues in gram-negative bacterial resistance: an update for the practicing clinician. *Mayo Clin Proc.* 2015;90(3):395-403.
5. Rossolini GM, Arena F, Pecile P, et al. Update on the antibiotic resistance crisis. *Curr Opin Pharmacol.* 2014;18:56-60.
6. Opal SM, Pop-Vicas A. Molecular mechanisms of antibiotic resistance in bacteria. In: Bennett JE, Dolin R, Blaser MJ, eds. *Principles and Practice of Infectious Diseases.* 8th ed. 2015:235-251.
7. Roberts RR, Hota B, Ahmad I, et al. Hospital and societal costs of antimicrobial-resistant infections in a Chicago teaching hospital: implications for antibiotic stewardship. *Clin Infect Dis.* 2009;49(8):1175-1184.
8. Barlam TF, Cosgrove SE, Abbo LM, et al. Implementing an Antibiotic Stewardship Program: Guidelines by the Infectious Diseases Society of America and the Society for Healthcare Epidemiology of America. *Clin Infect Dis.* 2016;62(10): e51-e77.

CHAPTER 43

SKIN AND SOFT TISSUE INFECTIONS

Erica S. Shenoy and David C. Hooper

GENERAL PRINCIPLES

1. If patients with skin or soft tissue infection are seen with signs of systemic toxicity, what laboratory studies should be undertaken?
   Blood cultures, cultures of drainage from skin infection site, complete blood cell count with differential, serum creatinine, bicarbonate, creatine phosphokinase, glucose, albumin, and calcium levels should be obtained (see Table 43.1).

2. What are clinical signs of potential severe deep tissue infection?
   - Pain disproportionate to physical findings
   - Skin findings: violaceous bullae, ecchymoses, cutaneous hemorrhage, sloughing, anesthesia
   - Rapid progression
   - Gas in tissue
   - Edema beyond the margin of erythema
   - Signs and symptoms of systemic involvement

Table 43-1. Evaluation of Cellulitis and Soft Tissue Infections

	STUDY	FINDING	COMMENTS
Microbiology	Culture and sensitivity	Identification of causative organism and antimicrobial susceptibility data to guide therapeutic choices	When possible, obtain before administration of antibiotics
Laboratory	CBC with differential	Leukocytosis with left shift suggests deep-seated or systemic infection Thrombocytopenia suggests bacteremia, TSS, or gas gangrene	*Clostridium sordellii*: associated with leukemoid reaction and hemoconcentration *C. perfringens*: associated with low hematocrit, elevated LDH, and intravascular hemolysis
	Serum creatinine	Elevation	Seen in group A streptococcal or clostridial myonecrosis, TSS
	Serum CPK	Elevation	Seen in rhabdomyolysis, clostridial or streptococcal myonecrosis, or necrotizing fasciitis
	Serum calcium	Decreased	Seen in staphylococcal or streptococcal TSS or necrotizing fasciitis
Radiology	CT or MRI	Localization of infections and extent of involvement	Useful in early diagnosis of necrotizing infections
	Ultrasound	Necrotizing fasciitis caused by group A streptococcus may reveal thickening of the fascia	CT preferred over ultrasound in adults to define extent of disease

CBC, Complete blood cell count; *CPK*, creatinine phosphokinase; *CT*, computed tomography; *LDH*, lactate dehydrogenase; *MRI*, magnetic resonance imaging; *TSS*, toxic shock syndrome.

Modified from Stephens DL, Fron LL. In the clinic: cellulitis and soft-tissue infections. *Ann Intern Med.* 2009; 150:ITC1–16.

Fig. 43.1 outlines the approach to management of nonpurulent and purulent skin and soft tissue infections (SSTIs).

3. Which common causative organisms have shown emerging antibiotic resistance?
   - *Staphylococcus aureus* (methicillin resistance with resistance to all β-lactams except ceftaroline)—Assume resistance because of high prevalence of methicillin-resistant *S. aureus* (MRSA), both community- and hospital-acquired.
   - *Streptococcus pyogenes* (erythromycin resistance)—Resistance to macrolides is increasing. In the United States, approximately 7% of isolates are resistant to macrolides, although rates as high as 48% have been reported in specific populations. In Europe, macrolide resistance is reported in the 2% to 32% range. The majority of isolates remain susceptible to clindamycin, and all are susceptible to penicillin.

CELLULITIS

4. What are the common presentation patterns of cellulitis caused by *Staphylococcus aureus* or *Streptococcus pyogenes*?
   - *S. aureus*—Cellulitis with associated furuncles, carbuncles, or subcutaneous abscesses; *S. aureus* infection is often associated with purulence.
   - *S. pyogenes*—Cellulitis that is more diffuse, can spread rapidly, and is less likely to have purulence.

5. What distinguishes impetigo from cellulitis?
   Impetigo is characterized by discrete purulent lesions, usually on the face, arms, and legs. Bullous and nonbullous forms exist. Whereas impetigo is superficial, cellulitis involves the deep dermis and subcutaneous fat.

6. Lack of response to initial therapy could signify what?
   - If a patient does not respond to initial therapy, consider the possibility of resistant strains, atypical organisms, deeper processes such as necrotizing fasciitis or abscess (which may require surgical intervention), as well as underlying conditions such as diabetes, chronic venous insufficiency, or lymphedema (which may slow the clinical response to antimicrobial therapy). Recurrences of cellulitis at the same site may also be slower to respond.
   - Timely administration of appropriate antibiotic therapy is essential. One study found that each hour of delay between documented hypotension and administration of antibiotics was associated with an average decrease in survival of 7.6% across all sources of infection; subgroup analysis for patients with SSTIs demonstrated a significant increase in the adjusted odds ratio of death. This same study found that time to initiation of effective antimicrobial therapy was the strongest predictor of hospital survival. Despite the impact of delayed therapy, the study found that the median time to effective therapy was 6 hours.

7. What risk factors predispose individuals to development of cellulitis?
   - Obesity
   - Previous episodes of cellulitis in the same location (may result in damage to lymphatics)
   - Toe-web abnormalities (i.e., maceration, tinea pedis)
   - Breach in skin barrier, such as ulcers, trauma, fungal infection, eczema
   - Surgical procedures that affect lymphatic drainage such as radical mastectomy with lymph node dissection or coronary artery bypass graft for which the saphenous vein has been harvested
   - Chronic medical conditions such as diabetes, arterial insufficiency, chronic venous insufficiency, chronic renal disease, neutropenia, cirrhosis, hypogammaglobulinemia

8. What organisms are associated with cellulitis in:
   - Cat or dog bites? *Pasteurella multocida, Capnocytophaga canimorsus*
   - Fresh water exposure? *Aeromonas hydrophila*
   - Saltwater exposure? *Vibrio vulnificus* and other vibrios
   - Exposure to fish farming and aquaculture? *Streptococcus iniae*
   - Exposure to meatpacking or shellfish? *Erysipelothrix rhusiopathiae*
   - Preorbital cellulitis in children? *Haemophilus influenzae*
   - Hosts with deficiencies in cell-mediated immunity? *Cryptococcus neoformans*
   - Combat trauma patient? *Acinetobacter baumannii* or other gram-negative bacteria
     See Table 43.2.

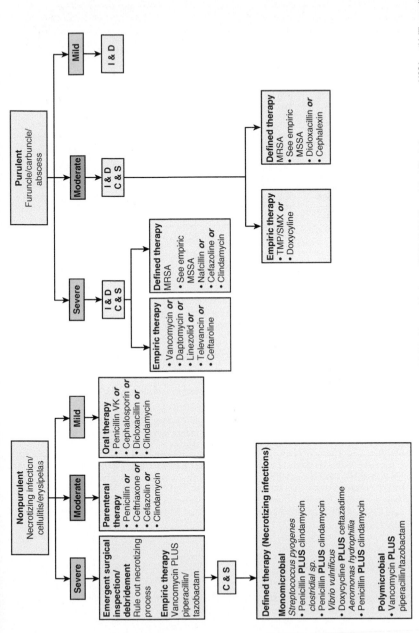

Figure 43-1. Management of skin and soft tissue infections. *C & S*, culture and sensitivity; *I & D*, incision and drainage; *MRSA*, Methicillin-resistant *Staphylococcus aureus*; *MSSA*, methicillin-sensitive *S. aureus*; *Penicillin VK*, Penicillin V-potassium; *SMX*, sulfamethoxazole; *TMP*, trimethoprim.

Table 43-2. Antimicrobial Therapy for Methicillin-sensitive *Staphylococcus aureus* and Methicillin-resistant *Staphylococcus aureus* Skin and Soft Tissue Infections

ORGANISM	ANTIBIOTIC	ADULT DOSING	PEDIATRIC DOSING
MSSA	Nafcillin or oxacillin	1–2 g IV every 4 h	100–150 mg/kg per day IV in four divided doses
	Cefazolin	1 g IV every 8 h	50 mg/kg per day in three divided doses
	Clindamycin	600 mg IV every 8 h or 300–450 mg PO every 6 h	25–40 mg/kg per day IV in three divided doses or 25–30 mg/kg per day PO in three divided doses
	Dicloxacillin	500 mg PO every 6 h	25 mg/kg per day PO in four divided doses
	Cephalexin	500 mg PO every 6 h	25 mg/kg per day PO in four divided doses
	Doxycycline, minocycline	100 mg PO every 12 h	Not recommended in children <8 years old
	TMP-SMX	1 or 2 DS tabs PO every 12 h	8–12 mg/kg (based on TMP component) IV in four divided doses or PO in two divided doses
MRSA	Vancomycin	30 mg/kg IV in two divided doses	40 mg/kg per day IV in four divided doses
	Linezolid	600 mg IV or PO every 12 h	10 mg/kg IV or PO every 12 h
	Clindamycin	600 mg IV every 8 h or 300–450 mg PO every 6 h	25–40 mg/kg per day IV in three divided doses or 30–40 mg/kg per day PO in three divided doses
	Daptomycin	4 mg/kg IV every 24 h	N/A
	Ceftaroline	600 mg IV every 12 h	N/A
	Doxycycline, minocycline	100 mg PO every 12 h	Not recommended in children <8 years old
	TMP-SMX	1 or 2 DS tabs PO every 12 h	8–12 mg/kg (based on TMP component) IV in four divided doses or PO in two divided doses

Note that doses may need to be adjusted for any abnormalities of renal function.

DS, Double strength; *IV*, intravenous; *MRSA*, methicillin-resistant *Staphylococcus aureus*; MSSA, methicillin-sensitive *Staphylococcus aureus*; *N/A*, not applicable; *PO*, oral; *TMP-SMZ*, trimethoprim/sulfamethoxazole.

Modified from Stevens DL, Bisno AL, Chambers HF, et al. Practice guidelines for the diagnosis and management of skin and soft tissue infections: 2014 Update by the Infectious Diseases Society of America. *Clin Infect Dis.* 2014;59(2):147–159.

CUTANEOUS ABSCESSES

9. How are abscesses managed?
   - Large abscesses should be incised and drained, with careful attention to the potential for loculated cavities (and the disruption of these cavities through probing of the pus pocket).
   - Once drained, the lesion can be left packed or unpacked, depending on its extent.
   - In the absence of multiple lesions, gangrene, impaired host defenses, fever, or systemic signs and symptoms of infection, once a cutaneous abscess is drained, systemic antimicrobial therapy may not be needed. A recent study found that in settings of high MRSA prevalence (~45%), patients treated with incision and drainage of uncomplicated abscess in addition to 7-day course of trimethoprim/sulfamethoxazole had higher cure rates.

10. What are the common organisms implicated in cutaneous abscesses?
    - Monomicrobial infection with *S. aureus* occurs in approximately 55% of cases.
    - Consider polymicrobial infection when there are predisposing conditions (i.e., diabetes mellitus, trauma resulting in a *dirty wound*) or based on the location of the abscess (i.e., perianal).

NECROTIZING SKIN AND SOFT TISSUE INFECTIONS

11. Is necrotizing fasciitis usually monomicrobial or polymicrobial?
    - Necrotizing fasciitis is both monomicrobial and polymicrobial. Organisms seen in monomicrobial infection include *S. pyogenes, V. vulnificus, A. hydrophila, S. aureus,* and anaerobic streptococci. In polymicrobial infections, an average of five different organisms can be cultured. Surgical procedures involving the intestinal tract, penetrating abdominal trauma, decubitus ulcer, perianal abscesses, infection at the site of injection drug use, and spread for a Bartholin abscess are associated with polymicrobial necrotizing fasciitis.
    - Necrotizing fasciitis is categorized as type I (usually mixed aerobic and anaerobic) and type II (usually caused by group A *Streptococcus* but also *S. aureus*).
    - *Vibrio* infections have been associated with saltwater exposures and ingestion of raw shellfish. Individuals with hepatic dysfunction are at greater risk for *Vibrio* infection.

12. Which organisms cause gas gangrene?
    - Clostridial gas gangrene, or myonecrosis, is caused by *Clostridium perfringens, Clostridium septicum, Clostridium histolyticum,* and *Clostridium novyi.*
    - Predisposing factors include penetrating trauma, crush injuries, and intravenous (IV) drug abuse.
    - *C. perfringens* is the most common cause of trauma-related gas gangrene. Symptoms usually develop within 24 hours of infection. *C. septicum* is the most common cause of spontaneous gas gangrene and is associated with neutropenia and gastrointestinal malignancies.
    - Antimicrobial therapy includes clindamycin and penicillin because 5% of strains of *C. perfringens* are clindamycin-resistant.
    - Rapid surgical débridement and excision of infected muscle is the most important determinant of outcome.

13. What is the appropriate antimicrobial therapy for necrotizing skin and soft tissue infections?
    - For mixed infection, ampicillin-sulbactam plus clindamycin plus ciprofloxacin or a third-generation cephalosporin. For patients with severe allergies to penicillin, clindamycin or metronidazole plus an aminoglycoside or fluoroquinolone can be substituted.
    - For streptococcal infections, including streptococcal toxic shock syndrome (TSS), treat with penicillin plus clindamycin. In patients with severe allergies to penicillin, vancomycin, linezolid, daptomycin, or quinupristin-dalfopristin can be substituted for penicillin.
    - The value of IV immunoglobulin (IVIG) in these circumstances has yet to be fully defined. One study showed no improved survival in patients with TSS randomly assigned to receive IVIG, whereas a retrospective cohort analysis did demonstrate improved outcomes. A more recent study in a pediatric population found no difference in outcomes for patients treated for TSS with and without IVIG.
    - For *S. aureus* infections, nafcillin, oxacillin, or cefazolin are drugs of choice for susceptible strains. If concern exists for methicillin resistance, vancomycin or clindamycin are options.

14. How should patients with allergies to penicillins and cephalosporins be managed?
    - The vast majority of patients with reported allergy to penicillin are not truly allergic and could tolerate a penicillin or cephalosporin. Based on a detailed allergy history, patients can be evaluated either by test dose (graded challenge), or penicillin skin testing, based on the nature of their prior reported reaction to penicillin or related agents. For example, patients with a history of Type I (IgE mediated) hypersensitivity reactions can receive third or fourth generation cephalosporins using a test dose procedure; however, if a penicillin, first-, or second-generation cephalosporin is needed, consultation with allergy specialists is recommended. Patients with a history of Type II to IV hypersensitivity reactions should avoid the use of penicillins or cephalosporins, and the involvement of allergy specialists is required, should either be clinically indicated in the setting of serious infection.

INFECTIONS AFTER ANIMAL BITES

15. Which organisms are commonly isolated after cat bites?
    Pasteurella spp., most commonly, but these infections are usually polymicrobial. Common organisms found in the oral cavity of cats include *Bartonella henselae, Moraxella* spp., staphylococci, streptococci,

Table 43-3. Major Pathogens Isolated From Cat and Dog Bites

	AEROBES	ANAEROBES
Cat bites	*Pasteurella* spp., *Streptococcus* spp., *Staphylococcus* spp., *Moraxella* spp.	*Fusobacterium* spp., *Bacteroides* spp., *Porphyromonas* spp.
Dog bites	*Pasteurella* spp., *Streptococcus* spp., *Staphylococcus* spp., *Neisseria* spp.	*Fusobacterium* spp., *Bacteroides* spp., *Porphyromonas* spp., *Prevotella* spp., *Capnocytophaga* spp.

Note: Most infections include a mix of aerobes and anaerobes.
From Oehler RL, Velez AP, Mizrachi M, et al. Bite-related and septic syndromes caused by cats and dogs. *Lancet Infect Dis.* 2009;9:439–447.

and anaerobes. Cats with outdoor exposure can additionally carry *Leptospira, Listeria,* and *Nocardia* spp. as well as *Francisella tularensis, Streptobacillus moniliformis, E. rhusiopathiae,* and *Coxiella burnetii,* but these organisms are uncommon causes of cat-bite infections (see Table 43.3).

16. **Which organisms are commonly isolated after dog bites?**
As in cat bites, *Pasteurella* spp. are most common, followed by staphylococci, streptococci, *Moraxella,* corynebacteria, *Neisseria,* and *Capnocytophaga canimorsus.*

17. **Which antibiotics should be administered after a cat or dog bite?**
Oral amoxicillin-clavulanate, with activity against both *Pasturella* and anaerobes, is a first choice; IV ampicillin-sulbactam or ertapenem can be chosen if IV therapy is required. In cases of invasive disease in patients with penicillin allergies, aztreonam has been reported to be successful.

18. **What are the infectious complications of animal bite wounds?**
    • Septic arthritis
    • Osteomyelitis
    • Abscess
    • Tendinitis
    • Bacteremia

19. **What are other considerations after animal bite wounds?**
    • Rabies prophylaxis—in the case of feral, wild, or unvaccinated domestic animal bites
    • Tetanus prophylaxis—in cases in which the last tetanus booster was greater than 5 years previously or unknown

INFECTIONS AFTER HUMAN BITES

20. **What are the common bacteria responsible for infections after human bites?**
Streptococci are found in 80% of human bite wounds. Other common organisms include staphylococci, *Haemophilus* spp., *Eikenella corrodens, Fusobacterium* spp., peptostreptococci, *Prevotella* spp., and *Porphyromonas* spp.

21. **What viruses can be transmitted by human bites?**
Herpesviruses, hepatitis B and C viruses, and HIV.

22. **Should antibiotics be administered after a human bite?**
Yes. Preemptive antibiotics should be given to all patients as early as possible after a human bite. Amoxicillin-clavulanate, administered for 3 to 5 days, with close follow-up, is recommended. Attention should be paid to wound-cleaning and the need for débridement as well as confirmation of tetanus vaccination status.

23. **What are the potential complications of human bite infections?**
    • Deep infection of the synovium, joint capsule, and bone in the case of closed-fist injuries. Early evaluation by a hand surgeon is recommended. Hospitalization for empiric IV antibiotics may be needed and should be directed at *S. aureus, Haemophilus* spp., *E. corrodens,* and β-lactamase–producing anaerobes.
    • Radiographs can be useful in identifying foreign bodies (e.g., retained teeth).

SURGICAL SITE INFECTIONS

24. How common are surgical site infections, and what factors are related to their incidence?
    - The development of a surgical site infections (SSI) depends on a variety of factors, including location and type of surgery; duration of the surgery; wound classification (clean, clean-contaminated, contaminated, or dirty); and a series of patient-related risk factors, including diabetes, obesity, smoking, skin colonization or nasal carriage with *S. aureus*, and use of systemic steroids, among other factors.
    - The most commonly isolated organism is *S. aureus*, although gram-negative bacteria are common for SSIs following abdominal and genitourinary procedures.

25. What techniques have been shown to reduce the risk of surgical site infections?
    - Proper skin preparation—Avoidance of preoperative use of a razor for removing hair at the incision site (clippers should be used if hair removal is needed), use of chlorhexidine-alcohol or iodophor-alcohol skin antiseptics
    - Surgical techniques—Gentle traction during surgery, effective hemostasis, removal of devitalized tissues, obliteration of dead space, irrigation of tissues, use of nonabsorbable monofilament suture material, closed-suction drains, and wound closure without tension
    - Maintenance of normothermia, provision of supplemental oxygen, and blood sugar control in diabetics (<200 mg/dL) during and after the surgical procedure have also been shown to reduce SSI risk.
    - Screening for *S. aureus* and decolonization prior to high-risk surgical procedures—For patients undergoing arthroplasty and cardiac surgery, programs that screen patients for *S. aureus* colonization and implement decolonization with chlorhexidine bathing and intranasal mupirocin have been associated with reduction of SSIs.
    - Antimicrobial prophylaxis—Preoperative administration of antibiotics within 1 hour before the incision is recommended. Cefazolin is a common choice, and should be administered within 30 to 60 minutes prior to incision. Vancomycin, which must be administered between 60 to 120 minutes prior to incision, is a common option in patients with penicillin allergy, as is clindamycin. Vancomycin should also be considered in the case of institutions where the rate of MRSA is high and in patients with known history of or current infection with MRSA.
    - SSIs are categorized as superficial incisional SSI, deep incisional SSI, and organ/space SSI.
    - SSIs are treated with incision and drainage; systemic antimicrobial therapy is often indicated.
    - Early SSIs, within 48 hours of the procedure, are often due to *S. pyogenes* or *Clostridium* species. Empiric therapy regimens, based on site of surgical procedure, are provided (see Table 43.4).

Table 43-4. Empiric Antimicrobial Therapy for Incisional Surgical Site Infections, by Site of Surgery

SURGICAL SITE	SINGLE-AGENT THERAPY	COMBINATION THERAPY
Intestinal or genital tract	Piperacillin-tazobactam Imipenem-cilastin Meropenem Ertapenem	Ceftriaxone + Metronidazole Ciprofloxacin + Metronidazole Levofloxacin + Metronidazole Ampicillin-sulbactam + Gentamicin OR Tobramycin
Surgery of trunk or extremity away from axilla or perineum	Oxacillin or nafcillin Cefazolin Cephalexin TMP/SMX Vancomycin	
Surgery of the axilla or perineum*		Metronidazole + Ciprofloxacin Metronidazole + Levofloxacin Metronidazole + Ceftriaxone

*Consider the addition of methicillin-resistant *Staphylococcus aureus* therapy with vancomycin.
TMP/SMZ, Trimethoprim/sulfamethoxazole.
Modified from Stevens DL, Bisno AL, Chambers HF, et al. Practice guidelines for the diagnosis and management of skin and soft tissue infections: 2014 Update by the Infectious Diseases Society of America. *Clin Infect Dis.* 2014;59(2):147–159.

KEY POINTS: SKIN AND SOFT TISSUE INFECTIONS

1. Selection of empiric antimicrobial therapy—In a patient with SSTI, consider host factors, including comorbidities, prior microbiologic history, and epidemiologic background.
2. Risk factors that predispose to cellulitis—Obesity, prior cellulitis in the same location, toe-web abnormalities, breach in skin barrier, surgical procedures that affect lymphatic drainage, diabetes, arterial insufficiency, chronic venous insufficiency, chronic renal disease, neutropenia, cirrhosis, and hypogammaglobulinemia are predisposing factors. Appropriate antimicrobial therapy for streptococcal TSS. Penicillin and clindamycin are first-line therapy for patients with severe allergies to penicillin; vancomycin, linezolid, quinupristin-dalfopristin, or daptomycin can be substituted for penicillin. For *S. aureus* TSS, use vancomycin if there is concern for MRSA.
3. Human bites—Always treat with preemptive antibiotics; involve surgical service early if complications, including deep infection, are suspected.
4. SSI rates—SSI rates depend on many factors, including location and type of surgery; duration of the surgery; surgical classification of the wound, peri- and intraoperative procedures, and a series of patient-related risk factors.

BIBLIOGRAPHY

1. Anaya DA, Dellinger EP. Necrotizing soft-tissue infection: diagnosis and management. *Clin Infect Dis.* 2007;44(5): 705-710.
2. Blumenthal KG, Shenoy ES, Hurwitz S, et al. Effect of a drug allergy educational program and antibiotic prescribing guideline on inpatient clinical providers' antibiotic prescribing knowledge. *J Allergy Clin Immunol Pract.* 2014;2(4): 407-413.
3. Blumenthal KG, Shenoy ES, Varughese CA, et al. Impact of a clinical guideline for prescribing antibiotics to inpatients reporting penicillin or cephalosporin allergy. *Ann Allergy Asthma Immunol.* 2015;115(4):294-300.e2.
4. Bebko SP, Green DM, Awad SS. Effect of a preoperative decontamination protocol on surgical site infections in patients undergoing elective orthopedic surgery with hardware implantation. *JAMA Surg.* 2015;150(5):390-395.
5. Bode LG, Kluytmans JA, Wertheim HF, et al. Preventing surgical-site infections in nasal carriers of Staphylococcus aureus. *N Engl J Med.* 2010;362(1):9-17.
6. Martin JM, Green M, Barbadora KA, et al. Erythromycin-resistant group A streptococci in schoolchildren in Pittsburgh. *N Engl J Med.* 2002;346(16):1200-1206.
7. Richter SS, Heilmann KP, Beekmann SE, et al. Macrolide-Resistant Streptococcus pyogenes in the United States, 2002–2003. *Clin Infect Dis.* 2005;41(5):599-608.
8. Sader HS, Farrell DJ, Flamm RK, et al. Antimicrobial activity of ceftaroline tested against Staphylococcus aureus from surgical skin and skin structure infections in US Medical Centers. *Surg Infect (Larchmt).* 2016;17(4):443-447.

CHAPTER 44

H1N1/INFLUENZA

Christopher Grace

INFLUENZA

1. **What is influenza?**
   Influenza is a respiratory illness caused by an RNA virus that comes in two forms that can infect humans: influenza A and influenza B. Although generally self-limited, influenza can cause significant morbidity and mortality, especially in those at risk (discussed later). Influenza is most common during the fall and winter months, due to increased indoor crowding and low humidity, though illness can continue through April and May in the Northern Hemisphere.

2. **How are influenza A strains designated?**
   Influenza A is described by two surface glycoproteins: hemagglutinin (H) and neuraminidase (N). The hemagglutinin, of which there are 18 structurally different types, allows attachment to host respiratory epithelium. The neuraminidase, of which there are 10 different types, acts as an enzyme facilitating release of newly replicated viruses from the infected cell. Humans are most often infected with influenza viruses having H1, H2, or H3 and N1 or N2.

   The H and N terminology is also used to name the influenza stains spreading yearly. Generally each year there are one or two influenza A strains and an influenza B strain circulating. During the recent influenza seasons, the circulating strains included A H1N1, A H3N2, and two strains of influenza B.

3. **What are the symptoms of influenza?**
   Influenza is an acute respiratory illness characterized by fever greater than 37.8°C (100°F) and cough. There may be associated sore throat, myalgias, arthralgias, fatigue, headache, nausea and vomiting, diarrhea, nasal congestion, and runny nose. The incubation period is generally 1 to 4 days. Not all patients have all these symptoms. Not all patients will have a fever at the time of clinical assessment (though they may be able to give a history of chills or sweats). The degree of illness may vary from quite mild to very severe. Severe influenza can result in hospitalization, require intensive care treatment, and result in death. It is important to keep in mind that influenza may
   - Cause an exacerbation of underlying chronic pulmonary or cardiac disease
   - Present as a pneumonia with infiltrates on chest x-ray
   - Be complicated by secondary bacterial infections
   - Present with more severe illness with respiratory difficulty, confusion, and a "sepsis-like illness" and multiorgan failure
   - Cause myocarditis, pericarditis, or trigger myocardial infarction

4. **Who is at risk for more severe or complicated influenza?**
   Influenza can be especially serious and life-threatening for patients with the risk factors listed here. These patients should be thoroughly assessed and consideration given to testing and treating during the influenza season.
   - Pregnant women
   - Children aged less than 5 years (especially <2 years)
   - Patients with asthma, chronic lung, heart, liver, and kidney disease
   - Immune-suppressed patients, including those with HIV, organ transplants, lymphoma and leukemia, receiving cancer chemotherapy or prolonged corticosteroids
   - Neuromuscular disorders
   - Obesity
   - Residents of nursing homes and other chronic-care facilities
   - Children and adolescents receiving long-term aspirin therapy (Reye syndrome)

5. **What complications can occur from influenza?**
   Centers for Disease Control and Prevention (CDC) estimates that from the 1976 to 1977 season to the 2006 to 2007 flu season, flu-associated deaths ranged from an estimated low of about 3000 to a high of about 49,000 deaths yearly. During the 2014 to 2015 influenza season, CDC estimated that about

40,435,474 (range 25,596,116–47,770,668) persons were infected, with an estimated 974,206 (range 859,853–1,173,760) hospitalizations. Rates of influenza-associated hospitalizations among people 65 and older caused about 758,000 hospitalizations.

Influenza can cause a primary viral hemorrhagic pneumonia characterized by progressive dyspnea and leukocytosis, potentially progressing to respiratory failure and an adult respiratory disease syndrome (ARDS) like clinical syndrome. Older patients and those with chronic cardiopulmonary illness may develop a secondary bacterial pneumonia. After a period of improvement, the patient appears to worsen with signs and symptoms of bacterial pneumonia, most often due to *Streptococcus pneumoniae*, *Haemophilus influenzae*, and *Staphylococcus aureus*. In addition, patients may experience exacerbations of chronic cardiopulmonary illnesses. Less common complications can include myositis, myocarditis, pericarditis, encephalitis, a toxic-shock-like illness, Guillain-Barre syndrome, and Reye syndrome.

6. What other infections can mimic influenza?
   The symptoms of influenza are very nonspecific and can be caused by a large array of viruses and bacteria. Since these pathogens can cause an illness similar to influenza, any febrile respiratory illness may be referred to as influenza-like illness (ILI). Causes of ILI, in addition to influenza, include respiratory syncytial virus (RSV), parainfluenza, rhinovirus and coronavirus (agents of the common cold), adenovirus, metapneumovirus, Group A *Streptococcus*, mycoplasma, chlamydia, and *Bordetella pertussis*.

7. How do you diagnose influenza?
   Influenza is often a clinical diagnosis. For those without risks for complications or requiring hospitalization, no further diagnostics are required. The most accurate way to confirm that a patient does or does not have influenza is to obtain a nasopharyngeal swab. The swab needs to be inserted through the nose to the pharynx. Testing by polymerase chain reaction (PCR) is most accurate. Testing by rapid influenza diagnostic tests (RIDT) is not very sensitive (50%–70%), but is reasonably specific (90%–95%). A negative RIDT is not helpful. A positive RIDT can be helpful, and most people with a positive RIDT have influenza A.

8. What is the approach to the patient with an influenza-like illness?
   During the winter or flu season, a person with an ILI should be assumed to have influenza until proven otherwise; see the flow diagram provided (Fig. 44.1). The approach to the patient with ILI can progress in a stepwise manner. The patient should be assessed for the degree of illness and presence of risk factors for complications. Those with mild symptoms (no shortness of breath and ability to maintain hydration) and no risks for complications do not need further testing and can be treated symptomatically. Those with moderate symptoms (some shortness of breath, difficulty maintaining hydration, signs and symptoms of pneumonia) should be tested and treated with antiviral medications. Those with severe symptoms (respiratory distress, altered mental status) need immediate assessment in the emergency department. Pregnant women with influenza, especially those in the third trimester, have a high rate of complications and should be emergently assessed by obstetrics or in the emergency department (Fig. 44.1).

9. How do you treat influenza?
   M2 channel blockers such as amantadine and rimantadine are not often used due to emergence of resistance and central nervous system toxicity. Neuraminidase inhibitors such as oseltamivir, zanamivir, and peramivir act by blocking the surface neuramidase (N). They are active against influenza A and B. Oseltamivir is oral and dosed at 75 mg twice daily for 5 days for treatment. Zanamivir is a oral spray (10 mg or two inhalations twice daily), has been approved for persons aged greater than or equal to 7 years, and is also given for 5 days. Peramivir is intravenous and can be used for persons unable to take oral or inhalational medications such as in the intensive care unit (ICU). It is given as a single 600 mg dose. Dosing of oseltamivir and peramivir must be modified for renal insufficiency. These agents have been shown to shorten the duration of influenza symptoms, but only modestly; if started within 48 hours of symptoms, the duration of the illness may be decreased by about 1 day. In the past, resistance has developed to the neuraminidase inhibitors but since 2009, 99% of influenza viral isolates have been susceptible.

10. How do you manage a patient admitted to the hospital with influenza-like illness?
    All patients with ILI during the fall/winter flu season admitted to the hospital should be presumed to have influenza until ruled out by nasopharyngeal PCR. Until that test result is back, they should be isolated in a private room, standard and droplet precautions instituted and treated with neuraminidase inhibitors. Consideration should be given to treating with antibiotics, such as ceftriaxone, to cover potential streptococcal, staphylococcal, and haemophilus superinfection. If the nasopharyngeal

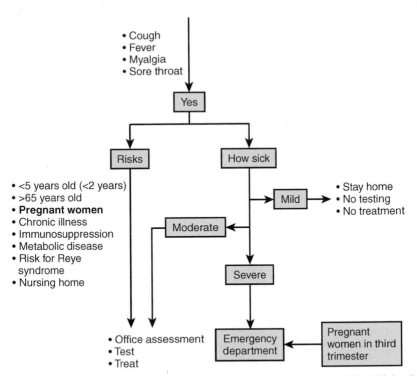

Figure 44-1. Approach to the patient with an influenza-like illness. When testing and treatment are being decided on, the patient's risk for complications and severity of illness need to be taken into account.

PCR returns negative, influenza treatment and isolation can be stopped. Keep in mind a negative RIDT does not rule out influenza.

11. **What are epidemics and pandemics?**
The hemagglutinin (H) and neuraminidase (N) undergo small changes (antigenic drift) in structure on a yearly basis, allowing the virus to partially evade our past immunologic response. These antigenic drifts cause the yearly epidemics. Larger changes (antigenic shift) in the H and N, due to genetic reassortment of genes from different influenza viruses infecting the same respiratory cell, occur infrequently. When these reassortments do occur, much of the population has no or limited immunity to the new strain. If these reassortment strains are able to be transmitted from person to person a pandemic can occur, as happened in 1918, 1956, 1967, and 2009. Pandemic refers to a new viral type and worldwide spread but not severity. The 1918 pandemic was very severe, with about an estimated 2.5% mortality, causing about 50 to 100 million deaths worldwide. In contrast, the 2009 pandemic was no more severe than a usual epidemic year, though it disproportionately affected younger adults and children.

12. **What have we learned from past pandemics?**
The influenza virus can mutate and reassort frequently and randomly, making occurrence of pandemics unpredictable. Over the past 300 years, there has been no regular periodicity with times between pandemics, varying from 8 to 42 years. Pandemics often unfold in waves of severity over several years, as occurred in 1918. Pandemics disproportionately affect the young as occurred in both 1918 and 2009. Pandemics may not follow seasonal (fall to winter) patterns, as occurred when the 2009 started in the spring.

13. **What is "bird" flu?**
Influenza is an avian virus that can infect humans, pigs, and other mammals. Viral strains that affect predominantly birds (aquatic fowl and domestic poultry) are referred to as bird flu and generally do

not infect humans. In 1997 a bird flu, H5N1, infected 18 people in Hong Kong, killing 6 of them. It reappeared in 2003 infecting persons in Vietnam, Cambodia, Laos, Thailand, Indonesia, China, Egypt, and central Asia. As of July 2016, there have been 854 confirmed human infections with H5N1 with 450 deaths—a 53% mortality! The great majority of these patients had extensive direct contact with infected poultry. There have been several limited episodes of human-to-human transmission, but no sustained transmission. It is still circulating. H5N1 continues to cause illness and death in the countries but has not attained the ability, yet to be easily transmitted to or between people. In March 2013, a new bird flu strain, H7N9, appeared in Southern China, most likely originating in the live animal markets in that area. As of February 2016, there have been 777 cases with 273 deaths, a 35% mortality. It is still circulating. Other strains of avian influenza, including highly pathogenic H5 strains, regularly affect domestic flocks in the United States, resulting in many millions of poultry deaths. In the United States, none of these strains have as yet infected humans.

14. What was the pandemic of 2009?

During the 2009 to 2010 influenza season, a large change in the H and N structure occurred leaving much of the population, especially those less than 65 years old, with inadequate immunity. This new structure was the result of a reassortment of bird, swine, and human influenza strains. It appeared to start simultaneously in Southern California and Mexico in the spring of 2009 and spread rapidly worldwide with the World Health Organization declaring a pandemic on June 11, 2009. Young adults and children were particularly affected. In Argentina, for example, pediatric hospitalization rates doubled. Of hospitalized children, 19% were admitted to the ICU, 17% required mechanical ventilation, and 5% died. In the United States, 45% of patients admitted to the hospital were under age 18 years. Seventy-three percent of patients had at least one underlying condition including asthma, diabetes, heart, lung and neurological diseases, and pregnancy. Fortunately the 2009 pandemic caused a "mild" pandemic as compared with that in 1918. Many countries, including Australia, Spain, and the United States, had more ICU admissions, need for mechanical ventilation, and deaths. Those admitted to ICUs often had extensive multifocal pneumonias on chest x-ray. In one study of those admitted to the ICU, 36% had pulmonary emboli on chest computerized tomography. Early in the pandemic, Spain noted that 91% of the patients admitted to the ICU had primary viral pneumonia, 75% had multiorgan failure, 75% required mechanical ventilation, and 22% needed renal replacement therapy. In the Australia and New Zealand experience, one-third of mechanically ventilated patients were treated with extracorporeal membrane oxygenation (ECMO), and 21% died. In Canadian experience, 81% of critically ill patients received mechanical ventilation for a median of 12 days. The 28-day mortality of these patients was 14.3%. Lung rescue therapies included neuromuscular blockade (28%), inhaled nitrous oxide (13.7%), high frequency oscillatory ventilation (11.9%), ECMO (4.2%), and prone positioning ventilation (3.0%). The 90-day mortality was 17.3%.

15. How should the patient admitted to the intensive care unit be managed?

Any patient admitted to the ICU with a respiratory illness during the influenza season should be presumed to have influenza, until proven otherwise by nasopharyngeal swab PCR. Patients may present with exacerbations of underlying cardiopulmonary diseases, primary viral pneumonia, and/or secondary bacterial pneumonias. All patients should be treated with a neuraminidase inhibitor and antibiotics. Antibacterial therapy should be directed toward primarily *S. pneumoniae, S. aureus*, and *H. influenzae*. Possible initial regiments may include ceftriaxone and vancomycin.

16. What infection control measures are needed?

Influenza is most often spread by large particle respiratory droplets created by patient coughing or sneezing. This mode of transmission generally requires close contact (3–6 feet), since these larger and heavier respiratory particles quickly fall out of the air. Hand contact with environmental surfaces contaminated with the virus can also transmit influenza when those hands come in contact with mucosal surfaces, such as touching your eye, nose, or mouth. There has been concern that influenza may be airborne transmitted by small particle aerosols, though it is not clear how much this mode of transmission contributes to community spread. For the office and hospital, the CDC recommend standard and droplet precautions that include:

- Placing the patient in a private room
- Persons entering the patient room wear a surgical mask
- Healthcare providers should wear gloves and gowns if contact with the patient's blood, body fluids, secretions (including respiratory), or excretions is expected.
- If participating in an aerosol-generating procedure such as intubation, extubation, bronchoscopy, or autopsy, a fit tested N95 respirator or a purified air-powered respirator (PAPR) should be used. All healthcare workers need to practice good hand hygiene before and after patient contact.

17. What is the influenza vaccine?

The influenza vaccine is made of inactivated surface hemagglutinin of the virus. Injected intramuscularly, it stimulates immunity against the influenza strains in the vaccine. The CDC and the World Health Organization (WHO) track influenza yearly, in order to determine the appropriate strains of influenza that should be incorporated into the seasonal vaccine. The most commonly used vaccine is a quadrivalent injection, which includes two strains of influenza A and two strains of influenza B. The previously marketed intranasal spray vaccine is no longer recommended for anyone. There is a high dose trivalent vaccine for those older than 65 years of age. It is felt this formulation is more antigenic, creates higher antibody levels, and hopefully is more protective of this older population. It causes slightly more arm discomfort than standard dose vaccine and is not quadrivalent, incorporating two influenza A strains, but only one influenza B strain.

Most influenza vaccines are made in chicken eggs. This process can take from 6 to 9 months and is dependent on adequate viral growth in the eggs; during the 2009 pandemic, the virus did not grow well in the eggs, thus delaying the distribution of the vaccine. The risk though for those with egg allergies is extremely low. Patients with a history of egg involving hives can receive the influenza vaccine. Patients with a history of egg-related angioedema, respiratory distress, light-headedness, recurrent emesis, or who required epinephrine or another emergency medical intervention may receive the influenza vaccine but for these patients, administration should be in an inpatient or outpatient medical setting under medical supervision.

New production methods have been developed that avoid egg-based growth methods. Cultured mammalian cells can be used to grow the virus, instead of eggs, for extraction of the hemagglutinin. These cell-based vaccines avoid egg allergies, speed up production, and may yield vaccines with more specific immunogenicity to the circulating strains, improving efficacy. Recombinant DNA technology uses an insect baculovirus expression system to manufacture the viral hemagglutinin used in the vaccine. A vaccine containing the oil-based adjuvant, MF59, has been approved for those older than 65 years of age. The mammalian cell-based, recombinant, and adjuvant technologies produce only trivalent vaccines.

Among adults aged 18 to 65 years, a 2012 meta-analysis found that the efficacy of the injection trivalent vaccine against confirmed influenza was 59% (95% CI = 51–67). For those older than 65 years of age, the vaccine is generally less protective. The influenza vaccine has reduced children's risk of pediatric ICU admissions due to influenza by 74%. For persons 50 years and older who received the influenza vaccine, their risk of hospitalization for influenza has been reduced by 57%.

18. Who should get the influenza vaccine?

The CDC recommends that all persons older than 6 months of age get yearly vaccinations. This is especially true for those at high risk for complications of influenza as outlined previously. All healthcare workers need to be vaccinated yearly, so as to remain healthy and not risk spreading influenza to the more vulnerable patients.

KEY POINTS: H1N1/INFLUENZA

1. Can cause severe respiratory illness requiring ICU care
2. May exacerbate underlying cardiopulmonary conditions
3. All patients admitted to hospital for presumed influenza should be treated with antiviral medications
4. Secondary bacterial pneumonias may develop and should be looked for and treated
5. All persons aged greater than 6 months should be vaccinated yearly

BIBLIOGRAPHY

1. Pleschka S. Overview of Influenza viruses. *Curr Top Microbiol Immunol.* 2013;370:1-20.
2. Grohskopf LA, Sokolow LZ, Broder KR, et al. Prevention and Control of Seasonal Influenza with Vaccines. Recommendations of the Advisory Committee on Immunization Practices—United States, 2016–17 Influenza Season. *MMWR Recomm Rep.* 2016;65(5):1-54.
3. Fiore AE, Fry A, Shay D, et al. Antiviral Agents for the Treatment and Chemoprophylaxis of Influenza. Recommendations of the Advisory Committee on Immunization Practices (ACIP). *MMWR Recomm Rep.* 2011;60(RR01);1-24.
4. Girard MP, Tam JS, Assossou OM, et al. The 2009 A (H1N1) influenza virus pandemic: a review. *Vaccine.* 2010;28: 4895-4902.
5. Kumar A, Zarychanski R, Pinto R, et al. Critically ill patients with 2009 Influenza A (H1N1) infection in Canada. *JAMA.* 2009;302(17):1872-1879.
6. Homsi S, Milojkovic N, Homsi Y. Clinical pathological characteristics and management of acute respiratory distress syndrome resulting from influenza A (H1N1) virus. *South Med J.* 2010;103(8):786-790.

CHAPTER 45

IMMUNOCOMPROMISED HOST

Kristen K. Pierce

1. **What is the initial approach to the immunocompromised host in the intensive care unit?**

   The approach in the intensive care unit (ICU) setting relies on several factors:

   - High index of clinical suspicion—Immune-compromised hosts often have atypical presentations of infection. For example, patients with severe immunocompromise may lack fever or abscess formation.
   - Understanding of the host's immune defect—Recognizing the deficient pathway (cell-mediated versus humoral) enables the physician to expand the differential diagnosis and has implications for empiric therapy.
   - Aggressive diagnostics—Blood work and cultures, imaging, bronchoscopy, and tissue biopsy, if indicated, are all essential in the initial workup of a suspected infection.
   - Early appropriate antimicrobial therapy—This is key when dealing with infections in the immunocompromised patient.

2. **What is the "net state of immunosuppression," and why is it important?**

   The concept of a net state of immunosuppression describes the infection potential in immunocompromised hosts. For example, a patient who underwent splenectomy 10 years ago after traumatic injury has a very different infection risk than does a patient with human immunodeficiency virus/acquired immunodeficiency syndrome (HIV/AIDS). This is important in understanding a patient's susceptibility to, and risk for, infection. The net state of immunosuppression is determined by the following characteristics:

   - Immunosuppressive medications—The degree of immunosuppression conferred by these medications will be influenced by their type, dose, and duration of therapy.
   - Presence of leukopenia—Long-standing neutropenia carries a different risk of infection as compared with acute-onset neutropenia. For example, acute neutropenia conveys an increased risk of infections with gram-negative and enteric organisms. As the duration of neutropenia continues, these patients are at increasing risk for invasive fungal infections.
   - Metabolic factors—Poor nutrition, hyperglycemia, and uremia all confer an increased risk for infection.
   - Concurrent infection with immunomodulating viruses such as cytomegalovirus (CMV), Epstein-Barr virus (EBV), hepatitis B and C, human herpes virus 6 (HHV-6), and HIV—These infections can weaken the host's defenses either by a low level of viral replication or by reducing the function of infected white blood cells. This leads to an increased risk for bacterial or fungal infection.
   - Anatomic factors—The presence of obstructing tumors, stents, central venous catheters, and endotracheal tubes can affect a host's risk for infection.

3. **How is immunosuppression measured?**

   Assessment can be based on the following:

   - Duration and level of neutropenia in those undergoing cytotoxic chemotherapy are used to determine the risk of infection and need for empiric antibiotic therapy. For example, patients with a longer duration of absolute neutropenia have a greater risk for invasive fungal infection compared with patients with acute neutropenia.
   - CD4 cell count in patients with HIV is an accurate measure of their immune function. A patient with HIV who has an absolute CD4 count of 700/mm^3 has a very different infection risk compared with someone whose CD4 counts are under 100/mm^3.
   - Treatment, type, and duration of therapy in patients receiving immunosuppression after solid organ, stem cell, or bone marrow transplantation (BMT). Also, the type of transplant (matched or unmatched donor) may be important. Patients who undergo stem cell transplantation or BMT from an allogeneic human leukocyte antigen–identical sibling or matched unrelated donor are at greatest risk for infection because they may require more immunosuppression.

4. **How does the timing of solid organ transplantation affect a patient's risk for infection?**

   See Table 45.1.

Table 45-1. Risk of Infection and Time From Transplantation

MONTHS AFTER TRANSPLANTATION	TYPE OF INFECTION
0–1	**Hospital Derived**
	Surgical site infection MRSA, VRE
	Catheter infections
	MRSA, VRE
	Candidal infections
	Ventilator-associated
	Aspiration
	Clostridium difficile colitis
	Donor-Derived Infections
	Reactivated HSV
	West Nile virus
	HIV
1–6*	**Opportunistic Infections**
	CMV
	PJP
	Cryptococcus
	Listeria monocytogenes
	EBV
	Adenovirus
	HHV-6
	Reactivation of Latent Recipient Infections
	Coccidioides immitis
	Mycobacterium tuberculosis
	Histoplasmosis
	Blastomycosis
	Reactivation of Latent Donor Derived
	HIV
	Hepatitis B or C
≥6	**Community Acquired**
	Pneumonia
	Urinary tract infections
	Fungal Infections
	Atypical molds
	Aspergillus
	Atypical Bacterial
	Nocardia
	Listeria
	Cryptococcus

(Continued on following page)

Table 45-1. Risk of Infection and Time From Transplantation *(Continued)*

MONTHS AFTER TRANSPLANTATION	TYPE OF INFECTION
	Late Viral Infections
	Polyomavirus infection
	Reactivated VZV
	CMV
	EBV

*Immunosuppression is greater when used as a bolus for antirejection rather than when used as initial induction therapy. Generally thought to be the time of greatest immunosuppression.

CMV, Cytomegalovirus; *EBV*, Epstein-Barr virus; *HHV-6*, human herpes virus 6; *HIV*, human immunodeficiency virus; *HSV*, herpes simplex virus; *IL*, interleukin; *MRSA*, methicillin-resistant *Staphylococcus aureus*; *PJP*, Pneumocystis jirovecii pneumonia; *TNF*, tumor necrosis factor; *VRE*, vancomycin-resistant enterococcus; *VZV*, Varicella-zoster virus.

Modified from Fishman JA, Issa NC. Infections in organ transplantation: risk factors and evolving patterns of infection. *Infect Dis Clin North Am.* 2010;24:273–283; Danovitch G. Immunosuppressive medications and protocols for kidney transplantation. In: Danovitch G, ed. *Handbook of Kidney Transplantation.* Philadelphia: Lippincott Williams & Wilkins; 2004:72–134. Modified from Fishman J. Infection in solid organ transplant recipients. *N Engl J Med.* 2007;357:2601–2614; Syndman DR. Epidemiology of infections after solid-organ transplantation. *Clin Infect Dis.* 2001;33(Suppl 1):S5.

5. Describe the timing of infection in hematopoietic stem cell transplant recipients.

   Pre-engraftment. Generally accepted as the first 2 to 4 weeks after transplantation and lasting until the engraftment of the transplant. During this period, patients are at risk for bacterial infections from their own endogenous bowel flora (*Escherichia coli*, *Klebsiella*, and *Pseudomonas*) and from skin flora such as *Staphylococcus* and *Streptococcus*. The longer the patient remains neutropenic, the greater the risk of developing invasive fungal infections Reactivation of latent viruses, such as CMV and herpes simplex virus (HSV), can lead to systemic infection.

   Early postengraftment. The period from the time of neutrophil engraftment until day 100. With the exception of those patients who still have indwelling catheters, bacterial infection is less common during this time period. Patients who have difficulties with engraftment or those in whom graft-versus-host disease (GVHD) may develop, requiring increased doses of steroids, are at risk for invasive fungal infections as well as viral infections (CMV and HSV).

   Late postengraftment. Ranging from around day 100 until immunity is restored. Patients are generally at risk for encapsulated bacterial infections *(Haemophilus influenzae, Streptococcus pneumoniae, Neisseria meningitidis),* fungal infections (*Candida* spp. and *Aspergillus* spp.), and late CMV infection.

6. What is the initial recommended workup of suspected infection in the immunocompromised host?

   History and physical. Clinical clues regarding unusual exposures can assist in creating a broad differential for suspected infection. Certain physical examination findings can be indicative of certain types of infection, and through physical examination, including visualization of the oropharynx, skin, and perirectal areas, looking for occult abscess is important.

   However, it is important to recognize that digital rectal examinations should not be performed in patients with neutropenia, nor should they be allowed to have rectal instillation of contrast for abdominal computed tomography (CT) scans, because of the risk of hematogenous dissemination of the patients' endogenous bowel flora.

   Questions that may provide clinical clues to source of infection include the following:

   - Type and duration of immunosuppressive medication
   - Duration of time since transplantation
   - Sick exposures—family members, coworkers
   - Recent travel, both in and outside of the country
   - Pets or animal exposures
   - Eating habits—raw fish, game meat
   - Hobbies—hunting, fishing, gardening
   - History of tuberculosis exposure

- Use of antimicrobial prophylaxis for viral or bacterial infection
- Insect exposures
- Food-borne illnesses
- Recent home renovations
- Recent unprotected sexual intercourse
  Blood cultures. Two sets should be obtained. If a patient has an indwelling central venous catheter a set should be collected from each lumen; at least one peripheral set should be obtained as well:
- Complete blood cell count with differential
- Serum creatinine, blood urea nitrogen
- Electrolytes
- Liver function tests
  Cultures should be obtained from other sites of potential infection: urine, sputum, and stool.
  Imaging. A chest radiograph is clinically indicated for those patients complaining of respiratory symptoms or with objective findings such as changes in oxygenation, chest pain, or cough. Abdominal imaging may be indicated for those with abdominal complaints: nausea, vomiting or diarrhea, abnormal liver function testing, or evidence of gram-negative bacteremia.

7. What infectious causes should be considered in a patient without a spleen who has suspected sepsis?
   Patients who have undergone splenectomy represent a special subset of the immune-compromised host. Whether from surgical removal or functional asplenia (radiation, Hodgkin disease), these patients are at risk from a fulminant sepsis syndrome, known as postsplenectomy syndrome (PSS) or overwhelming postsplenectomy infection (OPSI), which carries a mortality rate approaching 70%. PSS is characterized as a fulminant sepsis, meningitis, or pneumonia that occurs days to years after splenic removal. Although the risk of severe infection is highest in the first few years after removal, fatal cases of PSS have been well-documented even decades after the initial splenectomy. Encapsulated organisms such *N. meningitidis, H. influenzae,* and *S. pneumoniae* are the three most cited etiologic agents. In addition, *Capnocytophaga canimorsus* can lead to fulminant infection after dog bites. *Babesia,* in those with appropriate travel history, can cause severe disease in hosts without a spleen. *Salmonella* species are a common cause of illness in children with sickle cell disease and splenic dysfunction.

8. What is the initial treatment for a patient without a spleen who is seen with sepsis?
   In addition to aggressive supportive care, treatment of suspected postsplenectomy sepsis involves appropriate empiric antibiotic therapy directed at encapsulated organisms. Empiric antibiotic choices should include coverage for *Streptococcus,* allowing for concerns of penicillin resistance, β-lactamase-producing organisms, and broad gram-negative coverage, to include *Neisseria* and *H. influenzae.* Antibiotic allergy and local antibiotic resistance need to be taken into consideration when choosing an initial empiric regimen. However, combinations such as vancomycin and ceftriaxone or moxifloxacin or vancomycin and cefepime plus moxifloxacin would be reasonable starting regimens while awaiting microbiologic results.

9. What is the differential diagnosis in an immunocompromised patient who is seen with a central nervous system infection?
   Infections of the central nervous system (CNS) are a medical emergency. Prompt evaluation by lumbar puncture, imaging, and administration of empiric antibiotics are essential. The clinical presentation of disease may be more subacute in the immunocompromised patient. An understanding of the net state of immunosuppression of the patient can provide insight into creating a differential diagnosis of the nature of CNS infection based on clinical presentation. See Table 45.2.

10. What is the initial diagnostic approach to an immunocompromised patient who is seen with a suspected central nervous system infection?
    A prompt workup to determine the etiology of the infection is essential. However, empiric antimicrobial therapy should not be delayed during this process; antimicrobial therapy should be initiated immediately while investigation in ongoing.
    The workup should include the following:
- Imaging study
  - CT scan can reveal acute hemorrhage, mass effect, bony, or subdural lesions.
  - Magnetic resonance imaging can better evaluate the brain parenchyma, evidence and characteristics of mass lesions, brainstem and spinal cord lesions, edema.

Table 45-2. Differential Diagnosis of Suspected Central Nervous System Infection Based on Underlying Immune Defect

IMMUNE DEFECT	MENINGITIS	ENCEPHALITIS	MENINGOENCEPHALITIS
Impaired humoral immunity–B-cell dysfunction			
Multiple myeloma	*S. pneumoniae*	Echovirus	*L. monocytogenes*
Hyposplenism	*N. meningitides*	Poliovirus	*Cryptococcus*
Immunoglobulin deficiencies	*H. influenzae*		
B-cell lymphoma			
CLL			
Alcoholic liver disease			
Impaired cell-mediated immunity–T-cell dysfunction			
HIV/AIDS	*S. pneumoniae*	VZV	*Listeria monocytogenes*
Corticosteroid use	*N. meningitides*	HSV	*Cryptococcus*
Hodgkin	*H. influenzae*	CMV	
lymphoma	*Cryptococcus*	WNV	
Solid organ transplantation	Acute HIV infection	JC virus	
Stem cell transplantation			
Chronic renal failure			
Impaired granulocyte function			
ALL	*Streptococcus pneumoniae*	HSV	
BMT	*Staphylococcus aureus*[*]		
Chemotherapy-induced leukopenia	*Pseudomonas aeruginosa*[*]		
	Neisseria meningitides		
	Haemophilus influenzae		

[*]Especially in those with indwelling devices (i.e., catheters, pumps).
AIDS, Acquired immunodeficiency syndrome; *ALL*, Acute lymphocytic leukemia; *BMT*, bone marrow transplantation; *CLL*, chronic lymphocytic leukemia; *CMV*, cytomegalovirus; *HIV*, human immunodeficiency virus; *HSV*, herpes simplex virus; *JC*, John Cunningham virus; *VZV*, varicella-zoster virus; *WNV*, West Nile virus.
Modified from Cunha BA. Central nervous system infections in the compromised host: a diagnostic approach. *Infect Dis Clin North Am.* 2001;15:567–590; and Linden PK. Approach to the immunocompromised host with infection in the intensive care unit. *Infect Dis Clin North Am.* 2009;23:535–556.

- Lumbar puncture
  - Opening pressure
  - Cerebrospinal fluid (CSF)
- Cell count and differential
- Glucose, protein, and lactate
- Gram stain and bacterial culture
- Cryptococcal antigen
- Acid-fast smear and culture (if risk exists for *Mycobacterium tuberculosis*)
- Fungal smear and culture
- Polymerase chain reaction (PCR) for HSV, varicella-zoster virus (VZV), and other viral causes as clinically appropriate and influenced by seasonal and geographic variation—enterovirus, West Nile virus (WNV), eastern equine encephalitis (EEE), western equine encephalitis (WEE).
- Biopsy—If no definitive answer can be obtained from lumbar puncture, aspiration, or biopsy of CNS lesions may be required for definitive diagnosis.

11. Do special considerations exist for the treatment of meningitis and mass lesions in the immunocompromised host?
Although infection of the CNS is life-threatening, it is important to recognize that noninfectious mimics of CNS infections exist that should be taken into consideration as part of the differential diagnosis as well; however, these will not be discussed in detail here.
   Bacterial meningitis. Treatment in the immunocompromised host should include coverage for the usual bacterial pathogens (*N. meningitidis*, *H. influenzae*, and *S. pneumoniae*), with attention to the possibility of penicillin-resistant *S. pneumoniae*, *Staphylococcus aureus* (especially in those with indwelling lines or shunts), and also *Listeria monocytogenes*. Often, compromised patients with *Listeria* meningitis will be seen with subacute meningitis. However, the organism will usually grow in CSF cultures in 24 to 48 hours; thus empiric therapy should be continued until cultures are negative.
   Mass lesions. Several viral, fungal, and parasitic pathogens can present as mass lesions in an immunocompromised host and masquerade as tumor or bacterial abscess. Significant efforts should be made to establish a microbiologic or tissue diagnosis of CNS lesions because the differential is quite broad, making empiric therapy challenging and not recommended.

12. What is the definition of neutropenia?
Neutropenia is defined as an absolute neutrophil count (ANC) of less than 500 cells per cubic millimeter. The term may also be applied to those patients in whom an ANC decrease to less than 500 cells per cubic millimeter is expected within the next 2 days. Some patients will have a relatively normal ANC, yet still have profoundly impaired phagocytosis. These patients are said to have *functional neutropenia* and are still at risk for opportunistic infections, despite their normal counts.

13. Describe empiric therapy for the hospitalized patient with febrile neutropenia.
Patients with febrile neutropenia require empiric intravenous (IV) antibiotic therapy with an antipseudomonal β-lactam agent, such as meropenem, imipenem-cilastatin, piperacillin-tazobactam, or cefepime. Additional antibiotics (quinolones, vancomycin, daptomycin) may be added if concern exists for resistant organisms, vancomycin-resistant enterococcus (VRE), methicillin-resistant *S. aureus* (MRSA), or resistant gram-negative rods.

14. Describe the initial antibiotic regimen in a patient with febrile neutropenia who is allergic to penicillin.
The majority of patients who report an allergy to penicillin will tolerate cephalosporins and carbapenems. However, in those patients with an immunoglobulin (Ig) E–mediated immediate-type hypersensitivity reaction (hives, bronchospasm), these drug classes should be avoided. In this group of patients, alternative therapeutic options include ciprofloxacin and clindamycin or vancomycin and aztreonam.

15. What are the most common bacterial causes of community-acquired pneumonia in the immunocompromised host?
S. pneumoniae, *H. influenzae*, or *Moraxella catarrhalis* are the most common pathogens. In patients with cell-mediated immune defects, Legionnaires disease is the most common atypical pathogen. Compared with normal hosts, oral anaerobes as a result of oropharyngeal aspiration, *Mycoplasma*, and *Chlamydia* are less-common causes of infection in the compromised host. *Pseudomonas aeruginosa*, an unusual respiratory pathogen in normal hosts, has been implicated as a cause of community-acquired pneumonia in patients with cystic fibrosis or bronchiectasis and in patients living with HIV/AIDS.

16. What is the differential diagnosis for an immunocompromised patient with fever and pulmonary infiltrates?

   Respiratory compromise in the immunocompromised host carries with it a significant mortality rate with estimates between 30% and 90%. Although the physician must consider noninfectious causes of pulmonary infiltrates (Box 45.1), infectious causes require early recognition and treatment. The differential is based on understanding of the immune defect and characterization of the radiographic pattern of infiltrate, in conjunction with the timing of onset of symptoms. However, it is vital to recognize that no one radiographic appearance is pathognomonic for a specific infection (Table 16.3).

17. What is the role of bronchoalveolar lavage and lung biopsy in the diagnosis of pulmonary infiltrates?
   See Fig. 45.1.

18. Describe the clinical course of *Pneumocystis jiroveci* pneumonia infection and treatment.

   This organism was first associated with human disease in 1951 when it was discovered as the cause of severe pneumonitis in severely malnourished infants. Since that time, it has been associated with patients taking long-term steroids and those receiving certain chemotherapeutic regimens. However, it became famous as the major pathogen of patients with HIV infection.

   However, the advent of highly active antiretroviral therapy (HAART) has resulted in effective immune reconstitution, as well as effective prophylactic regimens, together resulting in a decreased susceptibility to infection in these patients. However, we now see an increase in *Pneumocystis jiroveci* pneumonia (PJP) infections among those receiving cytotoxic chemotherapy. Interestingly, in patients with HIV the clinical course is usually fairly indolent, with complaints of several weeks of cough and increasing dyspnea; at the time of presentation, the degree of hypoxemia is usually moderate, with little to no peripheral leukocytosis. This is in contrast with the population without HIV, in which the infection can present quite acutely with severe hypoxemia and respiratory failure. Chest radiographs often demonstrate bilateral or asymmetric interstitial infiltrates (more common in the population with HIV; see Table 45.4).

19. How is the diagnosis of *Pneumocystis jiroveci* pneumonia made?

   - **Bronchoalveolar lavage (BAL) specimens**—BAL with biopsy can make the diagnosis up to 90% of the time. BAL lavage alone is apt to make the diagnosis approximately 50% of the time in patients without HIV, but 90% of the time in those with HIV/AIDS because of the higher burden of organisms in this patient population.
   - **Sputum**—Induced (not expectorated) sputum can be useful for diagnosis, especially in patients with AIDS.
   - **Biopsy**—Histology will show pathognomonic frothy infiltrate that fills the alveoli; organisms can be seen in tissue sections as well. This infiltrate can be confused with hyaline membranes seen in acute respiratory distress syndrome (ARDS), although often the two disease states coexist.
     Serum markers include:
   - **Lactate dehydrogenase**—Often elevated in those with PJP, usually over 300 International Units/mL. Higher levels indicate that a larger amount of lung tissue may be involved.
   - **β-ᴅ-glucans**—Often positive in the setting of PJP infection, but not diagnostic.

Box 45-1. Noninfectious Causes of Pulmonary Infiltrates in Immunocompromised Host

- Radiation pneumonitis
- Lymphangitic spread of underlying malignancy
- Drug-induced lung toxicity
- Cryptogenic organizing pneumonia (COP) or bronchiolitis obliterans–organizing pneumonia (BOOP)
- Diffuse alveolar hemorrhage
- Acute respiratory distress syndrome (ARDS)
- Pulmonary edema
- Pulmonary embolism or infarction
- Idiopathic pulmonary fibrosis

Table 45-3. Radiographic Patterns of Pulmonary Disease in the Immunocompromised Host

| IMMUNE DEFECT | RADIOGRAPHIC PATTERN | Onset of Illness | |
		ACUTE	SUBACUTE OR CHRONIC
HIV	Consolidation	Bacterial	Bacterial
Long-term steroid use		*Streptococcus pneumoniae*	*Rhodococcus equi*
		Haemophilus influenzae	*Cryptococcus*
		*Legionella**	
	Reticulonodular		PCP
			Histoplasmosis
			Cryptococcus
			Mycobacterium avium
	Diffuse interstitial	Influenza	PCP
			CMV
	Discrete nodule		*Nocardia*
			Mycobacterium tuberculosis
			Endemic fungi
			Coccidioides
			Histoplasma
			Cryptococcus
Solid organ transplant recipient	Consolidation	Bacterial	
		S. pneumoniae	
		H. influenzae	
		*Legionella**	
		RSV	
		Influenza	
	Reticulonodular		*Nocardia*
			M. tuberculosis
	Diffuse interstitial	CMV	*Cryptococcus*
		RSV	Aspergillosis
		Influenza	
		PCP	
	Discrete nodules		*Aspergillus*
			M. tuberculosis
			Nocardia

(Continued on following page)

Table 45-3. Radiographic Patterns of Pulmonary Disease in the Immunocompromised Host *(Continued)*

IMMUNE DEFECT	RADIOGRAPHIC PATTERN	Onset of Illness	
		ACUTE	**SUBACUTE OR CHRONIC**
HSCT recipients	Consolidation	Bacterial	
		S. pneumoniae	
		H. influenzae	
		*Legionella**	
	Diffuse interstitial	Influenza	
		PCP	
		RSV	
		CMV	
		HSV	
	Reticulonodular		*Nocardia*
			Cryptococcus
			Histoplasmosis
			Aspergillus
	Discrete nodule		*Mycobacterium*
Chemotherapy-induced neutropenia	Lobar consolidation	Bacterial	
		S. pneumoniae	
		H. influenzae	
		*Legionella**	
	Diffuse interstitial	CMV	
		PCP	
	Reticulonodular		*Aspergillus*
			Histoplasmosis
			Coccidiomycosis
	Discrete nodule		*Aspergillus*

Legionella is usually rapidly progressive asymmetrical infiltrates.
Modified from Cunha B. Pneumonias in the compromised host. *Infect Dis Clin North Am.* 2001;15:591–612; and Linden PK. Approach to the immunocompromised host with infection in the intensive care unit. *Infect Dis Clin North Am.* 2009;23:535–556.
CMV, Cytomegalovirus; *HSCT,* Hematopoietic stem cell transplantation; *HSV,* herpes simplex virus; *RSV,* respiratory syncytial virus.

20. **When are steroids indicated in the treatment of *Pneumocystis jiroveci* pneumonia infection?**
    Steroids are recommended in addition to antibiotic therapy in patients who have a Pao_2 of less than 70 mm Hg on room air arterial blood gas or who have an A—a gradient of greater than 35 mm Hg. Steroids given in the first 72 hours of treatment can lessen the decreases in oxygenation and improve survival. Steroid dosing should consist of prednisone 40 mg daily (or equivalent) orally for 5 days then decreasing to 20 mg daily, to complete a total course of 21 days.

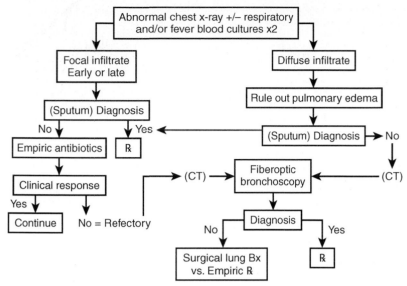

Figure 45-1. Diagnostic algorithm for evaluating pulmonary infiltrates in ill patients with cancer. *CT*, Computed tomography. (From White P. Evaluation of pulmonary infiltrates in critically ill patients with cancer and marrow transplant. *Crit Care Clin.* 2001;17:647–670.)

Table 45-4. Treatment of PCP Infection: Moderate to Severe Disease

DRUGS	DOSE	DURATION AND COMMENTS
TMP-SMX* IV and PO	15–20 mg/kg per day TMP† 75–100 mg/kg per day SMX†	Recommended duration: 21 days
Alternatives	3–4 mg/kg per day infused over ≥60 min	21 days duration
1. Pentamidine	4 mg/kg per day (max 300 mg/day)	
2. Primaquine *plus*	15–30 mg base/day	
Clindamycin	900 mg IV every 8 h	

*Some helpful conversions: 16 mg TMP per mL of Bactrim; **Bactrim DS** = 800 mg TMP/160 mg SMX; **Bactrim SS** = 400 mg TMP/160 mg SMX.

†Dosing is based on the TMP component.

Modified from Bartlett JG, Gallant JE, Pham PA. *Medical management of HIV Infection.* Durham, NC: Knowledge Source Solutions; 2009:449; and Rubin RH, Young LS. *Clinical Approach to Infection in the Compromised Host.* 4th ed. New York: Kluwer Academic/Plenum Publishers; 2002:265–289.

PO, Oral; SMX, sulfamethoxazole; TMP, trimethoprim.

21. What are the most common causes of esophageal disease in those undergoing cytotoxic chemotherapy and bone marrow transplantation?

    Esophageal disease from both infectious and noninfectious (i.e., GVHD, chemotherapy-induced mucositis) causes is common in this patient population. The normal mucosal barrier is often disrupted by chemotherapeutic agents, and this mucosal disruption can then become a portal of entry for bacteria. Most patients with esophageal disease are initially seen with dysphagia, odynophagia, nausea, or retrosternal pain.

    The most common causes of esophageal infection in this patient population are as follows:

    HSV Often presents with oropharyngeal ulcers, which can be quite friable and lead to gastrointestinal (GI) bleeding. The infection can have white exudates and is often mistaken for *Candida*. The ulcer appearance is not pathognomonic, has similar appearance to that of chemotherapy-induced mucositis, and is best diagnosed by culture or PCR test of the lesions. Oral trauma from nasogastric (NG) tubes or endotracheal tubes can lead to extension of infection from oral pharynx into lower respiratory tract. This can lead to dissemination and, in certain patients, development of HSV pneumonia.

    Candidal esophagitis—Most common cause of esophageal infections in compromised hosts. Classic manifestation is thick white plaques adherent to the posterior pharynx and buccal mucosa. Widespread use of azoles for prophylaxis has increased the risk of fluconazole-resistant candidal species. This is an important consideration in determining empiric antifungal therapy.

    CMV—Can cause infection throughout the entire GI tract. The ulcers do not have a unique appearance and may resemble those of HSV or chemotherapy-induced mucositis. Cultures and PCR specimens should be interpreted with caution because trauma and underlying illness may lead to mucosal shedding; biopsy samples of oral and esophageal lesions should be taken for clear diagnosis.

22. What is typhlitis, and how is it treated?

    Typhlitis, also known as neutropenic enterocolitis, is thought to ensue after a constellation of factors including mucosal injury of the bowel wall due to cytotoxic chemotherapy, impaired host defenses, and neutropenia. It is typically seen in patients with neutrophil counts less than $500/mm^3$; those affected often have abdominal pain, fever, nausea, diarrhea, and bloody diarrhea. The diagnosis carries a mortality rate of between 40% and 50%. Concomitant bacteremia, due to translocation of normal bowel flora, is common.

    The disease has a predilection for the cecum because of its relative lack of vascularization compared with the remainder of the colon; however, other sites of bowel involvement have been described. Radiographs of the abdomen are nonspecific, although they may demonstrate evidence of obstruction or free air. CT scans may reveal cecal wall thickening, pneumatosis, free air, or abscess formation. The use of rectal contrast or barium enemas should be avoided in patients with neutropenia because of the high risk of bowel wall perforation. Workup should include abdominal radiographs, CT scan of abdomen without rectal contrast, blood cultures, stool cultures including stool for *Clostridium difficile* testing, and surgical evaluation.

    Treatment includes IV volume resuscitation and broad-spectrum antibiotic therapy (see Box 45.2).

23. Describe some of the common causes of community-acquired bacterial enteritis in the immunocompromised patient.

    Patients with compromised immune systems are at risk for development of the same community infections as normal hosts, but they may be more severe. In addition, because of low neutrophil counts or loss of mucosal integrity, they may be more prone to development of bacteremia from

---

Box 45-2. Empiric Antibiotic Options for Suspected Typhlitis

Vancomycin and antipseudomonal carbapenem (meropenem or imipenem)
Or
Vancomycin and ceftazidime and metronidazole
Or
Vancomycin and aztreonam + metronidazole*

*One possibility for patients allergic to penicillin.
Regimen will vary according to antibiotic allergies, hospital formulary, and local resistance patterns.

their own endogenous bowel flora. Some of these infections can lead to dissemination outside the GI tract and lead to more severe disease in immunocompromised hosts.

Listeria. The common food-borne illness caused by this organism leads to outbreaks in immunocompromised and normal hosts alike. However, dissemination outside of the GI tract is increased in those with chronic lymphocytic leukemia, corticosteroid use, allogenic BMT, and pregnancy. Certain chemotherapeutic drugs such as fludarabine will increase this risk as well.

Salmonella. This is associated with a deficiency in cell-mediated immunity such as corticosteroid use and HIV infection. These hosts are at risk for disseminated *Salmonella* infection.

C. difficile. *C. difficile* has been associated with a higher mortality risk among BMT recipients compared with a normal host. Increased rates of infection among immunocompromised patients are likely due to frequent antibiotic therapy, increased rates of colonization, and frequent hospital admissions.

Cryptosporidium usually causes a mild diarrheal illness in those with normally functioning immune systems. However, in the immunocompromised host, it can lead to severe, protracted diarrheal disease, as well as biliary involvement. Further complicating this is that there is no effective therapy for cryptosporidium in this patient population.

24. Describe the most common causes of viral enteritis in the immunocompromised patient.
    - **CMV**—One of the more common pathogens in the transplant population. Diagnosis requires colonic biopsy. CT findings are nonspecific, and serologic markers such as antigenemia and viral load are unreliable indicators of disease limited to the GI tract.
    - **Adenovirus**—A common cause in both solid organ recipients and BMT recipients. The clinical picture is often that of diarrhea, although bleeding is not uncommon because the virus can lead to colonic ulceration. Dissemination outside of the GI tract can occur leading to pneumonitis, hepatitis, encephalitis, and cystitis.
    - **Rotavirus**—Usually seen in pediatric patients. It can lead to profuse watery diarrhea and is diagnosed by stool PCR testing.
    - **Enterovirus**—Presenting with watery diarrhea but can progress to meningoencephalitis. It is diagnosed by stool PCR testing.
    - **HSV**—Can lead to ulcerations in the upper and lower GI tract.

25. What is the best approach to manage highly active antiretroviral therapy for patients with human immunodeficiency virus in the intensive care unit?
    In patients with HIV receiving HAART, therapy should be continued whenever possible to prevent the development of resistance. This may not be possible in some patients when complications arise such as renal failure and/or liver disease, which are related to the HAART itself. Administering HAART to patients who can take nothing by mouth (NPO) can be challenging because some medications cannot be crushed for administration through an NG tube, and not all are available in liquid form. If HAART medications do need to be stopped, it is essential that all HAART be held at the same time. Discontinuation of only part of a patient's HAART regimen can lead to antiviral resistance and ensuing treatment complications down the road.

26. Should antirejection medications be altered for the solid organ transplant recipient with severe sepsis?
    In patients with life-threatening infections, withdrawal or reduction of immunosuppressive medications can be an effective treatment modality to assist in the treatment of infections. However, cessation of antirejection medications can lead to graft rejection and failure, and so changes in medications need to be considered on an individual basis. These decisions regarding medication adjustments should be carried out with the close assistance of the transplant team whenever possible.
    Here are some important facts to consider when considering reduction of immunosuppression:
    - Mortality associated with loss of allograft—Graft loss in heart or liver transplant recipients may be very different from graft loss in those who have undergone pancreas or kidney transplantation. If other modalities can be used (i.e., insulin or hemodialysis), then although not ideal, the graft may be able to be sacrificed in the setting of life-threatening infection.
    - Use of steroids—In the setting of acute infection, rapid withdrawal or taper of steroids may lead to adrenal insufficiency complicating the patient's hemodynamics. In addition, the use of steroids may be clinically indicated for treatment of the underlying infection or sequelae thereof (i.e., PJP or cerebral edema associated with toxoplasmosis).

KEY POINTS: IMMUNOCOMPROMISED HOST

1. The *net state of immunosuppression* is critical in assessing a patient's risk for infection.
2. The longer the duration of neutropenia, the greater the risk for invasive fungal disease.
3. Individuals without a spleen are at risk for infection with encapsulated organisms.
4. The greatest degree of immunosuppression in solid organ transplant recipients is 1 to 6 months after transplantation.
5. Early antimicrobial therapy is essential in patients with neutropenic fever.

BIBLIOGRAPHY

1. Baden LR, Maguire JH. Gastrointestinal infections in the immunocompromised host. *Infect Dis Clin North Am.* 2001;15:639-670, xi.
2. Bartlett JG, Gallant JE, Pham PA. *Medical Management of HIV Infection.* Durham, NC: Knowledge Source Solutions; 2009:449.
3. Bow EJ. Infections in neutropenic patients with cancer. *Crit Care Clin.* 2013;29:411-441.
4. Burnham JP, Kirby JP, Kollef MH. Diagnosis and management of skin and soft tissue infections in the intensive care unit: a review. *Intensive Care Med.* 2016;42:1899-1911. doi:10.1007/s00134-016-4576-0.
5. Cunha BA. Pneumonias in the compromised host. *Infect Dis Clin North Am.* 2001;15:591-612.
6. Cunha BA. Central nervous system infections in the compromised host: a diagnostic approach. *Infect Dis Clin North Am.* 2001;15:567-590.
7. Dropulic LK, Lederman HM. Overview of infections in the immunocompromised host. *Microbiol Spectr.* 2016;4(4). doi:10.1128/microbiolspec.DMIH2-0026-2016.
8. Fishman JA. Pneumocystis carinii and parasitic infections in the immunocompromised host. In: Rubin RH, Young LS, eds. *Clinical Approach to Infection in the Compromised Host.* 4th ed. New York: Kluwer Academic/Plenum Publishers; 2002:265-325.
9. Fishman JA. Infection in solid-organ transplant recipients. *N Engl J Med.* 2007;357:2601-2614.
10. Freifeld AG, Bow EJ, Sepkowitz KA, et al. Clinical practice guidelines for the use of antimicrobial agents in neutropenic patients with cancer: 2010 update by the Infectious Diseases Society of America. *Clin Infect Dis.* 2011;52:e56-e93.
11. Kotloff RM, Ahya VN, Crawford SW. Pulmonary complications of solid organ and hematopoietic stem cell transplantation. *Am J Respir Crit Care Med.* 2004;170:22-48.
12. Leather HL, Wingard JR. Infections following hematopoietic stem cell transplantation. *Infect Dis Clin North Am.* 2001;15:483-520.
13. Linden PK. Approach to the immunocompromised host with infection in the intensive care unit. *Infect Dis Clin North Am.* 2009;23:535-556.
14. Rubin RH, Schaffner A, Speich R. Introduction to the immunocompromised host society consensus conference on epidemiology, prevention, diagnosis, and management of infections in solid-organ transplant patients. *Clin Infect Dis.* 2001;33(suppl 1):S1-S4.
15. Sumaraju V, Smith LG, Smith SM. Infectious complications in asplenic hosts. *Infect Dis Clin North Am.* 2001;15:551-565.
16. Syndman DR. Epidemiology of infections after solid-organ transplantation. *Clin Infect Dis.* 2001;33(suppl 1):S5-S8.
17. Tasaka S, Hasegawa N, Kobayashi S, et al. Serum indicators for the diagnosis of pneumocystis pneumonia. *Chest.* 2007;131:1173-1180.
18. White P. Evaluation of pulmonary infiltrates in critically ill patients with cancer and marrow transplant. *Crit Care Clin.* 2001;17:647-670.

CHAPTER 46

HYPERTENSIVE CRISES

Abhishek Kumar and Varun Agrawal

1. **Which physiologic factors determine a person's blood pressure?**
   Arterial blood pressure (BP) is the product of cardiac output and systemic vascular resistance. The cardiac output is further determined by stroke volume and heart rate. Any factor, physiologic or pathologic, that increases these determinants of BP can cause hypertension. Increase in systemic vascular resistance as a result of humoral vasoconstrictors, such as angiotensin II or adrenergic hormones, is most commonly implicated in hypertensive crises.

2. **What is hypertensive crisis and how does one define "hypertensive emergency" and "hypertensive urgency"?**
   Hypertensive crisis is the condition of severe and uncontrolled increase in the BP with or without acute end organ damage. Systolic blood pressure (SBP ≥180 mm Hg) or diastolic blood pressure (DBP ≥120 mm Hg) is the defining feature of all hypertensive crises. In hypertensive emergency, there is evidence of end organ injury that warrants prompt treatment in the intensive care unit (ICU) with intravenous antihypertensives to lower the BP in minutes to hours. In hypertensive urgency, while there is no end organ injury, gradual lowering of the BP and outpatient follow-up are essential. "Malignant hypertension" and "accelerated hypertension" were previously used terms to define severe hypertension with papilledema and retinal hemorrhages, respectively, and are no longer preferred.

3. **What are the target organs affected in hypertensive emergency?**
   The following organ systems can be severely injured in hypertensive emergency and present as follows:
   - Kidney: Acute kidney injury caused by endothelial damage and fibrinoid necrosis of renal arterioles, proteinuria
   - Brain: Hypertensive encephalopathy, cerebrovascular accident (CVA), posterior reversible leukoencephalopathy syndrome (PRES)
   - Eye: Retinal hemorrhage, exudates, papilledema
   - Cardiovascular: Acute coronary syndrome, decompensated heart failure, aortic dissection, microangiopathic hemolytic anemia due to endothelial injury.

4. **What are the causes of hypertensive crises?**
   Common causes of hypertensive crises are listed in Table 46.1. Nonadherence to antihypertensive therapy or hypertension induced by drugs can be addressed by patient education and subsequent outpatient monitoring. Evaluation for secondary causes of hypertension may be pursued, especially if the patient has an atypical presentation of hypertension (age of onset <30 years), resistant hypertension (SBP >160 mm Hg despite being on three antihypertensives that includes a diuretic), or suggestive features such as electrolyte abnormalities or renal bruits.

5. **How should a patient with hypertensive crisis be clinically evaluated?**
   The treating physician needs to elicit symptoms of hypertensive organ damage such as shortness of breath, chest pain, back pain, focal neurologic deficits, seizures, headache, or altered consciousness. Evaluation of pulses in all extremities, thorough examination of the heart (for murmurs or gallops), lungs (for pulmonary edema), abdomen (for renal artery bruits), central nervous system (for focused neurologic deficits), and fundus (for hemorrhages, exudates or papilledema), needs to be performed. Cardiac enzymes, electrocardiogram, B-type natriuretic peptide, serum creatinine, urinalysis, complete blood count, and chest x-ray provide objective evidence of end-organ injury in hypertensive crises. Computed tomography (CT) brain and drug screen may be performed if indicated.

6. **What is the goal blood pressure in hypertensive emergency, and over what period is this to be achieved?**
   The Joint National Committee 7 guidelines recommend lowering the mean arterial BP by less than 25% in the first hour, and lowering the BP to 160/100 to 110 mm Hg in the next 2 to 6 hours with

Table 46-1. Common Causes of Hypertensive Crises

1. Essential hypertension (drug nonadherence, especially with clonidine or β-blocker cessation)
2. Renal:
   a. Renal parenchymal disease (chronic kidney disease)
   b. Renovascular disease (atherosclerotic renal artery stenosis or fibromuscular dysplasia)
3. Drugs:
   a. Prescription (e.g., antivascular endothelial growth factor agents, cyclosporine, glucocorticoid, erythropoietin, methylphenidate)
   b. Over-the-counter (e.g., pseudoephedrine, nonsteroidal antiinflammatory drugs, licorice)
   c. Illicit (e.g., tobacco, ethanol, cocaine, amphetamines, phencyclidine)
4. Endocrine:
   a. Adrenal causes: primary hyperaldosteronism, pheochromocytoma, hypercortisolism
   b. Hyperthyroidism
5. Central nervous system disorders: intracerebral bleed, intracranial hypertension
6. Autonomic dysfunction: baroreflex failure
7. Pregnancy: Pregnancy-induced hypertension or preeclampsia

subsequent gradual lowering in 24 to 48 hours. Excessive BP reduction is to be avoided, as this can worsen perfusion and organ injury as a result of impaired autoregulation in the cerebral, coronary, and renal arterial beds in hypertension. It is to be noted that hypertensive crises in aortic dissection are an exception to the previous stated targets, as the BP needs to be lowered to normal levels immediately.

7. What are the preferred antihypertensive drugs in hypertensive emergency?
   Intravenous short, rapid-acting titratable antihypertensive agents are preferred for reducing BP in hypertensive emergency. Intravenous dihydropyridine calcium channel blockers (nicardipine, clevidipine) and β-blockers (labetalol, esmolol) are commonly used agents in hypertensive emergency. Nicardipine and clevidipine are peripheral vasodilators and also improve coronary blood flow. β-blockers have a less vasodilator effect than calcium channel blockers, though labetalol does have mild α_1 blocking activity and is commonly used in pregnancy. Intravenous nitroglycerin and phentolamine are used in specific situations (vide infra). Currently, intravenous sodium nitroprusside is less preferred, as it may cause profound hypotension (due to arterial and venous vasodilator effect) and cyanide toxicity. Intra-arterial BP monitoring is recommended to titrate doses of these intravenous antihypertensive drugs.

8. Outline the management of hypertensive urgency in the hospital. Which antihypertensives are recommended for outpatient use after successful treatment of hypertensive crisis?
   As the complications of hypertensive urgency are not immediate, gradual reduction in the BP over 24 to 48 hours with long-acting oral medications can be done outside the ICU. While no specific antihypertensive agents has been proven beneficial, angiotensin-converting enzyme inhibitor (ACEi) or angiotensin II receptor blocker (ARB; to counteract the injurious effects of angiotensin II on the blood vessel wall) is commonly used in conjunction with diuretics or vasodilators (calcium channel blockers), as recommended in the hypertension guidelines. Outpatient follow-up with primary care physician, hypertension specialist, or nephrologist is essential. The patient needs to be educated on the need for drug adherence, regular outpatient follow-up, home monitoring of BP, and avoiding drugs that exacerbate hypertension.

9. What is the treatment of hypertensive crisis in a patient with adrenergic crisis, and how is pheochromocytoma evaluated?
   Adrenergic excess states present with palpitations, flushing, and signs of vasoconstriction. Catecholamine-associated hypertension is commonly due to pheochromocytoma or cocaine use as a result of increased adrenergic hormone secretion or central nervous system stimulation respectively. The treatment of choice is α_1-blocker intravenous phentolamine. Vasodilators such as nicardipine, clevidipine, or sodium nitroprusside may also be used. β-blockers are avoided without concomitant α-blocker because the unopposed peripheral α-receptor stimulation may worsen the hypertension. Benzodiazepines are used in cocaine toxicity to lower the central nervous system stimulation. Plasma fractionated metanephrines are an appropriate screening test for pheochromocytoma, and imaging with CT/magnetic resonance imaging (MRI) or meta-iodobenzylguanidine (MIBG) scan can help localize the site of excessive adrenaline production and plan surgical removal.

10. Which antihypertensive agent is used in a patient presenting with aortic dissection?
Hypertension in aortic dissection is to be treated as a hypertensive emergency to avoid progression of the dissection as a result of an intimal tear. The target BP is SBP less than 120 mm Hg and mean arterial pressure (MAP) less than 80 mm Hg, to be achieved within 5 to 10 minutes in the ICU. Beta-blockers (labetalol or esmolol) are the antihypertensives of choice, and these drugs also reduce myocardial contractility and heart rate that would further reduce wall shear stress. Intravenous nicardipine or nitroprusside may be added if BP is not at goal.

11. What is hypertensive encephalopathy, and how is it managed?
This is a form of hypertensive emergency in which patients present with symptoms and signs of cerebral edema when the BP exceeds the upper limit of cerebral vascular autoregulation. There is gradual onset of nausea, vomiting, headache, restlessness, and confusion. If not treated, the patient may develop seizures or coma. Focal neurologic symptoms are absent. Neuroradiologic findings are similar to that found in PRES. The goal of treatment is to lower MAP by 10% to 15% in the first hour and by less than 25% in the next 24 hours. Commonly used agents in hypertensive encephalopathy are nicardipine, fenoldopam, nitroprusside, labetalol, or clevidipine. Seizures are usually treated with phenytoin, which can be discontinued in 1 to 2 weeks.

12. How should hypertensive emergency be managed in a patient with cerebrovascular accident?
   - **Ischemic stroke**
     In a patient with acute ischemic stroke event and BP greater than 220/120 mm Hg who is not a candidate for fibrinolytic therapy, the goal of antihypertensive therapy is to lower the SBP by 15% in the first 24 hours. In the patient in whom fibrinolysis is indicated, SBP should be lowered to less than 185 mm Hg and DBP should be lowered to less than 110 mm Hg before fibrinolytic therapy is initiated. The patient needs to be closely monitored for neurologic deterioration associated with BP lowering.
   - **Intracerebral hemorrhage**
     In a patient with intracerebral hemorrhage and SBP between 220 and 150 mm Hg, acute lowering of SBP to less than 140 mm Hg within 1 hour is safe and can improve functional outcome by limiting the growth of the hematoma. Antihypertensive Treatment of Acute Cerebral Hemorrhage II (ATACH-2) was a randomized clinical trial in 2016 that demonstrated similar safety when the SBP was lowered to less than 110 mm Hg in patients with intracerebral hemorrhage. Intravenous nicardipine and labetalol (diltiazem or urapidil when labetalol was not available) were used in this trial.

13. What is posterior reversible leukoencephalopathy syndrome, and how is it diagnosed?
PRES is a clinical and radiologic syndrome with many etiologies besides hypertension, such as eclampsia, immunosuppressive medications, vasculitis, thrombotic thrombocytopenic purpura, hypercalcemia, or hypomagnesemia. The underlying cause is likely cerebral autoregulatory failure and endothelial dysfunction. Patients affected by PRES present with headache, visual changes, confusion, or seizure. Diffusion-weighted MR imaging demonstrates characteristic findings of symmetrical white matter edema in parieto-occipital areas of cerebral hemispheres not confined to a single vascular territory. PRES appears to be completely reversible after treatment within days to weeks, though radiologic recovery requires more time.

14. What is the management of hypertension crisis in a patient presenting with anginal chest pain and acute coronary syndrome?
Increased afterload in hypertensive crises raises the myocardial oxygen demand and thus may precipitate myocardial ischemia. Intravenous nitroglycerin and β-blockers (labetalol or esmolol) are the drugs of choice. Nitroglycerin increases coronary perfusion and decreases preload, while β-blockers reduce oxygen demand. Vasodilators such as sodium nitroprusside and hydralazine are to be avoided because of reactive tachycardia and decreased coronary blood flow to the affected heart muscle, but nicardipine can be given as this increases coronary blood flow. If the patient is in congestive heart failure and has pulmonary edema, intravenous loop diuretics are indicated.

15. What are the hypertensive disorders in pregnancy, and how is hypertensive crisis in pregnancy managed?
SBP greater than 160 or DBP greater than 110 mm Hg constitutes hypertensive crisis in pregnancy. Hypertensive crises in pregnancy may present in the setting of chronic hypertension, gestational hypertension, preeclampsia or hemolysis, elevated liver enzymes, and low platelets (HELLP syndrome). Preeclampsia is a severe form of hypertension with renal injury (proteinuria) that can lead

to significant maternal and fetal morbidity and mortality and thus needs to be promptly treated. Intravenous labetalol, hydralazine, or nicardipine are recommended drugs for use in hypertensive crises in pregnancy. ACEi or ARB is contraindicated in pregnant and nursing women. Close inpatient monitoring by a high-risk obstetrics team is essential, as delivery of the baby is the definitive treatment, especially beyond 34 weeks of gestation.

16. **How does renal artery stenosis cause hypertensive crises, and how should this be evaluated and treated?**
Renal artery stenosis (RAS) can be either due to atherosclerotic plaque (in the proximal artery) or fibromuscular dysplasia (in the distal artery). The resulting renal hypoperfusion causes severe renin-angiotensin-aldosterone activity and leads to hypertensive crises. RAS is suspected in patients with risk factors for atherosclerosis presenting with severe hypertension and acute diastolic congestive heart failure (known as flash pulmonary edema). Doppler ultrasound or CT angiography can identify RAS. There is no preferred drug therapy of hypertensive crisis in RAS, though the ACE inhibitor (or angiotensin receptor blocker) should be used carefully, with monitoring for acute kidney injury. Randomized trials have shown no difference between medical therapy and RAS angioplasty and stenting in BP or renal outcomes, though some patients with RAS and failure of medical therapy, flash pulmonary edema, or loss of renal function may be considered for angioplasty.

17. **What are the adrenal abnormalities that cause primary hyperaldosteronism, and how should these be distinguished and treated?**
Primary hyperaldosteronism (PHA) should be suspected in a patient with severe hypertension, hypokalemia, and metabolic alkalosis. Increased aldosterone secretion in PHA occurs either due to unilateral aldosterone-producing adenoma (APA) or bilateral idiopathic adrenal hyperplasia (IAH). Plasma renin activity below detection and plasma aldosterone greater than 20 ng/dL are diagnostic of PHA. CT abdomen or adrenal vein sampling (in a specialized center) are used to differentiate adrenal adenoma from hyperplasia. Definitive treatment of APA is surgical adrenalectomy, whereas IAH is medically managed with aldosterone antagonists (spironolactone or eplerenone) and potassium supplementation.

ACKNOWLEDGMENT

The authors wish to acknowledge Drs. Stuart L. Linas, MD, and Shailendra Sharma, MD, for the valuable contributions to the previous edition of this chapter.

KEY POINTS: HYPERTENSIVE CRISES

1. Hypertensive crises refer to acute presentation of severe hypertension (SBP ≥200 or DBP ≥120 mm Hg) where end organ injury may be present (hypertensive emergency) or be absent (hypertensive urgency). Hypertensive crises are associated with significant morbidity and mortality.
2. Hypertensive crises can result in damage to four major organ systems: eye, brain, heart, and kidney.
3. Hypertensive emergencies are managed in the ICU with short-acting titratable parenteral anti-hypertensives to lower BP immediately and limit target organ damage.
4. The preferred agents for hypertensive emergency are intravenous calcium channel blockers (nicardipine, clevidipine) or β-blockers (labetalol, esmolol). Nitroglycerin and phentolamine are used in specific situations.
5. Recommended mean arterial BP reduction in hypertensive emergency is less than 25% in the first hour, except in aortic dissection, where the goal BP is SBP less than 120 mm Hg within 5 to 10 minutes. In hypertensive urgency, BP is to be gradually lowered over 24 to 48 hours with ACE inhibitor, ARB, diuretics, or calcium channel blockers, and outpatient follow-up is vital.
6. Nonselective β-blockers are contraindicated in adrenergic crisis (pheochromocytoma or cocaine use), as these agents can worsen hypertension. α-blocker (phentolamine) or nicardipine may be used in this situation.
7. β-blocker (labetalol or esmolol) is the agent of choice for hypertension control in aortic dissection.
8. In a patient with acute coronary syndrome and hypertensive emergency, intravenous nitroglycerin and β-blockers (labetalol, esmolol) are the drugs of choice. Loop diuretics are to be used if the patient is in congestive heart failure and has pulmonary edema.

9. Blood pressure lowering is indicated in hypertensive emergency with acute ischemic stroke (especially if fibrinolytic therapy is being planned) or intracerebral hemorrhage, though goals and threshold for treatments vary considerably.
10. Hypertension complications in pregnancy (preeclampsia or HELLP syndrome) are managed by intravenous labetalol or hydralazine. Delivery of the fetus is to be considered if appropriate.

BIBLIOGRAPHY

1. Pimenta E, Calhoun D, Oparil S. Hypertensive emergencies. In: Jeremias A, Brown DL, eds. *Cardiac Intensive Care.* Philadelphia: Saunders Elsevier; 2010:355-367.
2. Padilla Ramos A, Varon J. Current and newer agents for hypertensive emergencies. *Curr Hypertens Rep.* 2014;16 (7):450.
3. Chobanian AV, Bakris GL, Black HR, et al. The Seventh report of the Joint National Committee on Prevention, Detection, Evaluation, and Treatment of High Blood Pressure. *Hypertension.* 2003;42(6):1206-1252.
4. Varon J. Treatment of acute severe hypertension: current and newer agents. *Drugs.* 2008;68(3):283-297.
5. Monnet X, Marik PE. What's new with hypertensive crises? *Intensive Care Med.* 2015;41(1):127-130.
6. Vaughan CJ, Delanty N. Hypertensive emergencies. *Lancet.* 2000;356(9227):411-417.
7. Jauch EC, Saver JL, Adams HP Jr, et al. American Heart Association Stroke Council, Council on Cardiovascular Nursing, Council on Peripheral Vascular Disease, Council on Clinical Cardiology. Guidelines for the early management of patients with acute ischemic stroke: a guideline for healthcare professionals from the American Heart Association/American Stroke Association. *Stroke.* 2013;44(3):870-947.
8. Hemphill JC 3rd, Greenberg SM, Anderson CS, et al. American Heart Association Stroke Council, Council on Cardiovascular and Stroke Nursing, Council on Clinical Cardiology. Guidelines for the Management of Spontaneous Intracerebral Hemorrhage: a Guideline for Healthcare Professionals from the American Heart Association/American Stroke Association. *Stroke.* 2015;46(7):2032-2060.
9. Vadhera RB, Simon M. Hypertensive emergencies in pregnancy. *Clin Obstet Gynecol.* 2014;57(4):797-805.
10. Greco BA, Freda BJ. What is the optimal treatment for patients with atherosclerotic renal artery stenosis? *Am J Kidney Dis.* 2014;64(2):174-177.
11. Funder JW, Carey RM, Mantero F, et al. The Management of Primary Aldosteronism: Case Detection, Diagnosis, and Treatment: An Endocrine Society Clinical Practice Guideline. *J Clin Endocrinol Metab.* 2016;101(5):1889-1916.

CHAPTER 47

ACUTE KIDNEY INJURY

Katharine L. Cheung

1. **How is acute kidney injury diagnosed?**
   Acute kidney injury (AKI) is a sudden decline in glomerular filtration rate (GFR) over a period of hours to days. Current clinical guidelines define AKI as a rise in serum creatinine of greater than or equal to 0.3 mg/dL within 48 hours or greater than or equal to 50% increase in 7 days, or urine output less than 0.5 mL/kg/h for 6 hours (Kidney Disease Improving Global Outcomes [KDIGO]). A rise in blood urea nitrogen (BUN) concentration may also reflect a decrease in kidney function (Table 47.1).

2. **What are the limitations of using creatinine or urine output to diagnose acute kidney injury?**
   The diagnosis of AKI is often delayed because the serum creatinine does not usually rise until 1 to 2 days after the injury at the earliest. In the setting of large volume resuscitation, a rise in serum creatinine concentration may be obscured. Serum creatinine may over- or underestimate kidney function because it is influenced by other factors, including, age, muscle mass, race, and catabolic rate. Trending the serum creatinine over time is useful to identify changes in renal function and to identify potential insults that preceded the rise in creatinine. While urine output may decrease closer to the injury, accurate and timely detection requires invasive monitoring with bladder catheterization, which increases the risk of infection. Newer methods of detecting real-time changes in GFR and therefore early detection of AKI such as the use of biomarkers are being developed but are not yet the standard of care.

3. **What are the limitations of using blood urea nitrogen to diagnose acute kidney injury?**
   BUN is also influenced by factors other than kidney function and may be elevated in states of increased urea production, such as corticosteroid use, high protein diet, and gastrointestinal bleeding.

4. **How do you measure renal function during acute kidney injury?**
   It is important to note that automated estimation of GFR by many laboratories is not accurate in the acute setting. It is only when the patient reaches a steady state that one can estimate GFR from serum creatinine concentration. One option is to perform a timed urine collection to measure creatinine clearance. This can be useful for antimicrobial dosing—for example, when achieving therapeutic levels is critical but supratherapeutic levels could worsen renal function.

5. **What features distinguish acute kidney injury from chronic kidney disease?**
   The definition of AKI relies in part on a baseline measurement of serum creatinine, which may be difficult to ascertain. Other clinical clues may assist in differentiating AKI from chronic kidney disease. Chronic renal failure is more likely than AKI to be associated with anemia, hypocalcemia, normal urine output, and small kidneys on ultrasound examination. A kidney biopsy may be warranted if the kidneys are of normal size.

6. **What are the potential etiologies of acute kidney injury?**
   The causes of AKI generally fall into the following categories: prerenal, intrarenal or parenchymal, and postrenal or obstructive (Table 47.2).

Table 47-1. Kidney Disease Improving Global Outcomes Classification of Acute Kidney Injury

	SERUM CREATININE CHANGES OVER 7 DAYS	URINE OUTPUT
Stage 1	1.5 × baseline OR increase by ≥0.3 mg/dL in 48 h	<0.5 mL/kg/h ≥6 h
Stage 2	2 × baseline	<0.5 mL/kg/h ≥12 h
Stage 3	3 × baseline	<0.3 mL/kg/h ≥24 h or anuria ≥12 h

Table 47-2. Differential Diagnosis of Acute Kidney Injury

PRERENAL	PARENCHYMAL	POSTRENAL
Effective volume depletion (e.g., hemorrhage, burns, diarrhea)	Tubular (e.g., ATN, antibiotics, myoglobin)	Ureter (e.g., nephrolithiasis, strictures, extrinsic compression)
Impaired cardiac function	Tubulointerstitial (e.g., allergic interstitial nephritis)	Bladder and prostate
Vasodilation (e.g., sepsis, cirrhosis)	Allergic interstitial nephritis (e.g., NSAIDs)	Urethra (e.g., trauma, strictures)
Renal vascular obstruction	Vascular (e.g., thrombosis, malignant HTN)	—
Renal vasoconstriction (e.g., acute hypercalcemia, norepinephrine, vasopressin, contrast media, hepatorenal syndrome)	Glomerular (e.g., anti-GBM, HUS)	—

Anti-GBM, Antiglomerular basement membrane; *ATN,* acute tubular necrosis; *HTN,* hypertension; *HUS,* hemolytic uremic syndrome; *NSAIDs,* nonsteroidal antiinflammatory drugs.

7. **How does examination of the urine help in the differential diagnosis of acute kidney injury?**
   Laboratory evaluation begins with careful examination of the urine. Concentrated urine is typical of prerenal causes but could also occur in patients on diuretics. An isotonic urine suggests parenchymal or obstructive causes. Typically the urine sediment of patients with prerenal azotemia demonstrates occasional hyaline casts or finely granular casts. In contrast, the presence of renal tubular epithelial cells with muddy and granular casts strongly suggests acute tubular necrosis (ATN), hematuria and red blood cell casts suggest glomerulonephritis, and white cell casts containing eosinophils suggest acute interstitial nephritis. Benign urine sediment is compatible with urinary obstruction. Crystals may be associated with intratubular obstruction.

8. **How does the measurement of urinary electrolytes aid in the differential diagnosis of acute kidney injury?**
   If the tubule is working well in the setting of decreased GFR, tubular reabsorption of sodium and water is avid, and the relative clearance of sodium to creatinine is low. Conversely, if the tubule is injured and cannot reabsorb sodium well, the relative clearance of sodium to creatinine is not low. Therefore, with prerenal azotemia, the ratio of the clearance of sodium to the clearance of creatinine, which is also called the *fractional excretion of sodium* (FENa; FENa = [Urinary sodium] / [Urinary creatinine] × [Plasma creatinine] / [Plasma sodium] × 100), is typically less than 1.0, whereas with parenchymal or obstructive causes of AKI, the FENa is generally greater than 2.0.

9. **What are the limitations to the fractional excretion of sodium test?**
   A low FENa test is less specific if the patient is not oliguric. Dye-induced ATN or ATN associated with hemolysis or rhabdomyolysis may be associated with a low FENa. Diuretic use in patients who have prerenal azotemia, adrenal insufficiency, chronic tubulointerstitial injury, or bicarbonaturia may have a relatively high FENa. In the last case, the fractional excretion of chloride, which is calculated in an analogous way, will be appropriately low (<1%). Finally, the early stages of AKI from glomerulonephritis, transplant allograft rejection, or urinary obstruction may be associated with a low FENa.

10. **What is the pathophysiology of acute tubular necrosis?**
    Renal ischemia, toxic injury to the kidney, or a combination of these insults can cause prolonged loss of renal function. Physiologically, decreased GFR must result from an alteration in glomerular hemodynamic factors, such as a decrease in the effective surface area or permeability of the glomerulus (Kf), a decrease in glomerular blood flow, or an abnormality in tubular integrity, including obstruction of tubular flow by cellular debris or back leak of ultrafiltrate through a porous tubule. In fact, each of these pathogenic features can be shown to be operant in some experimental models of AKI.

11. **How does acute tubular necrosis evolve?**
    The major mechanism by which renal failure is induced may be different from the primary mechanism by which it is maintained. For example, in ischemic AKI, decreases in renal and glomerular blood flow

may cause the initial loss of renal function. However, tubular necrosis, with its attendant obstructing debris and back leak of ultrafiltrate, maintains the low GFR. The tubular mechanisms are usually important in the maintenance of AKI from most causes seen clinically. Therefore pharmacologic efforts to improve renal blood flow are not, by themselves, generally effective in shortening the duration of AKI. Interestingly, modern ATN appears to recover much less quickly than when the syndrome was first described. This slow recovery may be related to repeated bouts of renal ischemia, which can be attributed to altered renal vasodilation related to the initial ATN insult. Therefore even mild degrees of hypotension should be avoided when treating patients with ATN.

12. How is acute tubular necrosis prevented?

ATN often occurs after surgery or during preexisting volume depletion. In these settings, nephrotoxic drugs, such as radiocontrast dye, aminoglycosides, amphotericin B, nonsteroidal anti-inflammatory agents, and some cancer chemotherapeutic agents (e.g., cisplatin, methotrexate), are far more potent in causing AKI. Optimizing volume status and establishing a relatively high rate of urine flow may minimize the risk of AKI. N-acetylcysteine theoretically scavenges free radicals generated in contrast administration, may prevent contrast induced nephropathy, and appears to be low risk. The generally accepted practice is to use the lowest dose possible of isosmotic contrast and give cautious volume expansion with sodium chloride or sodium bicarbonate before contrast administration. While contrast can be removed with hemodialysis, there is no evidence that this is beneficial, perhaps because the volume of contrast administered is minimal and delivery of contrast to the kidney is almost immediate. Mannitol, fenoldopam, and dopamine are not effective in preventing or managing AKI, and in some cases may be harmful.

13. What are the treatment options in acute tubular necrosis?

ATN is best treated, as previously discussed, by prevention. Because nonoliguric ATN is associated with lower mortality and morbidity rates than oliguric ATN, some excitement exists about the administration of high-dose loop diuretics in concert with low doses of dopamine. This therapy, which converts oliguric ATN in some patients to a nonoliguric state, certainly facilitates the management of volume. However, it is not clear whether these pharmacologic interventions actually improve the prognosis. Optimizations of fluid status and avoidance of and/or therapy for electrolyte disorders are the mainstays of conservative management of AKI.

14. Which critical electrolyte disorders accompany acute kidney injury?

The most common electrolyte disorders that accompany AKI include hyperkalemia, hypermagnesemia, hyperphosphatemia, hypocalcemia, and acidosis (Table 42.3). Of these disorders, hyperkalemia is the most common and probably the one that is usually most serious.

Hyperkalemia most commonly occurs with oliguric ATN or urinary obstruction. It is truly a medical emergency. A serum potassium level above 6.0 mEq/L mandates electrocardiography, to evaluate

Table 47-3. Electrolyte Disturbances in Acute Renal Failure

DISORDER	MECHANISM	FREQUENCY	CLINICAL IMPORTANCE
Hyperkalemia	Decreased K excretion Increased catabolism	Common, especially with oliguric AKI	Life threatening
Hypermagnesemia	Decreased Mg excretion	Common but not usually severe unless Mg is administered	Life threatening only if very severe
Hyperphosphatemia	Decreased phosphate excretion Increased catabolism	Common	Serious only if very severe
Hypocalcemia	Loss of 1,25-vitamin D_3 Calcium phosphate precipitation in tissues	Common but not usually severe	Life threatening if very severe
Acidosis	Decreased acid excretion Increased catabolism	Very common	Not usually life threatening

AKI, Acute kidney injury.

for peaked T waves, diminished P-wave amplitude, or prolonged QRS complex. Any of these findings warrants the use of immediate measures to correct hyperkalemia.

15. **What is the uremic syndrome?**
    The uremic syndrome is a symptom complex associated with renal failure. It may occur with chronic and acute renal failure and involves virtually all organs of the body. Major manifestations are nausea and vomiting, pruritus, bleeding disorder, encephalopathy, and pericarditis. In patients who desire aggressive measures, renal replacement therapy (dialysis) can be used to treat uremia. The pathogenesis of the uremic syndrome is still poorly understood; however, neither urea nor creatinine produces any of the known manifestations of uremia.

16. **What are the indications for nonconservative therapy for acute kidney injury?**
    Indications for nonconservative therapy, such as dialysis, include uremic signs or symptoms, fluid overload, intoxication with dialyzable toxin, and/or electrolyte abnormalities that are refractory to conservative management. It has become the standard of care to provide nonconservative therapy when the BUN level exceeds 100 mg/dL or the serum creatinine exceeds 10 mg/dL, especially in the setting of oliguric ATN. These latter guidelines are not absolute and must be interpreted in the light of other clinical features. A meta-analysis found no mortality benefit in early versus late initiation of dialysis for AKI in critical illness, but this has been challenged by a single-center, randomized trial that demonstrated reduced mortality with early initiation of dialysis. Further study is warranted to confirm these results. As with other intensive procedures, communication with patients and families is central to address the goals of care and whether nonconservative therapy (dialysis) is aligned with their goals.

17. **What are the options for nonconservative therapy of acute kidney injury?**
    The three main options for nonconservative therapy of AKI are hemodialysis, peritoneal dialysis, and continuous renal replacement therapy (CRRT). Each option has advantages and disadvantages (Table 47.4), and of course, variations exist of each of these modalities.
    Hemodialysis involves the pumping of blood through an artificial kidney that removes solutes primarily by dialysis along a concentration gradient; water is removed by ultrafiltration driven by a pressure gradient. Peritoneal dialysis involves the repetitive instillation and removal of fluid into and from the peritoneal cavity, respectively. Solute removal again results primarily by dialysis along a concentration gradient, and fluid removal occurs by ultrafiltration driven by an osmotic pressure gradient. Although this method is less efficient and less rapid than hemodialysis, no central venous access, anticoagulation, skilled technician, or expensive equipment is necessary.

Table 47-4. Dialysis Options in the Treatment of Acute Renal Failure

	INTERMITTENT HEMODIALYSIS	PERITONEAL DIALYSIS	CRRT
Access	Venous	Peritoneal catheter	Vascular
Anticoagulation	Yes	No	Yes
Efficiency	+++	+	+
Hours of staffing	~4–5 by dialysis RN	Minimal	24 hours often by intensive care unit nurse
Equipment	Vascular access, dialysis fluid, dialysis machine	Peritoneal catheter, peritoneal dialysis fluid, ± dialysis machine	Vascular access, large amounts of dialysis fluid, dialysis machine
Hemodynamic instability	Possible	Less likely	Possible
Advantages	Efficient and intensive	Little hemodynamic shift	Continuous management of volume status
Disadvantages	Vascular access infection	Peritoneal leaks, peritoneal catheter infection	Intensive monitoring, Immobilization of patient, vascular access infection

CRRT, Continuous renal replacement therapy.

18. What is continuous renal replacement therapy?

CRRT includes a number of treatments characterized by slow, gradual, continuous removal of fluid and electrolytes. Continuous venovenous hemodialysis (CVVHD) is the most widely used method. It involves solute removal by convection and fluid removal by hydrostatic pressure across high-flux membrane. Like conventional dialysis, CVVHD requires central venous access, anticoagulation, skilled staff, and complex equipment. Continuous arteriovenous hemofiltration and dialysis is a technically simple but less efficient form of CRRT. Although each of these techniques has advantages and disadvantages, in general, the expertise of the professionals working at the center is probably the most important factor. Because of the difficulty in orienting nursing staff to continuous dialysis methods, slow low-efficiency daily dialysis has been developed that provides dialysis over approximately one-half of the hours of the day. Of interest, the biocompatibility of the hemodialysis membrane appears to be an important factor in determining outcome, whereas the intensity of the dialysis prescription (i.e., blood flow, dialysate flow) does not appear to be an important factor in determining patient outcomes.

ACKNOWLEDGMENT

The authors wish to acknowledge Drs. Dinkar Kaw, MD, and Joseph I. Shapiro, MD, for the valuable contributions to the previous edition of this chapter.

KEY POINTS: ACUTE KIDNEY INJURY

1. Serum creatinine concentration may be insensitive to the loss of renal function particularly in the nonsteady state.
2. AKI due to ATN may be initiated by one mechanism and maintained by another different mechanism.
3. Results elicited by measures to prevent ATN are far superior to those yielded by efforts to provide treatment.
4. Urinalysis, microscopy, and urine electrolyte and creatinine estimation (fractional excretion) can provide important information about the cause of AKI.
5. Hyperkalemia is an important life-threatening complication of AKI requiring urgent management.
6. Renal replacement therapy, in the form of dialysis, may be indicated for correction of volume status, electrolyte imbalance, and acidosis, if conservative therapy fails.

BIBLIOGRAPHY

1. Basile DP, Anderson MD, Sutton TA. Pathophysiology of acute kidney injury. *Compr Physiol.* 2012;2(2):1303-1353.
2. Esson ML, Schrier RW. Diagnosis and treatment of acute tubular necrosis. *Ann Intern Med.* 2002;137:744-752.
3. Macedo E, Mehta RL. Continuous dialysis therapies: Core Curriculum 2016. *Am J Kidney Dis.* 2016;68(4):645-657.
4. Palevsky PM. Renal replacement therapy: indications and timing. *Crit Care Med.* 2008;36(suppl 4):S224-S228.
5. Perazella MA, Coca SG. Traditional urinary biomarkers in the assessment of hospital-acquired AKI. *Clin J Am Soc Nephrol.* 2012;7(1):167-174.
6. Sharfuddin AA, Weisbord SD, Palevsky PM, et al. Acute kidney injury. In: Skorecki K, Chertow GM, Marsden PA, et al. eds. *Brenner & Rector's The Kidney.* 10th ed. Philadelphia: Elsevier; 2016:958-1011.
7. Wierstra BT, Kadri S, Alomar S, et al. The impact of "early" versus "late" initiation of renal replacement therapy in critical care patients with acute kidney injury: a systematic review and evidence synthesis. *Crit Care.* 2016;20:122.
8. Wiseman AC, Linas S. Disorders of potassium and acid-base balance. *Am J Kidney Dis.* 2005;45:941-949.
9. Zarbock A, Kellum JA, Schmidt C, et al. Effect of early vs delayed initiation of renal replacement therapy on mortality in patients with acute kidney injury: The ELAIN Randomized Clinical Trial. *JAMA.* 2016;315(20):2190-2199.
10. Kidney Disease Improving Global Outcomes (KDIGO), Acute Kidney Injury Work Group. KDIGO Clinical Practice Guideline for Acute Kidney Injury. *Kidney Int Suppl.* 2012;2:1-138.

CHAPTER 48

RENAL REPLACEMENT THERAPY AND RHABDOMYOLYSIS

Stephanie Shieh and Kathleen D. Liu

RENAL REPLACEMENT THERAPY

1. **What are the indications for renal replacement therapy?**
   Indications can be grouped by using the AEIOU mnemonic:
   A: Acidosis (Metabolic): Refractory to bicarbonate administration.
   E: Electrolyte imbalances: Hyperkalemia refractory to medical therapy is the most common.
   I: Ingestions: Some drugs and toxins (and their toxic metabolites) can be cleared with dialysis, including aspirin, lithium, methanol, or ethylene glycol. A drug's dialyzability is dependent on many factors, including size, water solubility, and volume of distribution.
   O: Overload (Volume): Ultrafiltration (volume removal) with dialysis can relieve hypoxemia resulting from fluid overload in the setting of oliguria/anuria.
   U: Uremia: A constellation of varied symptoms due to the buildup of toxins from advanced renal dysfunction. Symptoms and signs of uremia can range from mild (anorexia, nausea, pruritus) to severe (encephalopathy, asterixis, pericarditis); patients may also have clinical platelet dysfunction (bleeding) due to uremia.

2. **List the different modes of renal replacement therapy.**
   Intermittent renal replacement therapies:
   - Intermittent hemodialysis (IHD)
     - Pure ultrafiltration (PUF): Fluid removal without convective or diffusive clearance
   - Hybrid therapies: Sustained low-efficiency (daily) dialysis (SLED)/Prolonged intermittent renal replacement therapy (PIRRT)
     - Sustained low-efficiency diafiltration (SLEDF)
     - Extended daily dialysis (EDD)
     - Slow continuous dialysis (SCD)
   - Continuous renal replacement therapies (CRRT):
     - Peritoneal dialysis (PD)
     - Slow continuous ultrafiltration (SCUF): Fluid removal without convective or diffusive clearance
     - Continuous venovenous hemofiltration (CVVH)
     - Continuous venovenous hemodialysis (CVVHD)
     - Continuous venovenous hemodiafiltration (CVVHDF)

3. **What are hybrid therapies?**
   This term refers to recently developed hybrid modes of dialysis that fall under the broader term PIRRT or SLED. Dialysis can be delivered through a variety of conventional IHD machines (an advantage over CRRT), usually with some minor modifications to allow for slower dialysate flow rates compared with IHD. Therapy is delivered intermittently but over a longer time period (6–12 hours per session) than conventional IHD (3–4 hours per session) and often on a daily basis. Thus hybrid therapies have many of the benefits of CRRT (e.g., more gentle fluid shifts and therefore better hemodynamic stability) without some of the disadvantages (see Question 5).

4. **When should continuous renal replacement therapies or hybrid therapy be considered?**
   CRRT or hybrid therapy should be considered in any critically ill patient with an indication for dialysis. CRRT or hybrid modalities tend to be better tolerated hemodynamically than intermittent dialysis because of slower rates of solute flux and fluid removal, although total fluid removal capacity can be even greater than intermittent dialysis due to the longer duration of therapy. Furthermore, in highly catabolic, critically ill patients, increased clearance with CRRT or hybrid modalities compared with IHD may allow for better control of azotemia, acidosis, and electrolyte abnormalities, including

hyperphosphatemia. Oftentimes, CRRT or hybrid modalities that utilize slower fluid rates are preferred in patients with increased intracranial pressure due to the concern over fluid and osmolar shifts that may exacerbate cerebral swelling. However, IHD is preferable to CRRT in patients with severe, life-threatening hyperkalemia and most ingestions (e.g., ethylene glycol) because clearance per unit time is faster with IHD compared with CRRT.

5. What are some disadvantages of continuous renal replacement therapies?
Because of its continuous nature, CRRT requires long-term relative immobilization of the patient, which can increase the risk for venous thromboembolism, pressure ulcers, and physical decon-ditioning. Continuous anticoagulation may be necessary to prevent filter clotting and subsequent blood loss, and this may increase the bleeding risk. CRRT frequently results in hypothermia, as blood is cooled during transit through the extracorporeal circuit; importantly, this can mask the development of a fever. Lastly, CRRT is highly labor intensive, typically requiring 1:1 nursing, and therefore costly.

6. Define hemofiltration, hemodialysis, and hemodiafiltration.
   • Hemofiltration: Plasma is forced from the blood space into the effluent via the application of pres-sure across a highly permeable membrane. This results in *convective* clearance of small and mid-dle-sized molecules through the physical property of solvent drag. This modality does not signifi-cantly change the concentration of serum electrolytes and waste products unless a replacement fluid is infused into the blood, effectively diluting out those solutes the physician wishes to remove (e.g., urea nitrogen and potassium) and increasing the concentration of those solutes in which the patient might be deficient (e.g., bicarbonate in a patient with acidemia).
   • Hemodialysis: Blood flows on one side of a semipermeable membrane, and the dialysate, which contains various electrolytes, flows along the other side, usually in the opposite (countercurrent) direction. A concentration gradient drives electrolytes and water-soluble waste products from the plasma compartment into the dialysate. The dialysis machine generates a pressure across the membrane to drive plasma water from the blood side to the dialysate side. Dialysis results in *diffusive* clearance, preferentially of small molecules.
   • Hemodiafiltration: This technique makes simultaneous use of hemofiltration and hemodialysis, resulting in both diffusive and convective clearance.

7. List the basic components of a prescription for intermittent hemodialysis and for continuous renal replacement therapies.
IHD:
   • Dialysis access: Arteriovenous fistula, arteriovenous graft, tunneled or temporary dialysis catheter
   • Treatment duration: For most patients with end-stage renal disease, this ranges between 3 and 4 hours. When a patient with acute renal failure or acute kidney injury (AKI) starts hemodialysis, initial sessions are shorter, with slower blood flow and dialysate flow rates to prevent disequilibrium syndrome.
   • Filter size and type: Biocompatible dialysis membranes are now routinely used.
   • Blood flow rate: Blood flow rates of up to 400 to 450 mL/min can be achieved with an arteriovenous fistula or graft and up to 350 mL/min with a tunneled or temporary catheter. Generally, the faster the flow, the more efficient the dialysis.
   • Dialysate flow rate: Typical flow rates range from 500 mL/min to 800 mL/min.
   • Dialysate bath: Concentrations of potassium, sodium, calcium, and bicarbonate can be customized on the basis of the patient's laboratory studies.
   • Ultrafiltration goal: This is the amount of fluid to be removed from the patient over the course of the session; determined by clinical assessment of the patient's volume status.
   • Anticoagulation: Clotting within the dialysis circuit can result in significant blood loss; heparin is typically used unless the patient has a contraindication.
CRRT:
   • As in IHD, the prescription includes dialysis access, filter size and type, hourly fluid balance, and anticoagulation. An alternative to heparin anticoagulation often used with CRRT is regional citrate anticoagulation, in which citrate is administered to chelate calcium, a critical cofactor in the clot-ting cascade. Arteriovenous fistulas and grafts are not typically used for CRRT, as the prolonged nature of the therapy can damage these types of access over time.
   • Blood flow rates are typically slower than in intermittent dialysis (150–250 mL/min).
   • Mode of therapy: CVVH, CVVHD, or CVVHDF
   • Dialysate or replacement fluid: The specific fluid is based on the metabolic parameters of the patient, including the patient's acid-base status and serum potassium concentration.

- Dialysate or replacement fluid flow rate: Dosing is weight-based and is typically prescribed to achieve a delivered dose of 20 to 25 mL/kg/h at a dose of 20 to 25 mL/kg/h. Studies have shown no mortality difference between patients with renal replacement therapy (RRT) administered at this rate or a higher rate (e.g., 35 mL/kg/h).

8. What kinds of laboratory tests should be ordered regularly for patients receiving continuous renal replacement therapies?
   Sodium, potassium, bicarbonate, calcium, and phosphate levels can change rapidly during CRRT. Hyperphosphatemia frequently occurs in IHD because of inefficient clearance of phosphate, but hypophosphatemia is more common during CRRT, given the continuous clearance of phosphate. Hypocalcemia and hypomagnesemia are also seen, especially when these cations are complexed with citrate (e.g., when citrate is used as an anticoagulant) or when a replacement fluid without these cations is infused into the patient (e.g., during CVVH). Patients with impaired lactate metabolism (e.g., because of severe sepsis or hepatic failure) may have high systemic lactate levels if the dialysate or replacement fluid contains lactate as a base equivalent. In these cases, high lactate levels or worsening acidosis should prompt the use of a bicarbonate-based dialysate or replacement fluid. The patient's acid-base status should be monitored by blood gas measurements.

9. What are nutrition considerations for patients with acute kidney injury receiving renal replacement therapy?
   - **Amino acids** are lost in both IHD and CRRT. Critically ill patients with AKI are often highly catabolic; many patients receiving CRRT will require at least 1.5 to 2 g/kg/day of protein or amino acids.
   - **Vitamins:** Water-soluble vitamins are lost in both IHD and CRRT. Replacement of these vitamins can be achieved with the daily administration of a vitamin complex specifically designed for patients receiving RRT. Fat-soluble vitamins are protein or lipoprotein-bound and are therefore not significantly cleared by CRRT or IHD.
   - **Trace minerals**, such as zinc, may be dialyzed with IHD or CRRT; the benefit of supplementation in this situation remains unproven. Aluminum-containing products, which were used in the past as phosphorus binders, should be avoided for any substantial period of time because of potential for aluminum accumulation resulting in central nervous system toxicity.

10. What are the complications of continuous renal replacement therapies?
    Among the most important risks of CRRT are the risks inherent in obtaining central venous access. In general, subclavian venous access should be avoided, given the risk of subclavian stenosis with an indwelling catheter, particularly among patients who might require long-term hemodialysis. Electrolyte abnormalities or hypovolemia may also develop with CRRT. Patients may have hypothermia because of heat loss, which may mask a febrile response to infection.

KEY POINTS: RENAL REPLACEMENT THERAPY AND RHABDOMYOLYSIS

Potential Advantages of Continuous Renal Replacement Therapies or Hybrid Therapies Over Intermittent Hemodialysis
1. Hemodynamic stability
2. Capacity for increased volume removal
3. Increased clearance of nitrogenous wastes
4. Improved control of acidosis
5. Fewer fluctuations in intracranial pressure

RHABDOMYOLYSIS

11. What causes rhabdomyolysis?
    Muscle ischemia, damage, and eventual necrosis lead to rhabdomyolysis. The various causes are grouped into physical and nonphysical causes in Box 48.1. Both groups of causes probably share a common pathway in which increased demand on muscle cells and their mitochondria, because of intrinsic deficiencies or extrinsic forces (i.e., decreased oxygen delivery or increased metabolic demands), leads to ischemia and eventual damage.

12. Discuss the symptoms and signs of rhabdomyolysis.
    The classic presentation of rhabdomyolysis, consisting of myalgias, weakness, and dark urine, is rare, and often only one or two of these symptoms are present. A history suggestive of muscle

---

Box 48-1. Major Causes of Rhabdomyolysis

Physical Causes
- Trauma and compression
- Occlusion or hypoperfusion of the muscular vessels
- Excessive muscle strain: exercise, seizure, tetanus, delirium tremens
- Electrical current
- Hyperthermia: exercise, sepsis, neuroleptic malignant syndrome, malignant hyperthermia

Nonphysical Causes
- Metabolic myopathies, including McArdle disease, mitochondrial respiratory chain enzyme deficiencies, carnitine palmitoyl transferase deficiency, phosphofructokinase deficiency
- Endocrinopathies, including hypothyroidism and diabetic ketoacidosis (due to electrolyte abnormalities)
- Drugs and toxins, including medications (antimalarials, colchicine, corticosteroids, fibrates, HMG-CoA reductase inhibitors, isoniazid, zidovudine), drugs of abuse (alcohol, heroin), and toxins (insect and snake venoms)
- Infections (either local or systemic)
- Electrolyte abnormalities: Hyperosmotic conditions, hypokalemia, hypophosphatemia, hyponatremia, or hypernatremia
- Autoimmune diseases: Polymyositis or dermatomyositis

HMG-CoA, 3-Hydroxy-3-methylglutaryl–coenzyme A.

---

compression, a physical examination demonstrating muscle tenderness, and laboratory tests confirming muscle damage (e.g., elevated creatine phosphokinase [CPK] level) lead to a strong presumptive diagnosis.

13. **What laboratory tests should be ordered to diagnose rhabdomyolysis?**
CPK activity is the most sensitive indicator of muscle damage; it may continue to increase for several days after the original insult. Hyperkalemia, hyperuricemia, and hyperphosphatemia also occur, as these substances are released from damaged muscle cells. Hypocalcemia develops as calcium is chelated and deposited in the damaged muscle tissue. Lactic acidosis and an anion gap metabolic acidosis can result from release of other organic acids from cells.

14. **What are the complications of rhabdomyolysis?**
The most immediate concern is hyperkalemia due to cell necrosis, particularly in the setting of AKI, which occurs through several mechanisms. Damaged myocytes release myoglobin and its metabolites, which precipitate with other cellular debris to form pigmented casts in renal tubules, obstructing urinary flow. Third-spacing of fluids, particularly at the site of muscle injury, can lead to both intravascular hypovolemia with impaired renal perfusion and compartment syndrome. Furthermore, precipitation of myoglobin in the kidney can initiate a cytokine cascade that leads to renal vasoconstriction, further exacerbating acute renal failure.
    Although patients usually have hypocalcemia, they rarely have symptoms. Caution should be exercised when treating hypocalcemia because patients often have rebound hypercalcemia during the recovery phase. Symptoms of hypocalcemia, such as tetany, Chvostek or Trousseau signs, or cardiac arrhythmias, should be treated promptly with intravenous calcium supplementation. Other immediate concerns include hypovolemia, particularly in the setting of crush injuries or other causes of compression injury.

15. **What treatment options are available?**
Supportive care, with intravascular volume repletion and prevention of continued renal insult, is the main strategy. In general, fluids should be instilled at a rate sufficient to result in an hourly urine output of 200 to 300 mL. Although limited clinical evidence supports this strategy, using sodium bicarbonate–based crystalloids to alkalinize the urine theoretically improves the solubility of myoglobin and decreases its direct tubular toxicity. The evidence supporting use of mannitol as well as diuretics is unclear, and currently both of these therapies are not routinely used in management of rhabdomyolysis. Allopurinol, dosed for the degree of renal impairment, reduces the production of uric acid, which can crystallize in the tubules along with myoglobin, but is also not routinely used in the management of rhabdomyolysis. Control of hyperkalemia, which may require the provision of dialysis, and treatment of symptomatic hypocalcemia are important parts of the treatment regimen.

16. **What kinds of prophylactic management options are possible?**
Guidelines for the treatment of catastrophic crush injuries (developed in response to natural disasters including earthquakes) recommend the initiation of volume resuscitation with crystalloid even before extrication. In the first 24 hours, up to 10 L of intravascular volume may be lost as sequestrated fluid in the affected limb. Administration of up to 10 to 12 L of fluid may be required during this period, with careful monitoring of urine output.

17. **What drugs need to be avoided in patients with rhabdomyolysis?**
Succinylcholine, a drug used for rapid muscle paralysis to achieve airway control, causes generalized depolarization of neuromuscular junctions and can cause hyperkalemia if the patient has abnormal proliferations of the motor end plates. Patients with rhabdomyolysis often have hyperkalemia, and therefore succinylcholine should generally be avoided, given the often lethal nature of these hyperkalemic events. In addition, medications that are known to be associated with rhabdomyolysis (e.g., 3-hydroxy-3-methylglutaryl–coenzyme A [HMG-CoA] reductase inhibitors) should be avoided, if possible.

KEY POINTS: RENAL REPLACEMENT THERAPY AND RHABDOMYOLYSIS

Management of Rhabdomyolysis
1. Volume resuscitation
2. Vigilance for hyperkalemia and treatment with dialysis or other supportive measures, if necessary
3. Treatment of symptomatic hypocalcemia
4. Alkalinizationof urine with sodium bicarbonate (limited data)

ACID-BASE INTERPRETATION

18. **Identify the normal extracellular pH, and define acidosis and alkalosis.**
The range for the normal extracellular pH in arterial blood is considered to be 7.37 to 7.43. Of note, the normal pH in venous blood is slightly lower (by 0.05 pH units on average); the lower venous pH results from the uptake of metabolically produced carbon dioxide in the capillary circulation. *Acidemia* is defined as an increase in the hydrogen ion concentration of the blood, resulting in a decrease in pH, and *alkalemia* is defined as a decrease in the hydrogen ion concentration in the blood, resulting in an increase in pH. Acidosis and alkalosis refer to processes that lower or raise the pH, respectively. These processes can be either metabolic or respiratory in origin and, occasionally, a combination of both.

19. **What information is necessary to properly interpret a patient's acid-base status?**
To accurately interpret a patient's acid-base status, an arterial blood gas analysis, serum electrolyte concentrations, and the serum albumin concentration are needed.

20. **What is the anion gap, how is it calculated, and why is it important in understanding a patient's acid-base status?**
The anion gap is defined as the difference between the plasma concentrations of the major cation (sodium) and the major *measured* anions (chloride and bicarbonate), expressed mathematically by the following equation:

$$\text{Anion gap} = [Na^+] - ([Cl^-] + [HCO_3^-])$$

A normal anion gap is generally considered to be 8 to 12 in a patient with a normal serum albumin concentration of 4.0 g/dL. In patients with hypoalbuminemia, the anion gap should be "corrected" by adding 2.5 to the calculated anion gap for every 1 g/dL decrease in albumin concentration from 4.0 g/dL. The anion gap is elevated in processes that result in an increase in the plasma concentration of anions that are not routinely measured in conventional chemistry panels, including lactate, phosphates, sulfates, and other organic anions (such as the degradation products of commonly ingested alcohols). Calculating the anion gap is critical when assessing a patient's acid-base status, because an elevated anion gap may alert the physician to the presence of a metabolic acidosis that might not be apparent on first glance of the arterial blood gas values. Accordingly, the anion gap should always be calculated when assessing a patient's acid-base status. Furthermore, the different diagnosis of a metabolic acidosis is largely influenced by the presence or absence of an elevated anion gap (see later).

21. Describe an approach to a comprehensive interpretation of a patient's acid-base status using the arterial blood gas and the serum chemistry values.
    1. Identify whether the patient has acidemia or alkalemia: If the pH is less than 7.37, the patient has acidemia, and if the pH is greater than 7.43, the patient has alkalemia. Importantly, a pH between 7.37 and 7.43 **does not** necessarily imply that the patient does not have an acid-base disturbance; rather it could suggest the presence of a mixed acid-base disorder.
    2. Determine whether the primary disturbance is respiratory or metabolic: If the patient has acidemia and the PCO_2 is greater than 40 mm Hg, then the primary process is respiratory; if the patient has acidemia and the serum bicarbonate concentration is less than 24 mEq/L, then the primary process is metabolic. If the patient has alkalemia and the PCO_2 is less than 40 mm Hg, then the primary process is respiratory; if the patient has alkalemia and the serum bicarbonate concentration is greater than 24 mEq/L, then the primary process is metabolic.
    3. Determine whether appropriate compensation for the primary disorder is present: To determine how the kidneys compensate for a primary respiratory process and vice versa, see Table 48.1. If the compensation is less than or greater than predicted, then another primary acid-base disturbance might be present. For example, in presence of a metabolic acidosis, if the PCO_2 is lower than expected, a concomitant primary respiratory alkalosis is present, whereas if the PCO_2 is higher than expected, a concomitant primary respiratory acidosis is present.
    4. Calculate the anion gap to look for the presence of an anion gap metabolic acidosis.
    5. Calculate the *delta-delta*: In the presence of an isolated anion gap metabolic acidosis, the serum bicarbonate concentration should fall by an amount that equals the degree to which the anion gap is raised. If this is not the case, another metabolic disorder (either a non–anion gap metabolic acidosis or a metabolic alkalosis) is present. This can be determined by calculating the delta-delta, which is mathematically expressed as follows:

$$\text{Delta–delta} = \frac{\text{Calculated anion gap} - \text{Normal anion gap}}{\text{Normal serum bicarbonate} - \text{Measured serum bicarbonate}}$$

Generally, 12 is used as the value of a normal anion gap, and 24 is used as the value for a normal serum bicarbonate. If the delta-delta is between 1 and 2, the disturbance is a pure anion gap metabolic acidosis. If the quotient is less than 1, a non–anion gap metabolic acidosis is also present, whereas if the quotient is greater than 2, a metabolic alkalosis is also present.

After all of these steps have been completed, the physician should have an assessment of all of the acid-base disorders present and should use the clinical information to determine the underlying cause(s).

22. List the differential diagnoses of the major acid-base disturbances.
    Each of the primary acid-base disturbances has a varied number of causes, and many acronyms have been generated to help the student or physician remember them. Of these, the most popular is the

Table 48-1. Appropriate Compensation for Primary Acid-Base Disturbances and Their Common Causes

PRIMARY ACID-BASE DISTURBANCE	SUBTYPE	EXPECTED COMPENSATION
Metabolic acidosis	Anion gap	Decrease in $PCO_2 = 1.2 \times \Delta HCO_3$ **or** $PCO_2 = (1.5 \times HCO_3) + 8 \pm 2$
	Non–anion gap	—
Metabolic alkalosis	—	Increase in $PCO_2 = 0.7 \times \Delta HCO_3$
Respiratory acidosis	Acute	Increase in $HCO_3 = 0.1 \times \Delta PCO_2$
	Chronic	Increase in $HCO_3 = 0.35 \times \Delta PCO_2$
Respiratory alkalosis	Acute	Decrease in $HCO_3 = 0.2 \times \Delta PCO_2$
	Chronic	Decrease in $HCO_3 = 0.4 \times \Delta PCO_2$

Box 48-2. Differential Diagnoses of the Primary Acid-Base Disturbances

Anion Gap Metabolic Acidosis

Common causes can be remembered with the *GOLDMARK* mnemonic:

Glycols (ethylene and propylene; propylene glycol is the carrier for certain medications, including intravenous lorazepam)

Oxoproline (acetaminophen ingestion)

L-lactate

D-lactate

Methanol

Aspirin

Renal failure (with accumulation of organic anions, including phosphates and sulfates)

Ketoacidosis (diabetes, alcoholic, starvation)

Non–Anion Gap Metabolic Acidosis

- Gastrointestinal loss of bicarbonate: Diarrhea, intestinal or pancreatic fistulas or drainage
- Renal dysfunction: Renal failure (leading to impaired ammoniagenesis) or renal tubular acidosis
- Dilutional: Caused by rapid infusion of bicarbonate-free fluids, such as normal saline
- Posthypocapnia
- Ureteral diversion

Metabolic Alkalosis

- Gastrointestinal loss of hydrogen ions: Removal of gastric secretions (vomiting, nasogastric tube suction)
- Renal loss of hydrogen ions: Primary mineralocorticoid excess, administration of thiazide or loop diuretics, posthypercapneic alkalosis, milk-alkali syndrome with associated hypercalcemia, congenital syndromes (Bartter syndrome and Gitelman syndrome)

Respiratory Acidosis

- Neuromuscular diseases: Guillain-Barré syndrome, myasthenia gravis, botulism, hypophosphatemia and hypokalemia, poliomyelitis, diaphragmatic dysfunction
- Central hypoventilation: Congenital central hypoventilation syndrome (Ondine curse), obesity hypoventilation syndrome, Cheyne-Stokes breathing
- Medications that depress respiratory drive: Narcotics, benzodiazepines, barbiturates, heroin
- Endocrine causes: Hypothyroidism
- Airway obstruction: Epiglottitis, chronic obstructive pulmonary disease, severe and late phase asthma
- Trauma leading to chest wall abnormalities or restrictive lung disease from severe kyphoscoliosis

Respiratory Alkalosis

- Central nervous system process: Stroke, infection, trauma, tumor
- Hypoxemia
- Hyperthermia
- Sepsis
- Liver disease
- Pain or anxiety (a diagnosis of exclusion)
- Medications: Medroxyprogesterone, theophylline, salicylates
- Pregnancy

MUDPILES acronym for the differential diagnosis of an anion-gap metabolic acidosis. However, the acronym of GOLDMARK has recently been used to reflect an update on a differential for anion gap metabolic acidosis (Box 48.2). If an anion gap acidosis is present, the osmolar gap should be measured and calculated; the presence of an osmolar gap in addition to an anion gap suggests a toxic alcohol ingestion, such as ethylene glycol, methanol, or ethanol. A more comprehensive differential diagnosis for each of the primary disturbances is presented in Box 48.2.

ACKNOWLEDGEMENT

The authors wish to acknowledge Dr. Brad W. Butcher, MD, for the valuable contributions to the previous edition of this chapter.

KEY POINTS: RENAL REPLACEMENT THERAPY AND RHABDOMYOLYSIS

Acid-base Disorders

1. An organized approach to the analysis of acid-base disorders is key.
2. The approach starts by determining whether the patient has acidemia or alkalemia; note that the presence of a normal serum pH does not imply that an acid-base disorder is not present.
3. Determine whether the primary process is metabolic or respiratory.
4. Determine whether there is appropriate componsation for the primary process.
5. Calculate the anion gap and the "delta-delta" to determine whether unrecognized metabolic disturbances exist, including gap and non-gap metabolic acidosis and metabolic alkalosis.

BIBLIOGRAPHY

1. Bellomo R, Cass A, Cole L, et al. Intensity of continuous renal-replacement therapy in critically ill patients. *N Engl J Med.* 2009;361:1627-1638.
2. Huerta-Alardin AL, Varon J, Marik PE. Bench-to-bedside review: rhabdomyolysis—an overview for clinicians. *Crit Care.* 2005;9:158-169.
3. Malinoski DJ, Slater MS, Mullins RJ. Crush injury and rhabdomyolysis. *Crit Care Clin.* 2004;20:171-192.
4. Golper TA. Sustained low efficiency or extended daily dialysis. Available at UptoDate.com. Accessed January 13, 2016.
5. McClave SA, Martindale RG, Vanek VW, et al. Guidelines for the provision and assessment of nutrition support therapy in the adult critically ill patient: Society of critical care medicine (SCCM) and American society for parenteral and enteral nutrition (A.S.P.E.N.). *JPEN J Parenter Enteral Nutr.* 2009;33:277-316.
6. Mehta AN, Emmett JB, Emmett M. GOLD MARK: an anion gap mnemonic for the 21st century. *Lancet.* 2008;372:892.
7. Palevsky PM. Prevention and treatment of heme pigment-induced acute kidney injury (acute renal failure). Available at UptoDate.com. Accessed August 04, 2017.
8. Palevsky PM, Zhang JH, O'Connor TZ, et al. Intensity of renal support in critically ill patients with acute kidney injury. *N Engl J Med.* 2008;359:7-20.
9. Vanholder R, Sever MS, Erek E, et al. Rhabdomyolysis. *J Am Soc Nephrol.* 2000;11:1553-1561.

HYPOKALEMIA AND HYPERKALEMIA

Alan C. Pao

CHAPTER 49

HYPOKALEMIA

1. **Is serum potassium concentration an accurate estimate of total body potassium?**
   No. The majority of potassium is distributed in the intracellular fluid (ICF) compartment, with only approximately 2% of the total body potassium in the extracellular fluid (ECF) compartment. Alterations in serum potassium concentration can result from changes in distribution of potassium between ECF and ICF compartments (internal potassium balance) or from changes in total body potassium (external potassium balance).

2. **What are the factors that dictate serum potassium concentration?**
   Plasma potassium concentration is tightly regulated between 3.5 and 5.3 mEq/L and is determined by internal and external balance. Insulin and catecholamines primarily regulate internal distribution of potassium. The kidneys, and to a lesser extent the gut, regulate external balance of potassium.

3. **Why is tight regulation of serum potassium concentrations so critical?**
   Although a small fraction of total body potassium is in the ECF compartment, changes in ECF potassium concentration, either by compartmental shifts or by net gain or loss, significantly alter the ratio of ECF to ICF potassium concentration, which determines the resting membrane potential of cells. As a consequence, small fluctuations in ECF potassium concentration can have profound effects on cardiac and neuromuscular excitability.

4. **When does serum potassium concentration falsely estimate total body potassium?**
   Transcellular shifts of potassium between ECF and ICF compartments can have profound effects on serum potassium concentration. Buffering of the ECF compartment, with reciprocal movement of potassium and hydrogen across the cell membrane, can raise serum potassium concentration in the case of acidemia and lower serum potassium concentration in the case of alkalemia. Two hormones that are known to drive potassium into the ICF compartment are insulin and catecholamines.

   The classic example of how serum potassium concentration falsely estimates total body potassium is a patient with diabetic ketoacidosis. Insulin deficiency and acidemia cause potassium to shift into the ECF compartment so that serum potassium concentration may be normal or high despite profound total body potassium depletion (due to osmotic diuresis and hyperaldosterone state). Only after treatment of insulin deficiency and acidosis does the total body potassium depletion become apparent.

5. **How do you estimate the total body potassium deficit?**
   It is difficult to predict accurately the total body potassium deficit on the basis of the serum potassium concentration, but in uncomplicated potassium depletion, a useful rule of thumb is as follows: For each 100 mEq deficit in potassium, serum potassium concentration should fall by 0.27 mEq/L. Thus, for a 70-kg patient, a serum potassium concentration of 3 mEq/L reflects a 300- to 400-mEq deficit, whereas a serum potassium concentration of 2 mEq/L reflects a 500- to 700-mEq deficit. In patients with acid-base disorders, this rule of thumb is not accurate because of compartmental shifts in potassium.

6. **What is the relationship between serum potassium and magnesium concentrations?**
   Magnesium depletion typically occurs after diuretic use, sustained alcohol consumption, or diabetic ketoacidosis. Magnesium depletion can cause hypokalemia that is refractory to treatment with oral or intravenous (IV) potassium. In the setting of severe magnesium and potassium depletion, magnesium and potassium should be replaced simultaneously. Magnesium depletion may cause renal potassium wasting by lowering intracellular magnesium concentration in the principal cells of the distal nephron where renal outer medullary potassium (ROMK) channels reside. Magnesium normally binds and

315

blocks the channel pore of ROMK to limit efflux of potassium from the cell and into the tubular lumen. When hypomagnesemia develops, intracellular magnesium falls, thereby releasing magnesium-dependent inhibition of ROMK and increasing distal potassium secretion into the urine.

7. **What are the key factors that stimulate urine potassium excretion?**
Key factors that stimulate urine potassium excretion include an increase in serum potassium concentration, an increase in sodium delivery to the distal nephron, an increase in aldosterone secretion, and an increase in renal tubular flow. An increase in sodium delivery to the distal nephron, combined with an increase in aldosterone secretion stimulate tubular reabsorption of sodium through the epithelial sodium channel (ENaO), which generates a negative potential across the distal tubule lumen and stimulates electrogenic potassium excretion through ROMK. An increase in renal tubular flow can also stimulate electrogenic potassium excretion through big potassium (BK) channels in the distal nephron.

8. **What are the causes of hypokalemia?**
   - Low potassium intake: Poor oral intake or total parenteral nutrition with inadequate potassium supplementation.
   - Intracellular potassium shift: Metabolic alkalosis, increased insulin availability, increased β_2-adrenergic activity, and periodic paralysis (classically associated with thyrotoxicosis).
   - Gastrointestinal (GI) potassium loss: Diarrhea.
   - Renal potassium loss: Diuretics, vomiting, states of mineralocorticoid excess (e.g., primary hyperaldosteronism, Cushing disease, European licorice ingestion, and renal artery stenosis), hypomagnesemia, high urine flow states (post acute tubular necrosis [ATN] diuresis and post obstructive diuresis), and familial hypokalemic alkalosis syndromes (Bartter, Gitelman, and Liddle syndromes).

9. **What are the clinical manifestations of hypokalemia?**
By depressing neuromuscular excitability, hypokalemia leads to muscle weakness, which can include quadriplegia and hypoventilation. Severe hypokalemia disrupts cell integrity, leading to rhabdomyolysis. Among the most important manifestations of hypokalemia are cardiac arrhythmias, including paroxysmal atrial tachycardia with block, atrioventricular dissociation, first- and second-degree atrioventricular block with Wenckebach periods, and even ventricular tachycardia or fibrillation. Typical electrocardiographic (ECG) findings include ST-segment depression, flattened T waves, and prominent U waves.

10. **Which drugs can cause hypokalemia?**
The most common drugs are diuretics: acetazolamide, loop diuretics, and thiazides. Penicillin and penicillin analogs (e.g., carbenicillin, ticarcillin, piperacillin) cause renal potassium wasting by increasing delivery of non-reabsorbable anions to the distal nephron, which results in potassium trapping in the urine. Drugs that damage renal tubular membranes such as amphotericin, cisplatin, and aminoglycosides can cause renal potassium wasting, even in the absence of a decrease in glomerular filtration rate (GFR).

11. **What is the diagnostic approach to a patient with hypokalemia?**
After eliminating spurious causes (such as leukocytosis), the diagnosis of true hypokalemia can be approached on the basis of spot urine potassium and urine creatinine concentrations, acid-base status, urine chloride concentration, and blood pressure (Fig. 49.1). A spot urine potassium to creatinine ratio (U_K+/U_{Cr}) less than 15 mEq K$^+$/g creatinine indicates an extrarenal cause of hypokalemia (e.g., poor oral intake, GI loss, or intracellular shift), whereas a spot U_K+/U_{Cr} greater than 15 mEq K$^+$/g creatinine indicates renal cause of hypokalemia (i.e., renal potassium wasting).

12. **Why is serum potassium concentration often low in patients with myocardial infarction or acute asthma?**
Both conditions activate the sympathetic nervous system and are associated with high levels of catecholamines, which induce shifting of potassium into the ICF compartment. If patients with myocardial infarction are also taking diuretics for hypertension, these patients may be at additional risk for catecholamine-induced hypokalemia because of concomitant total body potassium depletion. If patients with asthma are also acutely being treated with β_2-adrenergic agonists, additional potassium may be shifted into the ICF compartment and serum potassium concentration may be further lowered.

13. **How do you treat hypokalemia in the setting of potassium depletion?**
Oral replacement is the safest route, and administration of doses of up to 40 mEq three times daily is allowed. In most cases, potassium chloride is used because metabolic alkalosis and chloride depletion often accompany hypokalemia, such as in patients who are taking diuretics or who are vomiting.

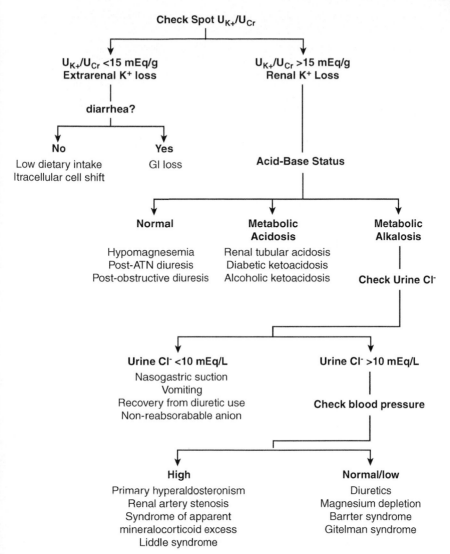

Figure 49-1. Algorithm for diagnosis of hypokalemia. *ATN,* Acute tubular necrosis; *Cl⁻,* chloride; *Cr,* creatinine; *GI,* gastro-intestinal; K⁺, potassium; *mEq/g,* milli-equivalents of potassium/gram of creatinine; *mEq/L,* milli-equivalents of chloride/liter of urine; *U,* urine.

In these settings, coadministration of chloride is important for the correction of both the metabolic alkalosis and hypokalemia. In other settings, potassium should be administered with alternative salt preparations. For example, in metabolic acidosis, replacement with potassium bicarbonate or bicarbonate equivalent (e.g., potassium citrate, acetate, or gluconate) can help alleviate the acidosis. Persons who abuse alcohol or who have diabetes with ketoacidosis often have concomitant phosphate deficiency and should receive some potassium in the form of potassium phosphate.

14. How do you treat hypokalemia in patients requiring loop diuretics?
    Maintaining positive potassium balance in patients requiring loop diuretics is important because hypokalemia increases the risk for cardiac arrhythmias. Increasing dietary or supplemental potassium intake is often inadequate for repletion of total body potassium stores. Administration of amiloride

(ENaC channel inhibitor) and spironolactone or eplerenone (mineralocorticoid receptor antagonist) can be used to limit the degree of renal potassium excretion.

15. **How do you treat hypokalemia in the setting of thyrotoxic periodic paralysis?**
In this condition, hyperthyroid patients develop painless muscle weakness and profound hypokalemia, classically after heavy exercise or ingestion of a carbohydrate-rich meal. Thyroid hormone increases tissue responsiveness to catecholamines and/or insulin, leading to enhanced shifting of potassium into the ICF compartment. In addition to potassium repletion, oral propranolol (nonselective β-blocker) at a dose of 3 mg/kg divided into three times a day is an effective treatment for an acute attack of thyrotoxic periodic paralysis

16. **When is intravenous potassium replacement necessary? What are the risks?**
In life-threatening situations such as severe muscle weakness, respiratory distress, cardiac arrhythmias, or rhabdomyolysis, or in situations when oral administration is not possible, potassium must be replaced intravenously. Infusion rates in the intensive care unit should be limited to 20 mEq/h to prevent the potentially catastrophic effect of a potassium bolus to the heart.

HYPERKALEMIA

17. **What are the causes of hyperkalemia?**
   - High potassium intake: Oral potassium replacement, total parenteral nutrition, and high-dose potassium penicillin, usually in the setting of renal failure.
   - Extracellular potassium shift: Metabolic acidosis, insulin deficiency, β-adrenergic blockade, rhabdomyolysis, massive hemolysis, tumor lysis syndrome, periodic paralysis (hyperkalemic form), and heavily catabolic states such as severe sepsis.
   - Low renal potassium excretion: Renal failure, decreased effective circulating volume (e.g., severe sepsis, congestive heart failure, cirrhosis), and states of hypoaldosteronism. States of hypoaldosteronism include decreased renin-angiotensin-aldosterone system (RAAS) activity (e.g., hyporeninemic hypoaldosteronism in diabetes, interstitial nephritis, angiotensin-converting enzyme (ACE) inhibitors, nonsteroidal anti-inflammatory drugs [NSAIDs]), decreased adrenal synthesis (e.g., Addison disease, heparin), and aldosterone resistance (e.g., high-dose trimethoprim, potassium-sparing diuretic agents).

18. **Which drugs can cause hyperkalemia?**
   - Drugs that release potassium from cells: Succinylcholine and rarely β-blockers.
   - Drugs that block RAAS, thereby decreasing renal potassium excretion: Spironolactone, ACE inhibitors, heparin (low molecular weight and unfractionated), and NSAIDs.
   - Drugs that block sodium and potassium exchange in cells: Digitalis.
   - Drugs that block sodium and potassium exchange in the distal nephron: Calcineurin inhibitors, amiloride, and trimethoprim.

19. **What are the clinical manifestations of hyperkalemia?**
The most serious manifestation of hyperkalemia involves the electrical conduction system of the heart. The correlation between serum potassium concentration and ECG changes depends on the rate of change of serum potassium concentration and the severity of hyperkalemia. ECG changes typically manifest when the serum potassium concentration exceeds 6 to 7 mEq/L in acute hyperkalemia, but more severe hyperkalemia may be required to elicit similar ECG changes in chronic hyperkalemia. Initially, the ECG shows peaked T waves and decreased amplitude of P waves, followed by prolongation of QRS waves. With severe hyperkalemia, QRS and T waves blend together into what appears to be a sine-wave pattern consistent with ventricular fibrillation. Profound hyperkalemia can lead to heart block and asystole. Other effects of hyperkalemia include weakness, neuromuscular paralysis (without central nervous system disturbances), and suppression of renal ammoniagenesis, which may result in metabolic acidosis.

20. **What degree of chronic kidney disease causes hyperkalemia?**
Chronic kidney disease per se is not associated with hyperkalemia until the GFR is reduced to approximately 75% of normal levels (serum creatinine concentration >3 mg/dL). Although more than 85% of filtered potassium is reabsorbed by the proximal tubule, urinary excretion of potassium is determined primarily by potassium secretion along the cortical collecting duct. Hyperkalemia usually results from a reduction in potassium secretion (due either to decreases in aldosterone concentration, as may occur in Addison disease, or to diabetes with hyporeninemic hypoaldosteronism) or from a reduction in sodium delivery to the distal nephron, as may occur in states of decreased circulatory volume.

21. How do states of decreased circulatory volume impair renal potassium excretion?

Renal potassium excretion is primarily dependent on adequate sodium delivery to the distal nephron and an increase in aldosterone secretion. In individuals with decreased circulatory volume (e.g., volume depletion, congestive heart failure, or cirrhosis), aldosterone secretion is increased, which stimulates expression of ENaC in the distal nephron. However, sodium reabsorption in more proximal elements of the kidney tubule can be so intense such that sodium delivery to ENaC is not sufficient and electrogenic sodium reabsorption stops. As a consequence, a negative potential across the distal tubule lumen fails to develop, and electrogenic potassium excretion through ROMK also stops.

22. What is pseudohyperkalemia?

Measurements in serum potassium concentration can be falsely elevated when potassium is released during the process of blood collection from a patient or during the process of clot formation in a specimen tube. These situations do not reflect true hyperkalemia. Potassium release from muscles distal to a tight tourniquet can elevate potassium concentration by as much as 2.7 mEq/L. Potassium release from leukocytes (white blood cell counts $>70,000/mm^3$) or platelets (platelet count $>1,000,000/mm^3$) during the process of clot formation in a specimen tube can also become significant and distort measurements of serum potassium concentration. In these circumstances, an unclotted blood sample (i.e., plasma potassium concentration) should be obtained.

23. What is the diagnostic approach to hyperkalemia?

The cause is often apparent after a careful review of history, medications, and basic laboratory values, including a chemistry panel with blood urea nitrogen and creatinine concentrations. Additional laboratory tests can be performed if clinical suspicion exists for any of the following:

- Pseudohyperkalemia (Look for high white blood cell or platelet counts.)
- Rhabdomyolysis (Look for high creatinine kinase concentration.)
- Tumor lysis syndrome (Look for high lactate dehydrogenase, uric acid, and phosphorus concentrations or low calcium concentration.)
- Hypoaldosterone state (Look for low plasma renin activity, serum aldosterone, or serum cortisol.)

24. What tests can be used to evaluate renal potassium excretion?

A 24-hour urine sample is not helpful in evaluating chronic hyperkalemia because daily urine potassium excretion reflects daily potassium intake under steady state conditions. The ratio between the urine potassium concentration and urine creatinine concentration (U_K+/U_{Cr}) from a spot urine sample can be calculated to estimate of the rate of renal potassium excretion. In cases of hyperkalemia due to extracellular shift or extra-renal K^+ gain, the kidneys should raise urine potassium excretion to a degree such that the U_K+/U_{Cr} greater than 200 mEq K^+/g creatinine. It is noteworthy that the transtubular potassium gradient (TTKG) has been used as an index for estimating the driving force for renal potassium secretion; however, it should no longer be used as a tool for evaluating renal potassium handling because one of the key assumptions in calculating the TTKG is not valid.

25. What are the indications for emergent therapy for hyperkalemia?

- ECG changes: Since cardiac arrest can occur at any point during ECG progression, hyperkalemia with ECG changes constitutes a medical emergency.
- Severe muscle weakness or paralysis.
- Severe hyperkalemia, typically above 6 to 7 mEq/L.

26. How do you treat hyperkalemia?

- Membrane stabilization: Calcium raises the cell depolarization threshold and reduces myocardial irritability. One or two ampules of IV calcium chloride result in improvement in ECG changes within seconds, but the beneficial effect lasts only about 30 minutes.
- Shifting potassium into cells: Administration of IV insulin with glucose begins to lower serum potassium concentrations in approximately 2 to 5 minutes and lasts a few hours. Correction of acidosis with IV sodium bicarbonate has a similar duration and time of onset. Nebulized β-adrenergic agonists such as albuterol can lower serum potassium concentration by 0.5 to 1.5 mEq/L, with an onset of 30 minutes and an effect lasting 2 to 4 hours.
- Removal of potassium: Loop diuretics can sometimes induce enough renal potassium loss in patients with intact renal function, but patients with persistent hyperkalemia typically have impaired renal function and require additional maneuvers to remove potassium from the body. Potassium-binding resins such as sodium polystyrene sulfonate can be administered acutely to remove potassium from the GI tract, although the effect is slow and may take up to 24 hours. It is important to note that sodium polysterene sulfonate should not be administered in sorbitol

because of an elevated risk for intestinal necrosis. Chronic use of potassium-binding resins should be reserved for the new class of oral potassium binding drugs (e.g., patiromer or ZS-9). These agents can be used to prevent hyperkalemia associated with RAAS blockade in individuals with diabetes, heart failure, or chronic kidney disease. Acute hemodialysis is definitive treatment for removing potassium from the body.

ACKNOWLEDGEMENT

The authors wish to acknowledge Drs. Stuart L. Linas, MD, and Shailendra Sharma, MD, for the valuable contributions to the previous edition of this chapter.

KEY POINTS: HYPOKALEMIA AND HYPERKALEMIA

What are the Circumstances Requiring Special Care in Monitoring Potassium Replacement?

1. Patients with defects in potassium excretion (e.g., renal failure, use of potassium-sparing diuretics or ACE inhibitors) must have their serum potassium concentrations monitored frequently when potassium is being replaced to prevent overcorrection.
2. Patients with diabetic ketoacidosis can present with normal or high serum potassium concentration despite having low stores of total body potassium. Treatment of insulin deficiency and acidosis in such patients can lead to severe hypokalemia and unmask profound deficits in total body potassium. Serum potassium concentration must be monitored frequently in the course of insulin therapy, and potassium supplementation should be started before serum potassium concentration falls below 4.0 mEq/L.
3. Patients with significant magnesium deficiency have renal potassium wasting and often must have their serum magnesium concentration corrected simultaneously when therapy for hypokalemia is initiated.

BIBLIOGRAPHY

1. Bronson WR, DeVita VJ, Carbone PP, et al. Pseudohyperkalemia due to release of potassium from white blood cells during clotting. *N Engl J Med.* 1966;274:369-375.
2. Chou TC. Electrolyte imbalance. In: Chou TC, Knilans K, eds. *Electrocardiography in Clinical Practice.* 4th ed. Philadelphia: Saunders; 1996:535-540.
3. Don BR, Sebastian A, Cheitlin M, et al. Pseudohyperkalemia caused by fist clenching during phlebotomy. *N Engl J Med.* 1990;322:1290-1292.
4. Hartman RC, Auditore JV, Jackson DP. Studies on thrombocytosis: 1 Hyperkalemia due to release of potassium from platelets during coagulation. *J Clin Invest.* 1958;37:699-707.
5. Huang CL, Kuo E. Mechanism of hypokalemia in magnesium deficiency. *J Am Soc Nephrol.* 2007;18:2649-2652.
6. Kamel KS, Halperin ML. Intrarenal urea recycling leads to a higher rate of renal excretion of potassium: an hypothesis with clinical implications. *Curr Opin Nephrol Hypertens.* 2011;20:547-554.
7. Kruse JA, Carlson RW. Rapid correction of hypokalemia using concentrated intravenous potassium chloride infusions. *Arch Intern Med.* 1990;150:613-617.
8. Lin SH, Lin YF. Propanolol rapidly reverses paralysis, hypokalemia, and hypophosphatemia in thyrotoxic periodic paralysis. *Am J Kidney Dis.* 2001;37:620-623.
9. Rhee EP, Scott JA, Dighe AS. Case records of the Massachusetts General Hospital. Case 4-2012. A 37-year-old man with muscle pain, weakness, and weight loss. *N Engl J Med.* 2012;366:553-560.
10. Rosa RM, Epstein FH. Extrarenal potassium metabolism. In: Seldin DW, Giebisch G, eds. *The Kidney.* New York: Lippincott Williams & Wilkins; 2000:1551-1552.
11. Rose B, Post TW. Hypokalemia. In: Rose B, Post TW, eds. *Clinical Physiology of Acid–Base and Electrolyte Disorders.* New York: McGraw-Hill; 2001:871-872.
12. Sterns RH, Cox M, Feig PU, et al. Internal potassium balance and the control of the plasma potassium concentration. *Medicine (Baltimore).* 1981;60:339-354.
13. Weiner ID, Wingo CS. Hypokalemia: consequences, causes, and correction. *J Am Soc Nephrol.* 1997;8:1183.
14. Welling PA. Roles and Regulation of Renal K Channels. *Annu Rev Physiol.* 2016;78: 415-435.
15. Whang R, Whang DD, Ryan MP. Refractory potassium repletion. *Arch Intern Med.* 1992;152:40-45.

HYPONATREMIA AND HYPERNATREMIA

Lowell J. Lo and Kathleen D. Liu

CHAPTER 50

1. **Why is sodium balance critical to volume control?**

   Sodium and its corresponding anions represent almost all of the osmotically active solutes in the extracellular fluid under normal conditions. Therefore the serum concentration of sodium reflects the tonicity of extracellular fluids. Serum osmolality is tightly regulated by thirst and antidiuretic hormone (ADH) secretion. Preservation of normal serum osmolality (i.e., 285–295 mOsm/L) guarantees cellular integrity by regulating net movement of water across cellular membranes.

2. **What is another name for antidiuretic hormone? What is its mechanism of action?**

   ADH is also called *arginine vasopressin* or simply *vasopressin*. ADH is a small peptide hormone produced by the hypothalamus that binds to the vasopressin 1 and 2 receptors (V1 and V2). Vasopressin release is regulated by osmoreceptors in the hypothalamus, which are sensitive to changes in plasma osmolality of as little as 1% to 2%. Under hyperosmolar conditions, osmoreceptor stimulation leads to stimulation of thirst and vasopressin release. These two mechanisms result in increased water intake and retention, respectively. Vasopressin release is also regulated by baroreceptors in the carotid sinus and aortic arch; under conditions of reduced effective arterial volume (either hypovolemia or hypoperfusion due to other reasons, such as heart failure), these receptors stimulate vasopressin release to increase water retention by the kidney. At very high concentrations, vasopressin also causes vascular smooth muscle constriction through the V1 receptor, increasing vascular tone and therefore the blood pressure. Accordingly, vasopressin is often administered parenterally as a vasopressor agent in patients with hypotension that is refractory to volume resuscitation.

3. **Does hyponatremia simply mean there is too little sodium in the body?**

   No. The serum sodium concentration is not a reflection of the total body sodium content; instead, it is more representative of changes in the total body water (TBW). With hyponatremia, defined as serum sodium level less than 135 mEq/L, there is too much TBW relative to the amount of total body sodium, thereby lowering its concentration. Despite this key observation, the serum sodium concentration is *not* a reflection of volume status, and it is possible for hyponatremia to develop in states of volume depletion, euvolemia, and volume excess. Assessing a patient's volume status is therefore the key step in identifying the underlying cause of hyponatremia (Fig. 50.1). Helpful physical findings include tachycardia, dry mucous membranes, orthostatic hypotension, increased skin turgor (associated with hypovolemia) or edema, an S_3 gallop, jugular venous distention, and ascites (present in hypervolemic states).

4. **Are *hyponatremia* and *hypo-osmolality* synonymous?**

   No. Hyponatremia can occur without a change in total body sodium or TBW in two settings. The first is pseudohyponatremia, which is a laboratory artifact in patients with severe hyperlipidemia or hyperproteinemia. This laboratory abnormality has been essentially eliminated by the use of ion-specific electrodes (rather than flame photometry) to determine the serum sodium concentration. The second setting occurs when large quantities of osmotically active substances (such as glucose or mannitol) cause hyperosmolar hyponatremia, a condition also known as *translocational hyponatremia*. In such states, water is drawn out of cells into the extracellular space, diluting the plasma solutes and equilibrating osmolar differences. In addition, the use of large quantities of irrigation solutions that do not contain sodium (but instead contain glycine, sorbitol, or mannitol) during gynecologic or urologic surgeries can also cause severe hyperosmolar hyponatremia, especially in the setting with concomitant acute kidney injury.

5. **How can hyponatremia develop in a patient with hypovolemia?**

   Hypovolemic hyponatremia represents a decrease in total body sodium in excess of a decrease in TBW. Simultaneous sodium and water loss can be due to renal (such as diuretic use) or extrarenal causes. Hypovolemia results in a decrease in renal perfusion, a decrement in the glomerular filtration rate, and an increase in proximal tubule reabsorption of sodium and water; all three mechanisms

Serum Na⁺ <135 mmol/L

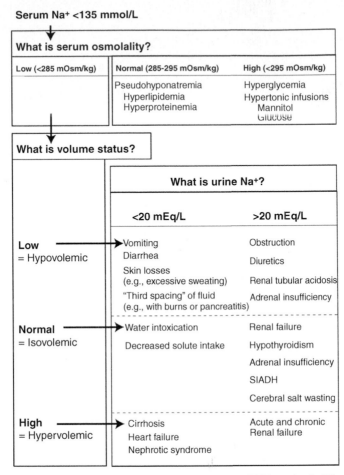

Figure 50-1. Diagnostic algorithm for hyponatremia. *Na⁺*, Sodium concentration; *SIADH*, secretion of antidiuretic hormone.

contribute to decreased water excretion. Furthermore, hypovolemia supersedes the expected inhibition of vasopressin release by hypo-osmolality and maintains the secretion of the hormone. In other words, the body protects volume at the expense of osmolality.

6. How does hypervolemic hyponatremia differ from hypovolemic hyponatremia?
   In hypervolemic hyponatremia, the kidneys are at the center of the problem because of either intrinsic renal disease or the renal response to extrarenal pathophysiology. Physical examination reveals edema and no evidence of volume depletion. Intrinsic renal disease with a compromised glomerular filtration rate (acute or chronic) prevents adequate excretion of sodium and water. Intake of sodium in excess of what can be excreted leads to hypervolemia (edema), whereas excessive intake of water leads to hyponatremia. In contrast, in congestive heart failure, hepatic cirrhosis, and nephrotic syndrome, the intrinsically normal kidney is stimulated to retain sodium and water in response to decreased effective arterial volume. The sodium and water retention along with daily relative hypo-tonic fluid ingestion from our diet leads to hypervolemia and hyponatremia. In general, hypervolemic hyponatremia due to an extrarenal cause is characterized by a low urine sodium concentration (≤10–20 mEq/L); this distinguishes it from hypervolemic hyponatremia due to intrinsic renal causes, where the urine sodium is greater than 20 mEq/L.

7. **What is the syndrome of inappropriate secretion of antidiuretic hormone?**
   Syndrome of inappropriate secretion of antidiuretic hormone (SIADH) is a common cause of euvolemic hyponatremia and is associated with malignancies, pulmonary disease, central nervous system disorders, pain, nausea, and many drugs. Common offending medications include hypoglycemic agents, psychotropics (including antipsychotics and antidepressants), narcotics, and chemotherapeutic agents. Endocrine diseases (hypothyroidism and adrenal insufficiency) are also considered causes of euvolemic hyponatremia, though in the case of adrenal insufficiency, mild volume depletion may also contribute to ADH secretion. Other causes of euvolemic hyponatremia include psychogenic polydipsia, a low-solute diet (beer potomania or the *tea and toast* diet), and reset osmostat.

8. **What diagnostic tests are useful in the evaluation of hyponatremia?**
   The physical examination is critical to the determination of volume status, as previously described. Serum electrolyte and serum and urine osmolality measurements are useful. High urine osmolality despite low serum osmolality suggests either hypovolemic hyponatremia or SIADH if the patient is in a euvolemic state. Very low urine osmolality suggests excessive water intake, as in psychogenic polydipsia or a low-solute diet. Measurements of thyroid-stimulating hormone and cortisol can be used to assess endocrine causes of hyponatremia. As mentioned previously, the urine sodium concentration can help distinguish renal and extrarenal causes of hypervolemic hyponatremia.

9. **Why do patients with diabetic ketoacidosis frequently have hyponatremia?**
   Diabetic ketoacidosis is an example of hyperosmotic hyponatremia. In general, the serum sodium concentration decreases by approximately 2.4 mEq/L for every increase of 100 mg/dL over normal glucose levels. In this setting, the serum sodium level should not be interpreted without an accompanying serum glucose measurement, and the appropriate correction should be made if the glucose exceeds 200 mg/dL.

10. **What is the difference between acute and chronic hyponatremia?**
    Acute hyponatremia: A distinct entity in terms of morbidity, mortality, and treatment strategies. Acute hyponatremia most commonly occurs in the hospital (frequently in the postoperative setting), in psychogenic polydipsia, and with ecstasy use.
    Chronic hyponatremia: Chronic hyponatremia is defined as hyponatremia lasting longer than 48 hours. The majority of patients who are seen by physicians or emergency departments with hyponatremia should be assumed to have chronic hyponatremia.

11. **What are the signs and symptoms of hyponatremia?**
    Hyponatremia is the most common electrolyte disorder in hospitalized patients, with a prevalence of approximately 2.5%. Although the majority of patients have no symptoms, symptoms often develop in patients with a serum sodium concentration less than 125 mEq/L or in whom the sodium has decreased rapidly. Gastrointestinal symptoms of nausea, vomiting, and anorexia occur early, but neuropsychiatric symptoms such as lethargy, confusion, agitation, psychosis, seizure, and coma are more common. Clinical symptoms roughly correlate with the amount and rate of decrease in serum sodium levels.

12. **What drugs, if any, are associated with hyponatremia?**
    Many drugs are associated with hyponatremia, but several warrant special note. Thiazide diuretics frequently cause hyponatremia by limiting the kidney's diluting capacity and promoting sodium excretion in excess of water. Of note, because loop diuretics directly impair the creation and maintenance of the medullary osmotic gradient, which limits the concentrating response to elevated levels of ADH, they are less likely to cause hyponatremia. Selective serotonin reuptake inhibitors and several chemotherapeutic agents cause hyponatremia, and this is thought to occur through SIADH. Nonsteroidal anti-inflammatory drugs block the production of renal prostaglandins and allow vasopressin to act unopposed in the kidney, which can lead to water retention. Tricyclic antidepressants and a number of anticonvulsants are also associated with hyponatremia. Lastly, the use of 3,4-methylenedioxymethamphetamine, or ecstasy, particularly in combination with consumption of large volumes of water, is associated with severe, life-threatening hyponatremia.

13. **Is there a standard therapy for hyponatremia?**
    Although controversy exists regarding treatment strategies, there is a consensus that not all patients with hyponatremia should be treated alike. Duration (acute vs. chronic) and the presence or absence of neurologic symptoms are the most critical factors in determining the therapeutic strategy. The prescribed therapy must take into consideration the patient's current symptoms and the risk of provoking

a demyelinating syndrome with overly rapid correction. The first priority is circulatory stabilization with isotonic fluids in patients with significant volume depletion. In patients with acute symptomatic hyponatremia, the risks of delaying treatment, which could lead to cerebral edema, subsequent seizures, and respiratory arrest, clearly outweigh any risk of treatment. Hypertonic (3%) saline solution should be given until symptoms subside. Consideration can also be made for concomitant administration of furosemide (which promotes free water excretion) or desmopressin (DDAVP, a synthetic vasopressin analog) (see Question 16). It is possible to calculate the expected change in serum sodium concentration on the basis of the volume of and rate at which hypertonic saline solution is infused, and this should be done before its administration. In contrast, the patient with asymptomatic chronic hyponatremia in high risk categories (e.g., alcoholism, malnutrition, concurrent hypokalemia, and liver disease) is at greatest risk for complications of the correction of hyponatremia—namely central pontine myelinolysis. Such patients may be best treated with water restriction. Vasopressin V2 receptor antagonists are newer agents (also known as *aquaretics* or *vaptans*) that are available in the United States for treatment of hypervolemic and euvolemic hyponatremia; these agents promote free water excretion and are useful in selected patients.

14. **What are some helpful guidelines for treatment of hyponatremia?**
   In patients with chronic asymptomatic hyponatremia, simple free water restriction (e.g., 1000 mL/day) allows a slow and relatively safe correction of the serum sodium concentration. This strategy, however, requires patient compliance, which may be particularly challenging in the outpatient setting. In selected patients who are behaviorally or physiologically resistant to free water restriction, administration of salt tablets, an ADH antagonist (e.g., demeclocycline, 600–1200 mg/day), the use of a V2 receptor antagonist, or a maneuver to increase urinary solute excretion, such as the ingestion of a high-solute diet, may be necessary.

   A difficult therapeutic dilemma is posed by patients with neurologic symptoms and hyponatremia of unknown duration. Such patients are at risk for development of a demyelinating disorder if treated too aggressively, yet the presence of symptoms is reflective of central nervous system dysfunction. These patients should be given treatment with hypertonic saline solution, and their serum sodium level should be monitored every 1 to 2 hours initially. The rate of increase should ideally not exceed 8 mEq/L in a 24-hour period. Acute therapy can be slowed once symptoms have improved or a *safe* serum sodium level (typically 120–125 mEq/L) is stably attained. (Note that if the serum sodium level is extremely low, this may be too aggressive a correction for the first 24 hours.)

15. **What is central pontine myelinolysis?**
   Central pontine myelinolysis is a rare neurologic disorder of unclear cause characterized by symmetric midline demyelination of the central pons. Extrapontine lesions can occur in the basal ganglia, internal capsule, lateral geniculate body, and cortex. Symptoms include motor abnormalities that can progress to flaccid quadriplegia, respiratory paralysis, pseudobulbar palsy, mental status changes, and coma. Central pontine myelinolysis is often fatal in 3 to 5 weeks; of the patients who survive, many have significant residual deficits. Alterations in the white matter are best visualized by magnetic resonance imaging. Central pontine myelinolysis is one of the most feared complications of therapy for hyponatremia. Risk factors include a change in serum sodium level of greater than 12 mEq/L in 24 hours, correction of serum sodium level to a normal or hypernatremic range, symptomatic and coexistent alcoholism, malnutrition, hypokalemia, and liver disease.

16. **How can the risk of central pontine myelinolysis be reduced for symptomatic patients who require 3% hypertonic saline treatment?**
   Using 3% hypertonic saline with DDAVP (synthetic vasopressin) may reduce the risk of overly rapid sodium correction, especially for patients with relatively lower urine osmolality (<400 mOsm/L). These patients must have their serum sodium level monitored very closely (q1–3 hours) to ensure that there is an improvement in serum sodium concentration while they are symptomatic, followed by a period with a slower rise or stabilization. The principle of DDAVP administration is that it avoids a transition to a low ADH state where overly rapid correction of hyponatremia may occur.

17. **Can hypernatremia also occur in hypovolemic, euvolemic, and hypervolemic states?**
   Yes, and these categories, based on physical examination, provide a useful framework for understanding and treating patients. Hypernatremia, defined as a serum sodium concentration greater than 145 mEq/L, occurs when too little TBW exists relative to the amount of total body sodium, thereby raising the sodium concentration. Given that even small rises in the serum osmolality trigger the thirst mechanism, hypernatremia is relatively uncommon unless the thirst mechanism is impaired or access to free water is restricted. As a result, hypovolemic hypernatremia tends to occur in the very young, the very old, and the debilitated. It is typically due to extracellular fluid losses accompanied by

inability to take in adequate amounts of free water. Febrile illnesses, vomiting, diarrhea, and renal losses are common causes.

Euvolemic hypernatremia can also be due to extracellular loss of fluid without adequate access to water or from impaired water hemostasis. Diabetes insipidus, either central (i.e., inadequate ADH secretion) or nephrogenic (i.e., renal insensitivity to ADH), results in the inability to reabsorb filtered water, which causes systemic hyperosmolality but hypo-osmolar (dilute) urine. Hypervolemic hypernatremia, although uncommon, is commonly iatrogenic or associated with excessive salt ingestion (seawater ingestion or an error in infant formula preparation). Sodium bicarbonate injection during cardiac arrest, administration of hypertonic saline solution, saline abortions, along with excessive salt ingestion are several examples of induced hypernatremia.

18. **What are the causes of diabetes insipidus?**
Central diabetes insipidus can result from trauma, tumors, strokes, granulomatous disease, and central nervous system infections, and it commonly occurs after neurosurgical procedures. Nephrogenic diabetes insipidus can be congenital, or it can occur in acute or chronic renal failure, hypercalcemia, hypokalemia, and sickle cell disease, or after treatment with certain drugs (e.g., lithium, demeclocycline).

19. **What are the signs and symptoms of hypernatremia?**
In awake and alert patients, thirst is a prominent symptom. Anorexia, nausea, vomiting, altered mental status, agitation, irritability, lethargy, stupor, coma, and neuromuscular hyperactivity are also common symptoms.

20. **What is the best therapy for hypernatremia?**
The first priority is circulatory stabilization with normal saline solution in patients with significant volume depletion. Once normotensive, patients can be rehydrated with oral water, intravenous 5% dextrose in water (D_5W), or even one-half normal saline solution. Overly rapid correction of long-standing hypernatremia can result in cerebral edema. Water deficit can be calculated with the formula in Question 21. Some investigators have suggested that in patients with long-standing hypernatremia, the water deficit should be corrected by no more than 10 mEq/L/day or 0.5 mEq/L/h. If the hypernatremia has occurred over a short period (hours), it can be corrected more rapidly, with the goal of correcting half of the water deficit in the first 24 hours. In addition to correcting the already established free water deficit, daily ongoing losses of free water in the urine and stool and from the respiratory tract and skin (particularly in patients with fever) should be replaced. In patients with central diabetes insipidus, a synthetic analog of ADH can be administered, preferably by the intranasal route.

21. **What are some helpful formulas for assessing sodium abnormalities?**
- **Serum osmolality** $= 2\,[Na^+] + Glucose/18 + Blood\ urea\ nitrogen/2.8 + Ethyl\ alcohol/4.6$
- **TBW** $= Body\ weight \times 0.6$ (for men)
- TBW $= Body\ weight \times 0.5$ (for women and the elderly)
- **TBW excess in hyponatremia** $= TBW\,(1 - [Serum\ Na^+]/140)$
- Expected change in serum sodium level after 1 L 3% saline solution $= (513\ mEq/L - Serum\ [Na^+])/(TBW + 1)$
- TBW deficit in hypernatremia $= TBW\,(Serum\ [Na^+]/140 - 1)$
- Expected change in serum sodium level after 1 L D5W $= (Serum\ [Na^+])/(TBW + 1)$

ACKNOWLEDGMENTS

The authors wish to acknowledge Drs. Brad W. Butcher, MD, Stuart Senkfor, MD, and Tomas Berl, MD, for the valuable contributions to the previous edition of this chapter.

KEY POINTS: HYPONATREMIA AND HYPERNATREMIA

Useful Diagnostic Tests in Hyponatremia
1. Serum osmolality measurement is useful in the diagnosis of hyponatremia.
2. Determination of volume status to distinguish between baroreceptor versus non-baroreceptor-related ADH secretion is necessary.
3. If urine osmolality is inappropriately high, it is easier to differentiate causes of euvolemic hyponatremia. High urine osmolality implies inappropriate levels of ADH or ADH-like hormones.
4. Urine sodium concentration needs to be interpreted with caution in cases of renal failure.

BIBLIOGRAPHY

1. Adrogué HJ, Madias NE. Hyponatremia. *N Engl J Med*. 2000;342:1581-1589.
2. Anderson RJ, Chung HM, Kluge R, et al. Hyponatremia: a prospective analysis of its epidemiology and the pathogenetic role of vasopressin. *Ann Intern Med*. 1985;102:164-168.
3. Berl T. Vasopressin antagonists. *N Engl J Med*. 2015;372:2207-2216.
4. Budisavljevic MN, Stewart L, Sahn SA, et al. Hyponatremia associated with 3-4-methylenedioxymethylamphetamine ("Ectasy") abuse. *Am J Med Sci*. 2003;326:89-93.
5. Elhassan EA, Schrier RW. Hyponatremia: diagnosis, complications and management including V2 receptor antagonists. *Curr Opin Nephrol Hypertens*. 2011;20:161-168.
6. Ellison DH, Berl T. The syndrome of inappropriate antidiuresis. *N Engl J Med*. 2007;356:2064-2072.
7. Hillier TA, Abbott RD, Barrett EJ. Hyponatremia: evaluating the correction factor for hyperglycemia. *Am J Med*. 1999; 106:399-403.
8. Lin M, Liu SJ, Lim IT. Disorders of water imbalance. *Emerg Med Clin North Am*. 2005;23:749-770.
9. Milionis HJ, Liamis GL, Elisaf MS. The hyponatremic patient: a systematic approach to laboratory diagnosis. *Can Med Assoc J*. 2002;166:1056-1062.
10. Moritz ML, Ayus JC. The pathophysiology and treatment of hyponatremic encephalopathy: an update. *Nephrol Dial Transplant*. 2003;18:2486-2491.
11. Sterns RH. Osmotic demyelination syndrome and overly rapid correction of hyponatremia. Available at http://www.uptodate.com. 2016. Accessed November 22, 2016.
12. Sterns RH. Disorders of plasma sodium–causes, consequences, and correction. *N Engl J Med*. 2015;372:55-65.
13. Verbalis JG. Disorders of water balance. In: Skorecki K, Chertow GM, Marsden PA, et al. eds. *Brenner and Rector's The Kidney*. 10th ed. Philadelphia: Elsevier; 2007:460-510.

VIII
GASTROENTEROLOGY

CHAPTER 51

UPPER AND LOWER GASTROINTESTINAL BLEEDING IN THE CRITICALLY ILL PATIENT

Leandra Krowsoski and Peter J. Fagenholz

1. How is gastrointestinal bleeding categorized anatomically?
   Gastrointestinal (GI) bleeding can occur anywhere along the GI tract. Upper gastrointestinal bleeding (UGIB) originates from a source proximal to the ligament of Treitz. Lower gastrointestinal bleeding (LGIB) occurs between the ligament of Treitz and the anus. Each broad category has its own distinct mechanisms of bleeding, natural history, and treatment.

2. What are the clinical signs of gastrointestinal bleeding?
   Clinical signs vary, depending on the location and rate of bleeding, which can range from occult to massive. Rapid bleeding from any location along the alimentary track can result in hemodynamic instability. Active or recent upper gastrointestinal (UGI) bleeding typically presents as bright red hematemesis, while coffee ground emesis is found with slower or resolved UGI bleeding. Examination of the stool often offers additional information about the bleeding source. Melena can occur with only 50 mL of blood and predicts an UGI source of bleeding in most cases (80% sensitivity). LGIB may present occultly or as melena or hematochezia. Melena tends to occur in slower bleeds with a longer transit time, such as those in the cecum.

3. Is nasogastric tube placement helpful?
   Sometimes—if there's no frank hematemesis, but blood is aspirated. The placement of a nasogastric tube (NGT) with the presence of bloody nasogastric aspiration has been shown to have a wide range of sensitivity (42%–84%) for diagnosing UGI bleeding without frank hematemesis and is not helpful in determining source if placement does not detect blood. However, positive nasogastric aspiration has been shown to be highly specific for predicting lesions at risk of re-bleeding.

4. What are risk factors of upper gastrointestinal bleeding? Lower gastrointestinal bleeding?
   A major risk factor associated with UGIB is infection with *Helicobacter pylori*. About half of all gastric ulcers and 80% of duodenal ulcers are caused by *H. pylori*. Other risk factors associated with UGIB are the use of nonsteroidal anti-inflammatory drugs (NSAIDs), antiplatelet medications, and anticoagulation. Similarly, medications have been identified as a prevalent risk factor in LGIB. Antiplatelet agents, anticoagulation, and NSAIDs have all been identified as predisposing agents in patients presenting with LGIB.

5. What are the most common causes of lower gastrointestinal bleeding?
   Approximately 20% to 25% of all GIB is attributed to a lower gastrointestinal (LGI) source. However, this number may not be accurate since patients with mild or occult LGIB may not present or be admitted to the hospital. The incidence of LGIB increases dramatically with age. The most common cause of arterial LGIB is colonic diverticula, followed by angiodysplasia and neoplasm. Colitis secondary to ischemia, infection, inflammatory bowel disease, and radiation as well as postsurgical bleeding represent most of the remaining instances.

6. What are the most common causes of upper gastrointestinal bleeding?
   More than half of all UGIB is the result of peptic ulcer disease (PUD). Bleeding from PUD accounts for up to 67% of all cases of UGIB. Esophagogastric variceal bleeding is the next most common source, followed by arteriovenous malformations, Mallory-Weiss tears, tumors, and erosions.

7. Which patients should be managed in the intensive care unit?
   There are several prediction rules that have been developed in order to risk stratify and guide the decision-making process for intensive care unit (ICU) admissions from the emergency department.

The BLEED study created criteria to predict which patients were at risk for re-bleeding, surgery, or mortality. Patients with visualized bleeding, hypotension, elevated prothrombin time (PT), labile mental status, or unstable comorbid conditions were more likely to develop in-hospital complications and require ICU level care. However, in a validation study, these criteria resulted in unnecessary ICU admissions and suggested that hematemesis or positive bloody NG aspirate with or without unstable comorbidities could accurately predict patients at risk of decompensation within the first 24 hours of admission who would benefit from ICU care.

8. Is there a way to predict who will need clinical interventions for upper gastrointestinal bleeding?
   The two scoring systems most commonly used in the emergency department are the Clinical Rockall Score (CRS) and the Glasgow-Blatchford Score (GBS). The CRS is a pre-endoscopic score that uses the clinical criteria of increased age, comorbidity, and shock to predict patients with UGIB at risk for re-bleeding and mortality. The GBS is based on clinical and lab criteria and is used to predict need for intervention such as blood transfusion or endoscopy. This score includes hemoglobin, blood urea nitrogen, systolic blood pressure, pulse rate, melena or syncope at presentation, and history of cardiac or hepatic failure. In a validation study, patients with UGIB who received a GBS score of 0 had no deaths or required interventions. These patients could then be safely worked up as outpatients.

9. Which patients will need clinical interventions for lower gastrointestinal bleeding?
   In LGIB, a study by Strate et al. demonstrated seven factors associated with severe bleeding. In patients with more than three of seven factors present, the risk of severe bleeding was increased with a likelihood of 80%. These factors were pulse rate greater than 100 beats per minute, systolic blood pressure less than 115 mm Hg, syncope, rectal bleeding within first 4 hours of presentation, aspirin use, more than two comorbid conditions, and nontender abdominal exam. These patients are more likely to require interventions.

10. Are there clinical findings associated with higher mortality in gastrointestinal bleeding patients?
    Higher mortality rates were found in patients presenting with an initial hemoglobin of less than 10 g/dL. As seen in the trauma literature, lactate is also useful in assessing acute blood loss. Elevated lactate greater than 4 mmol/L upon presentation in the emergency department was associated with a 6.4 fold increased risk of inpatient mortality in GIB patients.

11. When should patients be transfused in the setting of gastrointestinal bleeding?
    Ongoing massive hemorrhage is an indication for transfusion, but the appropriate transfusion strategy in nonexsanguinating patients is a topic of ongoing investigation. Villanueva et al. randomized patients to either a restrictive transfusion strategy, where patients were transfused red blood cells to a goal hemoglobin of 7 g/dL, or to a liberal transfusion strategy with a goal hemoglobin of 9 g/dL. Patients in the restrictive group had higher 6-week survival rates, lower rates of re-bleeding, and fewer overall complications. This study supports targeting a hemoglobin of 7 g/dL in patients without active cardiac ischemia. In LGIB patients, a target hemoglobin has not yet been identified and the decision to transfuse should be made based on the clinical status of the individual patient.

12. What is the role of proton pump inhibitors in acute upper gastrointestinal bleeding?
    In all patients with suspected UGIB, intravenous (IV) proton pump inhibitor (PPI) is recommended. In cases of bleeding due to PUD, initiation of PPI therapy prior to upper endoscopy is associated with decreased need for endoscopic intervention, reduced risk of re-bleeding, and lower likelihood of needing surgery. The recommended dose in a PPI-naïve patient is an 80-mg bolus of omeprazole followed by 8 mg/h for 72 hours (or equivalent PPI).

13. What additional medical interventions are used in cases of gastrointestinal bleeding?
    Other medical adjuncts include the use of somatostatin or octreotide. Both agents decrease splanchnic blood flow and acid production and are effective in variceal and nonvariceal bleeding. Although vasopressin similarly reduces splanchnic blood flow, and can be helpful in variceal bleeding as it reduces portal blood pressure, use has been limited because of the negative systemic effects. Finally, in patients with cirrhosis, prophylactic antibiotic therapy with ceftriaxone has been shown to improve survival.

14. How should coagulopathy be addressed?
    In patients receiving vitamin-K antagonists with minor bleeding, anticoagulation is reversed using oral vitamin K. IV vitamin K is preferred for large bleeds. Hemodynamic instability and international normalized ratio (INR) greater than 5 in an indication for reversal with prothrombin complex concentrate (PCC) or fresh frozen plasma (FFP). Although there is a theoretical benefit to the use of tranexamic acid (TXA), the benefit of its use in UGI bleeding is still unclear.

15. What is the first step in management of severe gastrointestinal bleeding?

Initial management of GIB should focus on the same ABCs as trauma management. Intubation can be considered for patients with severe UGIB for airway protection while IV access should be obtained with two large-bore catheters. With IV access in place, resuscitation should proceed with blood products as necessary to maintain hemodynamic stability and correct any coagulopathy present. As resuscitation is continued, the source of hemorrhage should be determined and further hemorrhage controlled either with upper endoscopy, colonoscopy, angiography, or surgery. The intervention is determined by the suspected source of bleeding and clinical condition of the patient.

16. Is there a way to temporize variceal bleeding emergently?

In cases of life-threatening exsanguinating variceal hemorrhage, balloon tamponade can be employed to temporize bleeding while awaiting upper endoscopy. Sengstaken-Blakemore and Minnesota tubes can be inserted nasally or orally and have a gastric and esophageal balloon.

17. How does balloon tamponade work?

When confirmed to be in correct position with auscultation over the stomach while irrigating the gastric port, the gastric balloon is inflated in 100 mL increments to a maximum of 500 mL while the pressure is measured. The tube is then pulled back against the diaphragm and secured against a traction device (such as a pulley device or helmet). If bleeding persists with the gastric balloon inflated and under traction, the esophageal balloon is then inflated to 35 to 40 mm Hg and clamped. Continued bleeding with both balloons inflated can be addressed by adding additional external traction on the tube to tamponade bleeding.

18. What complications can occur with balloon tamponade?

Complications such as pressure necrosis or esophageal rupture limit the length of time that these tubes can be used. When bleeding is controlled, the pressure should be reduced incrementally to the minimum pressure necessary to control bleeding and maintained in place for 24 hours.

19. How is endoscopy utilized in upper gastrointestinal bleeding?

Upper endoscopy is the first diagnostic tool used in patients with suspected UGIB and can also be used therapeutically. Interventions to achieve hemostasis include techniques like thermal coagulation, injection therapy, or metallic clipping and banding. Endoscopy is recommended within 24 hours of presentation for UGIB, but should be done as soon as possible in patients presenting with hematochezia or hemodynamic instability. Endoscopy performed within the first 13 hours of admission reduces mortality in patients with severe bleeding (GBS >12).

20. How is endoscopy utilized in lower gastrointestinal bleeding?

Colonoscopy is the initial recommended intervention to establish a bleeding source. Diagnostic yield is high, but is often limited by poor visualization due to rapid bleeding and inadequate bowel preparation. It can also be used therapeutically, with injection, thermal, and mechanical treatment. Timing is an ongoing debate—diagnostic yield is improved when performed early, but there is no difference in rates of re-bleeding, transfusion requirement, mortality, or length of stay in patients undergoing urgent colonoscopy within 12 hours versus 36 to 60 hours. Timing should therefore be based on the clinical situation, with urgent colonoscopy performed for severe bleeding. In cases of hematochezia with hemodynamic instability, UGI endoscopy should also be considered to rule out an UGI bleeding source.

21. Who is likely to re-bleed after upper endoscopic intervention?

After upper endoscopy and PPI infusion, the overall rate of re-bleeding in UGIB is 10% to 20%.

In PUD, location of the ulcer in the posterior duodenal bulb is a predictor of re-bleeding. Other risk factors of failure of endoscopic treatment in PUD include hypotension, age over 65, comorbid conditions, presenting hemoglobin less than 10 g/dL, fresh blood in the stomach on endoscopy, active bleeding from the ulcer at the time of endoscopy, and large ulcer size (>1 cm). More specifically, risk of re-bleeding and need for surgery can be predicted by the stigmata of recent hemorrhage seen during endoscopic intervention.

22. How does ulcer appearance predict risk of re-bleeding?

The Forrest Classification system describes the stigmata of bleeding. Type I ulcers have signs of active bleeding and the highest incidence of re-bleeding. Type II lesions show stigmata of recent bleeding such as a nonbleeding visible vessel or adherent clot and a slightly lower incidence of re-bleeding. The lowest incidence is present in ulcers without bleeding.

23. **What is the role of second-look endoscopy?**
    Second-look endoscopy for re-bleeding can achieve hemostasis in three-quarters of patients. Ulcer size of greater than 2 cm and re-bleeding presenting with hypotension were predictors of failure of retreatment with endoscopy. It can also be employed selectively in patients with lesion appearance most at risk of re-bleeding. However, routine second-look endoscopy in patients without re-bleeding is not recommended.

24. **What additional tests help localize bleeding?**
    When the source of GIB is unclear after endoscopy, one option in stable patients is a radionuclide 99mTc tagged red blood cell. It can detect bleeding rates of 0.1 mL/min and is considered most sensitive in identifying bleeding sites. Computed tomography (CT) angiography is another option in stable patients that can detect GIB with 85% sensitivity and 92% specificity. Studies in animal models have shown that bleeding can be detected at rates of 0.3 mL/min. Transcatheter angiography can be used for both diagnostic and therapeutic purposes. Visualization with angiography occurs with bleeding rates of 0.5 to 1.0 mL/min.

25. **What are the limitations of these imaging techniques?**
    The downside of each of these techniques, however, is that GI bleeding is often fitful, proceeding in a stop/start pattern, and imaging must be timed with active bleeding for visualization. Repeat imaging is often required. For bleeds that persistently recur, but repeatedly stop before being localized, "provocative angiography" that induces active bleeding with an agent like tPA may allow for the bleeding source to be both identified and treated.

26. **How can interventional radiology aid in management of nonvariceal upper gastrointestinal bleeding?**
    Transcatheter arteriography and intervention (TAI) has been technically and clinically successful for both localization and treatment of UGIB. Hemodynamic instability at the time of TAI correlates with positive findings on angiography; however, identification of active extravasation is not required for intervention. Rates of clinical success are similar in embolization after endoscopic identification of bleeding, but without active extravasation on angiography versus embolization of an actively bleeding site seen on angiography. In nonvariceal UGIB, the most likely site of bleeding is the gastroduodenal artery (GDA) and the celiac artery should therefore be selectively evaluated first and the GDA embolized if necessary. This should be followed by evaluation of the superior mesenteric artery (SMA) due to the collateralization via the pancreaticoduodenal arcade.

27. **How can interventional radiology aid in management of variceal upper gastrointestinal bleeding?**
    Endoscopy with variceal banding and pharmacotherapy are the mainstays of treating variceal bleeding; however, 10% to 20% of patients fail standard therapy. Transjugular intrahepatic portosystemic shunt (TIPS) is an option in these situations. Via the internal jugular vein, the radiologist accesses the hepatic vein under fluoroscopic guidance. A portal vein branch within the liver is catheterized and an expandable stent placed between the hepatic vein and portal vein branch to create a shunt that decompresses the portal vein. A successful procedure decreases the portal pressure to less than 12 mm Hg. Despite a success rate of 90%, 6-week mortality is as high as 35%.

28. **How can interventional radiology aid in management of lower gastrointestinal bleeding?**
    The SMA and inferior mesenteric artery (IMA) are the focus of TAI for LGIB. This method is rarely the first test in LGIB. It is generally employed when massive bleeding prevents adequate colonoscopy, or when colonoscopy is unable to locate the source of bleeding. Arteriography is most likely to localize a bleeding source when there is ongoing bleeding. Embolization is used and is typically more successful in treating focal bleeding, such as diverticular bleeds. Diseases with a wider blood supply, like angiodysplasias or tumors, are less successfully treated. The intermittent nature of LGIB often results in negative angiography. Provocative angiography, when anticoagulants or thrombolytic drugs are infused during imaging, can be employed after multiple bleeding episodes in a patient without an identified source.

29. **What is the difference between occult and obscure gastrointestinal bleeding?**
    Occult GIB is small volume bleeding that is not visible. This should be worked up in the typical manner discussed previously with upper and lower endoscopy. Obscure GIB is persistent bleeding that may be occult or may present as overt bleeding with the continued passage of blood, but does not have a defined source after upper endoscopy and colonoscopy. In this case, a small bowel source may be suspected and further evaluation of the small intestine is indicated. The most common cause of obscure overt bleeding in patients older than 40 years is angiodysplasia.

30. How should obscure gastrointestinal bleeding be worked up?

Capsule endoscopy is a noninvasive diagnostic option where a capsule is swallowed and travels through the small bowel via intestinal peristalsis while sending images wirelessly for examination. It is most successful when performed within 48 hours of the episode of bleeding. Push enteroscopy is performed transorally using a pediatric colonoscope, which is driven into the small intestine and can examine the first 90 to 150 cm. Balloon-assisted enteroscopy is the most common method of deep enteroscopy and allows the small bowel to be stabilized and pleated over the scope when inserted either via the mouth or rectum, providing even further visualization. Both push and deep enteroscopy are generally performed after a bleeding source is identified on capsule endoscopy.

31. What is the role of surgery in gastrointestinal bleeding?

In the modern era, with availability of endoscopy and angiography, the role of surgery has shifted to a salvage intervention when other therapy has failed. Even when endoscopy and radiologic studies and interventions fail to stop bleeding, they remain critical for localizing the site of bleeding prior to surgery whenever possible. Intraoperative localization is rarely possible, since bleeding is intraluminal and the surgeon can only examine the outside of the GI tract.

32. When is surgery indicated to treat lower gastrointestinal bleeding?

For localized LGIB refractory to endoscopic or angiographic intervention, segmental resection of the intestine involved in the bleeding is the usual treatment. One of the only scenarios in which surgery may be performed for incompletely localized GI bleeding is for massive LGIB with refractory hemodynamic instability. If UGIB and perianal or rectal sources can be ruled out, it may very rarely be appropriate to perform exploratory laparotomy with total abdominal colectomy (removing all the colon from the ileocecal valve to the peritoneal reflection) if no potential small bowel sources of hemorrhage (e.g., tumors or diverticulae, or a small intestine massively distended with blood) are identified. A complete algorithm for the treatment of LGIB is outlined in Fig. 51.1.

33. When is surgery indicated to treat upper gastrointestinal bleeding?

Timing of surgical intervention for UGIB is more contested. Recurrent bleeding is a prognostic factor of adverse outcomes. Re-bleeding in the elderly is particularly morbid. In current practice, endoscopy is still the first-line therapy in UGIB; however, trials have shown that early surgical intervention in elderly high-risk patients resulted in lower overall mortality. Therefore, surgical intervention for re-bleeding should be employed in carefully selected patients, while second-look endoscopy or angiography is recommended instead in most patients. An algorithm for the treatment of nonvariceal UGIB is outlined in Fig. 51.2 and variceal UGIB in Fig. 51.3.

34. What type of surgery should be performed?

The extent of the surgery performed for UGIB is also a topic of debate. When endoscopic or angiographic intervention fails, the minimal surgical intervention necessary to control bleeding is typically chosen. Gastric ulcers or arteriovenous malformations such as Dieulafoy's lesions can be controlled via local excision or small wedge resections. For peptic ulcer bleeding from a duodenal ulcer, minimal intervention involves suture ligation of the bleeding ulcer by applying sutures that control the GDA and the transverse pancreatic branch. More extensive ulcer operations incorporating vagotomy or gastrectomy may have slightly lower long-term risks of rebleeding, but have significantly higher short-term morbidity in the urgent scenarios in which surgery is now employed, and are thus rarely performed.

35. Are there any risk factors for gastrointestinal bleeding specific to intensive care unit patients?

Endoscopies performed within 3 days of admission to the ICU show gastric lesions in 75% to 100% of ICU patients. Only a small percentage of these lesions go on to lead to overt, clinically significant bleeding; however, the presence of this mucosal damage seen nearly universally demonstrated in critically ill patients shows that they are at increased risk for stress-related mucosal damage. The pathophysiology for this process is not fully understood, but may be in part caused by diminished blood flow, leading to mucosal ischemia. Presence of three or more comorbid diseases, liver disease, renal replacement therapy, coagulopathy, higher organ failure scores at the time of ICU admission, and mechanical ventilation were associated with clinically significant GI bleeding.

36. When should stress ulcer prophylaxis be used?

Stress ulcer prophylaxis has been shown to significantly reduce the risk of bleeding, is now considered standard of care in the ICU, and is recommended for patients with strong risk factors for stress-related mucosal disease (SRMD). This includes patients requiring mechanical ventilation, with coagulopathy, traumatic brain injury, and with major burn injury. ICU patients with multitrauma, sepsis, and acute

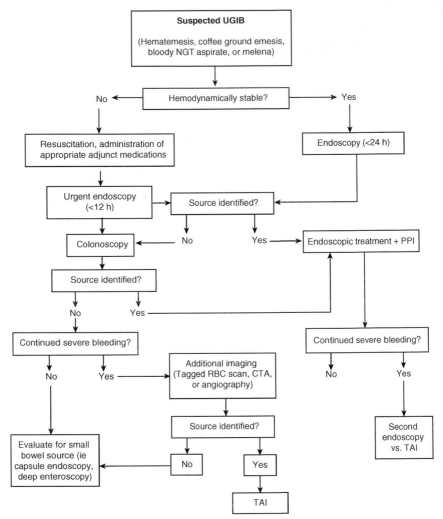

Figure 51-1. Suggested algorithm for treatment of upper gastrointestinal bleeding (UGIB). *CTA*, Computed tomography angiography; *NGT*, nasogastric tube; *PPI*, proton pump inhibitor; *RBC*, red blood cell; *TAI*, transcatheter arteriography and intervention.

renal failure as well as patients with an injury severity score of more than 15 and those requiring high-dose steroids should also receive prophylaxis.

37. **Are there side effects to the use of stress ulcer prophylaxis?**
    There is a question of overuse of stress ulcer prophylaxis leading to infectious complications—namely, nosocomial pneumonia and *Clostridium difficile.* Although some cohort and case-control studies suggest an increased risk of *C. difficile,* randomized controlled trials do not show any evidence that stress ulcer prophylaxis leads to an increased risk of nosocomial pneumonias or *C. difficile.* The benefit in reduced risk of bleeding outweighs the risk of infectious complications, and it is recommended that prophylaxis be continued while patients are mechanically ventilated, in the ICU, or unable to tolerate enteral nutrition.

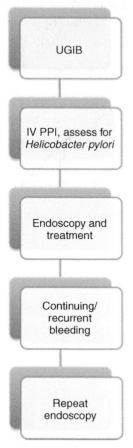

Figure 51-2. Nonvariceal upper gastrointestinal tract hemorrhage management algorithm. *IV,* Intravenous; *PPI,* proton pump inhibitor; *UGIB,* upper gastrointestinal bleeding.

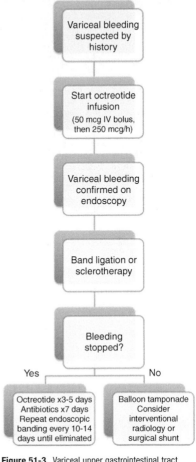

Figure 51-3. Variceal upper gastrointestinal tract hemorrhage management algorithm. *IV,* Intravenous.

ACKNOWLEDGMENT

The authors wish to acknowledge Drs. George Kasotakis, MD, and George C. Velmahos, MD, PhD, MSEd, for the valuable contributions to the previous edition of this chapter.

KEY POINTS: UPPER AND LOWER GASTROINTESTINAL BLEEDING IN THE CRITICALLY ILL PATIENT

1. Endoscopy is the mainstay of diagnosis and treatment in gastrointestinal tract bleeding and should be performed within 24 hours of presentation.
2. Transcatheter angiography and intervention is an option in patients who fail endoscopy.
3. GI bleeding is intermittent and diagnostic procedures may need to be repeated before a source of bleeding is identified.
4. Surgical intervention is reserved for patients who fail other interventions and every attempt should be made to localize bleeding before committing to surgery.

BIBLIOGRAPHY

1. Bardou M, Quenot JP, Barkun A. Stress-related mucosal disease in the critically ill patient. *Nat Rev Gastroenterol Hepatol.* 2015;12(2):98-107.
2. Chiu PW, Lau JY. What if endoscopic hemostasis fails?: alternative treatment strategies: surgery. *Gastroenterol Clin North Am.* 2014;43(4):753-763.
3. Darcy MD, Cash BD, Feig BW, et al. ACR Appropriateness Criteria® Radiologic management of lower gastrointestinal tract bleeding. Acute Trauma to the Foot. Available at: https://acsearch.acr.org/docs/69457/Nrrative/. Accessed March 10, 2017.
4. Guillamondegui OD, Gunter OL, Bonadies JA, et al. *Practice Management Guidelines for Stress Ulcer Prophylaxis* Chicago: Eastern Association for the Surgery of Trauma (EAST); 2008.
5. Kim BS, Li BT, Engel A, et al. Diagnosis of gastrointestinal bleeding: a practical guide for clinicians. *World J Gastrointest Pathophysiol.* 2014;5(4):467-478.
6. Krag M, Perner A, Wetterslev J, et al. Prevalence and outcome of gastrointestinal bleeding and use of acid suppressants in acutely ill adult intensive care patients. *Intensive Care Med.* 2015;41(5):833-845.
7. Laine L, Jensen DM. Management of patients with ulcer bleeding. *Am J Gastroenterol.* 2012;107(3):345-360.
8. Nable JV, Graham AC. Gastrointestinal bleeding. *Emerg Med Clin North Am.* 2016;34(2):309-325.
9. Nanavati SM. What if endoscopic hemostasis fails? Alternative treatment strategies: interventional radiology. *Gastroenterol Clin North Am.* 2014;43(4):739-752.
10. Qayed E, Dagar G, Nanchal RS. Lower gastrointestinal hemorrhage. *Crit Care Clin.* 2016;32(2):241-254.
11. Satapathy SK, Sanyal AJ. Nonendoscopic management strategies for acute esophagogastric variceal bleeding. *Gastroenterol Clin North Am.* 2014;43(4):819-833.
12. Strate LL, Gralnek IM. ACG Clinical guideline: management of patients with acute lower gastrointestinal bleeding. *Am J Gastroenterol.* 2016;111(4):459-474.
13. Villanueva C, Colomo A, Bosch A, et al. Transfusion strategies for acute upper gastrointestinal bleeding. *N Engl J Med.* 2013;368(1):11-21.
14. Zurkiya O, Walker TG. Angiographic evaluation and management of nonvariceal gastrointestinal hemorrhage. *AJR Am J Roentgenol.* 2015;205(4):753-763.

CHAPTER 52

ACUTE PANCREATITIS

Joseph D. Frasca and Mario J. Velez

1. **What is acute pancreatitis?**

   Acute pancreatitis is an inflammatory condition of the pancreas caused by the local release of pancreatic enzymes in response to recent acinar injury. Episodes of acute pancreatitis have a broad range of presentation and severity. They can be self-limited and without local complications or long-term sequelae, but can also be severe and associated with multiorgan failure and high-risk mortality. Clinically it is defined by the presence of two of the three following criteria: (i) epigastric pain or left upper quadrant pain, (ii) serum amylase and/or lipase greater than three times the upper limit of normal, and (iii) abdominal imaging consistent with the disease.

2. **What are the different degrees of severity in acute pancreatitis, and how are they defined?**

   The revised Atlanta Criteria (2013) characterize acute pancreatitis into three distinct severities: mild, moderately severe, and severe. Mild acute pancreatitis is defined by pancreatic inflammation (of any cause) without organ failure or local complications. Moderately severe acute pancreatitis is associated with transient organ failure of less than 48 hours and/or the presence of local complications. Local complications include, but are not limited to, pancreatic necrosis and/or pseudocyst formation. Finally, severe acute pancreatitis is defined as pancreatic inflammation with persistent organ failure (>48 hours). Organ failure is often defined by the presence of systemic shock (systolic blood pressure <90 mm Hg), hypoxemia (PaO_2 <60 mm Hg), renal failure (serum creatinine >2 mg/dL following resuscitation), and/or the presence of GI hemorrhage.

3. **What are the causes of acute pancreatitis?**

   Gallstone-related disease (40%–70% of cases) and excessive alcohol intake (25%–35% of cases) are the two most common causes of acute pancreatitis in the developed world. Alcohol-induced pancreatitis should be considered only in the setting of heavy alcohol use (>50 g/day) for at least 5 years. Beyond these etiologies, other causes of pancreatitis are rare and should be considered with caution. Primary and secondary hypertriglyceridemia can cause acute pancreatitis but should be considered only if serum triglyceride level is above 1000 mg/dL. Other potential causes include medications, trauma, inherited genetic mutations, and metabolic causes such as hypercalcemia and hyperparathyroidism. It is often difficult to identify a drug as the sole cause of pancreatitis. Some of the medications that have been implicated include angiotensin-converting enzyme inhibitors, furosemide, tetracycline, aminosalicylic acid, corticosteroids, procainamide, thiazides, metronidazole, ranitidine, 6-mercaptopurine, and azathioprine. Genetic mutations are becoming increasingly recognized and should be considered if other more common etiologies have been excluded, especially if a family history of pancreatitis is present. Endoscopic retrograde cholangiopancreatography (ERCP) causes pancreatitis in approximately 7% of all individuals who undergo this procedure.

4. **What are the presenting signs and symptoms of acute pancreatitis?**

   Acute pancreatitis is characterized by the sudden onset of abdominal pain, classically located in the epigastrium or left upper quadrant, and sometimes associated with nausea and/or vomiting. Radiation of pain from the epigastrium through to the back, chest, or flanks is a typical but not a necessary feature. Tachycardia related to pain or volume depletion and low-grade fever may be present. Two additional findings include the Grey Turner and Cullen signs. The Grey Turner sign is flank ecchymosis due to retroperitoneal hemorrhage. When present, it usually occurs 3 to 7 days after the onset of pain. The Cullen sign is periumbilical ecchymosis associated with both severe necrotizing pancreatitis and retroperitoneal hemorrhage.

5. **Are amylase and/or lipase measurements helpful in the diagnosis?**

   The most commonly used diagnostic markers are serum amylase and lipase. Although serum amylase levels have a high sensitivity in the first 24 hours, the specificity is very low. Elevated amylase levels are seen with many other conditions including bowel infarction, renal failure, perforated peptic ulcer, trauma to the salivary glands, and macroamylasemia. In contrast, serum lipase is more specific and more sensitive, making it the preferred laboratory parameter in diagnosing acute pancreatitis. A serum lipase greater than 3 times the upper limit of normal is a diagnostic criterion, but no correlation exists between the absolute level and the severity of pancreatitis. There is also no recommendation to trend the lipase levels, as this has no relation to clinical improvement or patient mortality.

6. **What is the role of imaging in the diagnosis of acute pancreatitis?**
Abdominal ultrasound should be performed in all patients presenting with acute pancreatitis. Ultrasound is noninvasive, relatively inexpensive, widely available, and can detect the presence of gallstone-related disease and other biliary abnormalities.
Computed tomography (CT) with oral and intravenous (iv) contrast has a high sensitivity and specificity for the diagnosis of acute pancreatitis. It is also helpful in detecting the development of early and late complications of disease. Features that may be identified on CT include evidence of inflammation (pancreatic parenchymal edema or peripancreatic fat stranding), peripancreatic or intrapancreatic fluid collections, degree of pancreatic perfusion, and the presence/extent of pancreatic necrosis.

7. **Should all patients have imaging studies done at the time of presentation?**
Abdominal imaging is useful in confirming the diagnosis of acute pancreatitis. It is currently recommended that all patients undergo a formal right upper quadrant ultrasound at the time of presentation to evaluate for choledocholithiasis or biliary pancreatitis. Imaging beyond an initial abdominal ultrasound on presentation is often reserved for patients failing to improve clinically within the first 48 to 72 hours. Patients citing continued abdominal pain, fever, or inability to initiate oral feeding should be sent for CT with IV contrast, as it provides a rapid and accurate assessment of disease severity.

8. **What if the patient cannot receive contrast for imaging?**
Magnetic resonance imaging (MRI) has a growing role in the diagnosis and management of acute pancreatitis and is a reasonable option in patients who cannot receive iodinated contrast for CT. Enhanced MRI requires the administration of gadolinium, which has been implicated in severe toxic side effects (nephrogenic systemic fibrosis) in patients with compromised renal function. Good correlation has been noted, however, when comparing magnetic resonance cholangiopancreatography (MRCP), with or without gadolinium contrast, to CT in the evaluation of acute pancreatitis. MRCP also has the added benefit of being able to better define the pancreatic and biliary ductal system in cases where there is suspicion for biliary pancreatitis.

9. **How do you determine the severity and prognosis of acute pancreatitis?**
Recognizing and differentiating mild from severe acute pancreatitis is important so that patients can be triaged to the appropriate treatment setting. Fortunately, most episodes of acute pancreatitis are mild and self-limiting, requiring only a brief hospitalization of less than 4 days. Most patients with mild pancreatitis usually begin oral feeding 48 hours after initial presentation and are discharged following an uneventful hospital course.
As already discussed, moderately severe pancreatitis, as defined by the revised Atlanta criteria (2013), includes the presence of local complications and/or transient organ failure that persists for less than 48 hours. If there is persistent organ failure beyond the initial 48 hours, it is considered severe disease.
Since the 1970s, several clinical scoring systems have emerged to help predict the degree of severity in acute pancreatitis. Although all are imperfect, they are considered superior to clinical judgment alone. The Ranson criteria (Table 52.1) was one of the earliest and most widely used scoring systems. The major disadvantage was that it required 48 hours to complete. The Acute Physiology and Chronic Health Evaluation (APACHE) II system, developed to evaluate critically ill patients, has also been used to differentiate mild acute pancreatitis from severe acute pancreatitis. The major disadvantage of this system is that many find it cumbersome, as it requires 12 physiologic measures to calculate. A CT severity index (Balthazar score) is used to predict severity of pancreatitis by radiographic features. The bedside index of severity in acute pancreatitis (BISAP) score (Table 52.2) integrates the systemic inflammatory response syndrome (SIRS) criteria and can be calculated relatively quickly on admission.

10. **What is the treatment for acute pancreatitis?**
The mainstay of treatment in acute pancreatitis, regardless of the degree of severity, is early aggressive volume repletion, pain control, nutritional support, correction of electrolyte abnormalities, and treatment of associated or causative conditions.
Adequate volume repletion in the form of an isotonic crystalloid fluid, such as lactated Ringer's, at a rate of 250 to 500 mL/h aims to restore perfusion to pancreatic microcirculation and prevent further cellular death. Inadequate volume repletion is associated with higher rates of pancreatic necrosis.

Table 52-1. Modified Ranson Criteria

	Etiology of Pancreatitis	
	ALCOHOLIC OR OTHER	BILIARY
At Initial Presentation		
Age (year)	>55	>70
White blood cell count (k/mm³)	>16	>18
Glucose (mg/dL)	>200	>220
Lactate dehydrogenase (U/L)	>350	>400
Aspartate (AST) (U/L)	>250	>250
During First 48 h		
Decrease in hematocrit (%)	≥10	>10
Elevation in blood urea nitrogen (mg/dL)	>5	>2
Serum total calcium (mg/dL)	<8	<8
Partial pressure of oxygen (mm Hg)	<60	NA
Base deficit (mmol/L)	>4	>5
Fluid sequestration (L)	>6	>4
PROGNOSIS	NUMBER OF CRITERIA MET	PREDICTED MORTALITY
	≤2	0.9%
	3–4	16%
	5–6	40%
	7–8	100%

NA, Not applicable.

Modified from Ranson JH, Rifkind KM, Roses DF, et al. Prognostic signs and the role of operative management in acute pancreatitis. *Surg Gynecol Obstet.* 1974;139:69–81; and Ranson JH. Etiological and prognostic factors in human acute pancreatitis: a review. *Am J Gastroenterol.* 1982;77:633–638.

11. How should patients with pancreatitis be fed?

Enteral feeding is the preferred method of nutritional support for all patients with pancreatitis. It is thought to help maintain the intestinal mucosal barrier and prevent bacterial translocation, which may be a major source of infection. No strong evidence exists that nasojejunal feeding is advantageous over nasogastric feeding. In fact, a recent systematic review found that nasogastric feeding was safe and well tolerated in patients with severe acute pancreatitis. Moreover, nasojejunal tube placement requires fluoroscopy or endoscopy and, as such, is usually a costly undertaking without proven benefit. Although there are concerns for aspiration in nasogastric feeding, this can usually be overcome by taking "aspiration precautions" and sitting the patient upright during continuous feeding. It is still not known if a low continuous rate compared with bolus feeding is optimal; however, checking gastric residuals is not usually helpful and now discouraged.

Total parenteral nutrition should be avoided in patients with acute pancreatitis based on observations from multiple randomized trials suggesting higher rates of infectious and line-related complications. A recent meta-analysis also found a decrease in infectious complications, organ failure, and mortality in patients with severe acute pancreatitis who were provided enteral nutrition as compared with parenteral nutrition.

Most experts would agree that immediate feeding is safe and well tolerated in patients with mild acute pancreatitis without nausea, vomiting, or ileus. Early feeding in this population results in a shorter hospital stay and can be initiated with a soft diet. The timing of initiation of feeding in severe pancreatitis is more controversial and without specific recommendations from evidence-based medicine.

Table 52-2. Bedside Index of Severity in Acute Pancreatitis Score

One point for each of the following if present:

BUN >25 mg/dL (8.9 mmol/L)

Impaired mental status

SIRS (two or more of the following):
- Pulse >90 beats/min
- Respiratory rate > 20/min or $PaCO_2$ > 32 mm Hg
- Temperature >38°C or <36°C
- WBC >12,000 or <4000 cells/mm^3 or >10% immature neutrophils (bands)

Age >60 years

Pleural effusion

BISAP Interpretation

BISAP SCORE	(MORTALITY %)
0–1	<2
2	2
3	5%–8%
4	13%–19%
5	22%–27%

BISAP, Bedside index of severity in acute pancreatitis; *BUN*, Blood urea nitrogen; *SIRS*, systemic inflammatory response syndrome; *WBC*, white blood cells.

Modified from Wu BU, Johannes RS, Sun X, et al. The early prediction of mortality in acute pancreatitis: a large population-based study. *Gut.* 2008;57:1698–1703.

12. **Do patients with pancreatic necrosis need antibiotics?**
As already stated, pancreatic necrosis is a serious local complication of acute pancreatitis. Recently there has been a notable paradigm shift in how to best manage both sterile and infected pancreatic necrosis, both ultimately favoring a more conservative approach. Prophylactic antibiotics are no longer recommended for sterile pancreatic necrosis in the absence of systemic infection. A meta-analysis of 11 prospective, randomized controlled trials evaluating the role of prophylactic antibiotics in sterile necrosis found that there was no benefit regarding mortality or preventing rates of infected necrosis in severe acute pancreatitis.

Instead, antibiotics are reserved for infected pancreatic necrosis, which usually has an onset of 10 to 14 days from initial presentation. Patients with infected pancreatic necrosis often show some clinical improvement following their initial admission and then rapidly decompensate with new fevers, pain, or hemodynamic compromise. New imaging in the form of CT with IV contrast can demonstrate air bubbles in pancreatic fluid collections, which can confirm the diagnosis. At this point, antibiotic selection becomes paramount. Carbapenems are the preferred agent, as they have high pancreatic penetration and broad-spectrum coverage. Quinolones, metronidazole, and high-dose cephalosporins are other options in cases where there is an allergy to carbapenems.

In addition to infected pancreatic necrosis, antibiotics are also used in signs of systemic complications or infections from pancreatitis like pneumonia or cholangitis.

13. **What is the role for surgery and/or endoscopic therapy in pancreatic necrosis?**
Asymptomatic pancreatic necrosis does not mandate intervention and will likely resolve over time. The previous notion that infected pancreatic necrosis required prompt surgical débridement has been refuted by long-term studies demonstrating lower patient mortality and complete resolution of infected necrosis with antibiotics alone.

Surgical débridement or endoscopic drainage with necrosectomy is now reserved for patients failing to respond to antibiotics. Retrospective reviews addressing the timing of intervention found that postponing endoscopic drainage or surgery until 4 to 6 weeks after the initial insult resulted in lower patient mortality compared with earlier intervention. As such, expert panels recommend delaying necrosectomy for at least 4 weeks in persistently symptomatic patients, while administering antibiotics and allowing the necrosis to organize.

14. **What are the comparative outcomes between endoscopic drainage and surgical débridement?**
Minimally invasive options for pancreatic necrosectomy are becoming increasingly favored over open surgical débridement, given their comparable success rates, lower rates of complications, and lower healthcare cost. The two alternative options to surgical débridement include an endoscopic approach, usually performed by gastroenterologists, and a percutaneous approach performed by interventional radiology. Percutaneous drainage without subsequent necrosectomy is an option for many patients and has been shown to reduce the need for surgery in about 50% of cases. This does not come without its own complications, however. Chronic cutaneous fistula development and recurrent infections have been described and are of concern with this approach.

There is now a growing focus in providing intraluminal drainage of large necrotic cavities with direct endoscopic necrosectomy. Centers with expertise in endoscopic ultrasound can provide intraluminal drainage of pancreatic cavities via a transgastric or transduodenal approach using a myriad of drainage catheters deployed directly into the pancreatic cavity. Direct endoscopic necrosectomy through specific stents is possible and has shown promising results. Studies have already shown that a step-up approach using minimally invasive drainage techniques followed by endoscopic necrosectomy results in a significant reduction of morbidity and mortality in necrotizing pancreatitis compared to primary surgical intervention.

It cannot be stressed enough that the management of persistently symptomatic pancreatic necrosis requires a multidisciplinary approach. Care should be individualized after consideration of all the available data, with input from multiple specialties. Regardless of the approach taken, the necrotic tissue should have enough time to organize with formation of a fibrous wall around the cavity. This allows the necrotic collection to be more amenable to drainage and resection. This process usually takes around 4 weeks, and follow-up imaging with CT scan should be used to confirm organization before any intervention is undertaken.

15. **Are there additional treatment options for acute biliary pancreatitis?**
Early ERCP has previously been the standard of care for all patients with suspected acute biliary pancreatitis; however, the timing of such intervention has been challenged by the literature. Studies have found a distinct, statistically significant benefit to performing ERCP only in the setting of biliary sepsis or retained common bile duct stones. In the absence of these events, there is no clear benefit from ERCP. In patients with biliary pancreatitis whose laboratory parameters (total bilirubin and alkaline phosphatase) improve, ERCP before cholecystectomy may be of limited value and/or harmful. Most experts would agree that ERCP in biliary pancreatitis should be performed only if there is clinical evidence of ongoing biliary obstruction or ascending cholangitis. If there is a question of a retained common bile duct stone in patients who improve clinically, an endoscopic ultrasound or MRCP can be performed to exclude that possibility.

16. **When is the optimal timing for cholecystectomy in patients with acute biliary pancreatitis?**
Studies have supported the notion that patients with mild gallstone pancreatitis should undergo cholecystectomy at the time of their index hospitalization. In fact, in cases where cholecystectomy is delayed beyond this time, the overall risk of developing recurrent pancreatitis within 90 days has been quoted close to 20%. In patients with more severe pancreatitis, cholecystectomy is typically delayed until resolution of acute illness and inflammation.

17. **What are pancreatic pseudocysts?**
Pancreatic pseudocysts are localized fluid collections surrounded by a wall of fibrous tissue that is not lined by epithelium. The fluid is often rich in amylase and other pancreatic enzymes. Pseudocysts can form as a result of pancreatic necrosis during an episode of pancreatitis or because of pancreatic duct disruption due to stenosis, calculus, or trauma. Pancreatic pseudocysts may be asymptomatic or present with pain, bleeding, infection, or rupture. Other complications include gastric outlet and/or biliary obstruction and thrombosis of splenic or portal veins with development of gastric varices. The diagnosis is usually made by CT scan.

18. **What is the best approach to the management of pseudocysts?**
Asymptomatic pseudocysts do not require intervention. The indications for pancreatic pseudocyst drainage are limited and related to complications from the cyst itself. These include biliary or luminal obstruction from large cysts or spontaneous infection of the cyst fluid.

Surgical, percutaneous, and endoscopic approaches have all been used to drain these collections. Endoscopic drainage has the advantage of being less invasive and more cost-effective, and is associated with lower lengths of stay than surgery. It is often limited by the position of the cyst or lack of expertise. The treatment modality for pancreatic pseudocysts should be based on a combination of factors including patient comorbidities, clinical status, site, characteristics of the lesion, and available local expertise.

ACKNOWLEDGMENT

The authors wish to acknowledge Drs. Neeraj K. Sardana, MD, Jon (Kai) Yamaguchi, MD, FACS, and David W. McFadden, MD, FACS, for the valuable contributions to the previous edition of this chapter.

KEY POINTS: ACUTE PANCREATITIS

Common Causes of Acute Pancreatitis

B: Biliary—gallstones, parasites, or malignancy
A: Alcohol
D: Drugs
T: Trauma, toxins
I: Idiopathic, ischemic, infectious, inherited
M: Metabolic—hyperlipidemia, hypercalcemia
E: ERCP
S: Smoking

BIBLIOGRAPHY

1. Banks PA, Bollen TL, Dervenis C, et al. Classification of acute pancreatitis—2012: revision of Atlanta classification and definitions by international consensus. *Gut.* 2013;62:102-111.
2. Banks PA. Acute pancreatitis: landmark studies, management decisions, and the future. *Pancreas.* 2016;45(5):633-640.
3. Freeman ML, Werner J, van Santvoort HC, et al. Interventions for necrotizing pancreatitis: summary of a multi-disciplinary consensus conference. *Pancreas.* 2012;8:1176-1194.
4. Gardner TB, Vege SS, Chari ST, et al. Faster rate of initial fluid resuscitation in severe acute pancreatitis diminishes in-hospital mortality. *Pancreatology.* 2009;9:770-776.
5. Jafri NS, Mahid SS, Idstein SR, et al. Antibiotic prophylaxis is not protective in severe acute pancreatitis: a systemic review and meta-analysis. *Am J Surg.* 2009;197:806-813.
6. Moretti A, Papi C, Aratari A, et al. Is early endoscopic retrograde cholangiopancreatography useful in the management of acute biliary pancreatitis? A meta-analysis of randomized controlled trials. *Div Liver Dis.* 2008;40:379-385.
7. Mouli VP, Sreenivas V, Garg PK. Efficacy of conservative treatment, without necrosectomy, for infected pancreatic necrosis: a systematic review and meta-analysis. *Gastroenterology.* 2013;144:333-340.e2.
8. Tenner S, Baillie J, DeWitt J, et al. American College of Gastroenterology Guideline: Management of Acute Pancreatitis. *Am J Gastroenterol.* 2013;108(9):1400-1415.
9. Villatoro E, Bassi C, Larvin M. Antibiotic therapy for prophylaxis against infection of pancreatic necrosis in acute pancreatitis. *Cochrane Database Syst Rev.* 2003;(4):CD002941.
10. Warndorf MG, Kurtzman JT, Bartel MJ, et al. Early fluid resuscitation reduces morbidity among patients with acute pancreatitis. *Clin Gastroenterol Hepatol.* 2011;9:705-709.

CHAPTER 53

HEPATITIS AND CIRRHOSIS

Zechariah S. Gardner and Jaina Clough

1. **What is hepatitis?**
   Hepatitis is defined as inflammation of the liver. It can be divided into infectious and noninfectious causes.

2. **What are liver function tests?**
   The term *liver function tests* (LFTs) commonly refers to alkaline aminotransferase (ALT), aspartate aminotransferase (AST), alkaline phosphatase, bilirubin, albumin, and protein. ALT and AST (transaminases) are enzymes found in hepatocytes, whereas alkaline phosphatase is found in cells in the bile ducts. Gamma-glutamyl transpeptidase (GGT) is an additional test that is used to determine whether alkaline phosphatase elevations originate from hepatobiliary sources. Prothrombin time is used to assess liver synthetic function.

3. **Elevations of which liver function tests are associated with hepatitis?**
   Hepatitis is a process of hepatocellular inflammation and damage that causes spillage of cellular elements into the blood. Hepatitis therefore results primarily in elevations in ALT and AST. Elevations can be modest in some forms of hepatitis (alcoholic) or extreme in others (acute viral hepatitis). Alkaline phosphatase levels can also be elevated in hepatitis, but elevations are generally less significant than those of the transaminases. Bilirubin can reach very high levels in hepatitis but usually lags behind the transaminases.

4. **What are the types of infectious hepatitis?**
   Hepatitis viruses primarily infect the liver and include hepatitis A, B, C, D, and E. Other nonhepatitis viruses can cause hepatitis, including cytomegalovirus, Epstein-Barr virus, and human immunodeficiency virus (HIV).

5. **What is hepatitis A, how is it diagnosed, what is the disease course, and what are some management techniques?**
   Hepatitis A is a disease caused by a RNA virus that is transmitted by the fecal-oral route, is endemic in the developing world, and occurs sporadically in the United States. Most childhood infections are asymptomatic. Adults are more likely to have acute symptoms. The incubation period is 2 to 6 weeks, after which patients develop fatigue, malaise, fever, and abdominal pain followed by jaundice. Transaminase levels are markedly elevated. Diagnosis is by a positive anti–hepatitis A virus (HAV) immunoglobulin (Ig)M antibody that denotes active infection and remains elevated for 3 to 6 months. HAV anti-IgG antibody positivity occurs later, remains elevated for decades, and indicates past infection or vaccination. Treatment is supportive. Significant morbidity and mortality are uncommon, but development of fulminant hepatic failure (FHF) can occur (<1%) and carries significant mortality (see Question 20). HAV vaccine is effective and widely available. It is recommended for individuals with chronic liver disease, child-care workers, and those traveling to endemic areas.

6. **What is hepatitis E?**
   Like HAV, hepatitis E virus (HEV) is an RNA virus that is transmitted by the fecal-oral route. It is endemic to Southeast Asia, Africa, India, and Central America. Infection in the United States is uncommon and is almost always associated with individuals who have recently traveled to endemic areas. It causes a self-limiting hepatitis similar to HAV infection but has a significantly higher tendency to progress to FHF in pregnant women. Laboratory tests for diagnosis include HEV IgG and IgM antibody testing, as well as HEV RNA polymerase chain reaction (PCR). A HEV vaccine is in the late stages of development but is not yet commercially available.

7. **What is hepatitis B?**
   Hepatitis B is a disease caused by a DNA virus that is transmitted through blood and body fluids. Risk factors include intravenous (IV) and intranasal drug use, unprotected sex with multiple partners, men who have sex with men, healthcare workers exposed to blood, children born to infected mothers,

incarceration, and spouses of infected individuals. Acute infection is most commonly asymptomatic but can cause constitutional symptoms including fatigue, malaise, nausea, vomiting, headache, arthralgias, myalgias, and low-grade fever, as well as jaundice, dark urine, clay-colored stools, and tender hepatomegaly. FFH occurs in 1% of infections. Other complications include a serum sickness–like syndrome (5%–10% of cases), glomerular nephritis with nephrotic syndrome, systemic vasculitis, and progression to chronic hepatitis B infection, which occurs in approximately 5% of cases. Some individuals go on to a carrier state in which they have persistent hepatitis B virus (HBV) in the liver without any significant inflammation. These individuals can be infectious and are termed "inactive carriers."

8. **How is hepatitis B diagnosed?**
   Serologic testing for hepatitis B is complicated by the fact that there are multiple blood tests routinely used to assess infection.
   - Hepatitis B surface antigen (HBsAg) is the lipid and protein layer that forms the outer shell of HBV. It is not infectious and is produced in excess during viral replication. It is the first viral antigen to become positive in the serum with acute infection, and its presence indicates active infection. It may be negative early in the acute infection, and it is also the first serum marker to be cleared by the host immune system, becoming undetectable 6 to 12 weeks after infection.
   - Hepatitis B surface antibody (HBsAb) is the antibody to HBsAg. It develops to detectible levels 6 to 8 weeks after infection and remains detectible for life. Positive HBsAb indicates past or resolving infection. Hepatitis B vaccine uses the surface particle, and vaccinated individuals will also be HBsAb positive.
   - Hepatitis B core antibody (HBcAb) is an antibody to a core viral protein. HBcAb can be measured as IgG or IgM and can also be reported as total, which includes both. IgM makes up the immune system's early response and is later replaced by IgG. Positive HBcAb IgM indicates early or chronic infection. Positive HBcAb IgG indicates past or chronic infection.
   - Hepatitis B early antigen (HBeAg) is a protein produced during viral replication, and detectible levels of this antigen indicate high levels of viral replication, increased infectivity, and higher risk of progression to fibrosis. It is positive during both acute infection and active viral phases of chronic infection.
   - HBV DNA can also be measured using PCR. Results can be used to determine eligibility for treatment of chronic HBV infection as well as to assess response to antiviral therapy.

9. **What is hepatitis C?**
   Hepatitis C is caused by a blood-borne RNA virus. It is transmitted primarily through contact with blood products from infected individuals. Risk factors include current or past IV drug use, healthcare workers exposed to blood, or transfusion of infected blood products (rare since routine screening was introduced in 1992). Sexual transmission can occur but is uncommon with hepatitis C virus (HCV). Most acute infections are asymptomatic, but 20% to 30% of infected individuals will have a self-limiting illness similar to other acute viral hepatitis infections. A majority (70%–85%) of those infected with HCV will go on to have chronic infection that can progress to cirrhosis and increases risk of hepatocellular carcinoma (HCC). It is currently estimated that more than 3 million individuals have chronic HCV in the United States, where it is the leading indication for liver transplantation.

10. **How is hepatitis C infection diagnosed?**
    Screening for infection is by serum testing for anti-HCV antibody. Antibody positivity occurs at 4 to 10 weeks and remains positive for life regardless of whether chronic infection develops. All positive antibody tests should be followed up with an HCV RNA PCR to determine whether active infection exists. Of those infected, 15% to 25% will spontaneously clear the virus and are not at risk for complications of chronic infection.

11. **What is the treatment for chronic hepatitis C infection, and who should be treated?**
    Until recently, pegylated interferon-α had been the backbone of regimens for the treatment of chronic HCV infections, often used in conjunction with ribavirin. Treatment was long, fraught with side effects, and only modestly successful in achieving sustained viral response (SVR). Since 2011 a number of direct-acting antivirals (DAAs) have been introduced which target viral proteins and disrupt replication. Now DAA-based interferon free regimens have been shown to be highly effective at achieving SVR with much shorter courses and without many of the side effects associated with interferon therapy. SVR reduces HCV related morbidity and mortality dramatically, and for this reason everyone with chronic HCV infection and access to DAAs should be considered for treatment. The timing of treatment

and selection of treatment regimen are guided by genotype, degree of fibrosis, history of prior treatment, and resistant-associated variants in the virus.

12. What extrahepatic conditions can be caused by hepatitis C infection?
    Some individuals with chronic hepatitis C infection can have other medical conditions that are thought to be due to the body's immune response to the HCV infection. These conditions are uncommon but are noted to occur at increased frequency in those infected with hepatitis C. They include diabetes mellitus, glomerulonephritis, mixed cryoglobulinemia, porphyria cutanea tarda, and non-Hodgkin lymphoma.

13. What is hepatitis D?
    Hepatitis D virus (HDV) or hepatitis delta virus is a small RNA viral particle that can cause infection only in the presence of HBV. It is blood borne, and IV drug use is the most common route of infection. Infection can occur either as coinfection when both HBV and HDV viruses are acquired together or as superinfection when HDV infection occurs in a patient with chronic hepatitis B infection. Concomitant infection with hepatitis B and D results in a higher likelihood of development of FHF, more rapid progression to cirrhosis, and higher rates of HCC.

14. What viral serologies should be tested in a patient with acute hepatitis?
    All patients with acute hepatitis should undergo testing for anti-HAV IgM, anti-HCV antibody, HBsAg, and HBcAb.

15. Who should be screened for hepatitis C virus infection?
    Because chronic hepatitis C infection is prevalent and treatment can reduce the morbidity and mortality associated with infection, screening is recommended for anyone who has used injection drugs, people who received clotting factors before 1987 or other blood products before 1992, patients undergoing hemodialysis, those with unexplained abnormal LFTs, healthcare workers with needle-stick injuries, individuals positive for HIV, and babies born to women positive for HCV. Patients with similar risk factors should be screened for HBV as well.

16. What are the risks associated with chronic hepatitis?
    Chronic hepatitis can develop with HBV, HCV, and HDV infections, as well as many nonviral causes of hepatitis. It is characterized by persistent liver inflammation. Chronic hepatitis is associated with the development of liver fibrosis and cirrhosis, and with increased risk for the development of HCC.

17. What are nonviral causes of hepatitis?
    There are many nonviral causes of hepatitis, which can be broken down into several broad categories including toxic or drug induced, autoimmune, and metabolic. The list of drugs and toxins that can cause liver injury is extensive. The two most common causes of drug- or toxin-induced liver injury are alcohol and acetaminophen. Metabolic causes of hepatitis include hemochromatosis, Wilson disease, and nonalcoholic fatty liver disease. Hepatitis can also develop as a result of other organ system dysfunction. An example of this is liver hypoperfusion in shock states, known as shock liver.

18. What is autoimmune hepatitis?
    Autoimmune hepatitis (AIH) is a chronic inflammatory liver disease caused by a host immune response to portions of the hepatocyte. This chronic inflammation can lead to progressive fibrosis and cirrhosis if left untreated. AIH can occur at any age but occurs most often in young women and is commonly associated with other autoimmune disorders. Circulating autoantibodies associated with AIH are antinuclear antibody, anti–smooth muscle antibody, and liver kidney microsomal antibody. Elevated Ig levels are also common. Liver biopsy is necessary for diagnosis of AIH. Treatment is with steroids alone or in combination with azathioprine, and remission can be achieved in 60% to 80% of cases.

19. How is alcoholic hepatitis managed?
    Alcoholic hepatitis can have a 1-month mortality rate as high as 30% to 50%. The Maddrey discriminant function score is a validated mechanism to score disease severity. It uses prothrombin time and total bilirubin to calculate a disease severity score with scores greater than or equal to 32, indicating severe disease. Data suggest that patients with severe disease benefit from treatment with a 4-week course of steroids or pentoxifylline if steroids are contraindicated. In addition, all patients with alcoholic hepatitis should be counseled to abstain from alcohol and should undergo nutritional assessment and receive aggressive nutritional therapy.

20. How is acetaminophen overdose diagnosed?

Acetaminophen poisoning is the most common cause of acute liver failure in the United States. It causes an acute hepatitis that is characterized by significant elevations of transaminases (>3000 IU/L). Hepatic injury is rapidly progressive, and early recognition is key. Early symptoms are nonspecific, and transaminases can be normal in the first 24 hours after ingestion. If there is suspicion of acetaminophen overdose, a serum level should be measured immediately and repeated 4 hours after ingestion or presentation. In addition, LFTs should be checked and patients should be screened for other co-ingested drugs.

21. How is acetaminophen overdose managed?

Patients presenting within 4 hours of ingestion should be given activated charcoal. Treatment is with N-acetylcysteine (NAC), which should be given to anyone with serum acetaminophen level 4 hours after ingestion above the treatment line on the modified Rumack-Matthew nomogram. Other candidates for NAC therapy include those whose time of ingestion is unknown and whose serum acetaminophen level is greater than 10 mcg/mL, those with an ingestion of greater than 150 mg/kg where no serum level is immediately available, and those with any evidence of hepatic toxicity after ingestion. Mortality is rare when NAC treatment is initiated within 12 hours of ingestion but increases as interval from ingestion to administration of NAC increases.

22. What is fulminant hepatic failure?

FHF or acute liver failure is a gastrointestinal emergency characterized by the rapid arrest of normal hepatic function. A defining feature of FHF is the rapid onset of hepatic encephalopathy. FHF can result from the most severe forms of most of the causes of hepatitis. This includes the viral hepatitides, drugs, toxins, AIH, and metabolic conditions affecting the liver. In addition to encephalopathy, FHF can result in coagulopathy, increased risk for infection, metabolic derangements including acute renal failure, electrolyte abnormalities, hypoglycemia, and pancreatitis. Significant cardiorespiratory and hemodynamic sequelae of FHF also occur that are characterized by hypotension resulting from low systemic vascular resistance, increased cardiac output, and tissue hypoxia.

23. What is the treatment and prognosis of fulminant hepatic failure?

Treatment for patients with FHF is supportive while allowing the liver time to regenerate. Mortality rates are high, and the only intervention with proven benefit is liver transplantation. Early referral to a transplant center should be considered when FHF is suspected. Some causes of FHF can be reversed with immediate treatment and should be assessed for early when FHF is suspected. These include acetaminophen, amanita mushroom poisoning, herpes simplex virus, acute fatty liver disease of pregnancy, and Wilson disease.

24. What is cirrhosis?

Cirrhosis is a progressive process of hepatic injury, subsequent fibrosis, and destruction of normal liver architecture. It may result from any chronic liver disease but is most commonly associated with viral hepatitis and alcoholic liver disease. Cirrhosis was the 12th leading cause of death in the United States in 2007.

25. What are the causes of cirrhosis?

The most common causes of cirrhosis are alcoholic liver disease and hepatitis C. Cryptogenic cirrhosis accounts for up to 18% of cases. Many cryptogenic cases may be due to nonalcoholic fatty liver disease. Other causes include hepatitis B, autoimmune hepatobiliary disease, hemochromatosis, extrahepatic biliary obstruction, Wilson disease, α_1-antitrypsin deficiency, and drug toxicity.

26. Describe the clinical presentation of cirrhosis.

Cirrhosis is often asymptomatic and discovered incidentally. Well-compensated cirrhosis can manifest as anorexia and weight loss, weakness, and fatigue. More progressive disease may present with the following signs: jaundice, pruritus, coagulopathy, increasing abdominal girth, splenomegaly, abdominal wall vascular collaterals (caput medusae), spider telangiectasia, palmar erythema, mental status changes, and asterixis. Advanced cirrhosis may present with severe complications such as upper gastrointestinal tract bleeding or hepatic encephalopathy.

27. How is cirrhosis diagnosed?

Liver biopsy provides the definitive diagnosis of cirrhosis and may be indicated when the clinical diagnosis is uncertain. Abdominal ultrasound findings of liver nodularity, irregularity, increased echogenicity, and atrophy are consistent with cirrhosis. LFTs (including prothrombin time and albumin), hepatitis serologies, autoantibodies, and a complete blood cell count may reveal the underlying causes of cirrhosis and the extent of liver dysfunction.

28. What are the major complications of cirrhosis?

The most common complication of cirrhosis is ascites, followed by gastroesophageal variceal hemorrhage and hepatic encephalopathy. Ascites and variceal hemorrhage are direct consequences of portal hypertension.

29. What is decompensated cirrhosis?

Patients who develop severe complications of cirrhosis including variceal bleeding, ascites, spontaneous bacterial peritonitis (SBP), hepatic encephalopathy, or hepatorenal syndrome (HRS) are said to have decompensated cirrhosis. Decompensated cirrhosis portends significantly worse prognosis than compensated cirrhosis.

30. What is portal hypertension?

Portal hypertension is defined as a portal pressure of greater than 12 mm Hg or a hepatic venous wedge pressure that exceeds the pressure of the inferior vena cava by greater than 5 mm Hg. The portal hypertension of cirrhosis is caused by the disruption of hepatic sinusoids, leading to increased resistance in the portal venous system. A compounding effect is increased portal flow due to vasodilation and increased cardiac output associated with cirrhosis. This leads to an imbalance of Starling forces, which results in fluid accumulation in the peritoneal cavity (ascites), as well as gastroesophageal varices.

31. What are other complications of cirrhosis?

Other complications of cirrhosis include altered hemodynamics, hyponatremia, immune compromise, and coagulopathy.

32. How is cirrhotic ascites diagnosed?

New-onset ascites should be assessed with diagnostic paracentesis to confirm cirrhosis as the cause and rule out SBP. The serum-ascites albumin gradient (SAAG) is the most important diagnostic parameter in determining the cause of ascites. A SAAG of greater than or equal to 1.1 g/dL indicates ascites from portal hypertension with a specificity of 97%. Ascitic fluid cell count, differential, and total protein should also be performed. Ascitic fluid culture should be obtained if any suspicion of SBP exists.

33. How is cirrhotic ascites managed?

Initial management focuses on dietary sodium restriction and abstinence from alcohol in alcohol-related liver disease. Diuretic therapy is the mainstay of medical management of ascites. Dual therapy with furosemide and spironolactone is the recommended starting regimen if renal function is stable. Large-volume paracentesis is used to relieve the discomfort of tense ascites. Serial paracentesis may be indicated for ascites refractory to medical therapy. Transjugular intrahepatic portosystemic shunt (TIPS) and liver transplantation should be considered in refractory cases. Surgically placed peritoneovenous shunts may be an option in patients who are not candidates for paracentesis, TIPS, or transplantation.

34. What is transjugular intrahepatic portosystemic shunt?

TIPS is a treatment for portal hypertension. It is reserved for patients with severe ascites or variceal bleeding who do not respond to medical therapy. Reduced portal pressure is achieved by a stent placed through the liver between the portal and hepatic circulation. TIPS is effective at reducing the sequela of portal hypertension but increases risk of developing hepatic encephalopathy.

35. What are the complications of cirrhotic ascites?

Ascites is associated with the complications of SBP and the HRS.

36. What is the mortality of cirrhotic ascites?

Cirrhotic ascites carries a 3-year mortality rate of 50%.

37. How is spontaneous bacterial peritonitis diagnosed and managed?

A positive ascitic fluid culture and absolute polymorphonuclear leukocyte (PMN) count of greater than or equal to 250 cells/mm^3 are diagnostic of SBP in the absence of an intraabdominal, surgically treatable source of infection. Empirical antibiotics should be initiated for SBP in any hospitalized patient with an ascitic fluid PMN count of greater than or equal to 250 cells/mm^3 or an ascitic protein level of less than 1 g/dL, or in a patient with clinical suspicion of SBP (i.e., fever, abdominal pain), regardless of PMN count. A third-generation cephalosporin is the initial antibiotic choice, ideally cefotaxime. Oral ofloxacin is an acceptable substitute in patients who are quinolone naïve and are clinically stable.

38. What are risk factors for spontaneous bacterial peritonitis, and how is it prevented?
Risk factors for SBP include prior SBP, variceal hemorrhage, and low-protein ascites. Prevention of SBP may be achieved with use of quinolones or a third-generation cephalosporin in patients with variceal hemorrhage. Oral quinolones may be used in patients who have had prior episodes of SBP. Antibiotic prophylaxis may be considered in those with low-protein ascites.

39. What is hepatorenal syndrome, and how is it managed?
HRS is renal dysfunction (creatinine level >1.5 mg/dL) that persists after 2 days of diuretic withdrawal and volume expansion in patients with cirrhosis and ascites. Type I HRS is rapidly progressive and fatal without treatment. Type II HRS progresses over months, with a median survival of 3 to 6 months. Type I HRS warrants an expedited referral for liver transplantation. Dialysis may be needed to bridge patients to transplantation. Medical therapies such as octreotide and midodrine may be used as temporizing measures as well.

40. What is variceal bleeding?
Variceal bleeding is upper gastrointestinal tract bleeding due to the rupture of gastroesophageal varices. It is the most common life-threatening complication of cirrhosis and occurs at a rate of 5% to 15% per year in patients with cirrhosis. Size of varices and severity of liver disease are the most important predictors of bleeding.

41. How is variceal bleeding prevented?
At the time cirrhosis is diagnosed, esophagogastroduodenoscopy (EGD) should be performed to screen for varices. If medium to large varices are present with a high risk of bleeding, nonselective β-blocker therapy or endoscopic variceal ligation (EVL) is recommended. For medium varices or small varices with a high risk of bleeding, nonselective β-blocker therapy is preferred with EVL reserved for patients intolerant to β-blocker therapy. Subsequent surveillance EGD is recommended to follow for development or recurrence of high risk varices.

42. What are other sources of upper gastrointestinal tract bleeding in patients with cirrhosis?
Portal hypertension also puts patients at risk of bleeding from portal hypertensive gastropathy and gastric antral vascular ectasia.

43. What is hepatic encephalopathy?
Hepatic encephalopathy is a syndrome of altered mental status in the setting of portosystemic shunting, either through collateral vessels or through surgically placed shunts. The mechanism is uncertain but may relate to changes in the blood-brain barrier that allow the passage of neurotoxic substances, including ammonia and manganese, into the brain. Another theory suggests that accumulation of circulating ammonia due to decreased hepatocyte function leads to encephalopathy.

44. How is hepatic encephalopathy diagnosed and managed?
Elevated serum ammonia levels indicate hepatic encephalopathy in patients with cirrhosis and altered mental status that cannot be explained by any other cause. Precipitating factors include gastrointestinal bleeding, infection, constipation, and metabolic disturbances. Treatment focuses on reducing intestinal production of ammonia, typically through the use of cathartics (such as lactulose) and antibiotics (such as neomycin and rifaximin). Low-protein diets are no longer recommended, as they do not appear to be effective at reducing encephalopathy and may contribute to malnutrition.

45. Describe the pulmonary syndromes associated with chronic liver disease?
Hepatopulmonary syndrome is a mismatch of ventilation and perfusion that results primarily from vasodilation of pulmonary capillaries. Arteriovenous communication in the lungs and pleura may occur as well. It is characterized by hypoxia and dyspnea that worsen with upright positioning (orthodeoxia and platypnea, respectively). Portopulmonary hypertension is the development of pulmonary hypertension in the presence of portal hypertension.

46. What is the model for end-stage liver disease?
Model for end-stage liver disease (MELD) is a validated statistical model initially developed to predict survival after TIPS that has been expanded to aid in estimating severity of liver disease and prognosis in non-TIPS patients. It uses serum bilirubin, serum creatinine, and International Normalized Ratio (INR) to calculate an overall score that can be used to estimate 3-month survival (MELD score calculator www.mayoclinic.org/meld/). MELD has been adopted by the United Network for Organ Sharing to prioritize patients for liver transplantation in the United States.

47. When should patients with cirrhosis be referred for liver transplantation?

Patients with cirrhosis should be referred for transplantation when they have their first major complication (ascites, variceal bleeding, hepatic encephalopathy) or evidence of significant hepatic dysfunction (MELD score ≥10, Child-Turcotte-Pugh [CTP] score ≥7). Type 1 HRS is an indication for expedited referral for liver transplantation.

KEY POINTS: HEPATITIS AND CIRRHOSIS

Hepatitis

1. Pregnant women are at significant risk for FHF with hepatitis E infection.
2. Everyone with chronic HCV infection and access to DAAs should be considered for treatment.
3. Steroids should be considered for the treatment of severe alcoholic hepatitis.
4. Some causes of FHF can be reversed with immediate treatment, including acetaminophen, amanita mushroom poisoning, herpes simplex virus, acute fatty liver disease of pregnancy, and Wilson disease.

Cirrhosis

1. Critical complications of cirrhosis include ascites, SBP, HRS, hepatic encephalopathy, and upper gastrointestinal tract bleeding due to gastroesophageal varices.
2. Management of variceal bleeding involves volume resuscitation, use of somatostatin or analogs, endoscopic treatment with sclerotherapy or EVL, and antibiotics to prevent SBP.
3. TIPS is reserved for refractory ascites or uncontrolled variceal bleeding. TIPS carries a high risk for encephalopathy.
4. Referral for liver transplantation is indicated in FHF when the MELD score is ≥10 or when major complications of cirrhosis develop. Type 1 HRS is an indication for expedited liver transplantation referral.

BIBLIOGRAPHY

1. Centers for Disease Control and Prevention. Hepatitis C information for health professionals. Available at http://www.cdc.gov/hepatitis/HCV/HCVfaq.htm#section2. Accessed July 15, 2011.
2. Córdoba J, López-Hellín J, Planas M, et al. Normal protein diet for episodic hepatic encephalopathy: results of a randomized study. *J Hepatol.* 2004;41:38-43.
3. Dienstag JL. Acute viral hepatitis. In: Fauci AS, Braunwald E, Kasper DL, et al., eds. *Harrison's Principles of Internal Medicine.* 17th ed. New York: McGraw-Hill; 2008.
4. Garcia-Tsao G, Sanyal AJ, Grace ND, et al. Practice Guidelines Committee of American Association for Study of Liver Diseases, Practice Parameters Committee of American College of Gastroenterology. Prevention and management of gastroesophageal varices and variceal hemorrhage in cirrhosis. *Am J Gastroenterol.* 2007;102:2086-2102.
5. Ghany MG, Strader DB, Thomas DL, et al. Diagnosis, management and treatment of hepatitis C: an update. *Hepatology.* 2009;49:1335-1374.
6. Ginés P, Quintero E, Arroyo V, et al. Compensated cirrhosis: natural history and prognostic factors. *Hepatology.* 1987;7:122-128.
7. Heidelbaugh JJ, Bruderly M. Cirrhosis and chronic liver failure: part I. Diagnosis and evaluation. *Am Fam Physician.* 2006;74:756-762.
8. Hézode C, Forestier N, Dusheiko G, et al. Telaprevir and peginterferon with or without ribavirin for chronic HCV infection. *N Engl J Med.* 2009;360:1839-1850.
9. Krajden M, McNabb G, Petric M. The laboratory diagnosis of hepatitis B virus. *Can J Infect Dis Med Microbiol.* 2005;16:65-72.
10. Lok ASF, McMahon BJ. Chronic hepatitis B. *Hepatology.* 2007;45:507-539.
11. Manns MP, Czaja AJ, Gorham JD, et al. Diagnosis and management of autoimmune hepatitis. *Hepatology.* 2010;51:2193-2213.
12. Murray KF, Carithers RL. AASLD practice guidelines: Evaluation of the patient for liver transplantation. *Hepatology.* 2005;41:1407-1432.
13. O'Shea RS, Dasarathy S, McCullough AJ, AASLD Practice Guidelines. Alcoholic liver disease. *Hepatology.* 2010;51:307-328.
14. Poordad F, McCone J, Jr, Bacon BR, et al. Boceprevir for untreated chronic HCV genotype 1 infection. *N Engl J Med.* 2011;364:1195-1206.
15. Rodríguez-Roisin R, Krowka MJ. Hepatopulmonary syndrome—a liver-induced lung vascular disorder. *N Engl J Med.* 2008;358:2378-2387.
16. Runyon BA, AASLD Practice Guidelines Committee. Management of adult patients with ascites due to cirrhosis: an update. *Hepatology.* 2009;49:2087-2107.
17. Rutherford A, Dienstag JL. Viral hepatitis. In: Greenberger NJ, Blumberg RS, Burakoff R, eds. *Current Diagnosis & Treatment: Gastroenterology, Hepatology, & Endoscopy.* New York: McGraw-Hill; 2009.

18. Sass DA, Shakil AO. Fulminant hepatic failure. *Liver Transpl.* 2005;11:594-605.
19. Xu J, Kochanek KD, Murphy SL, et al. Deaths: final data for 2007. *Natl Vital Stat Rep.* 2010;58:1-135.
20. Zhu FC, Zhang J, Zhang XF, et al. Efficacy and safety of recombinant hepatitis E vaccine in healthy adults: a large-scale, randomised, double-blind placebo-controlled, phase 3 trial. *Lancet.* 2010;376(9744):895-902.
21. Terrault NA, Bzowej NH, Chang KM, et al. AASLD guidelines for treatment of chronic hepatitis B. *Hepatology.* 2016;63(1):261-283.
22. Polson J, Lee WM. AASLD position paper: the management of acute liver failure. *Hepatology.* 2005;41:1179-1197. doi:10.1002/hep.20703. Available at: http://onlinelibrary.wiley.com/doi/10.1002/hep.20703/abstract;jsessionid=DF67 01258A4ABC857AE33149D24C9331.f03t01.

IX
ENDOCRINOLOGY

CHAPTER 54

DIABETIC KETOACIDOSIS AND HYPEROSMOLAR HYPERGLYCEMIC STATE

Joel J. Schnure and John L. Leahy

1. **What is diabetic ketoacidosis?**

   Diabetic ketoacidosis (DKA) is a serious, acute metabolic decompensation in persons with known or newly presenting diabetes. It is a consequence of a relative or an absolute insulin deficiency in combination with an excess of counter-regulatory hormones (primarily glucagon and catecholamines, but also cortisol and growth hormones). The classic triad of features is hyperglycemia (typically >250 mg/dL), anion gap metabolic acidosis, and ketosis. It is most commonly associated with type 1 diabetes, but also can occur with type 2 diabetes usually with another severe medical issue such as sepsis, bowel infarction, or cardiac or cerebrovascular event.

2. **Describe the tissue actions of insulin.**

   The major action of endogenously secreted or injected insulin is to lower the blood glucose level by increasing glucose uptake into the peripheral tissues, such as skeletal muscle and adipose, and by promoting glycogenolysis and stopping gluconeogenesis in the liver. Additionally, its anabolic effects inhibit adipose breakdown to free fatty acids and muscle breakdown to amino acids. The sensitivity of these actions differs in the various target tissues, with small amounts of insulin fully preventing triglyceride metabolism and the release of free fatty acids from adipose tissue, whereas larger amounts are needed to suppress hepatic glucose production and to promote glucose clearance into peripheral tissues.

3. **What is the pathogenesis of diabetic ketoacidosis in type 1 diabetes?**

   DKA usually starts with *absolute insulin deficiency* because of a broken or clogged insulin pump, missed injections, or damaged insulin from poor storage or excess heat exposure, or with *relative insulin deficiency* from a rise in tissue insulin requirements from infection, trauma, or other stresses. Glucose production from the liver increases, and glucose clearance into peripheral tissues is impaired, causing the blood glucose level to rise. Stress-related increases in counter-regulatory hormones exacerbate these effects. As the renal glucose threshold is passed, an osmotic diuresis occurs causing urinary losses of water and electrolytes. The ensuing dehydration further increases the level of catecholamines. Also, because glucagon and insulin levels are inversely related, the insulin deficiency causes hyperglucagonemia. The increased levels of catecholamines and glucagon, along with the insulin deficiency, promote excess release of fatty acids from the adipose tissue that further impairs insulin-mediated glucose uptake into peripheral tissues. The capacity of the liver for β-oxidation of the fatty acids is also exceeded, resulting in ketone production by the liver. This ketonemia and the resulting acidosis often cause nausea and vomiting; the patient's polydipsia therefore stops, worsening the dehydration. The patient is now in DKA with this whole process occurring over a 12- to 48-hour period. This sequence of events is depicted in Fig. 54.1.

4. **What is euglycemic diabetic ketoacidosis associated with sodium glucose transporter 2 inhibitors?**

   Sodium glucose transporter 2 (SGLT2) inhibitors are oral medications used for the treatment of type 2 diabetes that act by inhibiting the action of the SGLT2, which is expressed in renal tubules, and mediates 90% of the reabsorption of glucose from the glomerular filtrate to the plasma. SGLT2 is also expressed in islet α-cells and tonically inhibits glucagon secretion. The clinical effect of these agents is to cause glycosuria that improves blood glucose control and often promotes weight loss, and to lower blood pressure through the accompanying urinary excretion of Na and water. The result is a modest lowering of the insulin level that results in a small increase in free fatty acid release from the adipose tissue along with higher glucagon levels. A type of DKA has been described with these agents, which

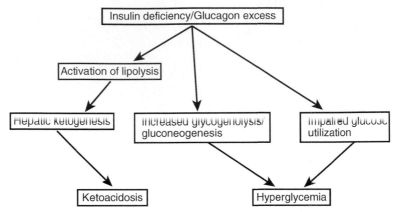

Figure 54-1. Pathogenesis of diabetic ketoacidosis. *(From Atlee J.* Complications in Anesthesia. *2nd ed. Philadelphia: Saunders; 2007.)*

is characterized by the usual metabolic defects of an anion gap metabolic acidosis, ketosis, and bicarbonate level less than 15 mEq/L, but without overt hyperglycemia. Many of these cases are patients with type 1 diabetes who were given these agents for weight loss. Alternatively, patients with type 2 diabetes have also been described. A common precipitating event is that the patient lowered their insulin doses often because of a viral gastroenteritis, so the insulin to glucagon ratio was decreased enough to promote the release of free fatty acids that are converted to ketones by the effect of the hyperglucagonemia to make the liver ketogenic. In contrast, hyperglycemia is not present or obvious because of the glycosuria. As such, a key diagnostic test for patients who are taking these agents and feel ill even without hyperglycemia, is urinary or serum ketones.

5. How does diabetic ketoacidosis cause an anion gap metabolic acidosis?
   The insulin deficiency and increased glucagon and catecholamines cause excess release of fatty acids from the adipose tissue and activation of metabolic pathways in the liver for conversion to ketoacids: acetoacetate, acetone, and β-hydroxybutyrate. Their accumulation results in the anion gap metabolic acidosis, which is characteristic of DKA. The *anion gap* is calculated by subtracting the serum concentration of the major anions (chloride and bicarbonate) from the main cation (sodium). A difference of more than 12 mEq/L along with a lowered bicarbonate level ($<$15 mEq/L) shows the presence of anions that are not identified in this calculation, thus the anion gap (in this case, the ketoacids).

6. How is type 1 diabetes diagnosed?
   Type 1 diabetes results from autoimmune-mediated destruction of islet beta-cells; therefore, patients present with signs and symptoms of insulin deficiency: exhaustion, weight loss, nocturia, the *polys* (polyuria and polydipsia), and sometimes DKA. It is usually diagnosed because of a typical clinical presentation, and can be confirmed with the use of specific markers for the autoimmune beta-cell destruction. The best known is decarboxylase-65 (GAD-65) antibody, which is directed against a beta-cell enzyme called glutamic acid decarboxylase. A positive test confirms type 1 diabetes, but a negative test does not rule it out. It is not necessary to perform GAD-65 antibody testing in all patients with newly identified type 1 diabetes, but it is most useful in those with elements of both type 1 and type 2 diabetes. In contrast, insulin or C peptide testing is not recommended, because insulin secretion is driven by glycemia, and the patient's hyperglycemia and short duration of diabetes mean that these measures are rarely absent in patients with new-onset type 1 diabetes.

7. Does diabetic ketoacidosis develop in persons with type 2 diabetes?
   Most series of persons with DKA show a 10% to 30% incidence of type 2 diabetes usually in association with an accompanying severe medical illness. The concept is that the added stress of the associated illness allows ketoacidosis to occur, in part because catecholamines are potent inhibitors of insulin secretion from the beta-cell. This accompanying illness also impacts the clinical course. Mortality rates are much higher in persons with DKA who are older than 50 years of age versus

younger patients, with the older group dying of sepsis, adult respiratory distress syndrome, shock, or cardiovascular collapse.

A form of type 2 diabetes also exists that is ketosis-prone, so-called *Flatbush diabetes* or *ketosis-prone type 2 diabetes*. These patients are mostly from minority populations (most studied are black and Latino) who have ketosis and sometimes DKA, often with obesity, but test negative for markers of type 1 diabetes. The defining clinical feature is being able to stop insulin months later, sometimes permanently. The pathogenesis is thought to be a heightened sensitivity for stress hormones to suppress insulin secretion that partially reverses with time.

8. What are the common precipitating events for diabetic ketoacidosis?
The most frequent initiating events for DKA are infection, insulin under-delivery, and newly presenting type 1 diabetes. Cardiovascular events and cerebrovascular accidents also occur, mostly in older patients. Insulin omission used to be mostly found in teenagers and young adults, but the growing use of insulin pumps in all ages means DKA from pump failure or catheter occlusion is age independent. Among infections, pneumonias, gastrointestinal tract viral infections, and urinary tract infections are the most common. Other causes are pancreatitis, drug abuse, or severe medical illness of any type. Even with all of the known causes, failure to identify a precipitating event is relatively common.

9. Describe the common signs and symptoms of diabetic ketoacidosis?
Patients typically describe 1 to 3 days of polyuria, nocturia, and thirst. Fatigue also occurs, and often a rapid weight loss reflects the catabolic effect of the insulin deficiency and volume depletion. As the ketonemia and metabolic acidosis progress, nausea and repeated vomiting may occur, exacerbating the dehydration. Abdominal pain is also common related to gastric distention from the metabolic acidosis or irritation from repeated vomiting. Patients may report shortness of breath from their Kussmaul respirations that can be mistaken for a pulmonary infection or a cardiac event. What is not usually reported is confusion or coma; fewer than 20% of patients are stuporous or show any confusion.

On exam, patients often show the Kussmaul breathing pattern of deep, sighing breaths as they attempt to compensate for the metabolic acidosis by lowering their pCO_2. Tachycardia is common. In contrast, the systolic blood pressure is rarely less than 100 mm Hg because of the osmotic effect of the hyperglycemia keeping fluid in the vascular space. Body temperature is usually normal even when an infection is present because the metabolic acidosis blunts the fever response. A distinguishing feature of DKA is the fruity sweet smell of the patient's breath from their exhaling the ketone acetone. The remainder of the physical examination is typically unremarkable except for a generalized abdominal tenderness.

10. How does the hyperosmolar hyperglycemic state differ from diabetic ketoacidosis?
Hyperosmolar hyperglycemic state (HHS) also is characterized by profound hyperglycemia but without ketoacidosis. The distinguishing clinical features of HHS are as follows:
- Occurs most often in the elderly and those with known type 2 diabetes
- Very high blood glucose levels of 600 mg/dL or greater
- Markedly elevated serum osmolarity of 320 mOsm/kg or greater
- Frequent occurrence of altered mental state or coma
- More serious hypotension and overt dehydration, including substantially larger electrolyte losses than DKA
- High mortality rate that averages 15% versus less than 2% in uncomplicated DKA

11. What is the pathogenesis of hyperosmolar hyperglycemic state?
A key pathogenic element of worsening hyperglycemia in type 2 diabetes is glucotoxicity: the effect of high glucose values to impair insulin secretion and promote worsening insulin resistance. However, the major difference from DKA is the presence of modestly higher circulating insulin that prevents much of a rise in free fatty acids (lipolysis) and thus blocks ketone production from the liver, but it is not enough to suppress hepatic glucose production or promote glucose clearance into peripheral tissues. Therefore, the main feature is hyperglycemia without ketoacidosis, although small amounts of urinary ketones and a modest widening of the anion gap can be seen. As such, the metabolic acidosis-induced vomiting and abdominal pain common in DKA—and which often get the patient to seek medical help—are lacking. Instead the worsening hyperglycemia and osmotic diuresis go on for much longer, typically many days or a couple of weeks, and the presentation is often insidious, manifesting in symptoms such as bed-wetting or modest confusion that may be unnoticed in the elderly. Thus the dehydration and urinary electrolyte losses are considerably worse than in DKA, and it is this dehydration that is the key feature leading to HHS by causing a fall in urine output and with

it, glycosuria. The blood glucose level now rises above the renal threshold to values that can exceed 1000 mg/dL. Serum osmolarity rises in parallel, and the resulting confusion or coma is usually why the patient is brought for medical attention. These events are depicted in Fig. 54.1.

12. **What are the common precipitating events in hyperosmolar hyperglycemic state?**
HHS occurs most often in patients with known type 2 diabetes, although it is the first evidence in 30% to 40% of patients. The most common cause is a medical crisis, such as infection or sepsis, cardio-vascular event, cerebrovascular accident, pancreatitis, or acute abdomen. Pharmaceuticals that raise glycemia also are sometimes at fault, with the best-known high-dose thiazides, corticosteroids, sym-pathomimetic agents, atypical antipsychotics, and β-blockers. Another common feature is caregivers having restricted the patient's access to water because of incontinence or bed-wetting.

13. **Describe the common signs and symptoms of hyperosmolar hyperglycemic state?**
Patients are usually brought for medical evaluation because of mood change, reduction in appetite, con-fusion, or coma. Particularly common are subtle behavior changes over several weeks, such as lethargy or less interaction with the family. Also hints to the precipitating cause or illness may be elicited. Useful history is a worsening of bed-wetting or incontinence to gauge the duration of the osmotic diuresis.
On examination, patients typically show some mental alteration from slow answers to questions or searching for words to obtundation or coma. Because of the advanced age of many of these patients and the potential for underlying central nervous system (CNS) pathologic conditions, they may have focal findings that mimic a stroke. In addition, these patients usually are seen with signs of severe volume depletion, such as marked hypotension, dry mucous membranes, and skin tenting. As with DKA, the absence of a fever does not exclude infection, especially because of the blunted fever response in elderly patients.

14. **Which initial laboratory tests are obtained in diabetic ketoacidosis and hyperosmolar hyperglycemic state?**
Laboratory testing at presentation includes a complete blood cell count, serum electrolytes, arterial blood gases, serum creatinine, serum ketones and/or β-hydroxybutyrate, a comprehensive metabolic panel (CMP), and urinalysis for signs of infection. In DKA, radiographs or scans, pan-cultures, drug screens, and serum brain natriuretic peptide, lactate, lipase, or markers of ischemic cardiac damage, are not usually obtained without a suggestive history or physical findings. In HHS, because of the advanced age of many patients and the insidious nature of the presentation, pan-testing is common, particularly in patients who are confused or comatose: urine and blood cultures, electrocardiogram, cardiac enzymes, and CNS imaging, especially if there are focal neurological findings. Hemoglobin A1c testing is very helpful to determine the diabetes control before the acute hyperglycemic event, or the chronicity of hyperglycemia in patients with new-onset diabetes.

15. **How and when to test for ketones.**
Testing for ketones in the serum or urine is done with the nitroprusside reaction that gives a semiquan-titative estimate of acetoacetate and acetone levels. However, it does not recognize β-hydroxybutyrate. Therefore, the severity of DKA may be underestimated if the ratio of β-hydroxybutyrate to the others is increased as can occur with lactic acidosis or alcohol. The common observation of the ketone reaction becoming more positive during therapy when the patient is clinically improving represents conversion of β-hydroxybutyrate to acetoacetate during metabolic breakdown of that ketone body. As such, it is recommended to test serum ketones only at presentation. Direct measures of serum β-hydroxybutyrate are commonly available, and have been advocated as a better diagnostic test for DKA than urine ketones; however, modest elevations can be seen with HHS or marked hyperglycemia without overt acidosis.

16. **How to interpret the complete blood count results in diabetic ketoacidosis and hyperosmolar hyperglycemic state.**
The white blood cell (WBC) count is usually elevated in DKA, sometimes to 20,000 or 25,000/mm^3, with a leftward shift because of stress hormone-induced demargination. The WBC count typically returns to the normal range after several hours to a day of treatment of the DKA. In contrast, hemo-globin and hematocrit values are typically normal unless a prior abnormality, such as chronic renal impairment, exists. Therefore a large decrease from the patient's pre-DKA baseline hemoglobin level should be evaluated for gastrointestinal bleeding or another source of internal or external hemorrhage.
The findings in HHS are more varied because of the older age of many of the patients and the presence of pre-existing comorbidities or severe precipitating illnesses. A stress-induced leukocytosis

is common, but unlike in DKA, it may persist for a few days because of the prolonged course of treatment in many patients. Dehydration is also more severe than in DKA, and a fall in hemoglobin level by 1 to 3 g with rehydration is often seen.

17. **What changes in serum sodium level occur in diabetic ketoacidosis and hyperosmolar hyperglycemic state?**
The osmotic diuresis in DKA and HHS results in large total-body reductions in volume and electrolytes. Impaired water intake is also a common feature both from the nausea and/or vomiting in DKA and the blunted thirst response of the elderly in HHS. Still, serum sodium is usually below normal in DKA because of the osmotic effect of the hyperglycemia drawing cellular and interstitial fluid into the vascular space. The sodium concentration of this fluid is much less than in blood (intracellular fluid is only 3–5 mEq), diluting the serum sodium concentration, an effect termed *pseudohyponatremia*. One can correct for this effect by adding 1.6 mEq/L of sodium to the measured value for every 100 mg/dL of glucose above the normal range of 100 mg/dL.
    The sodium concentration in HHS is a major contributor to the hyperosmolarity as it is often normal or above the normal range despite the marked hyperglycemia. This is because of the protracted diuresis of hypotonic urine that is a key pathogenic factor in HHS, resulting in a greater whole-body water deficit versus HHS. An additional feature in many patients is continued use of diuretics that exacerbate the urinary water loses.

18. **What are the changes in serum potassium in diabetic ketoacidosis and hyperosmolar hyperglycemic state?**
In DKA, the serum potassium level is altered by an adaption to the metabolic acidosis of an electroneutral shift of H^+ out of blood into cells in exchange for K^+ from cells back to blood. A formula to estimate the serum potassium at physiologic pH is 0.8 mEq of potassium for every 0.1 pH from 7.4. This explains the high level of concern over *normal* potassium levels in patients with acidosis and how treatment with bicarbonate could cause a hypokalemic crisis. In addition, serum potassium losses persist during early DKA therapy, which is related to the effect of insulin to drive potassium into cells, and additional urinary losses from the osmotic diuresis until the hyperglycemia is controlled. Thus DKA is characterized by large reductions in total-body potassium that are not accurately reflected in the initial serum potassium level.
    In HHS, the lack of significant acidosis means there is little K^+-H^+ exchange effect. Still, whole-body potassium losses typically exceed those seen with DKA, and there are the ongoing losses during treatment; therefore, the concern over low or low-normal potassium levels, and the need for potassium replacement, are equal to that of DKA.

19. How is the anion gap calculated and interpreted?
The anion gap is calculated by subtracting the serum concentrations of chloride and bicarbonate from the sodium concentration. A difference of greater than 12 mEq/L along with a lowered bicarbonate level (<15 mEq/L) shows the presence of an anion gap metabolic acidosis and is a defining feature of DKA. Other causes of anion gap metabolic acidosis are lactic acidosis, advanced renal failure, and ingestion of high-dose salicylates, methanol, or ethylene glycol. Some patients with DKA have a complex acid-base disorder that can include a metabolic alkalosis from the protracted vomiting or the marked dehydration, and/or a respiratory alkalosis from fever, pain, or an accompanying pulmonary or CNS illness.
    In HHS, the anion gap is often modestly increased from increased lactate because of the marked dehydration, but the bicarbonate level is greater than 15 mEq/L and the pH is greater than 7.3.

20. How is hyperosmolarity calculated in hyperosmolar hyperglycemic state?
The defining clinical feature of HHS is hyperosmolarity. The normal serum osmolarity is 275 to 295 mOsm/L. It is made up of the osmotic effects of serum sodium, potassium, glucose, and urea. However, urea traverses membranes relatively freely and thus does not contribute to the serum tonicity that is called the *effective osmolarity*, which is calculated by the following formula:

$$2 \times [Na(mEq/L) + K(mEq/L)] + Plasma\ glucose\ (mg/dL) / 18$$

    A relatively linear relationship exists between the effective osmolarity and mental state in HHS, with deficits beginning to occur at values above 320 mOsm/L and coma above 340 mOsms/L. As such, stupor or coma in a patient with hyperglycemia values below 320 mOsm/L warrants a careful work-up for causes of the mental status change. Also, mortality rises substantially with levels above 350 mOsm/L.

21. What are the goals of therapy in diabetic ketoacidosis?

The main pathogenic features of DKA are dehydration, insulin deficiency, and an excess of stress hormones that collectively cause the hyperglycemia and metabolic acidosis. Treatment goals are to

- reverse the ketogenesis and return the pH to normal;
- restore blood glucose control;
- correct the hypovolemia;
- replete the whole-body electrolyte stores;
- identify and reverse any precipitating illness;
- prevent the complications that can occur with DKA therapy.

22. Describe insulin therapy for diabetic ketoacidosis?

DKA is usually treated with a continuous intravenous (IV) infusion of regular insulin at 0.1 unit/kg per hour. Hourly intramuscular injections or 2-hour subcutaneous injections of a rapid-acting insulin at the same amounts as the IV insulin can be used when IV insulin is not possible. Once insulin is started, the blood glucose level should fall 50 to 70 mg/dL per hour; the initial fall may be greater related to the early large volume of fluid replacement. If it does not, the recommendation after 2 hours is to double the insulin dose hourly until that occurs. The insulin infusion rate is continued until the blood glucose falls below 200 mg/dL, and then is lowered by 50% along with switching the IV fluids to contain 5% dextrose (D5) or 10% dextrose to keep the blood glucose level between 100 and 200 mg/dL. The insulin infusion is also continued for another 6 to 12 hours to prevent recurrence of the ketoacidosis. A controversial issue is whether to give a bolus of insulin before starting the infusion because studies have not shown a benefit of the bolus approach, and in theory it could rarely cause hypoglycemia. It is still commonly used because many believe it gets therapy started while the patient is being fully evaluated, and that giving 10 units of Regular insulin rapidly IV gives up to an hour before the infusion must be started. A newer practice is to start the patient on subcutaneous basal insulin as soon as the DKA metabolic derangements start to improve, when the IV insulin infusion will still be continued for many hours, rather than when they are transitioned off the IV insulin; studies show less hyperglycemia and return of ketoacidosis following cessation of the IV insulin.

23. What is appropriate fluid therapy in diabetic ketoacidosis?

The osmotic effect of the hyperglycemia keeps the vascular space relatively fluid replete as the DKA develops. Administering insulin without fluid can reverse this effect and cause cardiovascular collapse. Unless an illness prevents aggressive fluid replacement, such as chronic renal failure with anuria or congestive heart failure, 1 L of normal saline solution is usually given, quickly followed by an isotonic saline solution or half-normal saline at 300 to 500 mL/h depending on the patient's sodium level. Potassium is added to the IV fluids as described below. Glucose is also added to the IV fluids once blood glucose is brought below 200 mg/dL to prevent hypoglycemia while the insulin infusion is continued for full reversal of the ketogenesis. The fluid deficit in DKA is up to 100 mL/kg, but larger volumes are often needed to restore euvolemia, because much of the infused volume over the first 5 to 6 hours is lost in the urine until glycemia is below the renal threshold. A common finding after closure of the anion gap is a subnormal serum bicarbonate and a raised chloride level. This hyperchloremic metabolic acidosis occurs because of the large amount of NaCl in the administered IV fluids, plus the loss of ketones in the urine equates to a loss of "bicarbonate equivalents" because bicarbonate is regenerated as the ketones are metabolized during the DKA therapy. Some institutions use IV fluids that contain small amounts of bicarbonate to minimize this effect. However, it is generally harmless and reverts to normal over a few days without therapy.

24. Describe potassium replacement in diabetic ketoacidosis?

Serum potassium stores are lowered 150 to 250 mEq in DKA. This depletion is usually not apparent in the initial serum potassium level because of the H^+-K^+ cellular shift, with the potential for severe hypokalemia and life-threatening arrhythmias with low or normal potassium levels at presentation without adequate replacement. Usually 20 to 40 mEq of KCl is included in all IV bags after the initial liter of run in the saline solution, except if the potassium level exceeds 5.5 mEq/L. In that case, potassium is added to the IV fluids as soon as the potassium level falls below 5.5 mEq/L. In addition, oral potassium supplements can be given to patients with a high risk of treatment-associated hypokalemia in the absence of severe nausea or vomiting. Because insulin drives phosphorus intracellularly, a common finding in DKA 12 to 24 hours after starting therapy is hypophosphatemia. Therefore, after the first few liters of IV fluid, some clinicians will replace the KCl with KPhos in 1 or 2 L of IV fluid. However, this is not supported by evidence-based outcomes, because trials of phosphate replacement in DKA have not shown a benefit. Many authors recommend phosphate replacement only for phosphate levels below 1 mmol/L.

25. **How are patients' conditions monitored during diabetic ketoacidosis therapy?**
Bedside fingerstick glucose, inputs and outputs, and vital signs are monitored hourly. Every 2-hour measures are serum glucose and electrolytes to monitor the K^+, Na^+, and anion gap. Once the anion gap is closed and the blood glucose falls below 200 mg/dL, a bedside glucose level is monitored every 1 to 2 hours, and electrolytes every 4 to 6 hours, to confirm reversal of the ketoacidosis as indicated by normalization of the anion gap.

26. **When is bicarbonate given?**
Studies have failed to show any benefit of bicarbonate therapy in patients with DKA. Concerns also exist that the rapid rise in pH could acutely lower the serum potassium. It is recommended that bicarbonate be given only with life-threatening acidosis, with most authors advocating a pH threshold of below 6.9, or when patients develop an inability to continue their respiratory compensation for the metabolic acidosis from tachypnea-induced extreme respiratory fatigue. Then, up to 100 mmol of sodium bicarbonate diluted in 400 mL sterile water plus 20 mEq KCl can be administered over a 2-hour period.

27. **How is the patient transitioned from the insulin infusion?**
Closure of the anion gap, along with clinical stability in terms of volume status and resolution of the marked hyperglycemia, and symptoms such as nausea or vomiting, signifies cessation of the DKA. The insulin and fluid-electrolyte infusions are continued for another 12 hours if possible as recurrence of ketoacidosis from turning off the infusion too fast is a common occurrence. The patient's usual therapy is then restarted—pump or injections—at the prior doses, or adjusted as needed on the basis on the hemoglobin A1c level at presentation and reported home blood glucose values. It is usually necessary to wait 2 to 3 hours after restarting the subcutaneous insulin before turning off the insulin infusion to allow adequate serum insulin levels from the subcutaneous insulin. However, administration of basal insulin near the time of the initiation of the IV insulin therapy for DKA facilitates the later transition off the insulin infusion.

28. **Is the treatment of diabetic ketoacidosis in children different?**
The general recommendations for diagnosis, therapy, and monitoring in children with DKA are similar to those for an older population. One difference is that children are treated in acute-care settings whereas, increasingly, uncomplicated DKA in adults is treated in emergency departments or monitored noncritical beds. The fluid and electrolyte replacement is also appropriate to the size and age of the child. Insulin infusion rates in preschool children are often started at 0.05 units/kg per hour, but in older children it is 0.1 unit/kg per hour as in adults. One issue of great concern in children is cerebral edema during the DKA treatment. Although uncommon, DKA-related cerebral edema occurs almost exclusively in children and is often fatal. Studies have shown some degree of brain swelling in virtually all children during DKA therapy, although the clinical syndrome of acute onset of altered mental state or frank coma is rare.

29. **Is the treatment of diabetic ketoacidosis in pregnancy different?**
Elements of the adaptive physiology of pregnancy have the potential to increase the risk of marked hyperglycemia and DKA in women with type 1 diabetes. Human placental lactogen, along with growth hormone and prolactin, markedly impair insulin sensitivity. There is also an accelerated lipolytic rate during normal pregnancy. In addition, the expanding abdominal girth causes rapid shallow breathing and a respiratory alkalosis that leads to a compensatory wasting of bicarbonate in the urine, lowering the patient's buffering capacity. Still, DKA is uncommon in pregnant patients, in part reflecting today's intensive diabetes management in pregnancy. When seen, DKA in a pregnant patient may be the first sign of diabetes or it may occur because of a broken pump or from an infection. The treatment is similar to that in nonpregnant patients, with mortality rates that are similarly low. On the other hand, older statistics that are still quoted suggest a high fetal loss rate: one review reported 9%.

30. **What are the goals of therapy in hyperosmolar hyperglycemic state?**
The main feature of HHS is extreme dehydration that results in marked hyperglycemia and hyperosmolarity-induced mental status changes. These patients frequently present with a precipitating illness that may be the main medical focus. As such, the primary goal is restoration of the

vascular volume and electrolytes. Although insulin is usually needed for full blood glucose control, volume replacement will improve most of the metabolic derangements, including inducing a marked fall in glycemia. The other major goal is to identify and start therapy for the precipitating illness. Because of the advanced age and comorbidities of many of these patients, plus their altered mental state and frequency of a serious accompanying illness, these patients are almost always treated in an intensive care unit (ICU) setting. The goals are as follows:

- Correct the hypovolemia for hemodynamic stability, and restore renal perfusion and glycosuria.
- Identify and reverse any precipitating illness.
- Recover blood glucose control.
- Slowly reverse the hyperosmolarity with a return to the patient's baseline mental state.
- Replete whole-body electrolyte stores.
- Prevent the complications that can occur with HHS therapy.

31. **What is appropriate fluid therapy in hyperosmolar hyperglycemic state?**
Because the fluid and electrolyte losses in HHS are typically greater than in DKA, patients are hypotensive or are in shock. The first priority is to restore adequate intravascular volume and renal perfusion followed by a gradual return to euvolemia and normal electrolyte stores. A liter or more of 0.9% saline solution is given quickly, especially to patients who have hypotension or are in shock unless a complicating issue exists, such as renal failure with anuria or congestive heart failure. Several methods are then used to determine whether to continue with 0.9% saline solution or reduce the osmotic load by switching to half-normal saline, with the more dilute fluid recommended when the corrected sodium is at or above the normal range, or for an effective osmolarity of greater than 330 mOsm/L. The rate of the fluid replacement is individualized so the serum osmolarity is lowered no more than 3 mOsms hourly to minimize the risk of cerebral edema. Another common guideline is to replace half of the patient's fluid deficit in the first 12 hours and the remainder over the next 12 to 24 hours, again to prevent rapid changes in tonicity changes that could precipitate cerebral edema. This is particularly important in pediatric patients with HHS who are at highest risk for cerebral edema; it is recommended that they receive no more than 50 mL/kg of saline solution over the first 4 hours, with correction of the remaining fluid deficit over 48 hours versus the 24 hours in adults. As in DKA, 20 to 40 mEq of potassium is added to each liter of IV fluids after the initial run in saline solution. Glucose-containing IV fluids are started earlier than in DKA, once the blood glucose falls below 250 to 300 mg/dL, along with titration of the insulin infusion to keep the blood glucose level between 100 and 200 mg/dL.

32. **How is the patient's water deficit calculated?**
The average fluid deficit in HHS is 100 to 200 mL/kg or 8 to 12 L. A patient's total body water deficit can be calculated with the use of the following assumptions and formula. Body water is 60% of the body weight in males and 50% in females. The patient's corrected sodium is calculated by adding 1.6 mEq/L of sodium to the measured value for every 100 mg/dL of glucose above the normal range of 100 mg/dL. This value, minus a normal sodium concentration of 140 mEq/L divided by 140, gives the percent deviation from the normal sodium concentration. Multiplying it by the patient's calculated total body water gives the fluid deficit. For instance, a 100 kg male with a glucose level of 800 mg/dL and measured sodium concentration of 145 mEq/L:

$$\text{Total body water} = 100 \times 60\% = 60\,\text{L}$$
$$\text{Corrected sodium} = 145 + (7 \times 1.6\,\text{mEq/L}) = 156\,\text{mEq/L}$$
$$\text{Fluid deficit} = (156 - 140)/140 = 11.6\% \times 60\,\text{L} = 6.9\,\text{L}$$

33. **Describe insulin therapy for hyperosmolar hyperglycemic state?**
Unlike in DKA, where immediate insulin replacement is required to reverse the ketoacidosis, in HHS, insulin therapy is secondary to restoration of the intravascular volume. Only after fluid support has been established and the patient is hemodynamically stable is insulin begun. It is administered as an IV infusion at 0.1 unit/kg, with or without an initial bolus as preferred by the caregivers. The goal of the combined fluid and insulin replacement is to lower the glucose level by 50 to 70 mg/dL per hour after the large drop from the initial fluid push. Thus the insulin infusion rate is adjusted hourly up or down until the blood glucose falls below 250 to 300 mg/dL, and then it is lowered by 50% along with switching the IV fluids to contain D_5, with continued hourly titration to keep the blood glucose level between 100 and 200 mg/dL. The clinical course of these patients often entails a lengthy ICU admission related to comorbidities, with maintenance of the insulin infusion until the patient is medically

stable. The patient's usual therapy is then restarted or changed as deemed appropriate. Unlike in DKA, some patients do not require long-term insulin therapy after HHS.

34. **What complications can occur in diabetic ketoacidosis and hyperosmolar hyperglycemic state?**
Today's aggressive fluid and potassium replacement along with the close monitoring of patients during the treatment of DKA and HHS has markedly reduced the risks of hypotension and shock related to the correction of hyperglycemia without adequate volume replacement, hypoglycemia, and severe hypokalemia. A key principle in comatose patients is protection of the airway and prevention of aspiration. Severe, and at times, life-threatening complications still can occur, sometimes in patients who have responded well to therapy but whose conditions then rapidly deteriorate, often with no identifiable cause: disseminated intravascular coagulation, acute respiratory distress syndrome, rhabdomyolysis, cerebral edema, and various thromboembolic events, such as pulmonary embolus, stroke, bowel infarction, or myocardial infarction. Some authors recommend prophylaxis against thromboembolic events, especially in severely dehydrated patients with HHS.

KEY POINTS: DIABETIC KETOACIDOSIS AND HYPEROSMOLAR HYPERGLYCEMIC STATE

1. Restore hemodynamic stability, and replete whole-body electrolyte stores with fluid replacement.
2. Recover blood glucose control with insulin therapy.
3. Identify and start therapy for any precipitating illness.
4. Prevent hypokalemia and hypoglycemia.
5. Closely monitor for the complications that can occur during or following therapy.

BIBLIOGRAPHY

1. Arora S, Henderson SO, Long T, et al. Diagnostic accuracy of point-of-care testing for diabetic ketoacidosis at emergency-department triage: β-hydroxybutyrate versus the urine dipstick. *Diabetes Care.* 2011;34:852-854.
2. Brooke J, Steill M, Ojo O. Evaluation of the accuracy of capillary hydroxybutyrate measurement compared with other measurements in the diagnosis of diabetic ketoacidosis: a systemic review. *Int J Environ Res Public Health.* 2016;13(9):837.
3. Canarie MF, Bogue CW, Banasiak KJ, et al. Decompensated hyperglycemic hyperosmolarity without significant ketoacidosis in the adolescent and young adult population. *J Pediatr Endocrinol Metab.* 2007;20:1115-1124.
4. de Veciana M. Diabetic ketoacidosis in pregnancy. *Semin Perinatol.* 2013;37:267-273.
5. Guenette MD, Hahn M, Cohn TA, et al. Atypical antipsychotics and diabetic ketoacidosis: a review. *Psychopharmacology (Berl).* 2013;226:1-12.
6. Hsia E, Seggelke S, Gibbs J, et al. Subcutaneous administration of glargine to diabetic patients receiving insulin infusion prevents rebound hyperglycemia. *J Clin Endocrinol Metab.* 2012;97:3132-3137.
7. Kitabachi AE, Murphy MB, Spencer J, et al. Is a priming dose of insulin necessary in a low-dose insulin protocol for the treatment of diabetic ketoacidosis? *Diabetes Care.* 2008;31:2081-2085.
8. Krane EJ, Rockoff MA, Wallman JK, et al. Subclinical brain swelling in children during treatment of diabetes ketoacidosis. *N Engl J Med.* 1985;312:1147-1151.
9. Morris LR, Murphy MB, Kitabchi AE, et al. Bicarbonate therapy in severe diabetic ketoacidosis. *Ann Intern Med.* 1986; 105:836-840.
10. Nyenwe EA, Kitabachi AE. The evolution of diabetic ketoacidosis: an update of its etiology, pathogenesis and management. *Metabolism.* 2016;65:507-521.
11. Pasquel FJ, Umpierrez GE. Hyperosmolar hyperglycemic state: a historical review of the clinical presentation, diagnosis, and treatment. *Diabetes Care.* 2014;37:3124-3131.
12. Peters AL, Henry RR, Thakkar P, et al. Diabetic ketoacidosis with canagliflozin, a sodium-glucose cotransporter 2 inhibitor, in patients with type 1 diabetes. *Diabetes Care.* 2016;39:532-538.
13. Rosenbloom AL. Hyperglycemic hyperosmolar state: an emerging pediatric problem. *J Pediatr.* 2010;156:180-184.
14. Skitch SA, Valani R. Treatment of pediatric diabetic ketoacidosis in Canada: a review of treatment protocols from Canadian emergency departments. *CJEM.* 2015;17:656-661.
15. Wolfsdorf JI. The international society of pediatric and adolescent diabetes guidelines for management of diabetic ketoacidosis: do the guidelines need to be modified? *Pediatr Diabetes.* 2014;15:277-286.
16. Umpierrez G, Korytkowski M. Diabetic emergencies – ketoacidosis, hyperglycemic hyperosmolar state and hypoglycaemia. *Nat Rev Endocrinol.* 2016;12:222-232.

CHAPTER 55

ADRENAL INSUFFICIENCY IN THE INTENSIVE CARE UNIT

Haitham Nsour

1. How is the adrenal gland function regulated during normal physiologic state?
   The adrenal gland glucocorticoid production is regulated by a negative feedback mechanism through the hypothalamic-pituitary-adrenal (HPA) axis. There is a normal circadian variation of total cortisol level. The percentage of free, biologically active, cortisol is dependent on protein binding to albumin and corticoid-binding globulin (CBG).

2. What are the pathophysiologic mechanisms contributing to the adrenal insufficiency during critical illness?
   Critical illness is associated with disruption of HPA axis making it "less sensitive to negative feedback" with elevated adrenocorticotropic hormone (ACTH) concentration and loss of normal circadian variation of cortisol.

   A rapid increase in cortisol levels occurs early during critical illness, often corresponding to an increase in ACTH levels suggesting possible activation of HPA axis. However, low ACTH levels are seen with prolonged critical illness. This dissociation between serum cortisol and ACTH levels is attributed to reduced cortisol breakdown leading to hypercortisolemia and ACTH suppression via negative feedback inhibition.

   Critical illness can lead to higher free cortisol levels due to reduced albumin and CBG.

3. What are the common causes of primary adrenal insufficiency?
   Autoimmune diseases (40% of cases), adrenal infections like tuberculosis (in nonwestern countries), cytomegalovirus (CMV) and systemic fungal infections, like histoplasma, in the setting of human immunodeficiency virus (HIV) or immunosuppression. Rarely, bilateral infiltrative diseases, tumor metastasis, or hemorrhage can result in primary adrenal insufficiency (PAI).

4. What are the diagnostic criteria of primary adrenal insufficiency in the noncritical care setting?
   The standard dose corticotropin (ACTH) 250 mcg stimulation test is the "gold standard" diagnostic test. Peak cortisol levels less than 18 mcg/dL at 30 or 60 minutes indicate PAI.

   Morning cortisol and serum ACTH levels may be used as screening or preliminary tests if the corticotropin stimulation test is not feasible. Morning cortisol less than 5 mcg/dL in combination with serum ACTH greater than 2-fold the upper limit of the normal reference range is suggestive of PAI (pending confirmatory testing).

   Testing should be deferred in patients with severe acute adrenal insufficiency symptoms or adrenal crises (AC).

5. Does glucocorticoid replacement with dexamethasone interfere with adrenocorticotropic hormone stimulation test?
   Yes. Dexamethasone has a long half-life and may cause prolonged suppression of the HPA axis limiting the value of subsequent ACTH testing.

6. What is the definition of acute adrenal insufficiency or adrenal crises?
   AC is a life-threatening medical emergency with at least two of the following signs and symptoms: hypotension (systolic blood pressure <100 mm Hg), nausea or vomiting, severe fatigue, fever, somnolence, hyponatremia (≤132 mmol/L) or hyperkalemia and hypoglycemia. Significant clinical improvement of AC is expected after the administration of parenteral glucocorticoid.

7. What are the laboratory abnormalities associated with primary adrenal insufficiency or acute adrenal crises?
   Hyponatremia is the most common (90%) secondary to natriuresis.
   Hyperkalemia and metabolic acidosis secondary to aldosterone deficiency.
   Changes in blood cell counts (anemia, mild eosinophilia, and lymphocytosis).

Hypoglycemia (more common in children).
Hypercalcemia (10%–20%) secondary to bone resorption.

8. What are the common precipitating factors of adrenal crises?
Gastrointestinal illness is the most common precipitant for AC. Other factors include surgical stress, infections, trauma, and noncompliance with maintenance glucocorticoid therapy or sudden withdrawal of steroids.

9. What are the mechanisms of shock in adrenal crises?
Hypotension in AC is multifactorial. Hypovolemia occur secondary to natriuresis, lack of fluid retention, and associated gastrointestinal symptoms, such as nausea and vomiting. Low cortisol levels will cause a loss of permissive effect of glucocorticoids on catecholamine action; hence, hypotension will be refractory to intravenous fluids (IVF) and inotropes without adequate glucocorticoid supplementation.

10. What is the recommended treatment approach of adrenal crises?
Treatment of suspected acute adrenal insufficiency or AC should never be delayed by diagnostic procedures. AC should be treated immediately with intravenous (IV) or intramuscular hydrocortisone 100 mg, followed by 100 mg every 6 to 8 hours until it is recovered. Isotonic (0.9%) sodium chloride should be given at an initial rate of 1 L/h until there is hemodynamic improvement. Dextrose infusion may be added in patients presenting with hypoglycemia. Rapid correction of hyponatremia should be avoided to avoid risk of central myelinosis.
The underlying etiology of AC (e.g., infection) should be sought and treated.

11. What are the causes of adrenal insufficiency secondary to hypothalamo-pituitary disease "central AI"?
The most common cause of central adrenal insufficiency (AI) is the exogenous glucocorticoid use leading to ACTH suppression. Pituitary gland tumors, infections, hemorrhage, or infiltrative diseases like sarcoidosis can lead to ACTH deficiency.
Pituitary dysfunction occurs in up to 30% of patients after head trauma.

12. What would be the dose and/or duration of steroid treatment that would result in adrenal suppression?
Short 5-day courses of high-dose steroids are associated with transient HPA axis suppression, which will normalize within 10 days after course completion. Prolonged adrenal suppression can be seen after long-term courses of steroids (dose equivalent $\geq$5 mg prednisolone/day). Those patients should receive adequate glucocorticoid supplementation therapy during acute illness to avoid acute AC.

13. What is critical illness-related corticosteroid insufficiency?
Critical illness-related corticosteroid insufficiency (CIRCI) is defined as inadequate corticosteroid activity for the severity of the illness of the patient. This arises due to dysfunction at any level of the HPA axis and corticosteroid resistance at the tissue level. CIRCI has replaced the previously used term "relative adrenal insufficiency."
Prior studies used a low basal cortisol of less than 10 mg/dL and less than 9 mg/dL rise from baseline (delta cortisol) after ACTH 250 mcg stimulation test as "predictors" of CIRCI. However, both tests have low sensitivity, and multiple other confounders can affect the level of serum cortisol during critical illness.

14. What are the clinical manifestations of critical illness-related corticosteroid insufficiency?
Hypotension refractory to IV fluid resuscitation and the use of vasopressors is a common manifestation. The other clinical manifestations of adrenal insufficiency (listed in question #5) may not be present, and the diagnosis of CIRCI should rely on a high level of suspicion.

15. Should we use the adrenocorticotropic hormone stimulation test to identify which subset of adult patients with septic shock should receive supplemental hydrocortisone therapy?
The latest Surviving Sepsis Campaign guidelines (2012 update) do not recommend using the ACTH stimulation test routinely in adults with septic shock. Intravenous hydrocortisone 200 mg/day should be added to treat adult septic patients if adequate fluid resuscitation and vasopressor therapy cannot restore hemodynamic stability. Hydrocortisone should be tapered when vasopressors are no longer required.
The addition of fludrocortisone 50 mcg/day remains optional as stress-dose hydrocortisone will provide adequate mineralocorticoid activity, in addition to glucocorticoid action.

16. What are the benefits of glucocorticoid supplementation (stress-dose steroids) in patients with septic shock?
The use of supplemental glucocorticoid therapy may reverse shock and attenuate the need for vasopressors. However, there has been no proven mortality benefit in all subsets of patients including

those who had biochemical evidence of a suboptimal response to critical illness based on ACTH-stimulation testing.

17. What are some of the medications that can predispose for adrenal insufficiency in the critical care setting?

Many of the medications used in intensive care unit (ICU) setting can interfere with HPA axis. Activation of the glucocorticoid metabolism by anticonvulsants, such as phenytoin, or antibiotics, such as rifampicin. Inhibition of cortisol synthesis by etomidate or antifungal medications (like ketoconazole, and—to a lesser extent—by fluconazole and itraconazole). Adrenal hemorrhage may occur secondary to anticoagulants. Exogenous use of glucocorticoids is one of the most common factors leading to adrenal insufficiency in the ICU setting.

18. What is the effect of etomidate on adrenal function and mortality in critically ill patients?

Etomidate use is highly associated with early-onset suppression of adrenal steroidogenesis for up to 72 hours even after a single dose. Although this effect may increase the risk of worsening hypotension, the effect of etomidate on mortality and prognostic outcomes remains unclear.

19. What is meant by "hepato-adrenal syndrome"?

Adrenal dysfunction is common in end-stage liver disease (ESLD) with or without sepsis, and these patients should be monitored carefully for symptoms and signs of adrenal insufficiency. Low cortisol production in ESLD is related to low cholesterol levels, which is the primary substrate of cortisol. Hypoalbuminemia in ESLD will also increase the free bioactive fraction of cortisol.

ACKNOWLEDGMENT

The authors wish to acknowledge Dr. Michael Young, MD, for the valuable contributions to the previous edition of this chapter.

KEY POINTS: ADRENAL INSUFFICIENCY IN THE INTENSIVE CARE UNIT

- An adrenal crisis is a life-threatening emergency that requires early recognition and immediate therapy with parenteral hydrocortisone and intravenous fluids.
- CIRCI should be considered in patients with persistent septic shock despite adequate fluid resuscitation and the use of vasopressors.
- Treatment of CIRCI with supplemental "stress-dose" glucocorticoid therapy should not be based on results of the ACTH stimulation test or a random cortisol level.
- Glucocorticoid supplementation therapy in CIRCI improves hemodynamics but does not have a survival benefit.
- Exogenous therapy with glucocorticoid is the most common cause of central adrenal insufficiency. These patients require adequate glucocorticoid supplementation during critical illness.

BIBLIOGRAPHY

1. Freund Y, Jabre P, Mourad J, et al. Relative adrenal insufficiency in critically ill patient after rapid sequence intubation: KETASED ancillary study. *J Crit Care.* 2014;29(3):386-389.
2. McPhee LC, Badawi O, Fraser GL, et al. Single dose Etomidate is not associated with increased mortality in ICU patients with sepsis: analysis of a large electronic ICU database. *Crit Care Med.* 2013;41:774-783.
3. Bruder EA, Ball IM, Ridi S, et al. Single induction dose of Etomidate versus other induction agents for endotracheal intubation in critically ill patients. *Cochrane Database Syst Rev.* 2015;1:CD010225. doi:10.1002/14651858. CD010225.pub2.
4. Boonen E, Vervenne H, Meersseman P, et al. Reduced Cortisol Metabolism during critical illness. *N Engl J Med.* 2013; 368:1477-1488.
5. Sprung CL, Annane D, Keh D, et al, CORTICUS study group. Hydrocortisone therapy for patients with septic shock. *N Engl J Med.* 2008;358:111-124.
6. Cooper MS, Stewart PM. Adrenal insufficiency in critical illness. *J Intensive Care Med.* 2007;22:348-362.
7. Bornstein SR, Engeland WC, Ehrhart-Bornstein M, et al. Dissociation of ACTH and glucocorticoids. *Trends Endocrinol Metab.* 2008;19(5):175-180.
8. Marik PE, Pastores SM, Annane D, et al. Recommendations for the diagnosis and management of corticosteroid insufficiency in critically ill adult patients: consensus statement from an international task force by the American College of Critical Care Medicine. *Crit Care Med.* 2008;36(6):1937-1949.
9. Dellinger RP, Levy MM, Rhodes A, et al. Surviving Sepsis Campaign: international guidelines for management of severe sepsis and septic shock, 2012. *Intensive Care Med.* 2013;39(2):165-228.

10. Husebye ES, Allolio B, Arlt W, et al. Consensus statement on the diagnosis, treatment and follow-up of patients with primary adrenal insufficiency. *J Intern Med.* 2014;275:104-115.
11. Bornstein SR. Predisposing factors for adrenal insufficiency. *N Engl J Med.* 2009;360:2328-2339.
12. Bornstein SR, Allolio B, Arlt W, et al. Diagnosis and treatment of primary adrenal insufficiency: an endocrine society practice guideline. *J Clin Endocrinol Metab.* 2016;101(2):364-389.
13. Puar TH, Stikkelbroeck NM, Smans LC, et al. Adrenal crises: still a deadly event in 21st century. *Am J Med.* 2016; 129(3):339.e1-e9.
14. Crowley RK, Argese N, Tomlinson JW, et al. Central hypoadrenalism. *J Clin Endocrinol Metab.* 2014;99(11):4027-4036.
15. Sprung CL, Annane D, Keh D, et al, CORTICUS Study Group. Hydrocortisone therapy for patients with septic shock. *N Engl J Med.* 2008;358:111-124.
16. Karagiannis AKA, Nakouti T, Pipili C, et al. Adrenal insufficiency in patients with decompensated cirrhosis. *World J Hepatol.* 2015;7(8):1112-1124.
17. Allolio B. Extensive expertise in endocrinology. Adrenal crises. *Eur J Endocrinol.* 2015;172:R115-R124.

CHAPTER 56

THYROID DISEASE IN THE INTENSIVE CARE UNIT

Annis Marney

1. What thyroid conditions require intensive care?
   - **Thyroid storm:** Life-threatening thyrotoxicosis (accounts for 1%–2% of admissions for thyrotoxicosis and carries 20%–30% mortality)
   - **Myxedema coma:** Life-threatening hypothyroidism (approximately 20% mortality)
   - **Note:** Nonthyroidal illness syndrome (NTIS), formerly known as euthyroid sick syndrome, is not life threatening

2. How do you diagnose thyroid storm?
   Thyroid storm often occurs in people with Graves disease who have stopped medication or whose underlying condition is undiagnosed. In addition, a precipitating factor often exists, such as severe infection, diabetic ketoacidosis, myocardial infarction (MI), cerebrovascular accident (CVA), heart failure, trauma, amiodarone therapy (short or long term), or a recent test involving iodinated contrast load (less than 6 weeks before presentation). It shares laboratory findings with thyrotoxicosis but is different from simple thyrotoxicosis in that it involves **fever**.
   Clinical symptoms include the following:
   - Fever greater than 102°F (38.9°C) (hallmark): most consider this the sine qua non of thyroid storm
   - Tachycardia
   - Tachypnea
   - Blood pressure not necessarily high or low
   - Cardiac arrhythmias, heart failure, and/or ischemia: common
   - Nausea, vomiting, diarrhea
   - Agitation, tremulousness, delirium
   - Jaundice: a particularly worrisome sign
     A scoring system has been developed by Burch and Wartofsky that can be used as a clinical guideline for severity of thyroid storm (Table 56.1). A score greater than 45 is considered truly indicative of thyroid storm, while 25 to 45 is suggestive of thyroid storm, and less than 25 unlikely to be thyroid storm. Laboratory findings include suppressed (undetectable, not just low) thyroid-stimulating hormone (TSH) and elevated serum total thyroxine (T_4) (TT_4), free T_4 (FT_4), total triiodothyronine (T_3) (TT_3), and free T_3 (FT_3).

3. How do you treat thyroid storm?
   Use common sense. First, support the patient as you would any critically ill patient and be sure to initiate cardiac monitoring. Next, reduce thyroid hormone production with thioureas. Finally, stop the release of preformed hormone by adding iodide. Simultaneously with these measures give β-blockade to slow the heart rate and reduce the conversion of T_4 to T_3 (Table 56.2).

4. How do you diagnose myxedema coma?
   Myxedema coma often occurs in people with undiagnosed or untreated hypothyroidism and is the end stage of a process that takes days to weeks. Often these people have had a precipitating event such as MI, CVA, acute infection, trauma, or hemorrhage. There may be a history of previous thyroid surgery or radioactive iodine ablation for hyperthyroidism, but because of mental status changes you may not get that history. Always look for an anterior neck scar for previous thyroid surgery.
   Clinical symptoms include the following:
   - Altered mental status (coma not strictly necessary, but altered mental status is)
   - Hypothermia (as low as 75°F [23.9°C] has been reported)
   - Dry, coarse skin
   - Gravelly, hoarse voice
   - Thick tongue
   - Thin scalp and eyebrow hair

Table 56-1. Thyroid Storm Scoring System

DIAGNOSTIC CRITERION	POINTS
Thermoregulatory/Temperature	
99–100	5
100–101	10
101–102	15
102–103	20
103–104	25
>104	30
Cardiovascular/Heart Rate	
100–110	5
110–120	10
120–130	15
130–140	20
>140	25
CNS Alteration	
Mild (agitation)	10
Moderate (delirium, psychosis)	20
Congestive Heart Failure Symptom	
Mild (pedal edema)	5
Moderate (bibasilar rales)	10
Severe (pulmonary edema)	15
Atrial fibrillation	10
Gastrointestinal	
Moderate (nausea, vomiting, diarrhea, and pain)	10
Severe (jaundice)	20
Precipitant History	
Absent	0
Present	10

CNS, Central nervous system.

Table 56-2. Supportive Care and Specific Medications for Thyroid Storm

INTERVENTION AND MECHANISM OF ACTION	DOSE	ROUTE
Supportive Care		
Isotonic fluids	Patient specific	IV
Oxygen	Patient specific	Nasal cannula if stable enough
Cooling blanket		Topical
Acetaminophen or other antipyretics	Adult dosing	Oral, rectal, or NG

(Continued on following page)

Table 56-2. Supportive Care and Specific Medications for Thyroid Storm *(Continued)*

INTERVENTION AND MECHANISM OF ACTION	DOSE	ROUTE
Thioureas: Reduce Thyroid Hormone Production		
Propylthiouracil	150 mg every 6 h	Oral, rectal, or NG
Methimazole (Tapazole)	20 mg every 8 h	Oral, rectal, or NG
Iodide: Reduce Hormone Production and T_4 to T_3 Conversion 2–4 h After Starting Thioamide (above)		
Saturated solution of potassium iodide	5 drops (250 mg) twice daily	Oral
Iopanoic acid	0.5 g twice daily	Oral or IV
Iohexol	0.6 g (2 mL of Omnipaque 300) twice daily	IV
β-Blockade: Reduce Heart Rate and Reduce Conversion of T_4 to T_3		
Propranolol	40–80 mg every 6 h	Oral
Propranolol	0.5–1.0 mg over 10 min every 3 h	IV
Esmolol (especially if patient has asthma and needs $β_1$-selective agent)	0.25–0.5 mg/kg bolus followed by 0.05–0.1 mg/kg per minute infusion	IV
Glucocorticoids: Support Circulation, Supplement Glucocorticoid Reserve Because of Increased Metabolism and Reduced Half-Life with Thyrotoxicosis, and Reduce T_4 to T_3 Conversion		
Dexamethasone	2 mg every 6 h × 48 h, then taper dose rapidly	Oral or IV
Hydrocortisone	100 mg every 8 h × 48 h, then taper dose rapidly	IV
Resin Binders: Remove T_4 in the Gut to Reduce Enterohepatic Circulation of Free T_4		
Cholestyramine or colestipol	20–30 g daily	Oral or NG

IV, Intravenous; *NG*, nasogastric.

- Pleural and cardiac effusions
- Delayed relaxation time of reflexes (Achilles = most sensitive)
  Laboratory findings include elevated TSH with low or low-normal serum TT_4, FT_4, TT_3, and FT_3.

5. How do you treat myxedema coma?
   Again, use common sense. First, support the patient as you would any critically ill patient and be sure to initiate cardiac monitoring and ventilatory support and secure intravenous access (avoid oral or nasogastric medications because of possible ileus, which is common in myxedema coma). Next, administer glucocorticoids. Thyroid hormone speeds metabolism throughout the body, including metabolism of glucocorticoids. If the patient has underlying or undiagnosed adrenal insufficiency (autoimmune, typically), administration of a thyroid hormone with a backdrop of adrenal insufficiency can precipitate adrenal crisis and is avoidable. Not every patient requires this, but it is impossible to differentiate acutely who does and who does not; therefore, everyone should get it. You can taper quickly once you determine who needs steroids. Finally, give a parenteral thyroid hormone (Table 56.3).
   Different schools of thought exist about T_3 therapy. It increases cardiac metabolic demands acutely, so it can be unwise in elderly patients already acutely ill. Many practitioners believe that patients can convert T_4 to T_3 on their own and thus administering T_3 is unnecessary and potentially dangerous.

Table 56-3. Supportive Care and Specific Medications for Myxedema Coma

INTERVENTION	DOSE	ROUTE
Supportive Care		
Isotonic fluids but avoid over-loading because of hyponatremia	Patient specific	IV
Oxygen	Patient specific	Nasal cannula if stable enough
Thyroid Hormone Replacement Therapy		
Levothyroxine (T$_4$)	300–400 mcg loading dose then 50–100 mcg daily (based on weight)	IV
Liothyronine (T$_3$) (controversial)	10 mcg every 8 h × 48 h	IV
Glucocorticoid Therapy: Support Circulation, Supplement Glucocorticoid Reserve Because of Possible Adrenal Insufficiency		
Dexamethasone	2 mg every 6 h × 48 h, then taper dose rapidly	IV
Hydrocortisone	100 mg every 8 h × 48 h, then taper dose rapidly	IV

IV, Intravenous.

6. How do you diagnose nonthyroidal illness syndrome?
   NTIS, formerly known as *euthyroid sick syndrome*, often occurs in patients who have severe, prolonged, critical illness and is essentially a laboratory abnormality to be monitored. It is not a primary thyroid disorder, but instead results from a resetting of the hypothalamic-pituitary-thyroid axis, as well as changes in peripheral thyroid hormone metabolism and transport induced by nonthyroidal illness. The laboratory abnormalities occur sequentially as follows:
   - Serum TT$_3$ and FT$_3$ levels are low (decreased conversion of T$_4$ to T$_3$ in peripheral tissues).
   - TT$_3$ and FT$_3$ levels are even lower. FT$_4$ level may be normal, decreased, or increased. TSH level is normal or slightly decreased.
   - FT$_4$ level is low and TSH is high (may transiently be significantly elevated in the teens and 20s). This is the recovery phase and can be prolonged. Normalization of laboratory values can take weeks to months.

7. Could these laboratory values be confused with central hypothyroidism or pituitary dysfunction, and how can you tell the difference?
   The laboratory results can be confusing, and you do have to take a careful history to be sure the patient has not had pituitary surgery or radiation therapy. Also, pituitary apoplexy could present with similar laboratory values, but the patient would have symptoms of severe headache and adrenal insufficiency as well. Only in cases where patients have symptoms that are concerning for apoplexy or a mass do you need to do magnetic resonance imaging (e.g., visual disturbance). Yes, sex hormones and insulin-like growth factor-1 levels may also be low, but this is likely the body's adaptive function and does not require therapy (also therapy with sex steroids and growth hormone have been proved not to help). Adrenal insufficiency that is clinically significant will cause symptoms, and testing for it can be tricky but may be necessary (see Chapter 55 on adrenal insufficiency in the ICU).

8. How do you treat nonthyroidal illness syndrome?
   Most often, you do not. However, there is a great deal of controversy in this area. The few studies that have been done show no benefit to giving T$_4$ in these patients. The recommendation is to recheck thyroid laboratory results in 4 to 6 weeks. It is possible that in cases of severely low T$_4$ and T$_3$ some patients may benefit from levothyroxine therapy, especially those with cardiac failure, but the evidence is far from conclusive.

ACKNOWLEDGMENT

The authors wish to acknowledge Dr. Michael Young, MD, for the valuable contributions to the previous edition of this chapter.

KEY POINTS: THYROID DISEASE IN THE INTENSIVE CARE UNIT

Thyroid Disorders

1. Thyroid storm is life-threatening thyrotoxicosis that often presents with a precipitating factor and carries a high mortality rate if not treated promptly and appropriately.
2. When thyroid storm is diagnosed or suspected, give appropriate supportive care and treat with antithyroid drugs, cold iodine, β-blockers, and stress doses of glucocorticoids, along with management of any precipitating factors.
3. Myxedema coma is life-threatening hypothyroidism that often has an identifiable precipitating cause and has a high mortality rate if not promptly and adequately treated.
4. When myxedema coma is diagnosed or suspected, first treat with stress doses of glucocorticoids followed by rapid repletion of the thyroid hormone and treatment of any precipitating causes.
5. NTIS is not a thyroid disorder but rather laboratory changes in serum TSH, T_4, and T_3 resulting from cytokines and inflammatory mediators produced in patients with nonthyroidal illnesses, and generally does not require treatment.

BIBLIOGRAPHY

1. Burch HB, Wartofsky L. Life threatening thyrotoxicosis. Thyroid storm. *Endocrinol Metab Clin North Am.* 1993;22:263-277.
2. DeGroot L. "Non-thyroidal illness syndrome" is functional central hypothyroidism, and if severe, hormone replacement is appropriate in light of present knowledge. *J Endocrinol Invest.* 2003;26:1163-1170.
3. Farwell AP. Thyroid hormone therapy is not indicated in the majority of patient with sick euthyroid syndrome. *Endocr Pract.* 2008;14:1180-1187.
4. Fliers E, Bianco AC, Langouche L, et al. Thyroid function in critically ill patients. *Lancet Diabetes Endocrinol.* 2015;3: 816-825.
5. Goldberg PA, Inzucchi SE. Critical issues in endocrinology. *Clin Chest Med.* 2003;24:583-606.
6. Kwaku MP, Burman KD. Myxedema coma. *J Intensive Care Med.* 2007;22:224-231.
7. Warner MH, Beckett GJ. Mechanisms behind the non-thyroidal illness syndrome: an update. *J Endocrinol.* 2010;205: 1-13.

X
HEMATOLOGY/ONCOLOGY

CHAPTER 57

BLOOD PRODUCTS AND COAGULATION

Rebecca Kalman, and Johnathan P. Mack

1. **What components of blood are available for transfusion?**
   Components available for transfusion include whole blood, packed red blood cells (PRBCs), fresh frozen plasma (FFP), platelet concentrates, cryoprecipitate, white blood cell concentrates, and clotting factor concentrates.

2. **What are packed red blood cells?**
   Red blood cells (RBCs) contain hemoglobin and serve as the primary oxygen-transporting agent to tissues. Packed RBCs (PRBC) are obtained by centrifugation of whole blood to remove most of the platelet-rich plasma, or by apheresis (a procedure in which whole blood is removed and separated into its components; the RBCs are kept and the remaining components are returned to the donor). The resulting product is called "packed" RBCs (PRBC), because of the high hematocrit (65%–80%). The volume of 1 unit of PRBCs is around 300 mL, and its shelf life ranges from 21 to 42 days, depending on the type of added storage solution. Transfusion of 1 unit of PRBCs typically raises the hemoglobin concentration by 1 g/dL or the hematocrit by 3%.

3. **What are the main red blood cell surface antigen systems?**
   The **ABO** system is one of the most important because antibodies to these antigens are "naturally occurring" (an individual will produce antibodies against the ABO antigens they lack without being exposed to foreign RBCs) and these antibodies can cause intravascular hemolysis. An individual's red cells may express A, B, both, or no surface A or B antigen, which determine that individual's ABO blood type. People carrying anti-A or anti-B antibodies cannot receive RBCs with the corresponding surface antigens, or immunologic destruction of the transfused red cells may occur. Consequently, type O individuals are considered *universal donors*, whereas AB individuals may donate RBCs only to other AB recipients.

   The RhD antigen is another important surface antigen that can be present (RhD-positive) or absent (RhD-negative) on the red cell membrane. This antigen is one of the most immunogenic, and the majority of individuals who are RhD-negative will develop antibodies to RhD when exposed to RhD-positive blood. This is not a problem for initial exposure, but hemolysis may occur with subsequent transfusions (Table 57.1) or lead to hemolytic disease of the fetus and newborn.

4. **What are blood typing, screening, and cross-matching?**
   Blood typing is a process that determines the ABO and RhD status of RBCs (usually collected from either a donor or potential transfusion recipient). **Blood antibody screening** is a procedure that tests the plasma for antibodies to non-ABO red blood cell antigens that could bind to transfused RBCs and lead to shortened RBC survival (hemolysis). **Cross-matching** is a process that verifies the compatibility between a specific donor's RBCs and a designated recipient's plasma. This has traditionally been accomplished by directly mixing the recipient's plasma with the donor's RBCs to ensure that hemolysis does not occur from undetected antibodies. "Electronic" cross-matching uses a computer system to confirm the ABO/RhD type of donor and recipient, and can replace a physical cross-match in select patients at a low risk of having red cell antibodies and with a negative screen. Compatible units identified with a cross-match are held for the designated patient.

5. **What are potential transfusion hazards?**
   The adverse events of blood component transfusions can be grouped into immunologic and nonimmunologic complications.
   Immunologic complications include the following:
   - Acute hemolytic transfusion reactions
   - Delayed hemolytic transfusion reactions
   - Febrile nonhemolytic reactions (FNHTR)
   - Allergic and anaphylactic reactions

Table 57-1. Compatible Donor-Recipient Combinations for Packed Red Blood Cells

PRBC		Donor					
		A	B	O	AB	RH+	RH-
RECIPIENT	A	×		×			
	B		×	×			
	O			×			
	AB	×	×	×	×		
	Rh+					×	×
	Rh-						×

- Transfusion-related acute lung injury (TRALI)
- Transfusion-associated graft-versus-host disease (TA-GVHD)
  Nonimmune-mediated complications include:
- Transmission of infectious agents (bacterial, viral, parasitic)
- Transfusion-associated circulatory overload
- Hypothermia
- Hypotensive transfusion reactions (bradykinin-mediated vasodilation)
- Metabolic complications, such as citrate toxicity (transient manifestations of hypocalcemia until citrate gets cleared in the liver) and hyperkalemia or hypokalemia

6. What is a febrile nonhemolytic reaction?

FNHTR is defined as a temperature increase above 38°C and an increase greater than or equal to 1°C during or within 4 hours of a transfusion, without other explanation. FNHTR can also manifest as chills or rigors without a temperature change. FNHTRs occur in fewer than 1% of all transfusions and are thought to arise from two mechanisms:
- recipient antibodies directed against donor white blood cells or platelets resulting in recipient cytokine production
- accumulation of cytokines in the transfused product (platelets only).

FNHTRs can be dramatic and uncomfortable for the patient but are generally not dangerous for the recipient. Since life-threatening important transfusion reactions can also manifest as a fever (acute hemolytic, septic, TRALI) any fever during transfusion should be taken seriously. Routine pretreatment with antihistamines and antipyretics is not recommended, as randomized trials have not demonstrated a reduction in transfusion reactions with this strategy. Patients having recurrent severe febrile reactions may benefit from leukoreduced blood products.

7. What is an acute hemolytic reaction?

Acute hemolytic reactions occur due to immunologic destruction of the transfused RBCs due to incompatibility with circulating antibodies present in the recipient's plasma. These reactions occur during or shortly after a transfusion. Acute reactions may occur when as little as 10 mL of blood is infused and can result in renal failure, shock, and even death. Associated mortality may be as high as 35%. The most common cause of acute hemolytic reactions is transfusion of ABO- or Rh-incompatible blood, resulting from identification errors. Serologic incompatibility undetected during pretransfusion testing is much less common.

8. What is a delayed hemolytic reaction?

Delayed hemolytic reactions occur when a recipient has been previously alloimmunized to a red cell antigen but does not have the antibody detectable in the plasma at the time of pre-transfusion testing. Re-exposure to the corresponding antigen via transfusion provokes anamnestic antibody production, and the transfused RBCs are immunologically destroyed. These reactions typically occur 2 to 14 days after a transfusion.

9. What are the classic findings in a hemolytic transfusion reaction?

In **acute hemolytic reactions**, fever (with or without chills), nausea/vomiting, tachycardia, back or flank pain, pain at the intravenous (IV) site, chest pain, dyspnea, hypotension, and red or brown urine may be present. *Disseminated intravascular coagulopathy* (DIC) and acute renal failure may develop in severe cases. Laboratory findings include hemoglobinuria and elevation of the indirect serum bilirubin and lactate dehydrogenase levels. The direct antiglobulin test is also positive. **Delayed hemolytic**

reactions may result in mild fever, although many are subtle. A slow drop in hematocrit and an increase in unconjugated bilirubin are common.

10. How should a hemolytic transfusion reaction be managed?

When an **acute hemolytic reaction** is recognized, the transfusion must be stopped immediately. The Blood Bank should be notified and transfusion forms and labels rechecked. Post-transfusion blood samples need to be sent along with the remaining blood component to the Blood Bank and a urinalysis should be performed. Treatment is supportive and includes administration of IV fluids, diuretics, inotropes, and close monitoring as needed. **Delayed reactions** often require no specific treatment.

11. What are the infectious risks of transfusion?

The risk of various transfusion-transmitted infections is shown in Table 57.2. Bacterial contamination of PRBCs is much less common than platelets due to storage conditions. Transmission of *Babesia* species is increasing in geographic areas where deer ticks are endemic. Transmission of other infectious agents (e.g., variant Creutzfeldt-Jakob disease agent) for which blood products are not routinely tested is possible, but even rarer.

12. What is transfusion-associated acute lung injury (TRALI)?

TRALI is the acute onset (within 6 hours) of noncardiogenic pulmonary edema after a blood component transfusion and is the most common cause of transfusion-related death in the United States. In addition to hypoxemia, criteria for diagnosis include bilateral infiltrates on chest radiograph and exclusion of pre-existing lung injury or circulatory overload. The most commonly accepted mechanism of TRALI is the "two-hit" mechanism: primed recipient neutrophils in the lung microvasculature are activated by human leukocyte antigen antibodies or human neutrophil antibodies in the transfused component. Activated neutrophils then cause pulmonary capillary leak. Transfusion should be stopped immediately when TRALI is suspected. Treatment is supportive and may require mechanical ventilation. Diuretics and steroids are not of benefit in the treatment of TRALI.

13. When should red cells be transfused to critically ill adults?

A growing body evidence suggests that a restrictive transfusion strategy (transfusion for hemoglobin concentration <7 g/dL) is as effective as a liberal transfusion strategy (transfusion for hemoglobin concentration <9 to 10 g/dL in many settings, including septic shock, upper gastrointestinal bleeding, and critically ill adults. It is also known from studies in populations with anemia who decline transfusions for religious reasons that perioperative mortality increases from 0% to 9% as the hemoglobin levels drop below 7 g/dL. Patients with acute myocardial infarction, unstable angina, stroke, and traumatic brain injury are an exception, and higher transfusion triggers may be needed. Other parameters, including patient age, chronic anemia, or acute blood loss, and vaso-occlusive disease should also be taken into consideration when individualizing transfusion triggers.

14. What are the most commonly used techniques of autologous transfusion?

- **Preoperative autologous blood donation.** Blood is collected as far in advance of surgery as possible (no later than 3 days before) and transfused perioperatively as needed. Advantages include the prevention of alloimmunization and transfusion-transmitted diseases, and a reduction in allergic and febrile reactions. Drawbacks include the increased risk of preoperative anemia and the likelihood of perioperative transfusion, increased cost, and waste of blood that is not transfused.
- **Acute normovolemic hemodilution.** This technique involves the collection of blood (typically 500 mL–1500 mL) from a patient immediately before surgery, and the restoration of circulating volume with crystalloids and/or colloids. The removed blood, which is anticoagulated and stored

Table 57-2. Risk of Transfusion-Transmitted Infections in the United States

TYPE OF INFECTION	APPROXIMATE RISK PER UNIT TRANSFUSED
Human immunodeficiency virus	1:1.5 million
Hepatitis B virus	1:850,000
Hepatitis C virus	1:1.15 million
Human T-lymphocyte virus	1:2.7 million
Bacterial contamination	1:2500 (platelets)

for up to 8 hours, is reinfused during or after surgery. Since intraoperative blood losses are diluted, fewer RBCs are lost for a given volume.

- **Intraoperative blood salvage (Cell Saver).** Blood is suctioned from the surgical field, anticoagulated, and then RBCs are separated by centrifugation. After washing, RBCs are re-infused through a filter. Blood salvage is contraindicated in the presence of hypotonic solutions in the surgical field, if hemostatic agents (topical thrombin, collagen-based products) or bone cement could be simultaneously aspirated, and in the setting of bacteremia or active cancer.

15. What else can be done to minimize blood loss and transfusion requirements?
    - **Antifibrinolytic agents** (ε-aminocaproic acid and tranexamic acid [TXA]) are synthetic lysine analogs that have been used extensively, particularly in cardiac and orthopedic surgery, to minimize blood loss and decrease transfusion requirements. A recent meta-analysis did not find an increased risk of myocardial infarction or renal dysfunction with their use. Aprotinin, an older-generation antifibrinolytic, was withdrawn from the market in 2008 when it was found to be associated with a higher risk for cardiovascular complications and death. A survival advantage for trauma patients given TXA has been demonstrated in a large, multicenter, prospective, randomized-controlled trial, particularly if given in the first 3 hours.
    - **Desmopressin** increases plasma levels of von Willebrand factor (vWF) and factor VIII, and is licensed for use in von Willebrand disease and hemophilia A. It can also be used to control bleeding in patients with uremic platelet dysfunction. Decreased efficacy with repeated doses (tachyphylaxis) occurs, likely due to depletion of endothelial vWF stores. Hyponatremia can develop following administration.
    - **Recombinant erythropoietin** is a hormone that stimulates erythropoiesis. Although it has been shown to reduce perioperative transfusion requirements when used preoperatively in cardiac and orthopedic surgery, an increased risk of thrombotic events has been observed. It's use in the critical care setting is largely limited to patients for whom allogeneic RBC transfusion is not possible (e.g., Jehovah's witness, antibody to common red cell antigen).
    - **Recombinant human factor VIIa** is licensed for use in patients with hemophilia. Interest in its use as a hemostatic agent led to studies of off-label use has been studied in a variety of settings, including trauma, cardiac surgery, liver disease, and intracranial hemorrhage. It has not been shown to improve survival, and in some studies it was associated with increased mortality and the risk of thromboembolism. The optimal use of recombinant factor VIIa remains to be defined outside of hemophilia, and restraint should be exercised in off-label use.
    - **Prothrombin complex concentrate** (PCC) is licensed for the urgent reversal of vitamin K antagonists (VKA) in the setting of acute major bleeding. PCC contains balanced concentration of factors II, IX, and X, proteins C and S, and variable levels of factor VII (minimal in 3-factor PCC, present in 4-factor PCC). Compared to plasma, PCC is given in small volumes ($\sim$150 mL vs. 1000–1500 mL). Vitamin K needs to be given with PCC for durable VKA reversal. PCCs contain heparin and should not be given to patients with heparin-induced thrombocytopenia.

16. What are the characteristics of an ideal oxygen carrier?
    - Effective O_2 carrying capacity and delivery to the peripheral tissues
    - Favorable interaction with nitric oxide
    - Universal compatibility (cross-matching elimination)
    - Minimal side effects
    - Easy storage, long shelf life, immediate availability
    - Cost-effective

17. What alternative oxygen carriers are available for use in the critically ill?
    Two types of oxygen carriers are available as alternatives to PRBC transfusion: *hemoglobin-based oxygen carrier* and *perfluorocarbons*, but neither of them is currently commercially available. The former has been associated with adverse outcomes in human studies, whereas the latter is currently undergoing phase III testing.

18. What is fresh frozen plasma?
    FFP is plasma obtained by centrifugation of a whole-blood donation or collected by apheresis and frozen within 8 hours of collection. It is stored at or below -18°C to preserve the labile coagulation factors (e.g., V and VIII). FFP is a source of all the coagulation factors present in blood, along with antithrombin III and proteins C and S, at near-physiologic concentrations. It can be stored for up to 12 months and has to be thawed before transfusion. It has to be matched for ABO system compatibility (Table 57.3) but not RhD compatibility. FP24 is plasma that is frozen within 24 hours of collection and has slightly reduced concentrations of labile clotting factors.

Table 57-3. Compatible Donor-Recipient Combinations for Fresh Frozen Plasma

FFP		Donor			
		A	B	O	AB
RECIPIENT	A	×			×
	B		×		×
	O	×	×	×	×
	AB				×

19. List the indications for FFP.
    - Treatment of bleeding due to a congenital or acquired clotting factor deficiency for which a concentrate is not available
    - Treatment of bleeding due to deficiency of multiple factors (severe liver disease, DIC, dilutional coagulopathy)
    - Emergent reversal of warfarin effect or vitamin K deficiency
    - Massive transfusion protocol
    - Treatment of antithrombin III deficiency
    - Replacement fluid in plasma-exchange procedure

20. What is cryoprecipitate?
    Cryoprecipitate is made by slowly thawing FFP at 1 to 6°C. The resulting precipitate, separated by centrifugation, is enriched in vWF, factor VIII, fibrinogen, factor XIII, and fibronectin. Compared to plasma, cryoprecipitate is lower in volume (10–15 mL per unit).

21. List the indications for cryoprecipitate.
    - Fibrinogen repletion (levels <100 mg/dL)
    - von Willebrand disease (type I disease)
    - Factor XIII deficiency

22. What types of platelet concentrates are available?
    Pooled platelet concentrates are platelet concentrates prepared from whole blood donation. Individual concentrates from 4 to 6 whole blood donations (and therefore multiple donors) are pooled to produce one platelet dose. Older Blood Bank terminology reflects this pooling process by referring to a platelet dose as "6 units," each "unit" referring to a concentrate from a single whole blood donation. **Single-donor platelets** are collected from an individual donor using a pheresis machine.
    The "dose" of platelets provided is approximately equivalent between pooled and single-donor platelets. For patients with platelet refractoriness due to anti-HLA or antihuman platelet antibodies, apheresis platelets are preferred.

23. What reactions are more common with platelet transfusion?
    Bacterial contamination is more common with platelet concentrates than other blood products due to storage conditions. Platelet concentrates are stored at room temperature since cold storage leads to rapid clearance from the circulation following transfusion. Room temperature storage favors the growth of bacteria compared to colder storage temperatures, and, as a consequence, platelet concentrates can only be stored for up to 5 days.
    Platelet concentrates can also cause FNHTR, allergic reactions, TRALI, volume overload, and can lead to HLA-alloimmunization. Small volumes of RBCs are present in platelet concentrates, but not enough to lead to significant hemolysis; however, RhD-exposure may rarely lead to anti-D production, and for female RhD-negative patients transfused platelets from an RhD-positive donor, prophylactic anti-D may be considered to reduce this risk.

24. What are the guidelines for platelet transfusion?
    Thresholds for platelet transfusion have generally been determined empirically and good quality clinical data guiding the use of platelet transfusions is lacking.
    Published guidelines for platelet transfusion in preparation for invasive procedures include:
    - Neurosurgery—100,000/microL
    - Other major surgery—50,000/microL

- Central line placement—20,000/microL
- Lumbar puncture—40,000 to 50,000/microL; 10,000 to 20,000/microL in patients with hematologic malignancies

  Prophylactic platelet transfusion to prevent spontaneous bleeding generally depends on the clinical scenario. Randomized clinical trials in patients with hematologic malignancies support the use of platelet transfusions to maintain a platelet count greater than 10,000/microL. Factors, such as the reason for the thrombocytopenia, bleeding history, and evidence of mucosal bleeding, should be taken into account.

25. Should platelets be transfused in the setting of active bleeding and recent antiplatelet agent use?

    Evidence to support platelet transfusion in this setting is lacking for most antiplatelet agents, and the transfusion of *multiple* platelet units should be avoided. A recent randomized study found increased harm with platelet transfusions given to patients with spontaneous intracerebral hemorrhage while on antiplatelet therapy.

26. What is the purpose of leukoreduction?

    Leukoreduced blood products have undergone a filtration process to reduce the number of leukocytes. Leukoreduction decreases the risk of FNHTR, HLA allo-immunization, and transmission of cytomegalovirus (CMV). The indications for leukoreduced blood products include:
    - History of FNHTR
    - Requirement for long-term transfusion support (platelets or PRBCs)
    - Solid-organ transplant recipient or candidate (excluding liver transplant)
    - Requirement for CMV-reduced risk blood products

27. Why are blood products irradiated?

    Irradiation reduces the risk of TA-GVHD, a fatal adverse reaction to blood transfusion that occurs when donor lymphocytes are able to proliferate in a susceptible host. Irradiation causes DNA damage and prevents cellular replication. The risk of transfusion-transmitted infections is not decreased with irradiation.

28. What is measured by prothrombin time? What is the international normalized ratio?

    The prothrombin time **(PT)** is a hemostatic screening test that is sensitive to abnormalities of factor VII (extrinsic pathway), X, V, II, and fibrinogen (common pathway). Prolonged PT is associated with liver disease, vitamin K deficiency, vitamin K antagonists, circulating lupus anticoagulants, factor inhibitors, and hypo- or dysfibrinogenemia.

    The international normalized ratio **(INR)** is a standardized method of reporting the PT, so that values from different laboratories can be compared. It was developed to monitor patients receiving oral warfarin therapy and may not accurately reflect the risk of bleeding, especially in liver disease.

29. What is measured by partial thromboplastin time?

    The partial thromboplastin time **(PTT)** is a hemostatic screening test that is sensitive to the abnormalities of factors XII, XI, IX, and VIII (the intrinsic pathway), as well as with the common pathway factors (X, V, II, and fibrinogen). Prolonged PTT is associated with factor deficiencies (e.g., hemophilia), factor inhibitors, the presence of heparin, and circulating lupus anticoagulants.

30. How does warfarin work?

    Warfarin (Coumadin) inhibits the conversion of vitamin K to its active form. This inhibition interferes with the hepatic synthesis of the vitamin K-dependent clotting factors (II, VII, IX, X, and proteins C and S). Warfarin therapy is routinely monitored using the INR.

31. How does unfractionated heparin work?

    Unfractionated heparin (UFH) is a mixture of different length polysaccharides that bind to and increase antithrombin activity, which exerts an anticoagulant effect by inactivating thrombin and activated factor X. The half-life of heparin is relatively short (1–2 hours), and after stopping an infusion, its effects dissipate within 2 to 4 hours. If urgent reversal is required, protamine can be given intravenously. Heparin therapy is monitored by serial PTT measurements or anti-Xa activity assay. Heparin can be administered to patients in renal failure.

32. What is low-molecular-weight heparin?

    Low-molecular-weight heparin (LMWH) is a fragment produced by the chemical breakdown of UFH. Like heparin, it exerts an anticoagulant effect by enhancing antithrombin-mediated inactivation of factor Xa. Unlike UFH, LMWH cannot bind and inactivate thrombin. The anticoagulant effect of LMWH is of longer duration than UFH, permitting once- or twice-daily dosing; however, this feature also complicates the management of bleeding complications. The half-life of LMWH is prolonged in renal failure. Reversal with protamine is less effective. The anticoagulant effect of LMWH can be evaluated using the anti-Xa activity assay.

33. What are the major differences between standard heparin and low-molecular-weight heparin?
    • LMWH has a longer half-life and can be administered once or twice daily.
    • LMWH provides a more predictable anticoagulant response; therefore it can be administered without monitoring.
    • LMWH is as effective as heparin but produces fewer bleeding complications at equivalent anti-thrombotic doses.
    • LMWH is associated with a reduced risk of heparin-induced thrombocytopenia

34. What are the direct oral anticoagulants?
    Direct oral anticoagulants (DOACs) are a relatively new class of anticoagulants that are orally administered with reliable pharmacodynamics, resulting in no need for monitoring of the anticoagulant effect. DOACs work by directly inhibiting either thrombin (dabigatran) or factor Xa (apixaban, edoxaban, rivaroxaban). The DOACs are approved for use in patients with nonvalvular atrial fibrillation, and the treatment and prevention of venous thromboembolism and have been demonstrated to be as effective as warfarin, with lower overall bleeding risk. Most of the DOACs rely on renal elimination and may accumulate in renal failure. The DOACs have not been adequately studied in pregnant patients or patients with antiphospholipid syndrome, and they should not be used in patients with prosthetic heart valves due to the increased risk of thrombosis. Until recently, effective reversal agents for DOACs were not available.

35. What are the specific antidotes available for direct oral anticoagulants?
    Idarucizumab is a monoclonal antibody fragment that binds to dabigatran, removing it from circulation. It is the only reversal agent currently licensed for use. Andexanet alfa is an inactivated form of factor Xa that binds to the Xa-inhibitors. Its clinical efficacy is being tested in clinical trials.

36. What is damage control resuscitation?
    The basic tenets of damage control resuscitation are to:
    • avoid crystalloid resuscitation
    • aim for permissive hypotension whenever possible
    • prevent coagulopathy through early use of blood products
    • aggressively break the vicious cycle of acidosis, coagulopathy, and hypothermia
        A key component of this damage control approach is early hemorrhage control. Prospective studies have demonstrated a survival benefit with ratio-based massive transfusion protocols, suggesting that FFP and platelets should be given early and in high ratios. However, controversy continues to exist regarding the optimal ratio. A randomized trial comparing a 1:1:1 ratio (i.e., 1 FFP/1 whole blood platelet/1 PRBC) did not demonstrate a survival benefit compared to a 1:1:2 ratio (i.e., 1 whole blood platelet/1 FFP/2 PRBCs) in patients with severe trauma and major bleeding.

ACKNOWLEDGMENT

The authors wish to acknowledge Drs. George Kastakis, MD, and Hasan B. Alam, MD, FACS, for the valuable contributions to the previous edition of this chapter.

KEY POINTS: BLOOD PRODUCTS AND COAGULATION

1. Controlling the bleeding is more important than replacing the losses.
2. Blood products carry significant risks; transfuse only when necessary.
3. Know the mechanism of anticoagulants and how they can be reversed.
4. Early use of blood component therapy can prevent the development of coagulopathy in massively bleeding patients.
5. Excessive crystalloid resuscitation can worsen coagulopathy.

BIBLIOGRAPHY

1. Baharoglu MI, Cordonnier C, Al-Shahi Salman R, et al. Platelet transfusion versus standard care after acute stroke due to spontaneous cerebral haemorrhage associated with antiplatelet therapy (PATCH): a randomized, open-label, phase 3 trial. *Lancet.* 2016;387:2605.
2. Brown CV, Foulkrod KH, Sadler HT, et al. Autologous blood transfusion during emergency trauma operations. *Arch Surg.* 2010;145:690.
3. Carson JL, Stanworth SJ, Roubinian N, et al. Transfusion thresholds and other strategies for guiding allogeneic red blood cell transfusion. *Cochrane Database Syst Rev.* 2016;10:CD002042.
4. Carson JL, Noveck H, Berlin JA, et al. Mortality and morbidity in patients with very low postoperative hemoglobin levels who decline blood transfusion. *Transfusion.* 2002;42:812.
5. Corwin HL, Gettinger A, Fabian TC, et al. Efficacy and safety of Epoetin Alfa in critically ill patients. *NEJM.* 2007; 357:965.
6. CRASH-2 trial collaborators, Shakur H, Roberts I, Bautista R, et al. Effects of tranexamic acid on death, vascular occlusive events, and blood transfusion in trauma patients with significant haemorrhage (CRASH-2): a randomised, placebo-controlled trial. *Lancet.* 2010;376:23.
7. Duchesne JC, Hunt JP, Wahl G, et al. Review of current blood transfusions strategies in a mature level I trauma center: were we wrong for the last 60 years? *J Trauma.* 2008;65:272-276. [discussion: 276-278].
8. Goodnough LT, Levy JH. The Judicious Use of Recombinant Factor VIIa. *Semin Thromb Hemost.* 2016;42:125.
9. Henry DA, Carless PA, Moxey AJ, et al. Anti-fibrinolytic use for minimising perioperative allogeneic blood transfusion. *Cochrane Database Syst Rev.* 2011;(1):CD001886.
10. Holcomb JB, Tilley BC, Baraniuk S, et al. Transfusion of plasma, platelets, and red blood cells in a 1:1:1 vs a 1:1:2 ratio and mortality in patients with severe trauma: the proppr randomized clinical trial. *JAMA.* 2015;313(5):471.
11. Holcomb JB, del Junco DJ, Fox EE, et al. The prospective, observational, multicenter, major trauma transfusion (prommtt) study: comparative effectiveness of a time-varying treatment with competing risks. *JAMA Surg.* 2013;148(2):127.
12. Hong H, Xiao W, Lazarus HM, et al. Detection of septic transfusion reactions to platelet transfusions by active and passive surveillance. *Blood.* 2016;127:496.
13. Kaufman RM, Djulbegovic B, Gernsheimer T, et al. Platelet transfusion: a clinical practice guideline from the aabb. *Ann Intern Med.* 2015;162(3):205.
14. Kennedy LD, Case LD, Hurd DD, et al. A prospective, randomized, double-blind controlled trial of acetaminophen and diphenhydramine pretransfusion medication versus placebo for the prevention of transfusion reactions. *Transfusion.* 2008;48:2285.
15. Ker K, Roberts I, Shakur H, et al. Antifibrinolytic drugs for acute traumatic injury. *Cochrane Database Syst Rev.* 2015;(5): CD004896.
16. Martí-Carvajal AJ, Solà I, González LE, et al. Pharmacological interventions for the prevention of allergic and febrile non-haemolytic transfusion reactions. *Cochrane Database Syst Rev.* 2010;(6):CD007539.
17. Sarode R, Milling Jr TJ, Refaai MA, et al. Efficacy and safety of a 4-factor prothrombin complex concentrate in patients on vitamin K antagonists presenting with major bleeding: a randomized, plasma-controlled, phase IIIb study. *Circulation.* 2013;128:1234.
18. Shih AW, Crowther MA. Reversal of direct oral anticoagulants: a practical approach. *Hematology Am Soc Hematol Educ Program.* 2016;2016:612.
19. Stramer SL, Notari EP, Krysztof DE, et al. Hepatitis B virus testing by minipool nucleic acid testing: does it improve blood safety? *Transfusion.* 2013;53(10 Pt 2):2449.
20. Stanworth SJ, Estcourt LJ, Powter G, et al. A no-prophylaxis platelet-transfusion strategy for hematologic cancers. *NEJM.* 2013;368(19):1771.
21. Vanderlinde ES, Heal JM, Blumberg N. Autologous transfusion. *BMJ.* 2002;324:772-775.
22. Zou S, Stramer SL, Dodd RY. Donor testing and risk: current prevalence, incidence, and residual risk of transfusion-transmissible agents in us allogeneic donations. *Transfus Med Rev.* 2012;26(2):119.

THROMBOCYTOPENIA AND PLATELETS

Jerome Crowley

CHAPTER 58

1. What is the role of platelets in hemostasis?

   Platelets attach to interrupted endothelium (collagen expressed in the sub-endothelium) and connect to other platelets to form a platelet plug. Platelets are also activated by thrombin, which is part of the coagulation cascade. Activated platelets *degranulate* and release fibrinogen and Factor V, furthering clot formation.

2. What is the most common congenital platelet deficiency?

   von Willebrand disease. The absence of von Willebrand factor disrupts the formation of platelet aggregates (see question 1).

3. Define thrombocytopenia.

   There is no strong evidence-based definition of thrombocytopenia; however, the following classification is used in multiple sources:
   Mild: 100,000 to 149,000 platelets/microliter
   Moderate: 50,000 to 99,000 platelets/microliter
   Severe: less than 50,000 platelets/microliter

4. What are the risks of thrombocytopenia?

   The principal risk is bleeding. While not supported by high-quality evidence, usual cut offs include:
   Periprocedural bleeding risk: Platelets less than 50,000/microliter
   For high-risk surgery (neurosurgery, or other cases where bleeding would be catastrophic) a cut off of less than 100,000/microliter is often used.
   Spontaneous bleeding risk is assumed to be significant for platelets less than 10,000/microliter.
   However, it is important to note that the absolute platelet number is less important than the functional quality of platelets (i.e., a patient with a normal platelet count, but dysfunctional platelets may be at a higher bleeding risk than a patient with thrombocytopenia). Certain causes of thrombocytopenia are actually associated with an *increased* risk of clot formation (heparin-induced thrombocytopenia, antiphospholipid syndrome, thrombotic microangiopathies, disseminated intravascular coagulation [DIC], paroxysmal nocturnal hemoglobinuria).

5. What are the basic underlying causes of thrombocytopenia?

   Thrombocytopenia can be caused by decreased platelet production (nutritional deficiencies, myelodysplastic syndromes leading to marrow replacement, infection), increased platelet destruction (autoimmune, thrombotic microangiopathy, prosthetic valves, extracorporeal bypass, disseminated intravascular coagulation), dilution (massive transfusion), or disordered platelet distribution (hypersplenism). Remember, these mechanisms can occur in isolation or in combination.

6. How prevalent is thrombocytopenia in critically ill patients, and what are the most common causes of thrombocytopenia in the intensive care unit?

   Thrombocytopenia has a prevalence of 30% to 50% of patients in the intensive care unit (ICU). Some of the most common causes of thrombocytopenia in the ICU are recent surgery and hemorrhage, blood transfusions, drug-induced thrombocytopenia, intravascular catheters, vascular grafts, aortic balloon pumps, sepsis, renal replacement therapy, DIC, liver failure, and myelodysplastic/metastatic disease. Most patients who have thrombocytopenia in the ICU have idiopathic thrombocytopenia (thrombocytopenia of critical illness).

7. What are the most common agents used in the intensive care unit that cause drug-induced thrombocytopenia?

   - Antibiotics: linezolid, vancomycin, β-lactams
   - Glycoprotein (GP) IIb/IIIa inhibitors: abciximab, eptifibatide, lotrifiban

- Histamine 2 (H_2) blockers: cimetidine, famotidine, ranitidine
- Antiseizure medications: valproic acid, phenytoin
- Heparin: unfractionated heparin and low-molecular-weight heparin (more likely with unfractionated heparin)

8. What is heparin-induced thrombocytopenia?

   Heparin-induced thrombocytopenia (HIT) is a prothrombotic complication of heparin administration (risk of 0.6% with unfractionated heparin and 0.3% with low-molecular-weight heparin in a recent large, multicenter trial of ICU patients). It results from an immune response triggered by the interaction of heparin with a specific platelet protein, platelet factor 4 (PF4). Certain patient populations are at higher risk than others for the development of HIT, with patients after cardiac surgery having a risk of HIT that can be greater than 2%. HIT with thrombotic complication has a mortality rate of 20%, with approximately 20% to 30% having permanent disability (i.e., amputations, stroke).

9. When should a patient have a work-up for heparin-induced thrombocytopenia?

   The diagnosis must be considered in any patient in whom thrombocytopenia develops, who has an unexplained fall in platelet count of 50%, or who has thrombotic complication 5 to 10 days (may be as late as 20 days) after heparin exposure.

10. How is heparin-induced thrombocytopenia diagnosed?

    Almost all the patients with HIT have circulating antibodies to complexes between PF4 and heparin. However, in most of the patients who have circulating antibodies, HIT does not develop clinically. Therefore, it is currently not indicated to screen patients without symptoms for these antibodies. Two different types of assays are available:
    - The *functional assays* measure heparin-dependent platelet activation by PF4-heparin antibody in vitro. One of the functional assays, ^{14}C-serotonin release assay (SRA), is considered the *gold standard* in diagnosis with a positive predictive value of almost 100% (but a negative predictive value of approximately 20%).
    - *Immunoassays* (such as enzyme-linked immunosorbent assay [ELISA]) measure the levels of antibodies in circulation (sensitivity 93%–97%, positive predictive value 93%–100%, specificity 86%–100%, and negative predictive value 88%–95%). ELISA is easy and rapid to obtain, but only 25% of the ELISA-positive specimens are SRA positive.

11. Is repeating heparin-induced thrombocytopenia testing useful?

    Testing should be repeated for negative but borderline ELISA results. The chances of a negative test turning positive 3 days later depend on the titer levels. Approximately 45% of high-titer negative (almost positive) may turn positive, whereas approximately 15% and 5% of the medium- and low-titer results, respectively, are likely to turn positive.

12. How is heparin-induced thrombocytopenia treated?

    The diagnosis of HIT requires immediate withdrawal of all heparin and treatment with anticoagulation agents. The Warkentin criteria may be used to determine the patient's pretest probability of HIT (Table 58.1). All patients (with or without thrombosis) with HIT must be anticoagulated, as the risk of thrombosis is greater than 50% without anticoagulation. Do not transfuse platelets unless clearly indicated, as platelet transfusion actually increases the amount of PF4 and may exaggerate the antigen response. If continued anticoagulation is required, a vitamin K antagonist (warfarin) should be initiated *after* the patient is fully treated with one of the following agents:
    - Danaparoid (low-molecular-weight glycosaminoglycan composed of heparan sulfate, dermatan sulfate, and chondroitin sulfate). This drug has mostly antifactor Xa activity with a limited antithrombin action. Dose is titrated to keep anti-Xa levels between 0.5 and 0.8 units/mL. There is no antidote for bleeding.
    - Recombinant hirudin (lepirudin [Refludan]) is a 7-kDa peptide that acts directly on circulating and clot-bound thrombin. Anticoagulant effects last about 40 minutes. It is given as a slow bolus (0.4 mg/kg) followed by continuous infusion at 0.15 mg/kg to maintain activated partial thromboplastin time (aPTT) between 1.5 and 2.5 times baseline. This is a good choice for patients who will need to get transitioned to warfarin. Lepirudin does not alter the interpretation of international normalized ratio (INR) as significantly as argatroban.
    - Argatroban is a 509-Da arginine-based direct thrombin inhibitor that inhibits both soluble and clot-bound thrombin. The half-life is 46.2 ± 10.2 minutes, and steady-state activity is achieved within 1 to 2 hours of continuous infusion. Dose is 2.0 mcg/kg per minute and adjusted to keep aPTT between 1.5 and 3 times baseline (maximum 10 mcg/kg per minute).

Table 58-1. Warkentin Criteria to Determine the Probability of Heparin-Induced Thrombocytopenia

CRITERIA	2 POINTS	1 POINT	0 POINT
Thrombocytopenia	>50% fall or platelet nadir of 20–100 × 10^9/L	30%–50% fall or platelet nadir of 10–19 × 10^9/L	<30% fall or platelet nadir of <10 × 10^9/L
Timing of platelet drop	Clear onset day 5–10 or <1 day (if heparin exposure within past 100 days)	Consistent with immune activation but not clear (e.g., missing data) or onset after day 10	Platelet count fall too early (without recent heparin exposure)
Thrombosis or other sequelae	New thrombosis, skin necrosis, post-heparin bolus acute reaction	Progressive or recurrent thrombosis, erythematous skin lesions, suspected thrombosis (not yet proved)	None
Other causes for thrombocytopenia	No other cause for platelet count drop evident	Possible other causes	Definite other cause present

Pretest probability score 6–8 = high; 4–5 = intermediate; 0–3 = low.

- Fondaparinux is a pentasaccharide factor Xa inhibitor that is given via the subcutaneous route. Dose is 7.5 mg once a day. It is renally cleared, so caution is advised in impaired renal function.

13. How should you monitor warfarin effect when it is coadministered with argatroban?
Chromogenic factor X assay can be helpful in determining when the patient is therapeutically anticoagulated with warfarin while receiving argatroban (which in itself elevates the INR value). Switch to the measurement of INR 3 hours after discontinuation of argatroban to be certain that a therapeutic level is maintained after discontinuation of argatroban.

14. What are different treatment options for patients with immune thrombocytopenic purpura?
Immune thrombocytopenia purpura (ITP) is caused by immunoglobulin G antibodies against the platelet GPs (GPIIb/IIIa and GP Ib/IX). Corticosteroids have been the mainstay of therapy for a long time, but alternative therapies are now commonly prescribed. These include intravenous gamma globulins (IVIG) and intravenous anti-D (IV anti-D). Both cause *Fc receptor blockade* as an important mechanism of acute platelet increase. IVIG works fast (24 hours) and can be used in Rh-negative patients and patients after splenectomy, whereas IV anti-D causes a slower rate of platelet increase (72 hours) and is relatively ineffective in Rh-negative patients and patients after splenectomy. However, it is effective in patients positive for the human immunodeficiency virus. Patients who initially respond to medical management but have a relapse within 1 to 3 months may be considered candidates for splenectomy. For refractory ITP, combination chemotherapies are used (cyclophosphamide, hydroxydaunomycin, Oncovin, and prednisone [CHOP]-like; vincristine–IVIG–Solu-Medrol) followed by maintenance therapy (using combinations of steroids, danazol, Imuran, CellCept, cyclosporin among others).

15. How do you differentiate between thrombotic thrombocytopenic purpura and hemolytic uremic syndrome?
Thrombotic thrombocytopenic purpura (TTP) and hemolytic uremic syndrome (HUS) share thrombocytopenia, hemolytic anemia, and thrombotic occlusions in terminal arterioles and capillaries. Differentiating clinical features are the presence of focal neurologic symptoms in TTP and renal impairment in HUS. In addition, the levels of plasma von Willebrand factor-cleaving protease are low in TTP and normal in HUS.

16. What are some causes of platelet dysfunction in the intensive care unit?
The principal causes of platelet dysfunction and thrombocytopenia in the ICU are due to drug side effects (e.g., aspirin, clopidogrel), uremia, and sepsis. Antibiotics, nitrates, local anesthetics, α- and β-adrenergic blockers, xanthine derivatives, diuretics, H_2 receptor blockers, and dextran are some examples of drugs that can impair platelet activity.

17. What is the difference between pooled platelets and a single apheresis unit?

Pooled platelets are collected from blood unit donations; however, each unit does not have enough platelets by itself so six units are combined (pooled) to make one "6-pack" of platelets. An apheresis is collected from a single donor. Both one apheresis and one "6-pack" are expected to raise platelet counts by 30,000/microliter. Advantages of the apheresis include the ability to match for HLA type and/or blood type with the downside being greater cost.

18. What is the indication for type-specific platelets?

While there is no absolute indication, human leukocyte antigen (HLA) type-specific platelets may be considered in patients with an inappropriate response to platelet transfusion that is suspected to be of immunologic origin.

19. What are the indications for platelet transfusion?

The platelet counts that should serve as a trigger for platelet transfusion continue to evolve. Although somewhat controversial, the following threshold levels have been proposed in the literature:

- Bleeding prophylaxis in a stable oncology patient: 10,000/mm^3
- Lumbar puncture in a patient with leukemia: 10,000/mm^3
- HIT without signs of hemorrhage: 10,000/mm^3
- Bone marrow aspiration: 20,000/mm^3
- Gastrointestinal endoscopy in cancer: 20,000 to 40,000/mm^3
- DIC: 20,000 to 50,000/mm^3
- Fiberoptic bronchoscopy: 20,000 to 50,000/mm^3
- Major surgery: 50,000/mm^3
- Thrombocytopenia resulting from massive transfusion: 50,000/mm^3
- Invasive procedures in cirrhosis: 50,000/mm^3
- Cardiopulmonary bypass: 50,000 to 60,000/mm^3
- Neurosurgical procedures: 100,000/mm^3
- Thrombocytopenia and bleeding (intracerebral, gastrointestinal, genitourinary, or retinal hemorrhage): 100,000/mm^3

There is no specific count at which bleeding is completely prevented. In addition to the count, the quality and function of the platelets are also important. However, life-threatening bleeding can occur with platelet counts less than 5000/mm^3 and spontaneous bleeding with counts less than 10,000 to 20,000/mm^3.

20. How does aspirin affect platelet function?

Aspirin irreversibly inhibits platelet cyclooxygenase, resulting in a functional defect that lasts the duration of the platelet's life span (8–9 days).

21. What laboratory test measures platelet function?

Bleeding time is a sensitive indicator of overall platelet function. Platelet function may also be assessed with thromboelastography.

22. How are platelet disorders managed?

The patient's drug regimen should be carefully scrutinized, eliminating or substituting medications implicated in thrombocytopenia. Platelet transfusion may be required (see answer to question 16). Uremia-associated thrombocytopenia can be treated with hemodialysis. Cryoprecipitate, 1-desamino-8-D-arginine vasopressin, and conjugated estrogens have also been used with good results.

ACKNOWLEDGMENT

The authors wish to acknowledge Drs. Chad T. Wilson, MD, MPH, and Hasan B. Alam, MD, FACS, for the valuable contributions to the previous edition of this chapter.

KEY POINTS: THROMBOCYTOPENIA AND PLATELETS

1. Thrombocytopenia is a common finding in intensive care unit patients, and the basic rule for management is to treat the underlying cause.
2. Transfuse platelets only if needed (question 16) or if the platelet count is less than 10,000/mm^3.
3. HIT is a relatively uncommon but potentially serious complication of heparin administration.

4. Platelet counts should be followed in all patients that are receiving heparin (unfractionated or low molecular weight). A drop in platelet count (>50% from baseline or below $100,000/mm^3$) is a reason to suspect HIT.
5. Most of the patients who have circulating antibodies to PF4 do not have clinical development of HIT. Therefore, screen patients for these antibodies only when clinically indicated.
6. All patients (with or without thrombosis) with HIT (type II) must be anticoagulated, as the risk of thrombosis is >50% without anticoagulation.

BIBLIOGRAPHY

1. AuBuchon JP. Platelet transfusion therapy. *Clin Lab Med.* 1996;16:797-816.
2. Chong BH, Eisbacher M. Pathophysiology and laboratory testing of heparin-induced thrombocytopenia. *Semin Hematol.* 1998;35:3-8.
3. Fuse I. Disorders of platelet function. *Crit Rev Oncol Hematol.* 1996;22:1-25.
4. Liumbruno G, Bennardello F, Lattanzio A, et al. Recommendations for the transfusion of plasma and platelets. *Blood Transfus.* 2009;7(2):132-150.
5. Lipsett PA, Perler BA. The use of blood products for surgical bleeding. *Semin Vasc Surg.* 1996;9:347-353.
6. Martel N, Lee J, Wells PS. Risk for heparin-induced thrombocytopenia with unfractionated and low-molecular-weight heparin thromboprophylaxis: a meta-analysis. *Blood.* 2005;106:2710-2715.
7. McCrae KR, Bussel JB, Mannucci PM, et al. Platelets: an update on diagnosis and management of thrombocytopenic disorders. *Hematology Am Soc Hematol Educ Program.* 2001;2001:282-305.
8. Aster RH, Bartolucci AA, Collins JA, et al. Platelet transfusion therapy. *Natl Inst Health Consens Dev Conf Consens Statement.* 1986;6:1-6.
9. Priziola JL, Smythe MA, Dager WE. Drug induced thrombocytopenia in critically ill patients. *Crit Care Med.* 2010;38 (suppl 6):S145-S152.
10. PROTECT Investigators for the Canadian Critical Care Trials Group and the Australian and New Zealand Intensive Care Society Clinical Trials Group, Cook D, Meade M, Guyatt G, et al. Dalteparin versus unfractionated heparin in critically ill patients. *N Engl J Med.* 2011;364:1305-1314.
11. Rebulla P. Platelet transfusion trigger in difficult patients. *Transfus Clin Biol.* 2001;8:249-254.
12. Selleng K, Warkentin TE, Greinacher A. Heparin-induced thrombocytopenia in intensive care patients. *Crit Care Med.* 2007;35:1165-1176.

CHAPTER 59

DISSEMINATED INTRAVASCULAR COAGULATION

Pavan K. Bendapudi and David Kuter

1. What is disseminated intravascular coagulation?

   Disseminated intravascular coagulation (DIC) is due to aberrant activation of the clotting cascade, leading to fibrin and platelet deposition in small vessels, which, along with concurrent activation of fibrinolytic mechanisms, leads to bleeding and/or thrombosis. Because they are consumed by the ongoing prothrombotic and fibrinolytic processes, coagulation proteins and platelets can become depleted, leading to simultaneous bleeding and clotting. DIC is a broad clinical entity, and different causes of DIC can lead to a spectrum of presentations. For example, DIC resulting from acute promyelocytic leukemia can present with uncontrolled bleeding, whereas purpura fulminans is a highly thrombotic subtype of DIC, which results from bacterial infection. DIC is also associated with conditions such as sepsis, pancreatitis, or trauma. DIC can be an acute or a chronic disorder, and the latter is seen mostly in obstetric and oncology patients. Hereafter, the discussion will focus primarily on acute DIC, the form most likely to be encountered in the critical care setting.

2. Why is disseminated intravascular coagulation important?

   DIC is a common cause of concurrent thrombocytopenia and prolonged clotting times (activated partial thromboplastin time [aPTT] and prothrombin time [PT]) in hospitalized patients. It can also be an independent predictor of mortality. DIC leads to fibrin and platelet deposition in small vessels, which can cause tissue ischemia and result in organ dysfunction (Fig. 59.1). The consumptive coagulopathy can also lead to clinically significant bleeding.

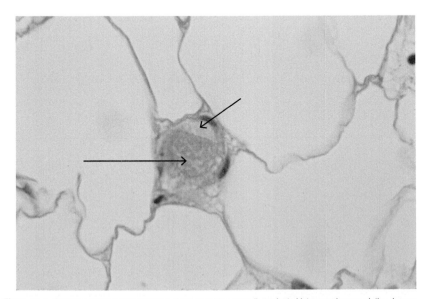

Figure 59-1. Microvascular thrombosis in skin of patient with severe disseminated intravascular coagulation. Lumen *(short arrow)* of blood vessel is partly occluded by fibrin/platelet thrombus *(long arrow)*.

3. What is the pathophysiology of acute disseminated intravascular coagulation?

Although the pathophysiology of DIC remains incompletely understood, it is thought to begin at the level of the microvasculature. As a result of the underlying illness (i.e., sepsis, trauma, or pancreatitis), tissue factor (TF) is expressed on the surface of inflamed endothelium and from damaged blood vessels released into circulation, after which it combines with Factor VIIa to produce thrombin via the extrinsic pathway. The thrombin activates platelets and cleaves fibrinogen, so platelets and fibrin are deposited in the microvasculature. Concurrently, fibrinolytic pathways are activated. As platelets and coagulation proteins are consumed, bleeding can occur as the result of a consumptive coagulopathy. Thus, DIC is characterized by simultaneous clotting and hemorrhage.

4. In critical care patients, what conditions are associated with disseminated intravascular coagulation?

- Sepsis
- Trauma
- Malignancy: adenocarcinoma, acute promyelocytic leukemia (incidence approaches 100%)
- Obstetric: hemolysis, elevated liver enzymes, and low platelets (HELLP) syndrome, retained uterine placental or fetal tissue, placental abruption or previa, amniotic fluid embolus
- Vascular: vasculitis, abdominal aortic aneurysm, cavernous hemangiomas
- Miscellaneous: burns, anaphylaxis, transfusion reaction, snake bite, acute pancreatitis, transplant rejection, intravenous anti-D immunoglobulin (Winrho)

5. How does disseminated intravascular coagulation present clinically?

In acutely ill hospitalized patients, DIC usually presents with prolongation of the PT and aPTT along with decreased fibrinogen and platelets; systemic bleeding and thrombosis may or may not be present. Typically, bleeding manifests as ecchymoses, purpura, petechiae; it also occurs at surgical incisions or insertion sites of vascular access catheters. Mucosal and urinary bleeding are common, while pulmonary, gastrointestinal (GI), and central nervous system (CNS) bleeding occur less frequently. Due to widespread intravascular coagulation, tissue ischemia can occur, resulting in cyanosis, delirium, oliguria, hypoxia, and frank tissue necrosis (Fig. 59.2).

6. What laboratory abnormalities are typical of acute disseminated intravascular coagulation?

No standard test exists for DIC, which remains a clinical diagnosis. Thrombocytopenia, prolongation of the PT, aPTT, and thrombin time, and hypofibrinogenemia are characteristic. Because fibrinogen is present in significant excess in plasma and is an acute phase reactant, decreased fibrinogen is an insensitive marker of DIC and should not be relied upon to make the diagnosis. Early in the course of DIC, the platelet count may be in the normal range, but it is often decreased from baseline. Platelet counts are rarely less than 20,000/microliter. D-dimer and fibrin degradation products (FDP) are almost always markedly elevated. The haptoglobin level is variably affected and is not helpful in confirming the diagnosis of DIC. Additionally, the presence of an abnormal "biphasic aPTT waveform" has been reported to be sensitive and specific for DIC, though this parameter is not standardly reported with the aPTT result at most centers.

7. Is the peripheral blood smear useful in the diagnosis of disseminated intravascular coagulation?

The peripheral blood smear from a patient with DIC typically shows mild to moderate thrombocytopenia; platelets may be very large and often accompanied by increased mean platelet volume. Additionally, red blood cells transiting microvascular beds obstructed by thrombi can be sheared, resulting in the presence of schistocytes (red blood cell fragments created by intravascular hemolysis, Fig. 59.3). However, the finding of schistocytes is neither sensitive nor specific and schistocytes are present in only 10% to 50% of cases of acute DIC. If present in DIC, there are usually only 1 to 4 per high-power field, in contrast to thrombotic thrombocytopenic purpura where they are much more abundant.

8. What conditions make interpretation of laboratory abnormalities in disseminated intravascular coagulation more difficult?

Fibrinogen is an acute-phase reactant. As such, it can be only mildly decreased or falsely normal in patients with acute DIC, especially if there is an underlying inflammatory disorder; therefore, comparison to a baseline value would be useful. Overall, hypofibrinogenemia is more specific than sensitive as a marker of DIC. Additionally, the D-dimer can be chronically elevated in cancer patients and in those with recent clots or liver disease (see below).

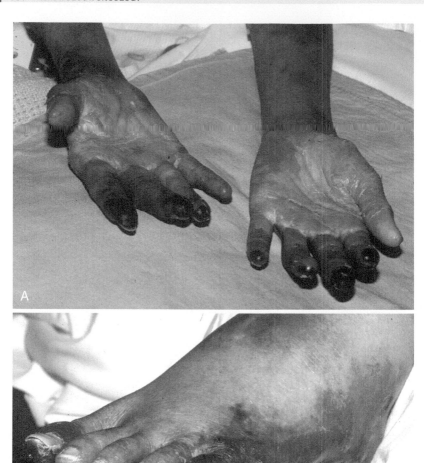

Figure 59-2. Ischemic necrosis of fingers (A) and feet (B) of patient with disseminated intravascular coagulation due to bacterial sepsis.

9. Why is it difficult to make the diagnosis of disseminated intravascular coagulation in patients with advanced liver disease?

The liver produces most coagulation proteins, and most cases of advanced liver disease are characterized by a prolonged PT and aPTT with decreased fibrinogen. The liver is also responsible for clearing D-dimers, which are therefore often elevated in liver disease. Additionally, the platelet count may be reduced in cirrhotic patients due to hypersplenism and reduced production of thrombopoietin by the liver. There is a general consensus that advanced liver disease alone does not lead to true DIC in the absence of other precipitating factors.

10. When and how is disseminated intravascular coagulation treated?

Because DIC tends to be secondary to other disorders, addressing the underlying disorder is the mainstay of treatment. Therapy is otherwise supportive. Blood products should be administered in cases of DIC complicated by clinically significant bleeding or a significantly elevated risk of bleeding

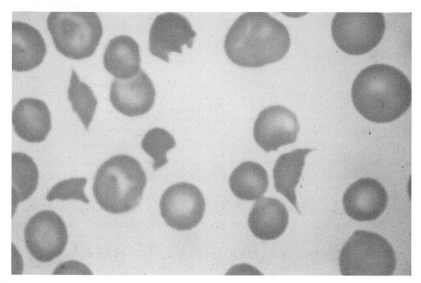

Figure 59-3. Schistocytes in peripheral blood smear of patient with severe acute disseminated intravascular coagulation. Note the absence of platelets as well.

(e.g., a patient with recent vascular surgery) but are not routinely required. Blood components should not be given solely in response to laboratory abnormalities. For cases of highly thrombotic (e.g., purpura fulminans) or hemorrhagic (e.g., acute promyelocytic leukemia) DIC, expert consultation is advised.

11. How should blood products be administered in cases of acute disseminated intravascular coagulation?
    Platelet transfusions should be reserved for patients with signs of clinical bleeding. Although there is no evidence to support a fixed platelet goal in DIC, a platelet goal of greater than 25,000/microliter with minor bleeding or greater than 50,000/microliter with major bleeding is reasonable in DIC. Cryoprecipitate may be administered to keep the fibrinogen level greater than 100 mg/dL. One dose (10-pack) of cryoprecipitate will raise the fibrinogen level by approximately 85 mg/dL in an averaged sized adult. Fresh frozen plasma (FFP) should be given only if clinically significant bleeding is present or if there is a significant risk for bleeding (e.g., for invasive procedures); it should not be used solely to "correct" a prolonged PT or aPTT. It should also be noted that international normalized ratio (INR) values of up to 1.7 are not associated with an increased risk of bleeding. Paradoxically, blood products are not associated with a worsening of DIC.

12. Are there special causes of disseminated intravascular coagulation that require specific treatment?
    HELLP syndrome is a peripartum form of DIC, resulting in clinically significant hepatic injury and hemolytic anemia. In addition to supportive care, treatment for HELLP includes either delivery of the fetus or dilatation and curettage to remove retained fetal or placental fragments. Acute promyelocytic leukemia (APL or APML) is almost always associated with DIC. In addition to appropriate transfusions for the treatment of DIC, the use of antifibrinolytic agents, such as amicar, may be indicated in cases with severe bleeding. Furthermore, these patients require the urgent initiation of chemotherapy, which should include all-trans-retinoic acid (ATRA). Finally, purpura fulminans is a thrombotic subtype of DIC that has been treated with infusions of protein C concentrate, although evidence supporting this practice remains sparse.

13. In what scenarios should heparin be considered for the treatment of disseminated intravascular coagulation?
    In cases of acute DIC characterized by clinically significant bleeding despite the administration of blood products or in thrombotic DIC with digital ischemia, heparin may be considered. Heparin should be employed with caution, as it can exacerbate bleeding. The rationale for using heparin is to limit microvascular clotting in DIC and thus correct the resultant consumptive coagulopathy. The use of

heparin requires that the platelet count be maintained at greater than 50,000/microliter and that there be no concurrent GI or CNS bleeding. Heparin is contraindicated in conditions that require surgical management, such as retained uterine placental tissue. In addition, its use should be avoided in patients with placental abruption.

14. **How should heparin be administered?**
No bolus dose should be given. A continuous infusion of unfractionated heparin, 5 to 10 U/kg per hour, is reasonable until the bleeding has lessened or stopped and/or the underlying clinical condition has been effectively treated. Heparin at these doses is unlikely to alter the aPTT, and patients in DIC can be relatively heparin-resistant due to the presence of acute phase reactants. Low-molecular-weight heparin and the newer direct acting oral anticoagulants have not been adequately studied for the treatment of acute DIC complicated by bleeding, and their use cannot currently be recommended.

15. **What other agents have been considered for use in disseminated intravascular coagulation?**
Fibrinolytic inhibitors, such as ε-aminocaproic acid (Amicar) and tranexamic acid, can be used to treat DIC-associated refractory bleeding by preventing systemic fibrinolysis. However, these inhibitors should be administered with caution in DIC as they can worsen systemic fibrin deposition. Combining their use with low-dose heparin infusion is one way to avoid converting a hemorrhagic patient into one with life-threatening thrombosis. Additionally, there is no role for recombinant VIIa or activated plasma-derived clotting factors in the treatment of DIC.

16. **How is the efficacy of disseminated intravascular coagulation treatment evaluated?**
Laboratory parameters, including the PT, aPTT, fibrinogen, and platelet count, should be followed and should return to baseline levels as the disorder is effectively treated. In addition, clinical bleeding should improve. The D-dimer should also decline with treatment but may remain persistently elevated due to other causes (unresolved clot, liver failure). The time course of recovery from DIC is usually linked to recovery from the underlying illness.

17. **What treatments are controversial in disseminated intravascular coagulation?**
Randomized trials in patients with DIC are lacking. Because DIC is associated with mortality in sepsis, recombinant activated Protein C (drotrecogin alfa) was approved in 2001 for use in severe sepsis with organ failure. However, the use of drotrecogin alfa is associated with an increased risk of bleeding, and the agent was withdrawn from the market in 2011 after follow-up studies failed to demonstrate efficacy.

18. **What new treatments may be available in the future for disseminated intravascular coagulation?**
A number of treatments directed against either the aberrant coagulation or fibrinolysis seen in DIC have been proposed. Recently, recombinant thrombomodulin (which operates in the same pathway as Protein C) has shown promising results in an unrandomized trial utilizing historical controls. Antithrombin concentrate has also been evaluated in small uncontrolled trials, but has not demonstrated benefit. Other agents that have been proposed for the treatment of DIC include recombinant tissue factor pathway inhibitor (failed to demonstrate efficacy in a Phase III trial), recombinant Factor VIIa (yet to undergo large randomized trials), recombinant hirudin (animal studies only), C1 esterase inhibitor (small human trials), and recombinant nematode anticoagulant c2 (animal studies only).

KEY POINTS: DISSEMINATED INTRAVASCULAR COAGULATION

1. Definition: Disseminated intravascular coagulation (DIC) is a syndrome involving the activation of both coagulation and fibrinolysis, resulting in the intravascular deposition of fibrin and the consumption of coagulation proteins and platelets, which commonly leads to bleeding (see question 1).
2. Importance: DIC can lead to organ dysfunction and is associated with high mortality (see question 2).
3. Diagnosis: No single laboratory test can be used to diagnose DIC. Instead, a combination of a prolonged aPTT and PT, decreased fibrinogen, decreased platelets, increased D-dimer or FDPs, and schistocytes on a blood smear in an appropriate clinical context may suggest the diagnosis (see questions 5, 6, 7).
4. Treatment: Management of DIC should focus primarily on treatment of the underlying disorder (see question 10).

BIBLIOGRAPHY

1. Abraham E, Reinhart K, Opal S, et al. Efficacy and safety of tifacogin (recombinant tissue factor pathway inhibitor) in severe sepsis: a randomized controlled trial. *JAMA.* 2003 Jul 9;290(2):238.
2. Abraham E, Reinhart k, Svoboda P, et al. Assessment of the safety of recombinant tissue factor pathway inhibitor in patients with severe sepsis: a muticenter, randomized, placebo-controlled, single-blind, dose escalation study. *Crit Care Med.* 2001;29:2081-2089.
3. Bick RL. Disseminated intravascular coagulation: Objective clinical and laboratory diagnosis, treatment, and assessment of therapeutic response. *Semin Thromb Hemost.* 1996;22:69-88.
4. Hermida J, Montes R, Páramo JA, et al. Endotoxin-induced disseminated intravascular coagulation in rabbits: effect of recombinant hirudin on hemostatic parameters, fibrin deposits, and mortality. *J Lab Clin Med.* 1998;131(1):77-83.
5. Levi M, Ten Cate H. Disseminated intravascular coagulation. *N Engl J Med.* 1999;341:586-592.
6. Schmaier AH. Disseminated intravascular coagulation. *N Engl J Med.* 1999;341:1937-1938.
7. Stouthard JM, Levi M, Hack CE, et al. Interleukin-6 stimulates coagulation, not fibrinolysis, in humans. *Thromb Haemost.* 1996;76(5):738-742.
8. Yamakawa K, Fujimi S, Mohri T, et al. Treatment effects of recombinant human soluble thrombomodulin in patients with severe sepsis: a historical control study. *Crit Care.* 2011;15(3):R123.
9. Toussaint S, Gerlach H. Activated Protein C for Sepsis. *N Engl J Med.* 2009;361:2646-2652.
10. Manios SG, Kanakoudi F, Maniati E. Fulminant meningococcemia. Heparin therapy and survival rate. *Scand J Infect Dis.* 1971;3(2):127-133.
11. Segal JB, Dzik WH. Paucity of studies to support that abnormal coagulation test results predict bleeding in the setting of invasive procedures: an evidence-based review. *Transfusion.* 2005;45:1413.
12. Asakura H, Ontachi Y, Mizutani T, et al. An enhanced fibrinolysis prevents the development of multiple organ failure in disseminated intravascular coagulation in spite of much activation of blood coagulation. *Crit Care Med.* June 2001;29(6):1164-1168.
13. Kitchens CS. Thrombocytopenia and thrombosis in disseminated intravascular coagulation (DIC). *Hematology.* 2009; 2009:240-246.
14. Bakhtiari K, Meijers JC, de Jonge E, et al. Prospective validation of the International Society of Thrombosis and Haemostasis scoring system for disseminated intravascular coagulation. *Crit Care Med.* December 2004;32(12): 2416-2421.

CHAPTER 60

COMA

M. Dustin Boone, Ala Nozari, Corey R. Fehnel

1. **How is consciousness defined?**
   Consciousness has classically been defined as a state of awareness of self and one's relationship to the environment. Consciousness has two components: arousal and content. Arousal is characterized by wakefulness/alertness. Content is composed of affective and cognitive functions, such as attention, memory, mood, and emotional state.

2. **Which central nervous system structures are responsible for arousal and content?**
   Arousal is mediated by the ascending reticular activating system (rostral pons, midbrain, thalamus, hypothalamus). Content depends on the integrity of the connections between the cerebral cortex and subcortical white matter. Fig. 60.1 illustrates the important central nervous system structures for consciousness.

3. **What is coma and how is it different from persistent vegetative state, minimally conscious state, and locked-in syndrome?**
   - *Coma* is a state of profound unresponsiveness where the patient is unaware of self and environment, and cannot be roused to respond to vigorous stimulation. It can be caused by structural and/or metabolic pathophysiologic processes. Psychogenic states of "coma" mimic true coma.
   - *Persistent vegetative state (PVS)* is a condition of partial arousal. Patients may briefly alert to sound or visual stimuli. They withdraw to noxious stimuli, but are unable to interact or respond voluntarily or in any purposeful way to stimuli. PVS is a chronic condition and thus is typically not assigned unless a patient's state of altered consciousness persists for more than 30 days.

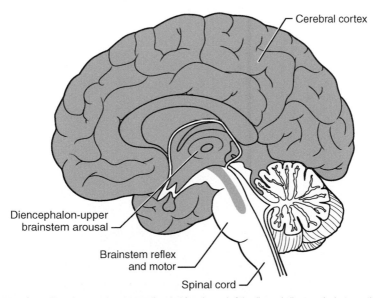

Figure 60-1. Coma: There is severe impairment of cortical function and of the diencephalic-upper brainstem activating systems. Patients are unarousable with eyes closed and have no purposeful responses, but brainstem activity is present. *(Reproduced with permission from Blumenfeld H. Brainstem III: internal structures and vascular supply. In Neuroanatomy Through Clinical Cases. 2010, Sinauer Associates, Inc. Chapter 14, Figure 14.16, p. 642.)*

- Patients in a *minimally conscious state (MCS)* exhibit deliberate or cognitively mediated behavior, may intermittently follow commands, or have intelligible but inconsistent verbal output. Patients may evolve to MCS from coma or PVS.
- Patients with *locked-in syndrome* have intact cognition but complete paralysis of voluntary muscles in most or all parts of the body. They traditionally have been able to communicate through code systems by blinking or repeated up-and-down eye movements; however, recent breakthrough technology has allowed some patients to communicate via a human-machine computer interface that allows patients to initiate computer commands with only their thoughts through the use of a surgically embedded microchip in the cerebral cortex (Table 60.1).

4. Describe the four steps involved with the neurologic assessment of the unconscious patient.
   1. Determine the level of consciousness
   2. Assess brainstem reflexes
   3. Evaluate motor responses
   4. Examine breathing patterns

5. Name two common scales that are used to quantitatively rate the severity of impaired consciousness.
   The Glasgow Coma Scale (GCS) and the Full Outline of Unresponsiveness Score (FOUR Score) (Table 60.2)

6. What are the limitations of the Glasgow Coma Scale?
   The GCS does not account for injury to the brainstem, nor does it distinguish patients with hemiparesis or aphasia. In addition, patients with the same GCS scores may have quite diverse clinical presentations from different combinations of sub scores. Thus, we recommend recording both total and sub-scores. The FOUR score has the advantage of including brainstem reflexes and respiratory patterns.

Table 60-1. Coma and Related States

ANATOMY	CEREBRAL CORTEX	DIENCEPHALON-UPPER BRAINSTEM AROUSAL SYSTEMS	BRAINSTEM REFLEX AND MOTOR SYSTEMS	SPINAL CORD CIRCUITS
Function Tested	Purposeful Response to Stimuli?	Behavioral Arousal, Sleep-wake Cycles?	Brainstem Reflexes?	Spinal Cord Reflexes?
Brain death	No	No	No	Yes
Coma	No	No	Yes	Yes
Vegetative state	No	Yes	Yes	Yes
Minimally conscious state	Yes, at times	Yes	Yes	Yes
Stupor, obtundation, lethargy, delerium	Yes, at times	Variable	Yes	Yes
Status epilepticus	Variable	Variable	Yes	Yes
Akinetic mutism, abulia, catatonia	Yes, at times	Yes	Yes	Yes
Sleep, normal and abnormal	Yes, at times	Yes	Yes	Yes
Locked-in syndrome	No	Yes	Yes	Yes

Reproduced with permission from Blumenfeld H. Brainstem III: internal structures and vascular supply. In *Neuroanatomy Through Clinical Cases.* Sinauer Associates, Inc. 2010. Chapter 14, Table 14.3, p. 643.

Table 60-2. Comparison of the Glasgow Coma Scale (GCS) and the Full Outline of Unresponsiveness Score (FOUR Score) for Grading of Coma

GCS	FOUR SCORE
Eye Opening Spontaneous 4 To speech 3 To pain 2 No response 1	**Eye Response** 4 Eyelids open, tracking or blinking to command 3 Eyelids open but not tracking 2 Eyelids closed but opens to loud voice 1 Eyelids closed but opens to pain 0 Eyelids remain closed with pain
Best motor response Obeys 6 Localizes 5 Withdraws 4 Abnormal flexion 3 Abnormal extension 2 No response 1	**Motor Response** 4 Thumbs up, fist or peace sign to command 3 Localizes to pain 2 Flexion response to pain 1 Extensor posturing 0 No response to pain or myoclonic status epilepticus
Best verbal response Oriented 5 Confused conversation 4 Inappropriate words 3 Incomprehensible sounds 2 No response 1	**Brainstem Reflexes** 4 Pupil and corneal reflexes present 3 One pupil wide and fixed 2 Pupil or corneal reflexes absent 1 Pupil and corneal reflexes absent 0 Absent pupil, corneal and cough reflex
	Respiration 4 Not intubated, regular breathing pattern 3 Not intubated, Cheyne-Stokes breathing pattern 2 Not intubated, irregular breathing pattern 1 Breathes above ventilator rate 0 Breathes at ventilator rate or apnea

7. **What are the major categories for coma etiology?**
   - Coma can be caused by *structural brain injury* involving the relay nuclei and connecting fibers of the ascending reticular activation system (ARAS), which extends from the upper brainstem through synaptic relays in the rostral intralaminar and thalamic nuclei to the cerebral cortex. The base of pons does not participate in arousal, and lesions such as central pontine myelinolysis do not usually profoundly impair consciousness. Instead, these lesions can interrupt all motor output except vertical eye movements and blinking (locked-in syndrome) that are initiated by nuclei in the mesencephalon.
   - *Mesencephalic and thalamic injuries*, for example, as a result of occlusion of the tip of the basilar artery, or bilateral thalamic injuries, may result in somnolence, immobility, and decreased verbal output characteristic for MCS.
   - *Bihemispheric injuries* involving the cortex, white matter, or both may also result in impaired arousal.
   - Acute *unilateral hemispheric* or *cerebellar mass* can lead to coma through destruction of the brain tissue and displacement of the falx cerebri and/or brainstem compression.
   - *Pathophysiologic brain states* resulting from generalized seizures, hypothermia, and poisoning or acute *metabolic and endocrine derangements* can also lead to coma. Typically, metabolic coma may spare the pupillary light reflex as it causes selected dysfunction of the cortex, whereas brainstem centers that control the pupils are spared. Hypoglycemia or nonketotic hyperosmolar coma, dysnatremia, thyroid storm, myxedema, fulminant hepatic failure, and acute hypopituitarism are examples in this category and should always be considered in a comatose patient. Asterixis, tremor, myoclonus, and foul breath may predominate the examination before these patients become unresponsive.
   - Malignant catatonia and *psychogenic unresponsiveness* also should be considered in all unresponsive patients.
   - *Acute muscle paralysis* (e.g., botulism or other toxins) also should be ruled out, because these patients may be awake and cognitively intact but unable to demonstrate responsiveness.

8. **Name common causes of structural brain injury in comatose patients.**
Structural brain injuries may be caused by the following:
- Bilateral cortical or subcortical infarcts (e.g., as a consequence of cardiac embolization or occlusion of major cerebral vessels)
- Bleeding (e.g., hemorrhagic contusions, epidural or subdural hematoma, subarachnoid hemorrhage)
- Infections (e.g., meningitis, cerebral abscess, subdural empyema, and herpes encephalitis)
- Neoplasm (primary tumors and metastases)
- Vasculitis and leukoencephalopathy, or lateral (acute midline shift of the brain of >1 cm) or downward herniation from mass effect or increased intracranial pressure (ICP) (e.g., massive brain edema, obstructive hydrocephalus)

9. **Describe the mechanisms of a toxic-metabolic coma.**
Depression of neuronal function can be caused by a reduction in the turnover of major neurotransmitters, such as acetylcholine, dopamine, and serotonin through the γ-aminobutyric acid–benzodiazepine chloride iodophor receptor complex. Moreover, toxins can result in hypoxia (e.g., through respiratory depression or aspiration) or hypoglycemia (e.g., ethanol, β-blockers, and salicylates) leading to coma. Seizures disrupt normal synaptic transmission through neurotransmitter depletion and other mechanisms termed "excitotoxicity." Glucose is the sole energy source for brain-profound hypoglycemia in the setting of insulin use, and is a common factor among diabetics.

10. **What are the initial steps in the evaluation and management of a comatose patient?**
The immediate approach to the comatose patient includes measures to protect the brain by providing adequate cerebral blood flow and oxygenation, reversing metabolic derangements, and treating potential infections and anatomic or endocrine abnormalities. Fig. 60.2 illustrates the initial steps in evaluating and managing a comatose patient.
- The clinician must ensure that the patient has a patent and protected airway and adequate breathing. Supplemental oxygen should be administered and the airway secured by intubating the trachea, if needed.
- Vascular access should be obtained and hypotension corrected with vasopressor agents or fluid administration, as required.
- Blood samples should be obtained to rule out infection and metabolic or endocrine abnormalities.
- Generalized seizures should be treated and metabolic abnormalities corrected as soon as possible.
- If the cause of coma is uncertain and hypoglycemia cannot be excluded, 50% dextrose should be administered. Empirical therapy for Wernicke encephalopathy or narcotic or sedative overdose should be considered, and thiamine, naloxone, or flumazenil administered if appropriate. Thiamine must be given before dextrose to prevent worsening of Wernicke encephalopathy.
- If increased ICP with mass effect is suspected, the patient should have mannitol, or hypertonic saline solution administered, and possibly hyperventilation as a bridge to specific neurosurgical decompressive measures.
- If meningitis is suspected, antibiotic treatment should be initiated, and then a computed tomography (CT) scan of the head performed to rule out mass effect or herniation, in combination with laboratory evaluation for coagulopathy or thrombocytopenia before lumbar puncture.

11. **When is brain imaging indicated in a comatose patient?**
An emergent noncontrast head CT should be obtained either for an unconscious patient with a structural cause of coma or for those patients without a clear cause of coma following the initial evaluation. A CT scan can identify several structural etiologies: (1) intracerebral hemorrhage; (2) brain masses compressing midline arousal pathways; (3) cerebral edema; (4) hydrocephalus; and (5) cerebral infarction.[a]

12. **List the differential diagnosis for a comatose patient. (Table 60.3.)**

13. **How can respiratory patterns help in the assessment of the comatose patient?**
Respiratory patterns and rate are often helpful in localizing structural causes of coma. Fig. 60.3 illustrates the various breathing patterns that might be seen depending on the location of the brain injury.

---

[a]Occlusion of the basilar artery may cause coma by infarction of the arousal system located in the pontomesencephalic tegmentum. If this is suspected, a CT angiogram may be useful in establishing the diagnosis.

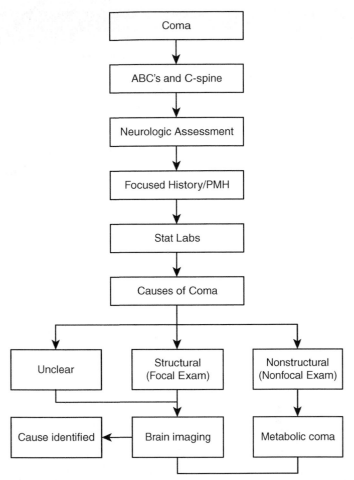

Figure 60-2. Emergency Neurologic Life Support (ENLS) protocol for initial evaluation. The ENLS committee recommends completing this algorithm within the first hour of evaluating a patient with coma. *ABC, airway, breathing, circulation; PMH, past medical history. (Reproduced with permission from Stevens RD, Cadena RS, Pineda J. Emergency neurologic life support: approach to the patient with coma.* Neurocrit Care. *2015;S2:69.)*

14. **What steps should be taken after the initial work-up and stabilization of the comatose patient?**
    - The comatose patient should be admitted to a specialized critical care unit for supportive care and to maximize the chance of recovery.
    - Cardiorespiratory support should be maintained as appropriate with attention to maintenance of cerebral oxygenation. Care should be taken for prevention of ventilator-associated pneumonia.
    - Electrolytes should be monitored closely and replaced as required. Early initiation of full enteral nutrition should be initiated whenever possible.
    - Other essential steps in the care of the comatose patient include measures to reduce the risk of infections, gastric ulcer prevention, thromboembolism prevention, physical therapy, splinting where appropriate, and skin care for pressure ulcer prevention.
    - Early tracheostomy may be considered if prolonged mechanical ventilation is deemed necessary.

Table 60-3. Etiologies of Coma

STRUCTURAL	TOXIC-METABOLIC
Trauma Subdural hematoma Epidural hematoma Parenchymal hemorrhage Diffuse axonal injury	Metabolic Encephalopathies Hypoglycemia Hypoxia/hyercapnia Diabetic ketoacidosis; hyperosmolar nonketotic hyperglycemia Hepatic encephalopathy Uremia Hyponatremia or hypernatremia Myxedema; thyrotoxicosis Adrenal failure Hypercalcemia Wernicke disease Sepsis
Neurovascular Intracerebral hemorrhage Subarachnoid hemorrhage Ischemic stroke	Drug/Medication Overdose Drugs of abuse (opioids, alcohol, methanol, ethylene glycol, amphetamines, cocaine) Sedative-hypnotics Narcotics Aspirin Acetaminophen SSRI Tricyclic antidepressants Antipsychotics Anticonvulsants
CNS infection Meningitis Encephalitis Abscess	Environmental Causes Heat stroke Hypothermia Carbon monoxide
Neuroinflammatory Disorders Acute disseminated encephalomyelitis Autoimmune encephalitis	
Neoplasms Metastatic Primary CNS Carcinomatous meningitis	
Seizures Nonconvulsive status epilepticus Postictal state	
Other PRES Osmotic demyelination syndrome Anoxic-ischemic encephalopathy	

CNS, Central nervous system; PRES, Posterior reversible encephalopathy syndrome; SSRI, selective serotonin reuptake inhibitors.
Modified with permission from Stevens RD, Cadena RS, Pineda J. Emergency neurological life support: approach to the patient with coma. *Neurocrit Care* S2:69, 2015.

15. Describe the natural history and prognosis of coma, persistent vegetative state, and minimally conscious state.

    The prognosis of coma is dependent on the underlying cause and other comorbidities. Metabolic and toxic disturbances can often be fully reversed and have, therefore, generally a better prognosis. Coma after traumatic brain injury (TBI) also has a better outcome than after anoxic brain injury. Coma often

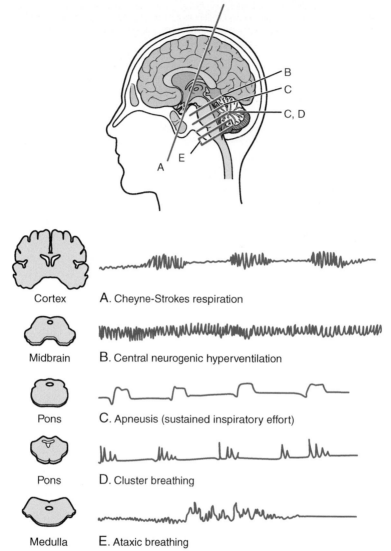

Figure 60-3. Respiratory patterns associated with structural lesions at various levels of the brain. *(Modified with permission from Frontera JA. Management of elevated intracranial pressure. In Decision Making in Neurocritical Care. 2009, Thieme. Chapter 15, Figure 15.4, p. 200.)*

evolves into PVS within a few weeks, but patients may remain in coma, PVS, or MCS permanently. The chance of meaningful recovery is minimal if PVS lasts more than 12 months after TBI, or more than 3 months in other cases. Typically, life expectancy is 2 to 5 years, but patients with MCS, particularly those who had TBI, have a better survival rate and an improved chance of functional recovery.

16. Can ancillary tests such as electroencephalography and magnetic resonance imaging be used as a prognostic tool?
No single test can fully prognosticate outcomes. Electroencephalography (EEG) patterns at 12 and 72 hours can be helpful in differentiating good versus poor outcomes. Magnetic resonance imaging (MRI)

injuries of the corpus callosum and dorsolateral brainstem are associated with poor recovery, but these patterns should be interpreted with caution in TBI patients. Functional MRI has demonstrated regions of preserved brain function and willful modulation of brain activity in some patients with PVS and MCS. The clinical significance of these findings has yet to be determined.

ACKNOWLEDGMENT

The authors wish to acknowledge Dr. Lee H. Schwamm, MD, FAHA, for the valuable contributions to the previous edition of this chapter.

KEY POINTS: COMA

1. Coma can be caused by a wide range of etiologies including: structural injury of the ARAS, metabolic and endocrine derangements, and pathophysiologic brain states.
2. After adequate oxygenation and circulation are ensured, it is important to identify the cause of coma and rapidly employ measures to correct potentially reversible conditions.
3. If the cause of coma is unknown, thiamine and dextrose should be administered early, and reversal of opioids, benzodiazepines, and neurotoxins should be considered. Infections, metabolic derangements, and structural injuries should be ruled out.

BIBLIOGRAPHY

1. Buettner UW, Zee DS. Vestibular testing in comatose patients. *Arch Neurol.* 1989;46:561-563.
2. Giacino JT, Ashwal S, Childs N, et al. The minimally conscious state: definition and diagnostic criteria. *Neurology.* 2002;58:349-353.
3. Giacino JT, Kalmar K. Diagnostic and prognostic guidelines for the vegetative and minimally conscious states. *Neuropsychol Rehabil.* 2005;15:166-174.
4. Giacino JT, Kalmar K. The vegetative and minimally conscious states: a comparison of clinical features and functional outcome. *J Head Trauma Rehabil.* 1997;12(4):36-51.
5. Hofmeijer J, Beernink TM, Bosch FH, et al. Early EEG contributes to multimodal outcome prediction of postanoxic coma. *Neurology.* 2015;85:137.
6. Levy DE, Caronna JJ, Singer BH, et al. Predicting outcome from hypoxic-ischemic coma. *JAMA.* 1985;253:1420-1426.
7. Liao YJ, So YT. An approach to critically ill patients in coma. *West J Med.* 2002;176:184-187.
8. Mercer WN, Childs NL. Coma, vegetative state, and the minimally conscious state: diagnosis and management. *Neurologist.* 1999;5:186-194.
9. Posner JB, Saper CB, Schiff N, et al. *Plum and Posner's Diagnosis of Stupor and Coma.* New York: Oxford University Press; 2007.
10. Ropper AH. Lateral displacement of the brain and level of consciousness in patients with an acute hemispheral mass. *N Engl J Med.* 1986;314:953-958.
11. Simeral JD, Kim SP, Black MJ, et al. Neural control of cursor trajectory and click by a human with tetraplegia 1000 days after implant of an intracortical microelectrode array. *J Neural Eng.* 2011;8(2):025027.
12. Stevens RD, Cadena RS, Pineda J. Emergency Neurological Life Support: Approach to the patient with coma. *Neurocrit Care.* 2015;(23 suppl 2):S69-S75.
13. Torbey MT. *Neurocritical Care.* 1st ed. New York: Cambridge University Press; 2010:227-241.
14. Wijdicks EF, Bamlet WR, Maramattom BV, et al. Validation of a new coma scale: the FOUR score. *Ann Neurol.* 2005; 58:585-593.
15. Wilson SL. Magnetic-resonance imaging and prediction of recovery from post-traumatic vegetative state. *Lancet.* 1998;352:485.
16. Zandbergen EG, de Haan RJ, Stoutenbeek CP, et al. Systematic review of early prediction of poor outcome in anoxic-ischaemic coma. *Lancet.* 1998;352:1808-1812.

CHAPTER 61

BRAIN DEATH

Jennifer Nelli, Ala Nozari, and Corey R. Fehnel

1. **What is brain death?**
   The Uniform Determination of Death Act (UDDA) has been adopted as law in most U.S. states. It defines as dead an individual who has sustained either:
   1. Irreversible cessation of circulatory and respiratory functions
   2. Irreversible cessation of all functions of the entire brain, including the brain stem
      A determination of death must be made with "accepted medical standards." The American Academy of Neurology (AAN) practice parameter for determining brain death in adults set forth "accepted medical standards" left open by the UDDA in 1995. In adults, there are no published reports of recovery of neurologic function after a diagnosis of brain death using the criteria presented in the 1995 AAN practice parameter. Brain death should be a diagnostic entity and never used as a prognostic statement about poor chances of recovery.

2. **When should the diagnosis of brain death be considered?**
   Active debate continues regarding minimum time of observation before determining brain death. The diagnosis is rarely, if ever, considered before the first 6 to 24 hours after injury. A variety of toxic and metabolic derangements associated with the onset of critical illness make brain and brainstem function difficult to assess in the hyperacute setting. Patients being considered for brain death uniformly have endotracheal tubes in place and are receiving mechanical ventilation. Sedatives, narcotics, and paralytics used for intubation must be allowed several half-lives of elimination. Pharmacokinetics are often prolonged in patients with multiorgan dysfunction who make up many of these patients.

3. **Who can perform a brain death examination?**
   Most states in the United States allow any physician to determine brain death. More recently, the majority of brain death determination has been done by neurologists, neurosurgeons, and intensive care specialists, as they may have specialized expertise. Brain death statutes vary by states within the United States, and certain hospital guidelines may require examiners to have specific expertise. Given the complexity of the examination, the examiner should have extensive experience with the brain death examination and full understanding of accepted standards.

4. **What prerequisites must be met before performing a brain death examination?**
   These are defined in Box 61.1.

5. **What findings should be present on brain death examination?**
   These are defined in Box 61.2.

Box 61-1. Prerequisites To Be Met Before Performing a Brain Death Examination

- Coma, irreversible and cause known.
- Neuroimaging explains coma.
- CNS depressant drug effect absent (if indicated, perform toxicology screen; if barbiturates given, serum level should be <10 mcg/mL).
- No evidence of residual paralytics (verify by electrical nerve stimulation if paralytics used).
- Absence of severe acid–base, electrolyte, endocrine abnormality.
- Normothermia or mild hypothermia (core temperature >36°C).
- Systolic blood pressure ≥100 mm Hg (with or without vasopressors).
- No spontaneous respirations.

CNS, Central nervous system.

Box 61-2. Key Findings on Brain Death Examination

- Pupils nonreactive to bright light, corneal reflex absent bilaterally.
- Oculocephalic reflex absent (test only if C-spine *cleared*).
- Vestibulo-ocular reflex absent (cold-water caloric testing).
- No facial movement to noxious stimuli at supraorbital ridge or temporomandibular joints.
- Gag reflex absent.
- Cough reflex absent to deep tracheal suctioning.
- Absence of motor response to noxious stimuli in all four limbs (spinally mediated reflexes are permissible; see Question 7).
- Apnea testing (see Question 9).

6. Can a patient make movements and still meet criteria for brain death?
   Yes. Spinally mediated reflexes and automatisms can be present in the setting of brain death. These movements are often misinterpreted by laypersons as signs of purposeful brain function. Careful neurologic examination can differentiate between reflexive movements and purposeful motor movements.

7. What are the common spinally generated movements?
   These are nonpurposeful movements *released* by lack of descending inhibition of primitive spinal motor reflex pathways. Deep tendon reflexes, abdominal reflexes, triple flexion or limb posturing are common spinally generated movements that may be present in patients meeting criteria for brain death.

8. What other movements may exist in brain-dead patients?
   Rare reports exist of facial myokymia, transient bilateral finger tremor, repetitive leg movements, ocular microtremor, and cyclic constriction and dilatation in light-fixed pupils. Many patients may retain plantar reflexes, either flexion or transient stimulation-induced toe flexion.

9. How do you perform apnea testing?
   Brain-dead patients must demonstrate an absence of respiratory drive. This is defined by an increase in $PaCO_2$ and no discernible respiration. Prerequisites for apnea testing include the following:
   - Normal blood pressure (systolic blood pressure >100 mm Hg)
   - Normothermia
   - Euvolemia
   - Eucapnia ($PaCO_2$ 35–45 mm Hg) and no prior evidence of CO_2 retention (i.e., chronic obstructive pulmonary disease, severe obesity)
   - Absence of hypoxia
     See Box 61.3.

10. Can brain-dead patients falsely trigger delivery of breaths on ventilators?
    Yes. Numerous case reports exist of ventilator autocycling in patients who in fact have no respiratory drive. Pressure-triggered ventilation in pressure support modes can be seen with endotracheal tube cuff leak and bronchopleural fistula. Flow-triggered ventilators can be initiated by cardiogenic oscillations. These potential confounders may be accounted for by switching between flow and pressure triggered ventilator modes. In patients who meet all brain death clinical criteria, yet continue to ventilate beyond the set ventilator rate, or breathe spontaneously, the patient should be closely observed off the ventilator circuit for evidence of spontaneous breathing. If no spontaneous breathing is present, then formal apnea testing may proceed as described above.

11. Is there a single ancillary test that can replace clinical diagnosis of brain death?
    No. Brain death remains a clinical diagnosis, and no ancillary test can replace a clinical determination of brain death. However, situations occur where the full brain death examination is not possible (e.g., apnea testing due to hemodynamic instability, severe facial trauma, prolonged sedative exposure). In these situations, *one* additional test may help to confirm the diagnosis. Ordering multiple ancillary tests is not advisable. No data support superiority of one test over another. Multiple tests increase the odds of indeterminate or false-positive results due to artifact.

12. What ancillary tests can help with diagnosing brain death?
    Testing can be divided into either cerebral arterial anatomic or flow studies versus studies of brain electrical activity. Common ancillary tests include cerebral angiography, transcranial Doppler ultrasonography, cerebral scintigraphy (technetium Tc 99m hexametazime), electroencephalography (EEG), and evoked potentials. See Box 61.4.

Box 61-3. Procedures for Apnea Testing

- Preoxygenate for at least 10 min with 100% oxygen to a PaO_2 >200 mm Hg.
- Reduce ventilation frequency to 10 breaths per minute to eucapnia.
- Reduce positive end-expiratory pressure (PEEP) to 5 cm H_2O (oxygen desaturation with decreasing PEEP may suggest difficulty with apnea testing).
- If pulse oximetry oxygen saturation remains >95%, obtain a baseline blood gas level (PaO_2, $PaCO_2$, pH, bicarbonate, base excess).
- Disconnect the patient from the ventilator.
- Preserve oxygenation (e.g., place an insufflation catheter through the endotracheal tube and close to the level of the carina and deliver 100% O_2 at 6 L/min).
- Look closely for respiratory movements for 8 to 10 min. Respiration is defined as abdominal or chest excursions and may include a brief gasp.
- Abort if systolic blood pressure decreases to <90 mm Hg.
- Abort if oxygen saturation measured by pulse oximetry is <85% for >30 s.
- Retry procedure with T-piece, continuous positive airway pressure 10 cm H_2O, and 100% O_2 12 L/min.
- If no respiratory drive is observed, repeat blood gas analysis (PaO_2, $PaCO_2$, pH, bicarbonate, base excess) after approximately 8 min. If there is any reason to abort the test because of instability of the patient's condition, draw an arterial blood gas sample immediately before reconnecting the ventilator.
- If respiratory movements are absent and arterial $PaCO_2$ is ≥60 mm Hg (or 20 mm Hg increase in arterial PCO_2 over a baseline normal arterial PCO_2), the apnea test result is positive (i.e., supports the clinical diagnosis of brain death).
- If the test is inconclusive but the patient is hemodynamically stable during the procedure, it may be repeated for a longer period of time (10–15 min) after the patient is again adequately preoxygenated.

Box 61-4. Ancillary Testing for the Determination of Brain Death

Cerebral Scintigraphy (Technetium Tc 99 m Hexametazime [HMPAO]):

- A noninvasive and safe measure of cerebral blood flow. Sodium pertechnetate technetium 99 m (15–21 mCi per adult) is given by intravenous bolus. A gamma camera then obtains anterior images every 3 s for a total of 60 s. External carotid flow is either digitally subtracted or excluded by forehead tourniquet. The isotope should be injected within 30 min of its reconstitution. Anterior and lateral planar image counts of the head should be obtained immediately, at 30–60 min, and then at 2 h. A positive scan reveals no radionuclide localization in the middle cerebral artery, anterior cerebral artery, or basilar artery territories of the cerebral hemispheres (hollow skull phenomenon).

Conventional Cerebral Angiography:

- Contrast medium is injected in the aortic arch under high pressure to reach both anterior and posterior circulations. A confirmatory test reveals absence of intracerebral filling beyond the carotid or vertebral arteries' entry to the skull. Patent external carotid (extracranial) circulation should be demonstrated.

Transcranial Doppler:

- Useful only if a reliable waveform is found. Abnormalities should include either reverberating flow or small systolic peaks in early systole. Complete absence of flow may not be reliable if inadequate insonation windows exist. All traditional cranial windows should be evaluated for flow. The orbital window can be considered to obtain a reliable signal. Prior craniotomy can complicate the study.

Electroencephalography (EEG):

- A positive EEG for brain death reveals a lack of reactivity to intense somatosensory or audiovisual stimuli. Isoelectric EEG or the finding of electrocerebral silence may be mimicked by conditions such as hypothermia, systemic hypotension, barbiturates, or other depressants. Hence, the patient should meet the same physiologic and hemodynamic standards during EEG as would be required during the brain death clinical examination.

Somatosensory-evoked Potential:

- A peripheral stimulus is given, typically at the median nerve, and a response is measured at the contralateral primary sensory cortex. Absence of transmission measured 20 ms (N20 response) after stimulation suggests brainstem dysfunction.

Brainstem Auditory Evoked Response:

- May be useful in evaluating patients in whom coma of toxic etiology is suspected (i.e., barbiturate coma). Brainstem and auditory short-latency responses that are absent in brain death but preserved in toxic and metabolic disorders can make this a useful test.

13. Are any blood tests helpful in establishing brain death?
No. Neuron-specific enolase and the glial protein S100 are the most studied. Neither marker is used for brain death determination. Clinical examination remains paramount. In cases where brain death is not being considered, serum markers may aid in determining prognosis after hypoxic ischemic injury.

14. What neuroimaging should be ordered to confirm brain death?
There is no requirement for a particular neuroimaging modality to diagnose brain death. However, a structural cause by brain imaging must be established as prerequisite for brain death diagnosis. Hence, computed tomography or magnetic resonance imaging of the head must be consistent with the diagnosis of brain death.

15. How many examinations are required to pronounce a patient brain dead?
Individual states have different guidelines and standards. Many states require only one full brain death examination. In states that require a second independent examination, organ donation rates may be adversely affected without any cases of incorrect brain death diagnoses being discovered.

ACKNOWLEDGMENT

The authors wish to acknowledge Dr. Lee H. Schwamm, MD, FAHA, for the valuable contributions to the previous edition of this chapter.

KEY POINTS: BRAIN DEATH

1. Brain death is the irreversible loss of both brain and brainstem function from a known cause.
2. Brain death is rarely determined before 6 to 24 hours from neurologic injury.
3. The brain death examination should be performed by an experienced and knowledgeable physician.
4. It is not uncommon for brain-dead patients to make spinally mediated reflexive movements that are not indicative of preserved brain function. Families should be educated about this.
5. Brain death is a clinical diagnosis.
6. Ancillary tests may be helpful in confirming brain death, but are not necessary or sufficient to make the diagnosis.

BIBLIOGRAPHY

1. Wijdicks EF, Varelas PN, Gronseth GS, et al. Evidence-based guideline update: determining brain death in adults: report of the Quality Standard Subcommittee of the American Academy of Neurology. *Neurology.* 2010;74:1911-1918.
2. Rosenberg JH, Alter M, Byrne TN, et al. Practice parameters for determining brain death in adults (summary statement): report of the Quality Standards Subcommittee of the American Academy of Neurology. *Neurology.* 1995;45:1012-1014.
3. Wijdicks EF, Rabinstein AA, Manno EH, et al. Pronouncing brain death: contemporary practice and safety of the apnea test. *Neurology.* 2008;71(16):1240-1244.
4. McGee WT, Mailloux P. Ventilator autocycling and delayed recognition of brain death. *Neurocrit Care.* 2011;14:267-271.
5. Imanaka H, Nishimura M, Takeuchi M, et al. Autotriggering caused by cardiogenic oscillation during flow-triggered mechanical ventilation. *Crit Care Med.* 2000;28:402-407.
6. Greer DM, Varelas PN, Haque S, et al. Variability of brain death determination guidelines in leading US neurologic institutions. *Neurology.* 2008;70:284-289.
7. Lustbader D, O'Hara D, Wijdicks EF, et al. Second brain death examination may negatively affect organ donation. *Neurology.* 2011; 76:119-124.
8. Stecker MM, Sabau D, Sullivan L, et al. American clinical neurophysiology society guideline 6: minimum technical standards for EEG recording in suspected cerebral death. *J Clin Neurophysiol.* August 2016;33(4):324-327.

CHAPTER 62

STATUS EPILEPTICUS

Jennifer Nelli, Corey Fehnel, and Ala Nozari

1. **What is the definition of status epilepticus?**

   The International League Against Epilepsy Commission on Classification and Terminology proposed a new definition of status epilepticus (SE) in 2015. They define SE as "a condition resulting either from the failure of the mechanisms responsible for seizure termination or from the initiation of mechanisms, which lead to abnormally, prolonged seizures." In this new definition, there are two operational time points for SE: T1, which occurs at 5 minutes, and T2, which occurs at 30 min. If the seizure exceeds T1, it should be considered continuous; if the seizure surpasses T2, there is a risk of lasting injury.

2. **What are the main causes of status epilepticus?**

   SE is often symptomatic of an underlying infectious or structural brain lesion, toxic or metabolic derangements, or low serum concentration of antiepileptic drugs (AED). Identification and treatment of the underlying disorder is therefore critical. Relapse of seizure in patients with known seizure disorder usually responds to a bolus of the maintenance drug. In younger patients, febrile illnesses are a common cause of seizures. Central nervous system (CNS) infections should be ruled out by performing a lumbar puncture.

3. **Describe the classification and clinical presentation of status epilepticus.**

   SE can be classified based on the presence or absence of prominent motor symptoms and the degree of impaired consciousness.

   1) Convulsive status epilepticus-repeated generalized tonic–clonic (GTC) seizures and postictal neurologic function between seizures.

   2) Nonconvulsive status epilepticus (NCSE) – continuous or fluctuating electrographic seizures without any motor manifestations lasting more than 5 minutes. Clinically, nonspecific signs such as altered mental status (including inattention), repetitive speech, impaired short-term memory, subtle eye movements, blinking and facial myokymia may be seen. Due to the subtle clinical features, EEG monitoring is essential for diagnosis.

   3) Focal motor or sensory status (a.k.a. epilepsia partialis continua) – repeated partial motor or sensory signs or symptoms of seizure not associated with altered consciousness or awareness.

4. **Why is treatment of status epilepticus a medical emergency?**

   Prolonged SE can lead to the development of pyrexia, deepening coma, and circulatory collapse. Aspiration is common and may result in respiratory failure with hypoxemia, systemic inflammatory response, and disseminated intravascular coagulation with multiple organ failure. Continuous seizures can result in rhabdomyolysis with risk for acute renal failure, lactic acidosis, and cardiac arrhythmias. Repetitive electric discharges can result in irreversible neuronal injury after as little as 5 to 20 minutes; cell death is common after 60 minutes. The highest mortality occurs in elderly patients and those with SE after a stroke or anoxia, whereas prognosis is more favorable among patients with prior history of epilepsy.

5. **Name general treatment measures for status epilepticus.**

   Initial interventions should focus on stabilizing the patient, including measures to establish an airway, provide oxygenation, and stabilize circulation. The seizure should be timed from its onset and vital signs should be monitored regularly. Supplemental oxygen should be provided, and intubation should be considered if respiratory assistance is needed. EEG monitoring should also be initiated. A finger stick blood glucose should be performed and IV access should be established to collect electrolytes, hematology, toxicology, and if appropriate, anticonvulsant drug levels. If glucose testing reveals a glucose less than 60 mg/dL, then adult patients should be given 100 mg of thiamine followed by 50 mL of 50% dextrose solution (D50W) IV.

6. **What are the first-line treatment options for generalized convulsive status epilepticus?**

   A benzodiazepine is the initial treatment of choice. If the seizure has not terminated on its own after 5 minutes, 0.1 mg/kg of IV lorazepam can be given at a rate no faster than 2 mg/min and in 4 mg doses to a maximal adult dose of 10 mg. If lorazepam is not available, a dose of 0.15 to 0.2 mg/kg of

IV diazepam may also be given to a max of 10 mg/dose; this may be repeated once more. If IV access has not been established, intramuscular midazolam may be administered at a dose of 10 mg for all patients weighing more than 40 kg.

7. What are the second-line treatments for SE?

Second-line therapy should begin when first-line therapy has been unsuccessful and seizure duration reaches 20 minutes. Historically, a phenytoin load with 18 to 20 mg/kg has been the standard treatment for SE when initial benzodiazepines have failed. Other drugs, such as fosphenytoin, valproate, and levetiracetam are used as possible alternatives. So far there is no clear evidence that any one of these options is superior. Studies are currently being conducted in an attempt to answer this question.

8. What are the third-line treatments for status epilepticus?

Again, there is no clear evidence to guide third-line therapy in SE. Only 7% of patients who have not responded to the above treatment will respond to a third-line drug. Therefore, if second-line therapy does not terminate the seizure activity, treatment should include repeating second-line therapies. Additional doses of 5 mg/kg phenytoin can be administered up to a total of 30 mg/kg. Alternatively, anesthetic doses of thiopental, midazolam, pentobarbital, or propofol may be administered. This should be done with continuous EEG monitoring. These treatments may result in respiratory depression and consideration should be given to inserting an endotracheal tube prior to beginning continuous therapy. Additionally, these drugs may be associated with hemodynamic changes and vasopressors may be required to support adequate blood pressure (Table 62.1).

Table 62-1. Drugs That Are Typically Used in the Treatment of Status Epilepticus

DRUG	LOADING DOSE	RATE OF ADMINISTRATION	MAINTENANCE DOSE	IMPORTANT ADVERSE EFFECTS
Diazepam	10–20 mg	Push	None	Hypotension, respiratory depression, sialorrhea
Lorazepam	4–8 mg	2 mg/min	None	Hypotension, respiratory depression, sialorrhea
Midazolam	0.2 mg/kg	0.4 mg/kg/h	0.75–10 mcg/kg/min	Hypotension, respiratory depression, metabolic acidosis
Phenytoin	18–20 mg/kg	50 mg/min	Additional doses of 5 mg/kg up to 30 mg/kg	Cardiac depression, arrhythmias, hypotension, Stevens-Johnson syndrome
Fosphenytoin	18–20 mg/kg Phenytoin equivalent	150 mg/min	IV bolus one-third of previous dose	Arrhythmias less frequent than with phenytoin
Phenobarbital	15–20 mg/kg	30–50 mg/min	1–4 mg/kg/day	Myocardial and respiratory depression, prolonged sedation
Pentobarbital	3 mg/kg	1–3 mg/kg/h	0.3–3 mg/kg/h	Myocardial and respiratory depression, prolonged sedation
Valproate	15–30 mg/kg	1.5–3 mg/kg/min	40 mg/kg/day in divided doses	Thrombocytopenia, hyperammonemia and hepatic toxicity, pancreatitis
Propofol	1–3 mg/kg	1–10 mg/kg/h	1–3 mg/kg/h	Hypotension, respiratory depression, hyperlipidemia, propofol infusion syndrome
Levetiracetam	20 mg/kg	Over 15 min	1500 mg twice daily	Psychosis and hallucination

9. Describe the management of seizures in patients with pre-eclampsia.
Magnesium sulfate remains the standard therapy in the prevention and treatment of eclampsia or SE. A loading dose of 4 g should be given followed by an infusion of 1 g/h for the next 24 hours with the aim to reach a therapeutic level of 3.5 to 7 mEq/L. Recurrent seizures should be treated with an additional bolus of 2 to 4 g over 5 minutes. Patients being treated with magnesium should be monitored for toxicity, including loss of patellar reflex and respiratory depression. Any evidence of toxicity should result in prompt discontinuation of the infusion. The most effective treatment of seizures related to eclampsia remains delivery of the fetus.

10. Describe the pathogenesis and treatment of postanoxic myoclonic status epilepticus.
Postanoxic myoclonus status is the occurrence of synchronous brief jerking in the limbs, face, or diaphragm that is correlated with epileptiform activity on EEG. It is typically encountered in comatose patients who have survived asphyxia or suffered a cardiac arrest. It typically indicates severe neurologic damage and portends a very poor prognosis. Myoclonic SE often consists of synchronous brief jerking in the limbs, face, or diaphragm and can be provoked by stimuli such as movement, touch, or sound. Myoclonic status typically is resistant to antiseizure medications, including phenbobarbital, phenytoin, and benzodiazepines. Some anecdotal evidence suggests that valproate may be effective in treating this syndrome.

11. What general measures should be considered after the seizure has been controlled?
It is important to establish the cause of the seizure once it is controlled and the patient's condition stabilized. Appropriate blood work and cultures should be completed. Lumbar puncture should be considered, if not already done, to rule out CNS infections and subarachnoid hemorrhage, and imaging with computed tomography or magnetic resonance imaging should be obtained to rule out structural CNS causes. Empirical antibiotics should be started if an infectious cause is suspected, and maintenance doses of anticonvulsants should be administered and adjusted on the basis of serum levels.

ACKNOWLEDGMENT

The authors wish to acknowledge Dr. Lee H. Schwamm, MD, FAHA, for the valuable contributions to the previous edition of this chapter.

KEY POINTS: STATUS EPILEPTICUS

1. SE has been defined as seizures lasting ≥5 minutes or recurrent seizure activity between which there is incomplete recovery of consciousness or function.
2. The most common cause of SE in a patient with known seizure disorder is low AED levels, whereas de novo SE is usually a manifestation of structural brain injury. Febrile seizures are the most common cause of seizures in children.
3. NCSE is difficult to diagnose due to lack of pronounced motor activity. Continuous EEG monitoring is essential for diagnosis.
4. Treatment for SE is directed at stabilizing the patient's condition, controlling the seizure, and identifying the cause. The underlying disease should be treated promptly.
5. Benzodiazepines are first-line therapy for the treatment of SE. Second-line therapy includes an antiepileptic drug (fosphenytoin, valproate, and levetiracetam). Third-line therapy includes repeating second-line therapies or administering anesthetic doses of thiopental, midazolam, pentobarbital, or propofol.

BIBLIOGRAPHY

1. Brophy GM, Bell R, Claassen J, et al. Guidelines for the evaluation and management of status epilepticus. *Neurocrit Care.* 2012;17(1):3-23.
2. Chen JW, Wasterlain CG. Status epilepticus: pathophysiology and management in adults. *Lancet Neurol.* 2006;5:246-256.
3. Trinka E, Cock H, Hesdorffer D, et al. A definition and classification of status epilepticus—Report of the ILAE Task Force on Classification of Status Epilepticus. *Epilepsia.* 2015;56(10):1515-1523.
4. Costello DJ, Cole AJ. Treatment of acute seizures and status epilepticus. *J Intensive Care Med.* 2007;22:319-347.
5. DeLorenzo RJ, Pellock JM, Towne AR, et al. Epidemiology of status epilepticus. *J Clin Neurophysiol.* 1995;12:316-325.
6. Fountain NB, Lothman EW. Pathophysiology of status epilepticus. *J Clin Neurophysiol.* 1995;12:326-342.

7. Huff JS, Fountain NB. Pathophysiology and definitions of seizures and status epilepticus. *Emerg Med Clin North Am.* 2011;29:1-13.
8. Kubota Y, Nakamoto H, Kawamata T. Nonconvulsive Status Epilepticus in the Neurosurgical Setting. *Neurol Med Chir (Tokyo).* 2016;56(10):626-631. doi:10.2176/nmc.ra.2016-0118.
9. Seinfeld S, Goodkin HP, Shinnar S. Status Epilepticus. *Cold Spring Harb Perspect Med.* 2016;6:a022830.
10. Falco-Walter JJ, Bleck T. Treatment of Established Status Epilepticus. *J Clin Med.* 2016; 5(5):E49.
11. Glauser T, Shinnar S, Gloss D, et al. Evidence-based guideline: treatment of convulsive status epilepticus in children and adults: report of the guideline committee of the american epilepsy society. *Epilepsy Curr.* 2016;16(1):48-61.
12. Silbergleit R, Durkalski V, Lowenstein D, et al, NETT Investigators. Intramuscular versus intravenous therapy for prehospital status epilepticus. *N Engl J Med.* 2012;366:591-600.
13. Bleck T, Cock H, Chamberlain J, et al. The Established Status Epilepticus Trial 2013. *Epilepsia.* 2013;(54 suppl 6):89-92.
14. Pritchard JA. The use of the magnesium ion in the management of eclamptogenic toxemias. *Surg Gynecol Obstet.* 1955;100:131-140.
15. Aya AG, Ondze B, Ripart J, et al. Seizures in the peripartum period: Epidemiology, diagnosis and management. *Anaesth Crit Care Pain Med.* 2016;(35 suppl 1):S13-S21.
16. Lucas MJ, Leveno KJ, Cunningham FG. A comparison of magnesium sulfate with phenytoin for the prevention of eclampsia. *N Engl J Med.* 1995;333:201-205.
17. Braksick SA, Rabinstein AA, Wijdicks EF, et al. Post-ischemic myoclonic status following cardiac arrest in young drug users. *Neurocrit Care.* 2016;26(2):280-283. doi:10.1007/s12028-016-0317-z.
18. Wijdicks EF, Parisi JE, Sharbrough FW. Prognostic value of myoclonus status in comatose survivors of cardiac arrest. *Ann Neurol.* 1994;35:239-243.
19. Bleck TP. Intensive care unit management of patients with status epilepticus. *Epilepsia.* 2007;(48 suppl 8):59-60.

CHAPTER 63

STROKE AND SUBARACHNOID HEMORRHAGE

Jennifer Nelli, Ala Nozari, and Corey R. Fehnel

1. **What is the definition of stroke?**
   Stroke is a sudden, focal neurologic syndrome due to cerebrovascular ischemia. Strokes are sudden, or apoplectic, by definition. A slow progression of neurologic symptoms should make the clinician consider alternative diagnoses. Stroke can be categorized as:
   - Ischemic stroke due to arterial occlusion
   - Hemorrhagic stroke (intracerebral or subarachnoid) due to vessel rupture

2. **What is the definition of subarachnoid hemorrhage?**
   Subarachnoid hemorrhage (SAH) is defined as bleeding into the subarachnoid space. Among the broadest classification of "stroke," it is the least common category.
   - Presents as a sudden-onset thunderclap headache and is typically described as "the worst headache of my life."
   - Other symptoms may include nausea, loss of consciousness, or focal neurologic deficits.
   - A relatively minor subgroup of patients will present with a sentinel headache prior to their SAH.

3. **What are the major types of ischemic strokes?**
   Table 63.1 and Box 63.1.

4. **What are the subtypes of primary hemorrhagic strokes?**
   Primary intracerebral hemorrhage (ICH) may be classified according to cause or location. Hypertensive hemorrhages more commonly involve deep brain structures because of the location of small arteries arising from large main trunk vessels that are most prone to hypertensive injury over time. Specific locations from most common to less common are the caudate, thalamus, pons, and cerebellum. Hemorrhages due to deposition of amyloid protein in the arterial wall, known as amyloid angiopathy, are lobar in location and spare the deep tissues. Although less common, ruptured aneurysms may present as intraparenchymal hemorrhages with minimal or no subarachnoid blood, and computed tomography (CT) or traditional transfemoral angiography should be considered when the hematoma overlies the sylvian cistern.

Table 63-1. Major Ischemic Stroke Types

ISCHEMIC STROKE TYPE	DEFINING CHARACTERISTIC
Transient ischemic attacks (TIAs)	Brief episodes of neurologic dysfunction lasting <1 h resulting from focal cerebral ischemia not associated with permanent cerebral infarction.
Major arterial vessel territory infarctions	(see Box 63.1).
Lacunar infarction	Small perforating vessel occlusions classically "pure" motor or sensory and lack cortical findings such as alterations of consciousness or corticosensory modalities (i.e., graphesthesia, stereognosis).
Watershed syndrome	Results from infarction at border zones between major arterial territories as the result of brain or hemispheric hypoperfusion. Weakness is more severe proximally >distally.

Box 63-1. Artery Infarction Syndromes

Anterior Circulation Syndromes

Carotid Artery Occlusion: Often associated with transient monocular blindness (amaurosis fugax) due to ophthalmic artery involvement. Key symptoms are reflected by MCA involvement and include contralateral hemiparesis of the face and arm more than the leg, as well as loss of corticosensory modalities. If dominant hemisphere is involved, aphasia is present. Nondominant hemisphere results in neglect. If patient has poor collaterals, this occlusion may produce hemiplegia of face, arm, and leg with gaze deviation and decreased level of arousal.

MCA: Proximal occlusions result in contralateral hemiparesis of the face and arm more than the leg, as well as loss of corticosensory modalities. If complete proximal occlusion occurs, symptoms may resemble the carotid artery syndrome. If dominant hemisphere is involved, aphasia is present. Nondominant hemisphere results in neglect. The MCA has two major branches:

Superior division: Results in anterior or Broca-type aphasia with more prominent motor symptoms of hemiparesis. Nondominant superior division occlusions spare language, but result in anosognosia and aprosody of speech.

Inferior division: Results in posterior or Wernicke-type aphasia with more prominent deficit of language comprehension and contralateral visual field loss. Nondominant hemisphere inferior division occlusions result in neglect, poor visual-spatial constructions, and sometimes agitation.

Posterior Cerebral Artery (PCA): Most commonly results in contralateral hemianopia. Detailed review of other features, which depend on laterality of the brain, is outside the scope of this chapter. Readers are instead referred to the bibliography.

Anterior Cerebral Artery (ACA): Weakness of foot and leg more than arm or face.

Posterior Circulation Syndromes

Basilar Artery

Top of the basilar: These patients are somnolent with small, poorly reactive pupils and multiple gaze palsies. The condition is sometimes associated with involuntary movements of the extremities (basilar fits) that may resemble convulsions or hallucinations. Patients may have quadriparesis and become "locked in."

Pontine syndromes: Bilateral or crossed findings and gaze palsies (i.e., internuclear ophthalmoplegia) are key to localizing infarcts to the pons. These patients often have fluctuating symptoms in the early hours of the onset of symptoms.

Vertebral Artery

Lateral medullary syndrome (Wallenberg): Vertigo, nystagmus, ipsilateral facial sensory loss, pharyngeal paresis, and Horner syndrome (autonomic dysfunction). Contralateral loss of pain and temperature to body and limbs.

Medial medullary syndrome: Ipsilateral tongue paresis (rarely seen), contralateral hemiparesis, and posterior column dysfunction due to the medial lemniscus.

Cerebellar Artery

Posterior inferior cerebellar artery: Vertigo, veering to ipsilateral side, ipsilateral limb ataxia, headache, and vomiting. Superior cerebellar artery and anterior inferior cerebellar artery infarction rarely occur in isolation because of robust collaterals.

5. What are the major types of subarachnoid hemorrhage?
   SAH may be caused by either traumatic or nontraumatic bleeding into the subarachnoid space. The most common cause of SAH is trauma. The most common cause of nontraumatic SAH is rupture of intracerebral aneurysms, which account for approximately 85% of these bleeds. The remaining 15% are due to a variety of other etiologies, most commonly perimesencephalic hemorrhage, dural arteriovenous fistula, vasculopathy/vasculitis, and congenital malformations.

6. What are the major treatment options for acute ischemic stroke?
   The last time the patient was known to be at his or her baseline is key to all acute stroke interventions. The major treatment options for acute ischemic stroke are medical, interventional, or surgical.
   1. Medical:
      Level I evidence supports initial medical management with intravenous tissue plasminogen activator (IV tPA). Patients who present within 3 hours of symptom onset and meet criteria are candidates for thrombolytic therapy (Fig. 63.1). Patients presenting between 3 and 4.5 hours after symptom onset may be candidates for extended-window IV tPA (Box 63.2). Patients treated with IV tPA were at least 30% more likely to have minimal or no disability at 3 months compared with placebo. The major risk of IV tPA treatment remains ICH.

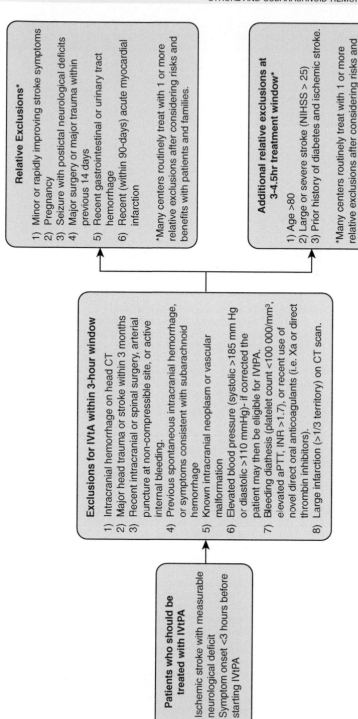

Figure 63-1. Inclusion and Exclusion Criteria for Patients with Ischemic Stroke who should be treated with IV tPA within 3 hours from symptom onset. *aPTT,* activated partial thromboplastin time; *BP,* Blood pressure; *CT,* computed tomography; *ECT,* ecarin clotting time; *IV tPA,* intravenous tissue plasminogen activator; *INR,* international normalized ratio; *PT,* prothrombin time; *TT,* thrombin time.

Box 63-2. Additional Exclusion Criteria for Extended-window Tissue Plasminogen Activator (Relative Exclusions at Many Stroke Centers)

- Age >80 years
- National Institute of Health Stroke Scale (NIHSS) score >25
- Taking an oral anticoagulant regardless of INR
- History of both diabetes and prior ischemic stroke

2. Endovascular:
   Thrombectomy is another treatment option for patients with large vessel proximal anterior circulation strokes. Among the subset of patients with proximal large vessel occlusions, time from last known well and favorable early CT score (ASPECTS score) determines eligibility. Patients successfully treated with endovascular therapy (generally within 7 hours of symptom onset) have dramatic reduction in disability at 3 months. Trials determining benefit of thrombectomy from use of imaging selection criteria are ongoing.

3. Surgical:
   Hemicraniectomy is a treatment option for patients presenting with very large territory strokes and risk for massive cerebral edema and herniation (so-called malignant middle cerebral artery [MCA] infarcts). Current data suggest a survival benefit from early decompressive surgery within 48 hours of stroke onset in persons under the age of 60 years. However, there is a risk of surviving with significant disability, especially in patients older than 60.

7. How should blood pressure (BP) be managed in acute ischemic stroke?
   Elevated BP is common during acute ischemic stroke. Extreme arterial hypertension is clearly detrimental, as it leads to encephalopathy, cardiac complications, and renal insufficiency. Current recommendations suggest not lowering the BP during the initial 24 hours of acute ischemic stroke unless the BP is greater than 220/120 mm Hg or there is a concomitant specific medical condition that would benefit from BP lowering. Patients being considered for fibrinolytic therapy should have their BP brought down to less than 185/110 mm Hg. Once intravenous rtPA is given, the blood pressure must be maintained below 180/105 mm Hg to limit the risk of ICH.

8. How should intracerebral hemorrhage be managed?
   1. Medical:
      Medical management is the mainstay of treatment with a focus on blood pressure control and rapid correction of coagulopathy if present. Current guidelines recommend that for patients with acute ICH presenting with an systolic blood pressure (SBP) between 150 and 220 mm Hg, without contraindication to acute BP treatment, acute lowering of SBP to 140 mm Hg is safe (class I evidence) and can be effective for improving functional outcome (class IIa evidence). For patients with SBP greater than 220 mm Hg, it may be reasonable to aggressively reduce BP with a continuous infusion and frequent BP monitoring (class IIb evidence). There is no data supporting the use of prophylactic antiepileptic drugs in spontaneous ICH. In fact, the early use of AEDs following acute ICH was strongly associated with severe disability and death. Continuous electroencephalogram (EEG) monitoring is probably indicated in ICH patients with decreased level of consciousness that is out of proportion to their injury.

   2. Surgical:
      Management of spontaneous supratentorial ICH remains controversial. However, cerebellar hemorrhages require emergent surgical decompression, which has been shown to provide durable benefit. Decompressive craniectomy with or without hematoma evacuation may provide a mortality benefit in patients with supratentorial ICH who are in a coma, have significant midline shift secondary to a large hematoma or have elevated ICP refractory to medical therapies.

9. What is the acute treatment of aneurysmal subarachnoid hemorrhage?
   Depending on the severity of the bleed, patients can present with a range of clinical symptoms (see Tables 63.2 and 63.3) which will affect their overall prognosis. SAH can lead to myocardial dysfunction, neurogenic pulmonary edema, and renal failure. Initial treatment should focus on providing emergency care and extraventricular drainage of CSF for acute hydrocephalus, if present. Once the patient is stabilized, the aneurysm should be secured by endovascular coiling or surgical clipping as quickly as possible to reduce the risk of rebleeding. Factors including the location of the aneurysm, its

Table 63-2. Hunt and Hess Classification

CATEGORY	CRITERIA
Grade 1	Asymptomatic, or minimal headache and slight nuchal rigidity
Grade 2	Moderate to severe headache, nuchal rigidity, no neurologic deficit other than cranial nerve palsy
Grade 3	Drowsiness, confusion, or mild focal deficit
Grade 4	Stupor, moderate to severe hemiparesis, possibly early decerebrate rigidity and vegetative disturbances
Grade 5	Deep coma, decerebrate rigidity, moribund appearance

From Hunt WE, Hess RM. Surgical risk as related to time of intervention in the repair of intracranial aneurysms. *J Neurosurg.* 1968;28:14–20.

Table 63-3. World Federation of Neurologic Surgeons Subarachnoid Hemorrhage Scale

WFNS GRADE	GCS SCORE	MOTOR DEFICIT
I	15	Absent
II	14–13	Absent
III	14–13	Present
IV	12–7	Present or absent
V	6–3	Present or absent

GCS, Glasgow Coma Scale; WFNS, World Federation of Neurosurgical Societies. Report of World Federation of Neurological Surgeons Committee on a universal subarachnoid hemorrhage grading scale. *J Neurosurg.* 1988;68:985–986.

morphology, and the patient's age may make endovascular coiling or surgical clipping preferable. All SAH patients are placed on oral nimodipine and undergo monitoring in the intensive care unit for delayed cerebral ischemia (vasospasm), which peaks at posthemorrhage day 4 and can last up to 14 days.

10. How should blood pressure be managed in aneurysmal SAH?
   BP should be strictly controlled until the aneurysm is secured. Parameters for blood pressure have not yet been defined; however, expert opinion suggests maintaining a systolic BP less than 140 mm Hg. Patients with secured aneurysms and signs of vasospasm should be allowed to autoregulate their BP to perfuse distal brain tissue.

ACKNOWLEDGMENT

The authors wish to acknowledge Dr. Lee H. Schwamm, MD, FAHA, for the valuable contributions to the previous edition of this chapter.

KEY POINTS: STROKE AND SUBARACHNOID HEMORRHAGE

Stroke
1. Ischemic stroke is a medical emergency where earlier treatment ("time is brain!") can dramatically improve functional outcome (current time limits are <4.5 hours for IV tPA and later for endovascular thrombectomy-eligible patients).
2. BP should *not* be treated in acute ischemic stroke unless it is greater than 220/110 mm Hg or SBP greater than 185/110 mm Hg if IV tPA is to be administered.
3. Cerebellar hemorrhages require emergent surgical decompression. Decompressive craniectomy may provide a mortality benefit in select patients with supratentorial ICH.
4. The classic presentation of SAH is a thunderclap headache. A minority of patients will present with sentinel headache preceding SAH.

BIBLIOGRAPHY

1. Jauch EC, Saver JL, Adams Jr HP, et al. Guidelines for the Early Management of Patients with acute Ischemic Stroke: a guideline for healthcare professionals from the American Heart Association/American Stroke Association. *Stroke.* 2013;44:870-947.
2. Yew KS, Cheng EM. Diagnosis of Acute Stroke. *Am Fam Physician.* 2015;91(8):528-536.
3. The National Institute of Neurological Disorders and Stroke rt-PA Stroke Study Group. Tissue plasminogen activator for acute ischemic stroke. *N Engl J Med.* 1995;333:1581-1587.
4. Hacke W, Kaste M, Bluhmki E, et al, for the European Cooperative Acute Stroke Study (ECASS) investigators. Thrombolysis with alteplase 3 to 4.5 hours after acute ischemic stroke. *N Engl J Med.* 2008;359:1317-1329.
5. Goyal M, Menon BK, van Zwam WH, et al. Endovascular thrombectomy after large vessel ischaemic stroke: a meta-analysis of individual patient data from five randomised trials. *Lancet.* 2016;387(10029):1723-1731.
6. Saver JL, Goyal M, van der Lugt A, et al. Time to treatment and outcomes from endovascular thrombectomy and outcomes from ischemic stroke: a meta-analysis. *JAMA.* 2016;316(12):1279-1288.
7. Broderick JP, Berkhemer OA, Palesch YY, et al. Endovascular Therapy is Effective and Safe for Patients with Severe Ischemic Stroke: Pooled Analysis of Interventional Management of Stroke III and Multicenter Randomized Clinical Trial of Endovascular Therapy for Acute Ischemic Stork in the Netherlands Data. *Stroke.* 2015;46(12):3416-3422.
8. Marler JR, Tilley BC, Lu M, et al. Early stroke treatment associated with better outcome: the NINDS rt-PA stroke study. *Neurology.* 2000;55:1649-1655.
9. Easton JD, Saver JL, Albers GW, et al. Definition and evaluation of transient ischemic attack: a scientific statement for healthcare professionals from the American Heart Association/American Stroke Association Stroke Council; Council on Cardiovascular Surgery and Anesthesia; Council on Cardiovascular Radiology and Intervention; Council on Cardiovascular Nursing; and the Interdisciplinary Council on Peripheral Vascular Disease. The American Academy of Neurology affirms the value of this statement as an educational tool for neurologists. *Stroke.* 2009;40:2276-2293.
10. Vahedi K, Hofmeijer J, Juettler E, et al. Early decompressive surgery in malignant infarction of the middle cerebral artery: a pooled analysis of three randomised controlled trials. *Lancet Neurol.* 2007;6:215-222.
11. Hankey GJ. Stroke. *Lancet.* 2016;389(10069):641-654. doi:10.1016/S0140-6736(16)30962-X.
12. Anderson CS, Huang Y, Wang JG, et al. Intensive blood pressure reduction in acute cerebral haemorrhage trial (INTERACT): a randomised pilot trial. *Lancet Neurol.* 2008;7(5):391-399.
13. Arima H, Huang Y, Wang JG, et al. Earlier blood pressure-lowering and greater attenuation of hematoma growth in acute intracerebral hemorrhage: INTERACT pilot phase. *Stroke.* 2012;43(8):2236-2238.
14. Hemphill JC 3rd, Greenberg SM, Anderson CS, et al. Guidelines for the management of spontaneous intracerebral hemorrhage: a guideline for healthcare professionals from the american heart association/american stroke association. *Stroke.* 2015;46(7):2032-2060.
15. Takeuchi S, Wada K, Nagatani K, et al. Decompressive hemicraniectomy for spontaneous intracerebral hemorrhage. *Neurosurg Focus.* 2013;34(5):E5.
16. Messé SR, Sansing LH, Cucchiara BL, et al, CHANT investigators. Prophylactic antiepileptic drug use is associated with poor outcome following ICH. *Neurocrit Care.* 2009;11(1):38-44.
17. Ropper AH, Samuels MA. Cerebrovascular diseases. In: *Adams and Victor's Principles of Neurology.* 9th ed. New York: McGraw-Hill; 2009:660-746.
18. Connelly Jr ES, Rabinstein AA, Carhuapoma JR, et al. Guidelines for the Management of Aneurysmal Subarachnoid Hemorrhage: a guideline for healthcare professionals from the American Heart Association/american Stroke Association. *Stroke.* 2012;43(6):1711-1737.
19. Macdonald RL, Schweizer TA. Spontaneous subarachnoid hemorrhage. *Lancet.* 2017;389(10069):655-666. doi:10.1016/S0140-6736(16)30668-7.
20. Hunt WE, Hess RM. Surgical risk as related to time of intervention in the repair of intracranial aneurysms. *J Neurosurg.* 1968;28:14-20.
21. Report of World Federation of Neurological Surgeons Committee on a universal subarachnoid hemorrhage grading scale. *J Neurosurg.* 1988;68:985-986.
22. Bogousslavsky J, Regli F. Unilateral watershed cerebral infarcts. *Neurology.* March 1986;36(3):373-377.

GUILLAIN-BARRÉ SYNDROME AND MYASTHENIA GRAVIS

Corey R. Fehnel and Ala Nozari

1. Name the key clinical distinctions between Gullian-Barré Syndrome and myasthenia gravis.
   Both conditions cause weakness. However, the pattern and associated signs with onset of symptoms are quite different, underscoring the distinct pathophysiology of the two conditions (Fig. 64.1).

2. What are the Guillain-Barré syndrome subtypes?
   There are numerous Guillain-Barré syndrome (GBS) subtypes: pure motor or motor-sensory variants, Miller Fisher variant, bulbar variant, and primary axonal GBS. Key distinctions relate to the peripheral nerves affected (for example, Miller Fisher variant preferentially affects cranial nerves). Symptom onset occurs over a range of a few days to 3 weeks.

3. What are the classic subtypes of myasthenia gravis?
   The disease is divided into ocular and generalized forms. Both forms can present similarly with extraocular, facial, and oropharyngeal muscle weakness presenting early in the course of the disease. The muscle weakness may present clinically as diplopia, ptosis, dysphagia, and hypophonia, respectively. The ocular form is restricted to the ocular muscles, whereas the generalized form may present initially with, and/or progress to, weakness of flexors and extensors of the neck and proximal muscles of the trunk.

4. Compare and contrast the pathophysiology of Guillain-Barré syndrome and myasthenia gravis.
   Both are autoimmune disorders (Table 64.1).

5. I am on call alone in the intensive care unit—how can I make the diagnosis of Guillain-Barré syndrome versus myasthenia gravis?
   Key clinical, laboratory, and diagnostic tests are as follows:
   - GBS presents with symmetric weakness, sensory dysesthesias, and hyporeflexia or areflexia. Mild cases may present with only mild weakness or as variants (e.g., ataxia, ophthalmoplegia, and hyporeflexia) without significant appendicular weakness. Fulminant cases may cause severe ascending weakness leading to complete tetraplegia with paralysis of cranial nerves and respiratory muscles (involvement of the phrenic and intercostal nerves).
   - **Perform a lumbar puncture**—Cerebrospinal fluid (CSF) analysis shows elevated protein level without pleocytosis (albuminocytologic dissociation). Elevated white blood cell count should make you consider alternative diagnoses.
   - **Order an electromyography (EMG)/NCS and consider an MRI**—Electromyogram and nerve conduction study results may be normal in the early acute period, but after 1 to 2 weeks reveal characteristic segmental demyelination and reduction of conduction velocity. Absence of F-waves may indicate early nerve root demyelination. In later stages, spine MRI may reveal diffuse enhancement of cauda equina and nerve roots.

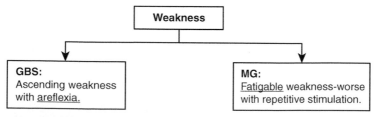

Figure 64-1. Clinical distinctions between Gullian-Barré syndrome (GBS) and myasthenia gravis (MG).

Table 64-1. Pathophysiology of Gullian-Barré Syndrome and Myasthenia Gravis

GBS	MG
Triggered by both humoral and cell-mediated autoimmune response with antibodies to gangliosides and glycolipids triggering *myelin disruption* in the peripheral nervous system. It is often preceded by an immune sensitizing event such as an upper respiratory tract infection or cytomegalovirus, herpes simplex virus, *Campylobacter jejuni,* or mycoplasma infections. A clear antecedent infection is, however, often difficult to identify.	A T-cell autoantibody against the *AChR* on the *postsynaptic* membrane. The antibodies produce a functional deficit of AChRs, as well as morphologic changes in the neuromuscular junction. Consequently, the effect of acetylcholine on the postsynaptic membrane is reduced, and the probability that a nerve impulse will result in a muscle action potential is reduced.

AChR, Acetylcholine receptor; GBS, Gullian-Barré syndrome; MG, myasthenia gravis.

- MG has the hallmark signs of fatigable muscle weakness and *no* sensory symptoms; often a history of better strength in the mornings that progressively worsens throughout the day can be elicited. Examination of sustained upgaze for greater than 30 seconds may reveal characteristic eyelid twitching, ptosis, or frank dysconjugate gaze and resultant diplopia. With ocular symptoms such as ptosis, an ice pack applied to the eyelid can speed synaptic transmission, which supports the diagnosis of MG. Edrophonium (Tensilon) is a very rapidly acting cholinesterase inhibitor and carries a small risk of heart block; a small test dose may be given in a monitored setting with access to external cardiac pacing pads.
- **EMG** is the current diagnostic test of choice in MG and reveals progressively smaller action potentials with repetitive nerve stimulation (decrement). Single-fiber EMG can be a more sensitive method, but requires great cooperation of the patient and is hence rarely employed for the patient in the intensive care unit (ICU).

6. Are serum autoantibodies to the acetylcholine receptor required for the diagnosis of myasthenia gravis?
No. Although they are often present and helpful, they are not required for the diagnosis. Acetylcholine receptor (AChR) antibodies are found in 80% to 90% of patients with generalized MG and 60% with ocular MG. Autoantibodies against the muscle-specific tyrosine kinase (MuSK) are found in 70% of patients with MG without AChR antibodies. Remaining patients without identified autoantibodies have what is termed *seronegative MG.*

7. What other conditions may mimic Guillain-Barré syndrome?
Other disorders that can cause subacute progressive, generalized motor weakness include hypophosphatemia, hypokalemia, acute intermittent porphyria, transverse myelitis, tick paralysis, and carcinomatous or lymphomatous meningitis. Severe peripheral neuropathies should also be considered.

8. What conditions mimic the bulbar weakness associated with myasthenia gravis?
- *Pyridostigmine toxicity* (cholinergic crisis): "Too much of a good thing" (pyridostigmine) can cause weakness and may be misdiagnosed as worsening of MG symptoms. Involuntary twitching and fasciculations may be observed with muscarinic side effects of excess salivation, lacrimation, miosis, blurred vision, diaphoresis, urinary incontinence, and diarrhea.
- *Lambert-Eaton myasthenic syndrome (LEMS):* LEMS presents in the opposite fashion of MG. Patients present with weakness that improves on repetitive stimulation of the muscle. Autoantibodies are directed presynaptically and prevent Ca^{++}-mediated release of synaptic vesicles. LEMS is most often a paraneoplastic disorder.
- *Thyrotoxicosis:* Presents with transient weakness and ocular findings. Hence, thyroid function tests are part of the initial evaluation of any patient with suspected MG.
- *Botulism:* Presents with blurred vision, midposition nonreactive pupils, dysphagia, and limb weakness.
- *Bulbar Onset Amyotrophic lateral sclerosis (ALS):* Though early-stage ALS can have protean manifestations, key differences are the presence of upper motor neuron signs such as spasticity and hyperreflexia not seen in MG.

9. What necessitates critical care for the Guillain-Barré syndrome patients?

Patients with GBS may need to be admitted to an ICU for close observation due to risk of neurogenic respiratory failure and autonomic instability. Dysautonomia results from excessive or insufficient sympathetic or parasympathetic activity and consists of rapid fluctuations in blood pressure, heart rhythm disturbances including sinus bradycardia, or even sinus arrest. Gastric motility can also be affected. Dysautonomia is more commonly seen with the demyelinating form, as opposed to the axonal form of GBS, and is usually present if the disease is severe enough to require mechanical ventilation.

10. When should a patient with Guillain-Barré syndrome or myasthenia gravis be endotracheally intubated?

The first clinical sign of neuromuscular respiratory failure is tachypnea. Respiratory failure in a patient with MG is referred to as "myasthenic crisis." Respiratory pattern may be rapid and shallow, and the patient may appear restless, diaphoretic, with or without increased accessory muscle and paradoxical abdominal movements during inspiration. Bedside pulmonary function testing is helpful; it may, however, be difficult to obtain reliable measurements in patients with facial weakness. Indications for intubation are not always clear, but the decision is supported by the presence of severe bulbar weakness with difficulty to handle secretions and protect airway, and rapidly evolving motor weakness. A vital capacity of less than 15 to 20 mL/kg and a maximum negative inspiratory pressure of less than −20 mm Hg can also indicate need for intubation. Because these patients often have facial weakness that prevents a tight seal around the lips, surrogate measures of vital capacity, such as having the patient count out loud as high as he or she can in one breath, may be useful (approximately 100 mL for each number counted slowly). Hypercapnia and respiratory acidosis are late signs of respiratory failure and should prompt rapid institution of ventilatory support. Hypoxia by pulse oximetry or arterial blood gas measurements are only very late signs of respiratory muscle failure, and if normal should not provide reassurance as to the stability of the condition of the patient with MG or GBS.

11. What are common triggers for myasthenia gravis exacerbation and myasthenic crisis?

MG exacerbations may occur spontaneously or may be precipitated by surgery, infection, pregnancy, or a number of drugs including aminoglycosides, erythromycin, β-blockers, procainamide, quinidine, and magnesium. It is helpful to familiarize yourself with a reliable web-based resource providing extensive lists of medications to avoid in among MG patients–some medications may surprise you!

12. What considerations regarding anesthesia and neuromuscular blockade should be kept in mind when performing endotracheal intubation in a patient with Guillain-Barré syndrome or myasthenia gravis?

Cranial and autonomic nervous dysfunction often predisposes these patients to an increased risk for aspiration. Aspiration precautions, including decompression of the stomach before the induction of anesthesia, should therefore be considered in all patients. A nondepolarizing neuromuscular blocking agent should be used whenever possible in both GBS and MG. Depolarizing neuromuscular blocking agents have been associated with an increased risk for hyperkalemia-induced cardiac arrest in immobilized or paralyzed patients with GBS. Patients with MG are sensitive to nondepolarizing neuromuscular blocking agents, but relatively resistant to depolarizing agents. As an example, the dose required to produce 95% depression of twitch height (ED95) for atracurium and vecuronium (nondepolarizing) is estimated to be 40% to 60% that of normal individuals. Short-acting agents are preferred, and if muscle weakness is excessive, intubation of the trachea can also be performed without neuromuscular blocking agents (e.g., with remifentanil and propofol bolus only). Patients with MG are more likely than normal patients to have a phase II block, and cholinesterase depletion with plasmapheresis or inhibition with pyridostigmine may prolong the blockade.

13. Which patients should I consider for early tracheostomy?

Early tracheostomy should be considered in GBS patients with severe weakness, particularly if it involves the bulbar musculature, as the course of the disease is more prolonged relative to MG. Intubation among MG patients is generally for shorter duration, providing underlying triggers are addressed and appropriate therapy is instituted.

14. Are there any specific therapies for Guillain-Barré syndrome?

Supportive therapy, mechanical ventilation, and measures to prevent aspiration are important. An arterial catheter may be placed to monitor blood pressure if hemodynamic instability is anticipated. Though debate remains, intravenous immunoglobulin (IVIG) is typically administered at a dose of 0.4 g/kg per day for 5 days. Side effects include anaphylaxis, aseptic meningitis, acute renal failure, and thromboembolic events. Patients who have immunoglobulin A (IgA) deficiency should receive IVIG that is also

IgA deficient to reduce the risk of adverse reaction. Early plasma exchange may augment the recovery and can reduce the residual deficit. Typically it consists of five exchanges of 50 mL/kg over a 90- to 120-minute period, with 5% albumin repletion. Side effects include hypovolemia and hemodynamic instability, vasovagal reactions, anaphylaxis, hemolysis, thrombocytopenia, bleeding, and hypocalcemia. Relative contraindications to treatment include sepsis, recent myocardial infarction, marked dysautonomia, and active bleeding. Steroids have been associated with worsening GBS.

15. What are the medical treatments for myasthenia gravis?

Acetylcholinesterase inhibitors represent the mainstay of symptomatic treatment. Pyridostigmine (Mestinon) is most commonly used, as it has few muscarinic side effects. Onset of action is within 15 to 30 minutes (oral administration) and peak effect within 1 to 2 hours. Usual daily doses are between 30 to 120 mg, divided into three to six administrations per day. Corticosteroids cause a reduction in the number of antibodies to the AChRs and are often used to initiate or maintain a remission. Care should be taken with sudden dose escalations of corticosteroids, as there may be an initial period of worsening before improvement. Azathioprine and cyclosporine are popular steroid-sparing agents, and more recently rituximab has been employed in refractory cases. Acute exacerbations require ICU care and are treated with IVIG or plasmapheresis. Cholinesterase inhibitors are often held in the critical care setting to avoid toxicity, and restarting them can be tricky, especially if the patient has reduced ability to handle oral secretions, which increase with use of these drugs. The oral dose of pyridostigmine is approximately 30 times the intravenous dose.

16. Who should undergo thymectomy?

Thymectomy is only used for MG patients, and there is now level I evidence favoring thymectomy as safe and effective. Hyperplasia of the thymus gland is seen in 65% of MG cases, whereas thymoma is seen in up to 15% of patients. Thymectomy should be performed electively and not during a myasthenic crisis.

17. What are other important components of the general care for patients with Guillain-Barré syndrome and myasthenia gravis?

In case of facial diplegia, the eyes should be protected from exposure keratitis. Aggressive skin care and measures to avoid pressure palsies of arms and legs are needed.

18. Describe the typical trajectory and outcomes associated with Guillain-Barré syndrome and myasthenia gravis.

GBS has a much more prolonged clinical course compared to MG. Recovery may not be complete for several months, and residual weakness and atrophy are present in up to 35% of patients. Prognosis for most MG patients is quite good and most patients are able to return to their regular lifestyle. However, a wide spectrum of disease severity exists and some patients require long-term corticosteroids and powerful immunomodulatory agents with frequent exacerbations.

ACKNOWLEDGMENT

The authors wish to acknowledge Dr. Lee H. Schwamm, MD, FAHA, for the valuable contributions to the previous edition of this chapter.

KEY POINTS: GUILLAIN-BARRÉ SYNDROME AND MYASTHENIA GRAVIS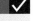

1. MG is an autoimmune disorder preferentially affecting ocular and bulbar musculature with antibodies directed against the postsynaptic acetylcholine receptors.
2. GBS is an acute inflammatory demyelinating polyneuropathy with progressive muscle weakness and areflexia.
3. An early sign of neuromuscular respiratory failure in GBS and MG is tachypnea. Hypercarbia, and especially hypoxia, develop *very* late and should not be used as intubation criteria.
4. Autonomic dysfunction with cardiovascular effects such as bradycardia, tachycardia, and heart block are life-threatening complications of GBS requiring critical care monitoring and support.
5. IVIG or plasmapheresis are the mainstays of treatment for GBS and myasthenic crisis. Steroids should not be used for GBS, but are a common component of MG therapy, along with other immunomodulatory agents.

BIBLIOGRAPHY

1. Asahina M, Kuwabara S, Suzuki A, et al. Autonomic function in demyelinating and axonal subtypes of Guillain-Barré syndrome. *Acta Neurol Scand.* 2002;105:44-50.
2. Goodfellow JA, Willison HJ. Guillain-Barré syndrome: a century of progress. *Nat Rev Neurol.* 2016;12(12):723-731.
3. Guillain-Barré Syndrome Steroid Trial Group. Double-blind trial of intravenous methylprednisolone in Guillain-Barré syndrome. *Lancet.* 1993;341:586-590.
4. Hughes RA, Hadden RD, Gregson NA, et al. Pathogenesis of Guillain-Barré syndrome. *J Neuroimmunol.* 1999;100:74-97.
5. Hughes RA, Raphaël JC, Swan AV, et al. Intravenous immunoglobulin for Guillain-Barré syndrome. *Cochrane Database Syst Rev.* 2006;(1):CD002063.
6. Lawn ND, Fletcher DD, Henderson RD, et al. Anticipating mechanical ventilation in Guillain-Barré syndrome. *Arch Neurol.* 2001;58:893-898.
7. Scherer K, Bedlack RS, Simel DL. Does this patient have myasthenia gravis? *JAMA.* 2005;293:1906-1914.
8. Gomez AM, Van Den Broeck J, Vrolix K, et al. Antibody effector mechanisms in myasthenia gravis-pathogenesis at the neuromuscular junction. *Autoimmunity.* 2010;43:353-370.
9. Jani-Acsadi A, Lisak RP. Myasthenic crisis: guidelines for prevention and treatment. *J Neurol Sci.* 2007;261:127-133.
10. Mao ZF, Mo XA, Qin C, et al. Course and prognosis of myasthenia gravis: a systematic review. *Eur J Neurol.* 2010; 17:913-921.
11. Wolfe GI, Kaminski HJ, Aban IB, et al., MGTX Study Group. Randomized Trial of Thymectomy in Myasthenia Gravis. *N Engl J Med.* 2016;375(6):511-522.

CHAPTER 65

ALCOHOL WITHDRAWAL

Joshua D. Farkas

1. **What is the single most important aspect of diagnosing alcohol withdrawal?**
   Although often difficult to obtain, an accurate drinking history is indispensable. Especially within electronic medical records, the diagnosis of "alcoholism" may remain on the chart long after the patient has quit drinking. The best sources of information are often a spouse, friends, or family. Pertinent details include the amount of alcohol consumed, the regularity, the time of the last drink, and what happened previously if the patient stopped drinking.

2. **What is the typical time-course of delirium tremens?**
   Delirium tremens typically begins within 2 to 4 days of alcohol cessation. Some cases have been reported to begin later, within a week of alcohol cessation. However, when patients develop delirium later on in their hospital course, it becomes increasingly likely that they are suffering from delirium due to another etiology (e.g., sleep deprivation, polypharmacy, sepsis).

3. **What are key clinical findings in delirium tremens?**
   Delirium tremens is marked by three features: (1) an acute confusional state, (2) increased sympathetic tone as manifested with tachycardia, hypertension, diaphoresis, miosis, and possibly fever, and (3) diffuse tremors. Unfortunately, delirium in general may be associated with autonomic deregulation, so the combination of confusion and sympathetic hyperactivity isn't diagnostic of delirium tremens.

4. **How should the diagnosis of delirium tremens be approached?**
   Although delirium tremens requires a compatible history and examination, it is largely a diagnosis of exclusion. Agitated delirium due to a variety of causes may mimic delirium tremens. Thus, alternative diagnoses must be considered. For example, a patient with alcoholism who presents with fever and agitated delirium requires a broad evaluation which may include neuroimaging and a lumbar puncture.

5. **What problem may occur in a severely agitated patient who is receiving frequent boluses of lorazepam?**
   Intravenous (IV) lorazepam may require 15 to 30 minutes to take full therapeutic effect. Therefore, after giving a dose of lorazepam, about 15 minutes should ideally be allowed to determine the therapeutic effect before redosing. However, when treating a severely agitated patient, there can be a tendency to give doses more frequently. This may lead to a phenomenon known as "dose-stacking," where several doses are given in short succession. When these doses eventually reach full effect, the patient may become overly sedated.

6. **What is a common pitfall resulting from a lorazepam infusion?**
   IV lorazepam contains 80% propylene glycol, which is more than any other commonly used medication. Prolonged infusion of lorazepam (especially at rates >10 mg/h) is likely to cause propylene glycol toxicity. Unfortunately, propylene glycol toxicity may manifest with agitation, seizures, and tachycardia – features that could easily be attributed to delirium tremens itself.

7. **Which is the benzodiazepine of choice for alcohol withdrawal?**
   Diazepam has unique pharmacokinetic advantages for alcohol withdrawal. IV diazepam has a very rapid onset (within 5 minutes), avoiding the risk of dose-stacking. Diazepam has a long duration of effect, which means that once symptom control is achieved, this will often persist for 1 to 2 days. Additional doses may be required, but it is less likely that the patient will revert into fulminant withdrawal (compared to lorazepam). The rapid-onset, extended-duration pharmacology of IV diazepam is ideal to gain symptom control rapidly and then maintain therapeutic effect.

8. **How should diazepam be dosed for alcohol withdrawal?**
   Diazepam is typically dosed with escalating IV doses as needed every 5 to 10 minutes (e.g., 10 mg, 10 mg, 20 mg, 20 mg, 20 mg, 40 mg, 40 mg, 40mg). Once a cumulative dose of about 200 mg has been reached, it may be time to consider switching to a second agent. A subset of patients does exist

who are refractory to benzodiazepines, but will respond to phenobarbital. Alternatively, if the patient responds favorably to diazepam, then this may be continued intermittently as needed (PRN).

9. **What does it mean if a patient becomes sedated following a low dose of benzodiazepine?**
Patients with alcoholism display cross-tolerance with benzodiazepines. Particularly among patients with delirium tremens, it is common to be resistant to very large doses of benzodiazpines. If the patient becomes sedated following a low dose of benzodiazepine, this strongly suggests that the patient does not actually have delirium tremens. Alternative diagnoses should be considered.

10. **Describe a common pitfall with the use of symptom scores to trigger therapy.**
A common practice is the use of symptom scores to trigger treatment with benzodiazepine. These scores may function poorly in complex patients and are therefore often not used in critically ill patients. For example, a patient with acute myocardial infarction could score higher due to diaphoresis, anxiety, and vomiting as a result of cardiac ischemia. In patients with multiple active problems, titrating medication based on clinical judgment may be preferable to using a symptom score.

11. **What is a trick to determine if a patient is simulating symptoms of delirium tremens?**
Occasionally, patients recovering from delirium tremens may intentionally simulate symptoms of alcohol withdrawal in order to receive additional doses of sedative. A useful sign of this may be a patient with marked extremity tremors, but no tongue tremor. It is easy to mimic tremoring of the extremities, but a fine tongue tremor cannot be feigned.

12. **Which agent is validated as second-line therapy after benzodiazepines?**
Several publications report success using phenobarbital as a second-line agent for patients refractory to benzodiazepine. Phenobarbital may be given in a dose of 130 to 260 mg intravenously as needed every 30 minutes. Some patience is required, as patients with severe withdrawal may require a large cumulative dose of phenobarbital (e.g., 500–1500 mg). There are no reports of phenobarbital "refractory" withdrawal; all patients should eventually respond to a sufficient dose.

13. **How might dexmedetomidine be utilized?**
Dexmedetomidine may treat agitation and sympathetic hyperactivation, but it will not prevent seizures. Thus, dexmedetomidine should never be used as the sole or primary medication to treat alcohol withdrawal. Dexmedetomidine does have the advantage of being titratable, which may reduce the risk of oversedation. For a severely agitated patient, adjunctive dexmedetomidine could be used to achieve symptom control more rapidly. Meanwhile, the benzodiazepine should be carefully titrated upwards, allowing the dexmedetomidine to be weaned off. There is no strong evidence supporting the use of dexmedetomidine in this setting.

14. **What is the final line of therapy?**
Intubation and treatment with a propofol infusion is highly effective for severe alcohol withdrawal. However, intubation and prolonged infusion of sedatives and opioids may ultimately aggravate the patient's delirium. If possible, complications may be minimized by avoiding intubation.

15. **Which medication class should generally be avoided in agitated patients with delirium tremens?**
Although antipsychotics are often used for treatment of agitation in the ICU, they should generally be avoided in the treatment of delirium tremens. Antipsychotics may mask the symptoms of delirium tremens without addressing the underlying pathophysiologic problem (deficiency of inhibitory GABA-receptor signaling). Furthermore, antipsychotics may lower the seizure threshold, which is especially dangerous since these patients are at increased risk of seizure.

16. **What other treatment should also be provided to patients with alcohol withdrawal?**
The possibility of Wernicke encephalopathy should be considered in any patient with alcoholism and confusion. This may be extremely difficult to diagnose, since the clinical examination is insensitive and often impossible in agitated patients. Failure to treat Wernicke encephalopathy may cause permanent neurologic disability. Thus, the safest approach is to empirically treat for possible Wernicke encephalopathy with thiamine. The ideal dose for this indication is unknown, with some authorities recommending high doses (e.g., 500 mg intravenously every eight hours).

17. **Describe a therapeutic dilemma that is often encountered 2 to 3 days after starting therapy for delirium tremens.**
Occasionally, patients may continue to experience confusion after a few days of therapy. The differential diagnosis here centers around undertreated delirium tremens versus multifactorial delirium (which may often be due to benzodiazepine toxicity!). This is critical to clarify. If the patient has undertreated

delirium tremens, then benzodiazepines are needed. However, if the patient has benzodiazepine toxicity, then benzodiazepines should be *avoided* and a low dose of antipsychotic might even be considered. Physical examination may help resolve this (e.g., evaluation for tremor and sympathetic hyperactivity).

18. What are some emerging therapies for alcohol withdrawal currently under investigation?
Earlier and more extensive use of phenobarbital is currently being investigated by some centers. One randomized controlled trial found that administering 10 mg/kg phenobarbital immediately upon arrival in the emergency department reduced subsequent symptom severity and decreased the likelihood of patients requiring ICU admission. Possible advantages of phenobarbital may include that it is uniformly successful (unlike benzodiazepines, to which some patients are refractory) and that it is particularly effective in preventing seizures.

19. Can protocols improve the management of delirium tremens?
Observational studies suggest that a protocolized approach to delirium tremens may improve care. Validated protocols involve escalating doses of IV diazepam, followed by escalating doses of IV phenobarbital, followed by intubation with propofol. Protocols may encourage providers to use adequate medication doses and to escalate to more powerful therapies earlier. This may also avoid a disorganized approach with excessive polypharmacy.

20. What is the best treatment for seizures related to withdrawal?
First-line therapy is IV benzodiazepine, as for seizures in general. Most seizures will resolve, often spontaneously. Scheduled doses of benzodiazepine should be considered to prevent recurrence. Rarely, status epilepticus may occur. Unfortunately, traditional antiepileptic drugs (e.g., phenytoin) do not seem to be as effective for this type of seizure. For status epilepticus which is refractory to benzodiazepine, intubation followed by propofol infusion may be necessary.

21. Can alcohol be used to prevent delirium tremens?
Ongoing alcohol intake will generally prevent delirium tremens. This may be considered in extremely rare circumstances when a patient is at very high risk of withdrawal, competent to make decisions, and adamant about having no intention to quit drinking. For example, this may be preferable compared to the patient leaving against medical advice.

ACKNOWLEDGMENT

The authors wish to acknowledge Drs. Bruce A. Crookes, MD, FACS, and William Peery, MD, for the valuable contributions to the previous edition of this chapter.

KEY POINTS: ALCOHOL WITHDRAWAL

1. Delirium tremens typically occurs 2 to 4 days after cessation of drinking.
2. Diagnosis requires exclusion of other causes of delirium and clarification of the patient's drinking history.
3. Benzodiazepines are the first-line therapy for delirium tremens, with IV diazepam having an attractive pharmacokinetic profile.
4. Phenobarbital is an emerging therapy for patients who fail to respond favorably to benzodiazepine.

BIBLIOGRAPHY

1. Horinek EL, Kiser TH, Fish DN, et al. Propylene glycol accumulation in critically ill patients receiving continuous intravenous lorazepam infusions. *Ann Pharmacother.* 2009;43:1964.
2. Hack JB, Hoffmann RS, Nelson LS. Resistant alcohol withdrawal: does an unexpectedly large sedative requirement identify these patients early? *J Med Toxicol.* 2006;2:55.
3. Moore PW, Donovan JW, Burkhart KK, et al. Safety and efficacy of flumazenil for reversal of iatrogenic benzodiazepine-associated delirium toxicity during treatment of alcohol withdrawal, a retrospective review at one center. *J Med Toxicol.* 2014;10:126.
4. Rosenson J, Clements C, Simon B, et al. Phenobarbital for acute alcohol withdrawal: a prospective randomized double-blind placebo-controlled study. *J Emerg Med.* 2013;44:592.
5. Duby JJ, Berry AJ, Ghayyem P, et al. Alcohol withdrawal syndrome in critically ill patients: protocolized versus nonprotocolized management. *J Trauma Acute Care Surg.* 2014;77:938.
6. Gold JA, Rimal B, Nolan A, et al. A strategy of escalating doses of benzodiazepines and phenobarbital administration reduces the need for mechanical ventilation in delirium tremens. *Crit Care Med.* 2007;35:724.

XII
Surgery and Trauma

CHAPTER 66

BURNS AND FROSTBITE

T.J. Henry and Yuk Ming Liu

1. **What are the most common types of burn injuries?**
   The most common types of burn injuries are thermal burns from open flame and from liquid scalding. For children (5 and under), scald burns are the most common. The other types of burns are contact burns (direct contact with hot object), chemical exposure, and conduction of electricity.

2. **What are the two types of pathophysiologic destruction that occur in burn injuries?**
   Coagulative necrosis and liquefactive necrosis. Flame, scald, and contact burns all induce cellular damage by the transfer of energy (heat) and induce coagulative necrosis. Chemical exposure and electrical burns cause direct cytotoxic disturbance to the cellular membranes in addition to the transfer of energy and can cause coagulative and liquefactive necrosis.

3. **What are the Jackson zones of injury?**
   Zone of coagulation—Irreversibly damaged cells that become necrotic from the direct injury.
   Zone of stasis—The area immediately surrounding the zone of coagulation that sustained a modest degree of insult. There is decreased tissue perfusion from vessel leakage and vascular damage. Depending on the wound environment and relative concentrations of vasoconstrictors and local inflammatory agents, can either survive or become necrotic.
   Zone of hyperemia—Area surrounding the zone of stasis that has clearly viable tissue, exhibits vasodilation, and is the area that begins the healing process.
   See Fig. 66.1.

4. **How are thermal injuries classified?**
   Thermal injuries are classified based on the degree of injury to the epidermis, dermis, subcutaneous fat, and underlying soft and bony tissues.
   First degree—The injury is localized to the epidermis (most sunburns); the area is painful, erythematous, blanches with gentle pressure, but retains an intact epidermal barrier.
   Second degree—Also termed a "partial thickness injury"; there is injury to the epidermis and part of the underlying dermis. The dermis consists of a superficial papillary region and a deeper

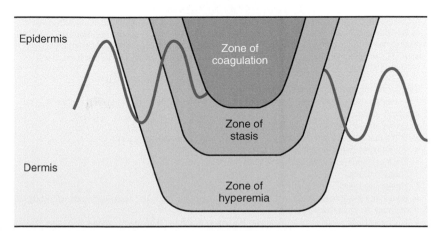

Figure 66-1. Zones of Injury after a Burn. The zone of coagulation is the portion irreversibly injured. The zones of stasis and hyperemia are defined in response to the injury. *(From Jeshke MG, Williams FN, Gauglitz GG, et al. Burns. In: Townsend CM, Beauchamp RD, Gauglitz GG, et al., eds. Sabiston Textbook of Surgery. 19th ed. Philadelphia: Elsevier Saunders; 2012.)*

reticular region. The burns are typically very painful, form blisters, and have varying degrees of moistness and blanching (depending upon how deep the reticular layer is affected). But they will heal the majority of time without surgical intervention from the retained epidermal structures in hair follicles and sweat glands.

Third degree—Also termed a "full thickness injury" because the entire epidermis and dermis are destroyed. Typically described as white and leathery in appearance and is asensate (nerve endings are completely destroyed). The base of this injury will not be able to regenerate itself and must either heal by wound edges and contraction (must be very small and will form a severe scar) or by excision and grafting.

Fourth degree—Injury deeper than the skin; affecting the fat, muscle, and/or bone

5. **How do you estimate the size of a burn injury?**
The rule of nines. For an adult patient, every body part is roughly 9% (head, right upper extremity, left upper extremity, chest, abdomen, upper back, lower back, anterior right lower extremity, posterior right lower extremity, anterior left lower extremity, posterior left lower extremity) plus 1% for genitalia. For a child, the torso and upper extremities are the same, but the head is much larger, respectively, and divided into anterior and posterior (each 9% now) and the lower extremities are smaller and only 14% each. This is the total body surface area (TBSA) injured and used to calculate the initial resuscitation requirements. First-degree burns are not included in the estimation. See Fig. 66.2.

6. **What are the initial steps to managing care for a burn patient?**
Stop the burning process! Patients should be removed from the source of injury, burning clothing should be extinguished, and chemical exposure should be rinsed away. Burn patients should be treated like any trauma victim and have a thorough examination of any life-threatening injuries first, utilizing advance trauma life support (ATLS) principles of Airway, Breathing, Circulation, Disability, and Exposure.

7. **How do you identify inhalation injuries?**
A history of fire in an enclosed space is a very strong risk factor for inhalation injury. Any of the following physical exam findings should make you suspicious of an inhalation injury and warrant further evaluation by direct laryngoscopy and bronchoscopy: face and/or neck burns, singeing of eyebrows or nasal hair, carbon deposits in the mouth or nose, erythema of the oropharynx, hoarseness, or carboxyhemoglobin levels greater than 10%. Inhalational injuries can result in severe upper airway edema and intubation should never be delayed.

8. **What are the initial fluid requirements of a burn patient?**
Burn patients have severe intravascular volume depletion from increased capillary permeability. During the first 24 hours after injury, the burn patient will require a considerable amount of intravenous fluids. The Parkland Burn Formula is the most widely used resuscitation formula: 2 to 4 mL/kg per TBSA injured (do NOT include first-degree burns in TBSA). Half of this volume is given over the first 8 hours and the second half is given over the remaining 16 hours. This formula is an *estimate* of the total amount of fluid the patient will require. The rate of actual fluid administration should be adjusted on the actual hemodynamic status of the patient and monitoring of the urine output (goal should be 0.5 mL/kg per hour of urine output for adults and 1 mL/kg per hour for children). Lactated ringer's solution is the crystalloid of choice for resuscitation of burn patients.

9. **Who should be referred to a verified burn center?**
The American Burn Association recommends that patients with the following injuries require referral to a burn center:
- Partial-thickness burns greater than 10% TBSA
- Burns that involve the face, hands, feet, genitalia, perineum, or major joints
- Third-degree burns in any age group
- Electrical burns, including lightning injury
- Chemical burns
- Inhalational injury
- Burn injury in patients with pre-existing medical disorders that could complicate treatment, prolong recovery, or affect mortality
- Any patient with a burn and concomitant trauma in which the burn injury poses the greatest risk of morbidity or mortality. In such cases, if the trauma poses the greater immediate risk, the patient may be initially stabilized in a trauma center before being transferred to a burn unit.
- Burned children in hospitals without qualified personnel or equipment for the care of children
- Burn injury patients who will require special social, emotional, or rehabilitative intervention

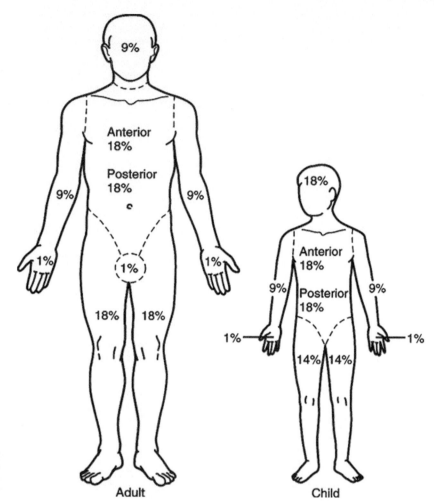

Figure 66-2. The Rule of Nines. *(From Cinat ME, Vanderkam, VM. Introduction to Fires and Burns. In: Ciottone GR, ed. Disaster Medicine. 1st ed. Philadelphia, PA: Mosby Elsevier; 2006:790–795.)*

10. Describe initial wound care for a burn patient.
   Stop the burning process! Using room temperature water to cool down the affected area is appropriate for the first 15 minutes following the injury. However, after this time period the patient may have considerable difficulty maintaining normothermia and every effort should be made to decrease heat loss from the exposed tissue. Clean, dry dressings (preferably in a nonstick form; Saran Wrap works great) should be placed and will also help control pain by covering the exposed nerve endings. Damp dressings or ice packs should never be used.

11. How should you assess circumferential extremity injuries?
   All circumferential extremity injuries need to be assessed for adequate distal circulation and perfusion. Because of the increased capillary permeability and edema that will develop in the extremity, there is a chance to develop compartment syndrome. Physicians must be diligent in assessing distal circulation and performing escharotomies if the extremity is showing signs of compartment syndrome (increased pain with passive motion, tightness, numbness, decreased pulses). Escharotomy may be indicated to release compartments.

12. What are the two postburn metabolic phases?
    The first 48 hours after a severe thermal injury is termed the *ebb phase* and is characterized by massive release of inflammatory molecules, impaired glucose tolerance with hyperglycemia, decreased cardiac output, increased systemic resistance, and the beginning of protein breakdown. By about 5 days postinjury, the *plateau phase* (or flow phase) begins and is characterized by hyperdynamic circulation and a hypermetabolic state. This hypermetabolic state accompanied by increased cortisol, cytokines, catecholamines, basal energy requirements, impaired glucose metabolism, and insulin sensitivity has been shown to persist far past the closing of wounds and even for up to 3 years postinjury!
    In major burns, there is up to a 50-fold increase in catecholamines, corticosteroid levels, and inflammatory mediators. This increases the resting metabolic rate to greater than 140% of normal. The cardiac output (although initially low) can increase to 1.5 times that of baseline. Protein catabolism occurs at an alarming rate and can lead to severe muscle wasting with decreased strength, inability to heal, and failure to rehabilitate. There is stimulation of gluconeogenesis and glycogenolysis that results in hyperglycemia and insulin resistance.

13. After the burn patient has been adequately assessed and resuscitated, how do you care for the wounds?
    Second-degree injuries should be dressed in a way to reduce evaporative heat loss, protect rejuvenating epithelium, minimize bacterial colonization, and provide comfort for the underlying painful wound. This can be accomplished through multiple types of dressings, each with their own advantages and disadvantages, including topical antimicrobials, cotton gauze, elastic wraps, biologic dressings, or synthetic coverings. Third-degree injuries will need to undergo excision and grafting for adequate and timely healing.

14. What are some special considerations for electrical injuries?
    Electrical injuries are typically divided into low voltage and high voltage. Most household currents range from 110 to 220 V, are considered low-voltage injuries, and are very similar to thermal burns only affecting local tissues and without transmission to deeper tissues. For high-voltage injuries (typically anything around or >600 V), the current is carried through the tissues with the least resistance (nerves, vessels, and muscles) and the majority of the injury is actually hidden from the surface. The skin has a relatively high resistance and is mostly spared. There must be a high index of suspicion for underlying tissue destruction and all patients should be evaluated for any cardiac dysrhythmias, as well as other associated trauma ("blown back," falling, explosions, other blunt traumas, severe contractions resulting in fractures, etc.). Muscle damage also results in release of myoglobin, which is filtered in the glomeruli and can lead to obstructive nephropathy. Robust intravenous fluid administration is required to maintain urine output approximately 2 mL/kg per hour.

15. How do you treat chemical burns?
    Stop the burning process! The concentration, type of chemical, and length of exposure time determine the degree of tissue damage. For dry powder, brush the powder away, remove clothing, and irrigate with copious amounts of water. For liquid chemicals, immediately remove any affected clothing and then irrigate with copious amounts of water. Never try to neutralize the agent with another weak acid or base. That reaction is an exothermic reaction and creates heat and can further injure the patient. Multiple liters of water (sometimes 15–20) is the best way to rinse off and dilute the chemical down to a normal pH. Continue to check the pH and irrigate the wound until a stable pH of 7 to 7.5 is reached.

16. What is the process of injury for alkali burns? For acid burns?
    Alkali burns involve saponification of fat, massive extraction of water, and creation of alkaline proteinates that contain hydroxide ions and penetrate deep into tissues. Acid burns induce hydrolysis and protein breakdown; this typically results in eschar formation and the acid does not penetrate as deep into the tissues, as compared to the same "strength" of alkali.

17. What is different about hydrofluoric acid?
    It is the strongest inorganic acid known and produces dehydration and corrosion of tissue with free hydrogen ions. The ions can form complexes with bivalent cations (calcium and magnesium) to form insoluble salts and ultimately lead to calcium chelation, hypocalcemia, and life-threatening arrhythmias. In addition to copious amounts of water to irrigate the surface affected, calcium gluconate gel should be applied topically. These wounds are typically very painful and the gel should be continually

Table 66-1. Topical Antimicrobials

TOPICAL ANTIMICROBIAL	Spectrum of Activity			ADVANTAGES	DISADVANTAGES
	GRAM +	GRAM −	FUNGAL		
Bacitracin	X			Ease of application, painless, cheap	Can cause allergic reaction
Mafenide acetate (sulfamylon)	X	X	X	Penetrates eschar; good broad spectrum coverage	Large area of use may cause metabolic acidosis (carbonic anhydrase inhibitor)
Mupirocin	X (MRSA)			Most effective staphylococcal coverage	Expensive; very narrow coverage
Silver nitrate solution	X	X	X	Can easily resoak dressing without removal; effective against all microorganisms	Hyponatremia (hypotonic solution); stains contacted areas; may cause methemoglobinemia
Silver sulfadiazine (silvadene)	X	X	X	Broad coverage, painless	Mild inhibition of epithelialization; may cause transient leukopenia

MRSA, methicillin-resistant *Staphylococcus aureus*.

applied and changed at 15-minute intervals until the pain subsides and there is sufficient fluoride ion removal.

18. What are some of the advantages and disadvantages of topical antimicrobials?
Topical antimicrobial application has vastly improved the care of burn patients and decreased systemic infections. Burn wounds quickly become colonized with many types of bacteria and if left untreated will allow the proliferation of microorganisms and allow them to penetrate the tissues and progress to systemic infections. Thankfully, this is not very common with the routine use of different types of topical antimicrobials. Some of the antimicrobials have a broad range of activity against gram-positive and gram-negative organisms (silver sulfadiazine [silvadene], mafenide acetate [sulfamylon], and silver nitrate), while some of the antimicrobials have a more narrow spectrum, but are very easy to apply and work well on minor injuries (bacitracin, neomycin, and mupirocin [bactroban]). See Table 66.1.

19. What are the different types of freezing injuries?
Frostnip and frostbite. Frostnip is characterized by intense vasoconstriction and subsequent pallor and numbness. Ice crystals may form on the skin surface, but no deep tissue ice crystal formation occurs, and with rewarming, there is no long-term tissue damage. Frostbite is a combination of ice crystal formation in tissues and microvascular occlusion with thrombosis. There are varying degrees of damage to the epidermis, dermis, subcutaneous tissues, and deeper muscle and bone involvement.

20. How do you treat frostbite?
All damp clothing should be removed and replaced with warm blankets. The patient should be monitored and assessed for systemic hypothermia and other injuries. The frostbite injuries should be rapidly rewarmed with circulating water, preferably in a hospital setting, and ensuring no refreezing of the extremity. Avoid dry heat, rubbing, or massage of the injured area. If the injury is less than 24 hours, strong consideration should be given to urgent angiography and potential catheter-directed thrombolysis.

ACKNOWLEDGMENT

The authors wish to acknowledge Drs. Shawn P. Fagan, MD, and Jeremy Goverman, MD, FACS, for the valuable contributions to the previous edition of this chapter.

KEY POINTS: BURNS AND FROSTBITE

1. Stop the burning process! Completely evaluate for other injuries.
2. Thermal injuries are classified by the depth of damage to the epidermis and dermis and have characteristic appearances:
   - First degree—red, no blisters
   - Second degree—blisters with blanching redness and appear moist
   - Third degree—white, leathery, dry in appearance
3. Quick estimation of the size of burns by the rule of nines and begin aggressive fluid administration with the Parkland formula for TBSA >20%, but tailor ongoing administration using urine output and markers of resuscitation.
4. Burns cause a substantial increase in metabolism and require proper nutrition and physical rehabilitation.
5. Early excision of necrotic tissue, daily wound care, and topical antimicrobials are the mainstay of treatment to decrease systemic infection.
6. Frostbite injuries should undergo rapid rewarming with circulating water and, if applicable, potentially catheter-directed thrombolysis, in particular, for extremities and within 24 hours.

BIBLIOGRAPHY

1. *Advanced Trauma Life Support Student Course Manual.* 9th ed. Chicago: American College of Surgeons Committee on Trauma; 2012.
2. American Burn Association. *Advanced Burn Life Support Providers Manual.* Chicago: American Burn Association; 2005.
3. American Burn Association. *National Burn Repository: Report of data from 1999-2008.* 2009. Available at: http://ameriburn.org/education/publications/.
4. Bruen KJ, Ballard JR, Morris SE, et al. Reduction of the incidence of amputation in frostbite injury with thrombolytic therapy. *Arch Surg.* 2007;142:546-551.
5. Herndon DN, Tompkins RG. Support of the metabolic response to burn injury. *Lancet.* 2004;363:1895-1902.
6. Jackson DM. The diagnosis of the depth of burning. *Br J Surg.* 1953;40(164):588-596.
7. Jeschke MG, Chinkes DL, Finnerty CC, et al. Pathophysiologic response to severe burn injury. *Ann Surg.* 2008;248: 387-401.
8. Jeshke MG, Williams FN. Burns. In: Townsend CM, Beauchamp RD, eds. *Sabiston Textbook of Surgery.* 19th ed. Philadelphia: Elsevier Saunders; 2012:521-545.
9. Kirkpatrick JJ, Enion DS, Burd DA. Hydrofluoric acid burns: a review. *Burns.* 1995;21:483-493.
10. Ryan CM, Chang PH. Cold Injury, Frostbite, and Hypothermia. In: Cameron JL, ed. *Current Surgical Therapy.* 11th ed. Philadelphia: Elsevier; 2014:1139-1143.
11. Williams FN, Jeschke MG, Chinkes DL, et al. Modulation of the hypermetabolic response to trauma: temperature, nutrition, and drugs. *J Am Coll Surg.* 2009;208:489-502.

THORACIC TRAUMA (FLAIL CHEST, AND PULMONARY AND MYOCARDIAL CONTUSION)

Noelle N. Saillant and D. Dante Yeh

1. **What is the significance of blunt chest injuries?**
   Blunt chest trauma is the result of the transfer of energy to the rigid structure of the thorax. Thoracic injury and its complications are responsible for up to 25% of blunt trauma mortality.

   Thoracic injuries may involve disruption of the chest wall with rib fractures and flail segments and injury to the underlying organs such as the lung and heart.

2. **What are the most common injuries in patients sustaining blunt chest trauma?**
   Overall, rib fractures are the most common injury after chest trauma. Pulmonary contusion is also a common occurrence in 40% to 60% of patients with blunt chest trauma. Associated pneumothorax and hemothorax is seen in 20% of bluntly injured patients.

   The incidence of blunt cardiac injury (BCI) depends on the criteria and diagnostic modality used, but is reported to be present in 20% to 78% of all blunt thoracic trauma patients.

3. **Are there age-related differences in injury pattern of the chest?**
   Blunt chest trauma patterns are different at the extremes of age. In young patients, chest injury is typically the consequence of high-energy mechanisms. Due to the increased elasticity and compliance of the youthful bony thorax, significant injury may occur to the underlying lung parenchyma in absence of rib fracture. Underlying lung injury with pulmonary hemorrhage and contusions are the prominent cause of respiratory failure in this age group. In contrast, patients over the age of 65 have a calcified but frail bony wall, thus rendering them susceptible to rib fractures and flail injuries after low-energy injury.

4. **What is a flail chest, and how is it diagnosed?**
   Radiographically, flail chest is defined as fractures of three or more consecutive ribs or costal cartilages fractured in two or more places (Fig. 67.1). The term may also apply to a costochondral disruption associated with a sternal fracture or when the fracture fault crosses the axillary line leading to a flail segment of the entire anterior chest. Although flail chest may be seen on radiography, imaging does not account for the muscular stabilization of the chest wall and the dynamic mechanics of breathing. The diagnosis is made by *clinical* examination of the spontaneously breathing patient. A true flail segment will move paradoxically, with the chest wall collapsing inward during inspiration and billowing out with exhalation. Importantly, patients receiving positive pressure through mechanical ventilation usually do not demonstrate the classic paradoxical movements.

5. **How do rib fractures and flail segments alter chest wall mechanics?**
   A clinical flail segment may alter the mechanical dynamics of ventilation, leading to increased work of breathing, decreased ventilation and in severe cases, compromised gas exchange. However, respiratory dysfunction usually does not result from paradoxical chest motion alone, but rather is compounded by underlying pulmonary injury and splinting from pain.

6. **What is a pulmonary contusion?**
   Pulmonary contusion is a bruise of the lung, with alveolar and interstitial hemorrhage and destruction of the pulmonary parenchyma. The subsequent inflammation leads to asymmetric edema, atelectasis, and poor mucus clearance from the airways. Pulmonary contusion and hemorrhage lead to shunt-related hypoxemia and loss of pulmonary compliance. This is usually manifested clinically as progressive respiratory failure developing over the first 6 to 24 hours, with the nadir of respiratory function occurring approximately 72 hours after injury.

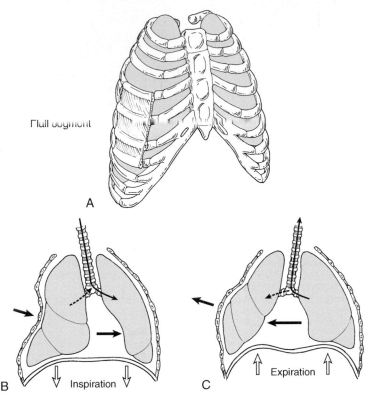

Flail segment

A

B   Inspiration   C   Expiration

Figure 67-1. Diagram illustrating respiratory dysfunction with flail chest. (A) Flail segment of the right chest lead to an unstable portion of the chest wall. (B) During inspiration the flail segment moves inward while the chest expands. (C) During exhalation the flail segment moves outward while the chest wall recoils.

7. What are the radiographic findings associated with pulmonary contusion?

Pulmonary contusions are diagnosed radiographically. Although initial chest radiographs may be unremarkable, a nonsegmental infiltrate typically develops over a 6-hour period. If the contusions are visible on the initial chest radiograph, the injury is likely to be more severe, and enlargement of the contused area on the radiograph over the next 24 hours is a poor prognostic sign. Classic radiograph patterns include irregular consolidations or a diffuse patchy pattern (Fig. 67.2). Even after development of chest radiograph findings, plain radiographs may underestimate the severity

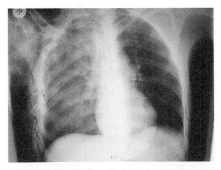

Figure 67-2. Radiograph of a patient with a pulmonary contusion.

of the contusions. Computed tomography (CT) scan is more sensitive for diagnosis of pulmonary contusions and can quantify the volume of lung involved. However, "occult" pulmonary contusions seen only on CT are rarely of clinical importance.

8. Describe the causes of blunt cardiac injury.
BCI typically occurs in the setting of a rapid deceleration mechanism commonly seen in motor vehicle collisions and occasionally in falls or crush injury. The abrupt pressure fluctuation leads to shearing forces in the chest and compression of the heart between the spine and sternum. While sternal fractures are commonly considered a marker of force applied to the heart, BCI can occur in absence of bony injury. A rare cause of BCI, termed *commotio cordis*, occurs when a projectile strikes the chest (e.g., baseball). Such a strike may cause cardiac arrest if it occurs during a period of electrical susceptibility in the cardiac cycle during the 10 to 30 ms before the peak of the T wave.

9. What are the clinical manifestations of blunt cardiac injury?
The right side of the heart has the most anterior surface area and therefore is the most commonly injured chamber. Injuries may include rupture of the interventricular septum, a valve, or the ventricle. Patients with a ruptured chamber will rarely reach the hospital alive. Less commonly, injury to coronary arteries occurs that may lead to myocardial infarction.

10. Describe clinical features that could suggest blunt cardiac injury.
Specific signs such as cardiac arrhythmias, murmurs, or precordial thrills are clear indications that warrant evaluation of heart injury. In very severe cases, patients may present with distended jugular veins and hypotension as signs of cardiogenic shock. However, clinical suspicion is critical as BCI is commonly clinically silent, and the diagnosis may be missed unless the clinician conducts further testing. Electrocardiography (ECG), echocardiography, and cardiac enzymes may support the diagnosis.

11. What is the role of electrocardiography in diagnosis of blunt cardiac injury?
ECG findings associated with BCI include ventricular or atrial arrhythmias, bundle-branch block, and ST-wave abnormalities. The prevalence of abnormal ECGs in patients with BCI ranges from 40% to 83% in the literature. The ECG will not conclusively rule in or rule out BCI.

12. What is the role of troponins in blunt cardiac injury?
Cardiac troponins are more specific than creatine kinase myocardial bound (CKMB) for myocardial cellular injury. In the setting of an abnormal ECG, troponin levels are unlikely to affect clinical management. However, in those patients with a nonspecific sinus tachycardia, measuring cardiac troponin levels in 6 hours from the time of injury can effectively rule out a significant cardiac contusion.

13. How is echocardiography used in the diagnosis of blunt cardiac injury?
Transthoracic echocardiography (TTE) provides rapid visualization of the heart and is a useful diagnostic tool for BCI. It can be used to identify anatomic abnormalities (e.g., valvular injury, pericardial effusion), ventricular dyskinesia, shunting of blood, and intracardiac thrombi. It provides necessary information in patients who manifest hemodynamic instability or abnormal screening tests (ECG, cardiac enzymes), but has lower sensitivity in the patient whose condition is stable. Transesophageal echocardiography (TEE) provides better visualization of wall motion abnormalities and valvular injuries than TTE, albeit in a more invasive fashion. It has superior sensitivity to TTE for injuries that require therapeutic intervention and can be performed with relative ease at the bedside or concurrent with other surgical procedures. Either form of echocardiography is indicated only if the patient is hemodynamically unstable.

14. Does imaging modality alter rates of detection of chest injuries?
The advancement of modern imaging and increased use of CT has doubled the detection of injury in blunt chest trauma. Although many CT findings do not alter clinical care, a recent prospective, multicenter analysis of 5912 trauma patients who had both a radiograph and a chest CT showed that 14% of those occult injuries identified by CT alone led to insertion of a chest tube, mechanical ventilation, or surgery.

15. What is the relationship among rib fractures, flail chest, pulmonary contusions, and blunt cardiac injury?
Pulmonary contusions and cardiac contusion may occur in the setting of minimal to no rib fractures in the compliant rib cage. Flail chest, however, indicates that the chest wall sustained a large force; therefore, more than 90% of patients with flail chest have associated intrathoracic injuries, underlying

pulmonary contusions, and potential BCI. These patients may also have a concomitant hemothorax, pneumothorax, or both. Patients with flail chest are also more likely to have head injury and intra-abdominal injury.

16. What are the patient risk factors for adverse outcomes after blunt thoracic injury?
    The greatest patient risk factors for mortality in blunt chest trauma are age 65 years or greater, the presence of medical comorbidities (especially cardiopulmonary disease), and sustaining three or more rib fractures. The elderly are affected disproportionately by respiratory embarrassment, with respiratory failure and pneumonia being the predominant cause of mortality. Profound morbidity may result from the loss of efficient respiratory mechanics, pain-related chest wall splinting, and underlying lung injury. An oxygen saturation less than 92% on room air, a tidal volume under 1.4, and an incentive spirometry (IS) volume under 15 mL/kg are markers of impending respiratory compromise.

17. What is the relationship between pulmonary contusions and acute respiratory distress syndrome?
    Patients with pulmonary contusions are at higher risk than other patients for the development of pneumonia and acute respiratory distress syndrome (ARDS). The volume of lung parenchyma involved as determined by CT scan is a risk factor for the development of ARDS, with patients having contusion volumes of greater than 20% at the highest risk. In these patients, ARDS has been shown to develop in approximately 80%.

18. What is the mortality rate and cause of death for patients with flail chest and pulmonary contusions?
    The overall mortality rate of patients with blunt chest trauma is 16% with either a pulmonary contusion or flail chest. The rate of death increases to 42% when patients had both injuries. Although these patients have severe thoracic injury, the most common cause of death in patients with flail chest and pulmonary contusions is brain injury.

19. What are the immediate management strategies for flail chest or pulmonary contusions?
    All trauma patients should be assessed and treated according to the principles of Advanced Trauma Life Support (ATLS). The primary survey verifies the ABCs (airway, breathing, and circulation) and is paramount to the diagnosis and treatment of immediate life-threatening injuries. The unstable patient with chest trauma may present with respiratory failure requiring endotracheal intubation and mechanical ventilation. Tube thoracostomy may be indicated in cases of hemothorax or pneumothorax. Stable patients with chest trauma require close monitoring of the respiratory status, aggressive lung physiotherapy, early mobilization, and adequate nutrition.

20. What is the optimal approach to the diagnosis of blunt cardiac injury?
    After the initial ATLS workup, life-threatening conditions of BCI should be identified through physical examination, ECG, and bedside ultrasound (i.e., focused abdominal sonography for trauma [FAST]). An ECG is routinely performed in trauma patients with complaints of chest pain, history of heart disease, or other symptoms and signs suggestive of active cardiac pathologic condition. If the FAST is negative or equivocal for hemopericardium in patients with significant arrhythmias or unexplained hemodynamic instability, a formal TTE should be performed. In cases of continued diagnostic uncertainty, patients may require TEE.

21. Describe the standard management of blunt cardiac injury.
    For asymptomatic patients with minimal or no associated injuries, negative or minimal ECG findings, and normal troponin levels, discharge from the hospital after several hours of observation is supported. Patients who are elderly, have a history of cardiac disease, or are hemodynamically unstable require continuous cardiac monitoring for at least 24 hours. The use of antiarrhythmic agents in patients with myocardial contusion is controversial and should occur in consultation with cardiologists. Also, consultation of cardiothoracic surgeons should occur in suspected cases of surgically amenable injuries.

22. Is follow-up needed in patients with blunt cardiac injury?
    Long-term prognosis of patients with BCI is good, and functional recovery of the heart should be expected. As such, follow-up is not routinely required in patients with an uneventful cardiac course in the hospital. For those patients with a complicated course, a follow-up echocardiography is warranted to exclude formation of an aneurysm, cardiac thrombus, or valve anomaly.

23. What are the options for pain control in chest wall trauma?
    Adequate pain control is fundamental to the management of rib fractures to decrease chest wall splinting and alveolar collapse by permitting patient mobilization, deep breathing, and secretion clearance. Enhanced pulmonary toilet decreases the risk of developing for pneumonia. Analgesia is best

achieved through multimodal therapy. Opioids may be administered through oral, intermittent intravenous bolus, and patient-controlled analgesia (PCA) dosing, but must be balanced against the risk of oversedation, hypoventilation, and depression of cough and respiratory efforts. Delirium is an unintended, morbid side effect of opioid treatment in the elderly with potentially serious morbidity. Regional blocks of the intercostal, intrapleural, and paravertebral spaces or thoracic epidural analgesia (TEA) are additional adjuncts for pain control in appropriately selected patents. Spine fractures, coagulopathy, or antiplatelet medications may preclude the use of these interventions.

Retrospective studies of trauma patients with rib fractures have shown inconsistent benefits of epidural analgesia compared with other analgesic modalities. A recent systematic review and meta-analysis of randomized controlled trials failed to show a benefit of epidural analgesia on mortality, intensive care unit (ICU) and hospital length of stay (LOS), despite small randomized controlled trials showing some evidence to the contrary. Bulger et al. found that the incidence of nosocomial pneumonia was reduced (18% vs. 38%) by epidural analgesia compared with parenteral opioids. Despite the lack of clear evidence, the use of epidural and paravertebral blocks is supported by the 2016 Western Trauma Association expert consensus guidelines for the management of rib fractures.

24. What is the optimal fluid management strategy in patients with blunt chest trauma?
Judicious fluid resuscitation is required during the initial resuscitation of the patient with blunt chest trauma, as the injured lung is prone to edema while at the same time significant secondary injury can result from under transfusion of fluids. Increased permeability of pulmonary capillaries occurring early after pulmonary contusion predisposes the patient to the development of tissue edema and worsening gas exchange. The use of colloid solutions for patients with pulmonary contusion has been advocated by some, with the aim of maintaining plasma oncotic pressure and possibly withdrawing water from the contused lung, though no randomized trials exist that demonstrate a clear benefit from colloid administration in this setting. Current opinion on fluid replacement is in favor of ensuring adequate resuscitation to ensure end-organ perfusion followed by avoidance of further unnecessary fluid administration. This may be best achieved with early use of invasive monitoring or echocardiography to guide fluid replacement.

25. Which respiratory therapy procedure(s) should be used for patients with significant blunt chest trauma?
Nonintubated patients with blunt chest trauma should be maintained with aggressive pulmonary toilet. Lung expansion therapy using IS, deep breathing, and coughing is critical to reduce secretions, prevent atelectasis, and avoid the need for intubation. All patients should have pain assessed and receive maximal lung expansion therapy on a frequent schedule. Underlying reactive lung disease should be optimized as well. Chest physiotherapy consists of postural drainage, enhanced coughing maneuvers, chest vibration, and percussion. However, prospective studies are lacking for efficacy, and chest percussion is obviously not well tolerated in patients with thoracic trauma. Nasotracheal suctioning is reserved for patients unable to effectively mobilize their secretions.

26. Is there a benefit to high-flow oxygen in chest trauma?
High-flow oxygen combines an air/oxygen blender that traverses a heated circuit, and humidification applied to a patient through a nasal cannula. Oxygen flow rates of 60 L/min can be achieved with some mild positive end-expiratory pressure (PEEP) effect. Although there is a lack of randomized trial data, small retrospective studies have associated high-flow oxygen with decreased ICU and hospital LOSs. Furthermore, it has been correlated with a reduced incidence of ventilator-associated pneumonias and decreased rates of unplanned re-intubation. Although further research is needed, high-flow oxygen may be a first-line option for the patient with decreasing, but adequate pulmonary reserve.

27. Is there a role for noninvasive ventilatory strategies in patient with chest wall and pulmonary trauma?
Recent studies have shown that a significant number of patients with flail chest and/or pulmonary contusion can be safely and effectively managed with aggressive pulmonary care, including face mask oxygen, continuous positive airway pressure (CPAP), and chest physiotherapy. CPAP restores functional residual capacity, improves compliance, and stabilizes the flail segment until the underlying pulmonary contusion resolves. CPAP, compared with intermittent positive pressure ventilation, has also been shown to lower mortality and nosocomial infections in patients who required mechanical ventilation. Noninvasive ventilation is particularly attractive for the patient who initially does not require emergent intubation and may decrease the need for subsequent intubation. Contraindications include frank shock or head injury due to concern for aspiration. If noninvasive ventilation is implemented, then close monitoring is essential as patients may fail and require endotracheal intubation.

28. Do all patients with flail chest require mechanical ventilation?
    In a recent 2015 retrospective analysis of the National Trauma Database, up to 59% of patient with a flail injury require mechanical intubation. Early initiation of mechanical ventilation is essential in patients with refractory respiratory failure, shock, or other serious traumatic injuries.

29. What is the optimal mode of ventilation for patients with flail chest or pulmonary contusion?
    When required, mechanical ventilation should be tailored to maintain normal oxygenation while minimizing secondary lung injury. In patients with ARDS, lung protective ventilation strategies using a volume- and pressure-limited approach have resulted in reductions in mortality. This strategy is aimed at reducing further ventilator trauma. Many of the newer modes of ventilation are consistent with a lung protective strategy and have shown promising results, but data are lacking showing superiority.

30. What is the role of positive end-expiratory pressure in the management of blunt chest trauma?
    Providing a constant pressure throughout the respiratory cycle may recruit atelectatic lung regions and prevent the cyclic opening and closing of the alveoli, thereby reducing additional lung injury. Identifying optimal PEEP is complex, but in general the goal is to select a PEEP level that prevents derecruitment and allows for FiO_2 reduction. PEEP can have significant physiologic effects relevant to the trauma patient. Most notably, PEEP can significantly reduce venous return in the patient with hypovolemia. This can worsen hemodynamics in the setting of hemorrhagic shock. PEEP may also exacerbate ventilation-perfusion mismatch in patients with asymmetric pulmonary injury.

31. What are the indications for surgical stabilization of flail chest injuries?
    Prospective evidence in support of surgical rib fixation has emerged in recent trials comparing surgical options with medical management. Surgical fixation appears to decrease the likelihood of respiratory failure, pneumonia, and ICU LOS, although the data interpretation is limited by potential selection bias, heterogeneous patient populations, and variations in timing of interventions. In intubated patients, surgical stabilization is associated with decreased duration of mechanical ventilation and decreased need for tracheostomy. Proposed indications for rib fracture repair include flail chest; painful, movable rib fractures refractory to conventional pain management; chest wall deformity or defect; rib fracture non-union; and during thoracotomy for other traumatic indication (in stable patients). A variety of fixation methods have been proposed, including pins, plates, wires, and struts. Despite these reported benefits, stabilizations are seldom performed.

32. What is the long-term morbidity in flail chest injuries?
    Few long-term follow-up studies regarding disability after flail chest injury are available. Outcomes in patients with flail chest injuries with or without pulmonary contusion are difficult to delineate without accounting for the presence of other injuries. Patients with flail chest consistently report symptoms of chest tightness, pain, and decreased activity level. In a prospective study of 28 patients surviving severe chest injury, Livingston and Richardson found severe pulmonary dysfunction with pulmonary function tests (PFTs) at 40% to 50% of predicted within 2 weeks of hospital discharge, but a trend of marked improvement that continued out to at least 18 months after discharge, with PFTs 65% to 90% of predicted. Only 5% of patients met criteria for pulmonary disability.

ACKNOWLEDGMENT

The authors wish to acknowledge Drs. Susan R. Wilcox, MD, and Edward A. Bittner, MD, PhD, for the valuable contributions to the previous edition of this chapter.

KEY POINTS: THORACIC TRAUMA (FLAIL CHEST, AND PULMONARY AND MYOCARDIAL CONTUSION)

1. Blunt chest trauma is associated with 25% of trauma mortality.
2. Clinical suspicion is key to diagnosing BCI, as it may be clinically silent.
3. Echocardiography, transthoracic, or transesophageal, is a useful diagnostic tool in hemodynamically unstable patients with suspected BCI.
4. Asymptomatic patients with negative ECG findings and normal serum troponin levels may be safely discharged home after a short observation period.

5. Elderly patients with multiple rib fractures are at high risk for pulmonary complications.
6. Pulmonary contusions increase the risk for developing pneumonia and ARDS.
7. Management of flail chest or pulmonary contusion includes immediate assessment of airway, breathing, and circulation and, for stable patients, monitoring the respiratory status, pain control, lung physiotherapy, and early mobilization.
8. Fluid management for patients with pulmonary contusion entails adequate resuscitation to ensure end-organ perfusion followed by restriction of unnecessary fluid administration and diuresis, if necessary.
9. Lung protective ventilation should be used when patients with a flail chest or pulmonary contusion requiring mechanical ventilation.
10. Surgical rib fixation may be considered in carefully selected patients.

BIBLIOGRAPHY

1. Al-Hassani A, Abdulrahman H, Afifi I, et al. Rib fracture patterns predict thoracic chest wall and abdominal solid organ injury. *Am Surg.* 2010;76:888-891.
2. Bastos R, Calhoon JH, Baisden CE. Flail chest and pulmonary contusion. *Semin Thorac Cardiovasc Surg.* 2008;20: 39-45.
3. Battle CE, Hutchings H, Evans PA. Risk factors that predict mortality in patients with blunt chest wall trauma: a systematic review and meta-analysis. *Injury.* 2012;43:8-17.
4. Bulger EM, Edwards T, Klotz P, et al. Epidural analgesia improves outcome after multiple rib fractures. *Surgery.* 2004;136:426-430.
5. Carrier FM, Turgeon AF, Nicole PC, et al. Effect of epidural analgesia in patients with traumatic rib fractures: a systematic review and meta-analysis of randomized controlled trials. *Can J Anaesth.* 2009;56:230-242.
6. Hernandez G, Fernandez R, Lopez-Reina P, et al. Noninvasive ventilation reduces intubation in chest trauma-related hypoxemia: a randomized clinical trial. *Chest.* 2010;137:74-80.
7. Kiraly L, Schreiber M. Management of the crushed chest. *Crit Care Med.* 2010;38(suppl 9):S469-S477.
8. Livingston DH, Shogan B, John P, et al. CT diagnosis of rib fractures and the prediction of acute respiratory failure. *J Trauma.* 2008;64:905-911.
9. Nirula R, Mayberry JC. Rib fracture fixation: controversies and technical challenges. *Am Surg.* 2010;76:793-802.
10. Simon B, Ebert J, Bokhari F, et al. Practice management guideline for "pulmonary contusion—flail chest." *J Trauma.* 2012;73(5):S351-S361.
11. Langdorf MI, Medak AJ, Hendey GW, et al. Prevalence and clinical import of thoracic injury identified by chest computed tomography but not chest radiography in blunt trauma: multicenter prospective cohort study. *Ann Emerg Med.* 2015;66(6):589-600.
12. Bulger EM, Arneson MA, Mock CN, et al. Rib fractures in the elderly. *J Trauma.* 2000;48(6):1040-1047 [discussion: 1046-1047].
13. Bergeron E, Lavoie A, Clas D, et al. Elderly trauma patients with rib fractures are at greater risk of death and pneumonia. *J Trauma.* 2003;54(3):478-485.
14. Brasel KJ, Moore EE, Albrecht RA, et al. Management of rib fractures: A Western Trauma Association: Critical Decision algorithm. *J Trauma Acute Care Surg.* 2017;82:200-203. doi:10.1097/TA.0000000000001301.
15. Gaunt KA, Spilman SK, Halub ME, et al. High flow nasal cannula in a mixed adult ICU. *Respir Care.* 2015;60(10):1383-1389.
16. Pieracci F, Lin Y, Snyder M, et al. A prospective, controlled clinical evaluation of surgical stabilization of severe rib fractures. *J Trauma Acute Care Surg.* 2016;80(2):187-194.
17. Dehghan N, de Mestral C, McKee M, et al. Flail chest injuries: A review of outcomes and treatment practices from the national trauma data bank. *J Trauma Acute Care Surg.* 2014;76:462-468.
18. Marasco SF, Davies AR, Cooper J, et al. Prospective randomized controlled trial of operative Rib fixation in traumatic flail chest. *J Am Coll Surg.* 2013;216:924-932.
19. Cataneo AJ, Cataneo DC, de Oliveira FH. Surgical versus nonsurgical interventions for flail chest. *Cochrane Database Syst Rev.* 2015;(7):CD009919.
20. Bansal MK, Maraj S, Chewaproug D, et al. Myocardial contusion injury: redefining the diagnostic algorithm. *Emerg Med J.* 2005;22:465-469.
21. Chirillo F, Totis O, Cavarzerani A, et al. Usefulness of transthoracic and transoesophageal echocardiography in recognition and management of cardiovascular injuries after blunt chest trauma. *Heart.* 1996;75:301-306.
22. O'Connor J, Ditillo M, Scalea T. Penetrating cardiac injury. *J R Army Med Corps.* 2009;155:185-190.
23. Prêtre R, Chilcott M. Blunt trauma to the heart and great vessels. *N Engl J Med.* 1997;336:626-632.
24. Schultz JM, Trunkey DD. Blunt cardiac injury. *Crit Care Clin.* 2004;20:57-70.
25. Velmahos GC, Karaiskakis M, Salim A, et al. Normal electrocardiography and serum troponin I levels preclude the presence of clinically significant blunt cardiac injury. *J Trauma.* 2003;54:45-50 [discussion: 50-51].

CHAPTER 68

ACUTE ABDOMEN AND PERITONITIS

Alita Perez-Tamayo and William E. Charash

1. **What is an acute abdomen?**
   Any intra-abdominal process that classically presents with sudden, severe pain. Urgent intervention is warranted, often (but not always) surgical. Peritonitis (see below) may or may not be part of the "acute abdomen" process.

2. **What is peritonitis?**
   Inflammation of the thin membrane lining the abdominal cavity and covering the abdominal organs, also known as the peritoneum. The presence of peritonitis may be accompanied by symptoms of systemic sepsis. Peritonitis may be subdivided into two broad categories. Spontaneous (or primary) bacterial peritonitis occurs without any known source of contamination. Secondary bacterial peritonitis originates from visceral pathology or from external sources, such as iatrogenic introduction or penetrating injury.

   Peritonitis may be generalized across the abdomen, suggesting a diffuse process. When it is localized over a portion of the abdomen, it may suggest a focal or contained process. As a result, not all localized peritonitis necessarily requires immediate surgical intervention.

3. **How does peritonitis manifest itself clinically?**
   Peritonitis often presents as an acute abdomen. Aside from the findings of pain, tenderness, and distention, peritonitis is characterized by rebound tenderness, involuntary guarding, and in severe states, rigidity. Most physical findings of abdominal tenderness occur with displacement of the tissue. One of the distinguishing features of peritonitis is tenderness to changes in velocity of the tissue. This is called rebound tenderness. Historical features suggestive of rebound tenderness include discomfort with sudden movement. Tenderness to percussion is a form of rebound tenderness. Further, involuntary muscle guarding can often be appreciated as a wave of muscular contraction detected by the examiners finger following percussion.

   Physical findings of systemic infection can be present and may include fever, chills, tachycardia, diaphoresis, tachypnea, oliguria, and altered mental status. Due to the significant surface area of the peritoneum, peritonitis will generate significant third space fluid losses. Without proper resuscitation, these patients are susceptible to hypovolemia and circulatory collapse.

4. **What are some causes of acute abdomen in the critical care setting that require invasive intervention?**
   1. **Inflammatory: can include bacterial causes (e.g., diverticulitis, appendicitis, cholecystitis, infected pancreatic necrosis, intra-abdominal abscesses) or chemical (e.g., perforated gastric ulceration).** Perforations that are contained, in the absence of diffuse peritonitis, may be managed nonoperatively. One caveat is that necrotizing pancreatitis, particularly with ascites, may manifest as severe peritonitis with a systemic inflammatory response syndrome indistinguishable from diffuse abdominal sepsis. Distinguishing this from infected pancreatic necrosis presents a diagnostic challenge. Surgical consultation is recommended.
   2. **Vascular: mesenteric ischemia (e.g., thrombus, embolus, hypoperfusion), even in the absence of necrosis.**
   3. **Mechanical: typically obstructive conditions (e.g., incarcerated hernias, malrotation, small or large bowel obstruction).**
   4. **Traumatic: can be penetrating or blunt traumas, causing uncontrolled hemorrhage or bowel perforations.**

5. **Name some causes of acute abdomen that are initially treated medically but may ultimately require surgery.**
   Clostridium difficile colitis, inflammatory bowel disease, Ogilvie's syndrome, pancreatitis, diverticulitis, acute pelvic inflammatory disease, and nephrolithiasis.

6. Which causes of acute abdomen should not require surgery?
   Spontaneous bacterial peritonitis, regional gastroenteritis, ruptured ovarian follicle.

7. List thoracic conditions that can cause abdominal pain.
   Lower-lobe pneumonia, pulmonary embolism, pleuritis, empyema, ruptured esophagus, lower rib fractures, pericarditis, and myocardial infarction.

8. How does the initial evaluation of abdominal pain differ in critically ill patients?
   The history and physical examination, a mainstay of abdominal evaluation, is often limited as a consequence of the critically ill patient's depressed level of consciousness. In a critical care setting, multiple organ systems may be failing, leading to a broader differential of causes. Nonspecific findings such as unexplained sepsis, hypovolemia, and abdominal distension may suggest an acute abdomen.

9. Which laboratory tests are helpful in the setting of abdominal pain?
   An elevated hemoglobin or hematocrit may suggest third space fluid losses with hemoconcentration. A low hematocrit may indicate preexisting anemia or active hemorrhage. Elevated white blood cell (WBC) count, especially with left shift, suggests an inflammatory process. A low WBC count may be present if there is a viral process or gastroenteritis, or in the case of overwhelming sepsis. Metabolic acidosis on an arterial blood gas, or an elevated lactate, may indicate an ischemic abdominal process. It is important to note that an elevated lactic acid level does not always indicate an abdominal source, it rather can also reflect under-resuscitation. Elevated amylase and/or lipase may suggest pancreatitis. Amylase may also be elevated with gastric or intestinal pathology. Liver function tests can be helpful if a hepatobiliary process is suspected.

KEY POINT: ACUTE ABDOMEN AND PERITONITIS

Elevated amylase with normal lipase—consider penetrating peptic ulcer or a small intestinal process.

10. What imaging studies can aid in the diagnosis?
    1. Oral and intravenous contrast-enhanced abdominal/pelvic computed tomography (CT) scanning provides the greatest yield. The patient must be stable enough for transport. Contrast may also jeopardize renal function. Renal protection with intravenous (IV) fluid hydration is recommended for high-risk patients.
    2. Upright (or semi-upright) chest x-ray can demonstrate free air under diaphragm (hollow viscus perforation). Abdominal x-ray can demonstrate bowel distention with air/fluid levels (obstruction) or free air in decubitus positioning.
    3. Abdominal ultrasound can demonstrate free peritoneal fluid and in some cases, may diagnose the cause of the abdominal pain (e.g., cholecystitis, appendicitis).
    4. Angiography or CT-angiography can reveal occlusive vascular disease or active hemorrhage. Again, this requires a certain amount of hemodynamic stability and carries the risk of contrast-induced nephropathy.

11. What causes *Clostridium difficile* colitis?
    The pathogenic changes seen in *C. difficile* colitis (also known as pseudomembranous colitis) are a result of Toxin A and B production within the colon of the patient. *C. difficile* is the leading cause of nosocomially transmitted diarrhea and is spread in the fecal to oral route. Overgrowth of this bacteria occurs with concurrent depletion of normal flora, typically secondary to antibiotic use. Many of the contributing factors are within the control of the healthcare system. Risk factors for severe colitis include age greater than 60 years, residence in a chronic care facility, gastric acid suppression, immunosuppression, significant medical comorbidities, and duration/spectrum of antibiotic coverage.

12. How can *Clostridium difficile* colitis be prevented?
    Prevention is key. The spores that clostridia species form are resistant to the standard hand sanitizers that are routinely used. Contact precautions, with a gown and gloves, should be used when an active infection is suspected. Healthcare workers must wash their hands with soap and water after contact with patients and contaminated surfaces. Secondarily, healthy gut flora

decreases the risk of colitis if exposure occurs. Antibiotics alter this flora, and should always be used judiciously.

KEY POINTS: ACUTE ABDOMEN AND PERITONITIS

Prevention of *Clostridium Difficile* Infection
Every one of us must take ownership of this nosocomial epidemic! Wash your hands with soap and water!

13. How is *Clostridium difficile* colitis treated?
    Discontinue the inciting antibiotic as soon as possible. If antibiosis is still required, narrow the spectrum of coverage. Antibiotic therapy should then also be directed at *C. difficile*, with either metronidazole (IV or oral) or vancomycin (orally ± rectally). Do not use antimotility agents. There is new developing research in the use of probiotics for prevention and fecal transplants for cure of active infections.
    Surgical treatment with a subtotal colectomy with ileostomy is indicated for patients with fulminant colitis. Diffuse or persistent peritoneal signs, failure of improvement with antibiotic therapy, and signs of multiorgan failure all indicate the need for surgery.

14. What is Ogilvie syndrome?
    Ogilvie syndrome, also known as acute colonic pseudo-obstruction, is a massive dilation of the colon with an obstructive pattern, in the absence of mechanical obstruction. It is most prevalent in late middle age and is seen in association with a wide spectrum of illnesses including myocardial infarction, neurologic diseases, cancer, severe infections, metabolic alterations, surgery, and trauma.

15. How is Ogilvie syndrome treated?
    Initial treatment includes fasting, intravenous fluids, correction of electrolyte imbalances, and decreasing narcotic use. Patients should be ambulated, if possible. A rectal tube may also be helpful. A water-soluble enema and fluoroscopy may be diagnostic and therapeutic.
    If there is no resolution in 48 hours, or if cecal diameter exceeds 10 to 12 cm, pharmacologic treatment with 2.5 mg neostigmine given over 3 minutes may be therapeutic. You must rule out a mechanical cause of large bowel obstruction prior to administration of neostigmine. It is important to take into account the patient's cardiac and hemodynamic status as profound bradycardia and heart block may be encountered secondary to administration of neostigmine.
    Alternatively, or if this is not successful, colonoscopic decompression is indicated. This requires significant skill, as air insufflation must be avoided. Surgery is indicated in cases of actual or imminent perforation or in patients who have not responded to maximum nonsurgical measures.

16. What is intra-abdominal hypertension?
    Intra-abdominal hypertension (IAH) is defined as a sustained or repeated intra-abdominal pressure of at least 12 mm Hg.

17. How is intra-abdominal hypertension monitored?
    Most commonly by transducing the pressure in the urinary bladder. This can be done by aseptically inserting a needle (connected to a typical intensive care unit [ICU] pressure transducer) into the sampling port of a Foley catheter drainage tube, with a clamp placed distally from the side port. The pubic symphysis is used as a zero reference.
    Alternatively, the Foley tubing itself can be used as a manometer. As urinary specific gravity is close to 1, the height of the fluid column in centimeters needs to be multiplied by 0.74 to convert to mm Hg. A fixed volume (20–50 mL) of fluid is instilled into the urinary bladder to ensure a continuous column of fluid. With either method, the operator should observe respiratory variation in the measured pressure to confirm that one is transducing pressure within the abdomen.

18. What is abdominal compartment syndrome?
    Intra-abdominal pressure sustained above 20 mm Hg with associated end-organ dysfunction (renal dysfunction, ventilator failure, or intestinal ischemia).
    The acute abdomen, peritonitis, abdominal surgery, trauma, retroperitoneal bleeding, the systemic inflammatory response syndrome, and over-resuscitation with fluids are all risk factors for abdominal compartment syndrome.

KEY POINT: ACUTE ABDOMEN AND PERITONITIS

Abdominal Compartment Syndrome
Consider this diagnosis in all patients with organ failure and abdominal distention.

19. How is abdominal compartment syndrome managed?

    The goal is to decrease IAH. Consider decreasing intra-abdominal contents by minimizing intake, as well as nasogastric tube or rectal tube placement. Avoid over-resuscitation with IV fluids. Optimize sedation and analgesia. Neuromuscular blockade may be used, if necessary. Prolonged requirement for neuromuscular blockade should prompt invasive intervention. Percutaneous catheter drainage of free intra-abdominal fluid, air, abscess, or blood may be effective if more conservative measures are proving to be ineffective. Surgical decompression is indicated when a patient has refractory end organ dysfunction, despite the management above. The open abdomen that is created is then typically managed with some form of negative pressure dressing until it is safe to definitively close the abdomen.

20. How is acalculous cholecystitis managed?

    The definitive treatment for cholecystitis is a cholecystectomy. However, patients with acalculous cholecystitis are often unfit for surgery due to their comorbidities. Percutaneous cholecystostomy is a minimally invasive alternative that is appropriate for most critically ill patients.

21. When should an abdominal abscess be suspected?

    The presence of an abdominal abscess should be considered in patients with fever, leukocytosis, and/or sepsis who have sustained blunt abdominal trauma, are recovering from abdominal surgery, or are undergoing medical treatment for complex peritonitis.

22. Describe the management of nonocclusive mesenteric ischemia.

    Nonexclusive mesenteric ischemia is most commonly a result of bowel hypoperfusion secondary to splanchnic vasoconstriction. To ensure adequate blood flow, intravascular volume status must be optimized through IV fluids or blood products, depending on the cause of hypovolemia. Broad-spectrum IV antibiotics, bowel rest, and nasogastric tube (NGT) decompression is initiated. Vasopressin and alpha-adrenergic drugs should be avoided. Beta-adrenergic agonism might be required. Surgery is reserved for patients with transmural necrosis or perforation. Thus far, there has not been a proven benefit to heparin or vasodilator infusions.

23. How is occlusive mesenteric ischemia managed?

    The strategy described above for nonocclusive mesenteric ischemia should be already employed. Once occlusive mesenteric ischemia is diagnosed, emergent intervention is necessary. Primary percutaneous embolectomy or thrombolysis may be an option when perforation and necrosis are not suspected. Emergent laparotomy is indicated if bowel gangrene or perforation is suspected. Necrotic bowel should be resected and restoration of blood flow via embolectomy or mesenteric revascularization should be performed. A second-look laparotomy is often planned following the initial surgery. The provider should consider anticoagulation in this population pre- and postoperatively.

24. Does the differential diagnosis in immunocompromised patients with acute abdomen vary from immunocompetent patients?

    Immunocompromised patients may suffer from the same diseases as immunocompetent patients. However, they may present with atypical symptoms such as altered mental status and tachycardia and lack the classic signs of an acute abdomen because of their blunted immune response. However, in this patient population, the differential diagnosis should be expanded to include cytomegalovirus infection, opportunistic infections, neutropenic enterocolitis, and drug toxicity.

25. Which antibiotics should be used for intra-abdominal infections?

    Empiric broad-spectrum antimicrobial therapy should be administered as soon as possible in the critically ill patient. It is good practice to obtain urine, sputum/bronchial lavage, and blood cultures prior to administration of antibiotics. Antibiotics with broad-spectrum activity against gram-negative organism in combination with metronidazole should be used for patients with high-severity community-acquired intra-abdominal infection. For infection that is hospital-acquired, the regimen should be based by local microbiologic results. Methicillin resistant *Staphylococcus aureus* (MRSA) and enterococcus coverage is often appropriate in this population. Antifungal therapy should be considered in esophageal and gastric perforations, as well as in the immunocompromised population. As culture sensitivities result, coverage of the antibiotic treatment should be narrowed.

26. What should the duration of antibiotic treatment be?

Antibiotic duration varies with severity of the infection and whether source control/drainage was achieved. In complicated intra-abdominal sepsis, if the contaminated material is cleared from the abdominal cavity, a 4- to 5-day course of antibiosis is sufficient, given resolution of fever and leukocytosis. Treatment for surgically treated uncomplicated acute appendicitis should be prophylactic only and not last more than 24 hours. Acute stomach and proximal jejunal perforation with source control within 24 hours in the absence of acid-reducing therapy or malignancy require only 24 hours of coverage for aerobic gram-positive cocci.

27. What is the significance of diarrhea following abdominal aortic aneurysm (AAA) repair?

Evacuation of the colon (with or without bloody mucous) in the immediate postoperative period is highly concerning for ischemic colitis. Bedside procto-sigmoidoscopy should be immediately performed to assess for mucosal edema, sloughing, or necrosis. The majority of affected patients do not have symptoms of abdominal pain and a minority have blood in their stool.

Melena or hematochezia in a patient with a more distant history of AAA repair could signify aorto-enteric fistula.

28. How does the management of small bowel obstruction differ from large bowel obstruction?

Small bowel obstructions may be managed expectantly with nasogastric tube decompression, bowel rest, and IV fluids. The obstruction is often due to adhesive disease which responds well to bowel decompression. Even if pursing nonsurgical management, serial abdominal exams are indicated. Surgery is appropriate if the small bowel obstruction fails to resolve or if there is a closed-loop obstruction.

A large bowel obstruction may require more urgent surgical intervention. The obstruction in large bowel is often due to the presence of a tumor narrowing the lumen distally. Also, a competent ileocecal valve does not allow for relief of colonic pressure. The built-up pressure may result in gangrene and/ or perforation, particularly of the cecum.

29. What cecal diameter is worrisome for impending perforation?

An acute distension to 12 to 14 cm puts a patient at risk for ischemic necrosis and perforation.

KEY POINTS: ACUTE ABDOMEN AND PERITONITIS

Follow cecal diameter with serial abdominal x-rays. Acute cecal distention to greater than 12 cm in the setting of worsening abdominal exams may demand immediate intervention.

---

30. When should surgery be considered for acute pancreatitis?

There are three major indications for surgical intervention in acute pancreatitis. Hemorrhage can occur secondary to erosion into a regional blood vessel or due to splenic rupture following splenic vein thrombosis. Necrosis or perforation of an adjacent hollow viscus may also occur. Open debridement of the pancreas is indicated in the setting of infected pancreatic necrosis or symptomatic sterile necrosis. Debridement for necrotizing pancreatitis in the absence of infection is rarely undertaken because of the high morbidity and mortality of operative intervention without compelling evidence of benefit. The goal of surgical debridement is to excise the necrotic tissue, preserve viable pancreas, prevent adjacent organ damage, and minimize fistula formations. Abdominal decompression through midline laparotomy or catheter drainage of significant fluid collections may be required if abdominal compartment syndrome develops, but should be avoided if possible.

31. When is early surgical consultation warranted?

Surgery should be consulted if there is reasonable suspicion that a patient's condition will ultimately require surgical management, even if surgical intervention is not yet required. A worsening abdominal exam with increasing distension and development of peritoneal signs may signal the need for surgical involvement. An open collaborative relationship between consulting services should be fostered.

ACKNOWLEDGMENT

The authors wish to acknowledge Dr. Sarah Pesek, MD, for the valuable contributions to the previous edition of this chapter.

BIBLIOGRAPHY

1. Bhangu A, Søreide K, Di Saverio S, et al. Acute appendicitis: modern understanding of pathogenesis, diagnosis, and management. *Lancet.* 2015;386(10000):1278-1287.
2. Bobo LD, Dubberke ER. Recognition and prevention of hospital-associated enteric infections in the intensive care unit. *Crit Care Med.* 2010;38(suppl 8):S324-S334.
3. Champagne BJ, Darling RC 3rd, Daneshmand M, et al. Outcome of aggressive surveillance colonoscopy in ruptured abdominal aortic aneurysm. *J Vasc Surg.* 2004;39(4):792-796.
4. Cheatham ML. Abdominal compartment syndrome. *Curr Opin Crit Care.* 2009;15(2):154-162.
5. Chen EH, Mills AM. Abdominal pain in special populations. *Emerg Med Clin North Am.* 2011;29(2):449-458.
6. De Giorgio R, Knowles CH. Acute colonic pseudo-obstruction. *Br J Surg.* 2009;96(3):229-239.
7. Frossard JL, Steer ML, Pastor CM. Acute pancreatitis. *Lancet.* 2008;371(9607):143-152.
8. Heinlen L, Ballard JD. Clostridium difficile infection. *Am J Med Sci.* 2010;340(3):247-252.
9. Kolkman JJ, Mensink PB. Non-occlusive mesenteric ischaemia: a common disorder in gastroenterology and intensive care. *Best Pract Res Clin Gastroenterol.* 2003;17(3):457-473.
10. Renner P, Kienle K, Dahlke MH, et al. Intestinal ischemia: current treatment concepts. *Langenbecks Arch Surg.* 2011; 396(1):3-11.
11. Rodriguez JR, Razo AO, Targarona J, et al. Debridement and closed packing for sterile or infected necrotizing pancreatitis: insights into indications and outcomes in 167 patients. *Ann Surg.* 2008;247(2):294-299.
12. Solomkin JS, Mazuski JE, Bradley JS, et al. Diagnosis and management of complicated intra-abdominal infection in adults and children: guidelines by the Surgical Infection Society and the Infectious Diseases Society of America. *Surg Infect (Larchmt).* 2010;11(1):79-109.
13. Stoker J, van Randen A, Laméris W, et al. Imaging patients with acute abdominal pain. *Radiology.* 2009;253(1):31-46.
14. Trevisani GT, Hyman NH, Church JM. Neostigmine: safe and effective treatment for acute colonic pseudo-obstruction. *Dis Colon Rectum.* 2000;43(5):599-603.

CHAPTER 69

ORGAN DONATION

Benjamin T. Suratt and Kapil Patel

1. Who governs the rules and regulations for organ donation?
   - The Organ Procurement and Transplantation Network (OPTN) is a system for operating and monitoring the unbiased allocation, through established medical criteria, of organs donated for transplantation and maintaining a recipients' waiting list (including the listing and delisting of recipients).
   - The United Network for Organ Sharing (UNOS) is a nonprofit organization awarded the contract by the Department of Health and Human Services in 1986 to implement the OPTN.
   - Organ Procurement Organizations (OPO) serve specific regions in the country for clinical services including working with hospital staff to maintain donor-organ function, working with UNOS to match donor organs with recipients, coordinating organ recovery surgery, and giving compassionate and professional support to donors' families.

2. Who can be a potential organ donor?
   Potential for organ or tissue donation has few absolute contraindications: human immunodeficiency virus (HIV) infection, active hepatitis B virus infection, active visceral or hematologic neoplasm, or active bacterial infection, with no age limitation (see below). Appropriateness for donation is assessed when the occasion arises. The majority of cases that are considered for organ donation occur within the intensive care unit (ICU). Despite severe organ shortage, no set universal protocol exists for organ donation. It is at the discretion of the intensivist to consider cases for organ donation. If a case is considered, then the next step is to notify the local OPO, which will then gather data and discuss the critical care management with the regional organ donation specialist, usually an intensivist.
   The general rule for the possibility for organ donation is that there should be no evidence of end-organ damage (e.g., acute tubular necrosis, myocardial depression, or pneumonia), with the final decision per the accepting transplant center.

3. Should high-risk behavior associated with human immunodeficiency virus, seronegative, patients be considered organ donors?
   The Public Health Service has identified persons at risk of having HIV infection based on behavioral risks. Pooled HIV incidence estimates were calculated for each category of high-risk donor behavior and used to determine the risk of "window period" HIV infection. The estimated risk per 10,000 donors, using nucleic acid testing (NAT), is 4.9 for injection drug users, 4.2 in men who have sex with men, 2.7 in commercial sex workers, 0.9 in incarcerated donors, 0.6 in donors exposed to HIV-infected blood within the past 12 months, 0.3 in donors engaging in high-risk sex within the past 12 months, and 0.035 in hemophiliacs. Routine testing using NAT is OPO-dependent based on availability of turn-around time of results and relatively high cost. Ultimately, it is the decision of the transplant team and recipient to weigh the risk versus benefit.

4. Should hepatitis C or B seropositive patients be considered for organ donation?
   Donors who are seropositive hepatitis C are suitable organ donors for recipients positive for hepatitis C virus. On the contrary, patients' positive with hepatitis B virus core-antibody and negative for surface antigen are considered acceptable organ donors for all recipients. Given small risk for transmission, oral antiviral agents are used postoperatively for 1 year.

5. Does malignancy exclude the possibility of organ donation?
   Over the past four decades, the Israel Penn International Transplant Tumor Registry has collected transplantation outcomes data for organs for donors with known or incidentally discovered non-central nervous system malignancies. Although this registry has been collected from voluntary reporting of index cases of transmission and may therefore fail to appreciate the entire at-risk population of recipients who did not develop malignancy, it suggests that choriocarcinoma (93%), melanoma (74%), and lung cancer (43%) have high transmission rates. Therefore, patients with these malignancies are considered unacceptable for organ donation. In addition, renal cell carcinoma appears to have a

transmission rate of 63%, except in low-grade tumors (<2.5 cm) free of extracapsular or vascular invasion and excised prior to transplantation, which showed no risk of cancer transmission. Patients with central nervous system malignancies with the certain risk factors (high-grade tumors [III–IV], or prior craniotomy, systemic chemotherapy/radiation therapy, or ventriculoperitoneal or ventriculoatrial shunts) carry a 53% chance of donor tumor transmission compared to 7% in the absence of risk factors.

In 2003, the consensus conference of the American Society of Transplant Surgeons approved the use of organs from donors with T1 colon cancer and a minimum of 1-year disease-free interval for white male donors and 5 years for female donors, independent of race. However, organs are not recommended for transplantation in the African American men with early stage colon due to the aggressive nature of colon cancer in this population. Organs from donors with early stage breast cancers (ductal carcinoma in situ and lobular carcinoma in situ) are approved transplantation due to a low transmission rate of cancer in the setting.

6. Are outcomes following transplantation of organs procured from bacteremic donors worse?
   There appears to be no increase in morbidity, mortality, or graft dysfunction following transplantation of organs from donors found to be bacteremic at the time of organ procurement, as long as transplanted recipients receive appropriate antibiotics for approximately 7 to 14 days following transplantation.

7. Which organs can be donated?
   • Organs: kidney, heart, lung, liver, pancreas, and the intestines. Of note, combined organ transplantations (kidney-pancreas, heart-lung, other transplant) can be performed.
   • Tissue: corneas, the middle ear, skin, heart valves, bones, veins, cartilage, tendons, and ligaments.

8. What is the current standard for organ donation?
   Organ transplantation is guided by the overarching ethical requirement known as the "dead donor rule," which simply states that patients must be declared dead before the removal of any vital organs for transplantation. Most organ donation occurs in the setting of donors who are declared brain dead. However, despite efforts to promote organ donation, an enormous shortage of available organs for transplant continues to exist. As a result, efforts have been undertaken to expand the settings in which organs may become available (i.e., donation after cardiac death [DCD]; see later). See Boxes 69.2, 69.3, and 69.4 and Tables 69.1 and 69.2.

9. What are the currently acceptable deceased organ donation pathways?
   1. Donation after brain death (DBD) follows the confirmation of death by neurological criteria (Box 69.1). See also Boxes 69.2, 69.3, and 69.4 and Tables 69.1 and 69.2. In DBD, donors are declared dead but given continued support as needed prior to organ procurement to improve donor organ viability (see below).

Box 69-1. Brain Death Criteria

• Unresponsiveness or coma
• Core body temperature (≥32°C)
• Absence of cerebral motor responses to pain in all extremities
• Absence of brainstem reflexes, that is, pupillary, oculocephalic *(doll's eyes)*, vestibulo-ocular (cold calorics), corneal, gag, and cough reflexes
• Apnea test (see Boxes 69.2, 69.3, and 69.4)
• Exclusion of conditions that may confound clinical assessment of brain death, that is, metabolic or endocrine abnormality or drug intoxication

---

Box 69-2. Prerequisites for Performing the Apnea Test

Core body temperature ≥36.5°C
Systolic blood pressure ≥90 mm Hg (may use intravenous fluids or dopamine to achieve)
Eucapnia ($PaCO_2$ approximately 40 mm Hg) if possible
Normoxemia (PaO_2 ≥200 mm Hg) if possible (typically 10 min at an FiO_2 of 1.0 will achieve)

FiO₂, Fraction of inspired oxygen.

Box 69-3. Apnea Test

1. Patient is disconnected from the ventilator.
2. Oxygen cannula is placed at the level of carina, and 100% oxygen is delivered at a rate of 6 L/min.
3. Patient is observed for respiratory movements (e.g., chest or abdominal excursions).
4. Arterial PaO_2, $PaCO_2$, and pH are measured after approximately 8 min.
5. Patient is reconnected to the ventilator.

Box 69-4. Interpretation of Apnea Test Results

Confirmatory results: No respiratory movements witnessed with resultant arterial PCO_2 ≥60 mm Hg (or 20 mm Hg increase in PCO_2 over pretest baseline)

    Contradictory results: Any evidence of respiratory movements (regardless of PCO_2 level)

    Inconclusive results: No respiratory movements and PCO_2 ≤ 60 mm Hg. Apnea test may be repeated within 10 min.

    If cardiovascular or pulmonary instability occurs during the test (i.e., systolic blood pressure ≤90 mm Hg, dysrhythmia, or arterial oxygen desaturation), arterial blood gas value is immediately obtained, and the patient is reconnected to the ventilator. Alternative confirmatory testing to determine brain death (see Table 69.1) is then performed at the discretion of physician.

Table 69-1. Confirmatory Brain Death Testing

ELECTROENCEPHALOGRAPHY	NO ELECTRICAL ACTIVITY FOR A PERIOD OF 30 MIN
Cerebral angiography	No intracerebral filling at the level of the carotid bifurcation or circle of Willis Patent external carotid circulation
Transcranial Doppler sonography	No diastolic or reverberating flow Systolic-only or retrograde diastolic flow Small systolic peaks in early systole
Somatosensory evoked potential	Bilateral absence of response to medial nerve stimulation
Cerebral scintigraphy (technetium Tc 99 m brain scan)	No uptake of radionuclide in brain parenchyma *(hollow skull phenomenon)*
Magnetic resonance imaging	Not yet determined

---

2. Controlled DCD follows the planned withdrawal of life-sustaining treatments and subsequent confirmation of death using cardiorespiratory criteria. In DCD, only donors that are declared dead within 60 minutes of care withdrawal undergo organ procurement (immediately following cardiac death) to reduce donor organ injury. Potential donors who survive longer than 60 minutes following withdrawal of care are excluded from organ donation and receive usual comfort care measures until death.
3. Uncontrolled DCD follows an unexpected cardiac arrest and death is confirmed using cardiorespiratory criteria after resuscitation efforts have been unsuccessful. However, given ethical issues within the United States, uncontrolled DCD is being performed internationally.

10. Is donation after cardiac death ethically appropriate?

A national conference on DCD in 2005 concluded that it is "an ethically acceptable practice of end-of-life care, capable of increasing the number of deceased-donor organs available for transplantation." This national conference affirmed the ethical propriety of DCD as not violating the "dead donor rule."

Table 69-2. Comparison of Donation After Brain Death and Donation After Cardiac Death

	DONATION AFTER BRAIN DEATH	DONATION AFTER CARDIAC DEATH
Cause of illness (e.g., anoxic, trauma, stroke)	Severe irreversible brain injury Does meet criteria of brain death	Severe irreversible brain injury Does not meet criteria of brain death
Organ procurement process	Physician (non–transplant team) declares brain death	Family elects withdrawal of life support
	Referral to OPO	Referral to OPO
	Await OR time for organ procurement	Withdrawal of life support in the OR or ICU
	Transplant team retrieves organs	Physician (non–transplant team) declares cardiac death
	Heart, lungs, kidneys, liver, pancreas, and/or intestines are transplantable	Transplant team waits 5 min after cardiac death is declared before procuring organs
		Transplant team retrieves organs
		Kidney, pancreas, and liver are generally transplantable

ICU, Intensive care unit; *OPO*, organ procurement organizations; *OR*, operating room.
Modified from Organ Donation After Cardiac Death. Madison, WI, University of Wisconsin Organ Procurement Organization; 2009.

11. **What is the probability of death within 60 minutes in a controlled donation after cardiac death?**
The University of Wisconsin developed a tool for assessing the probability of donor death within 60 minutes of the withdrawal of care using donor response to a 10-minute cessation of mechanical ventilation (Table 69.3). Using these criteria, they were able to predict organ suitability for DCD in 83.7% of the cases in 60 minute period and 74.4% of the cases in 120 minute period. Time frame is dependent on transplant team and hospital policy.
    Prospectively validated criteria were used to develop criteria predictive of death within 60 minutes by the UNOS DCD consensus committee (Table 69.4).
    Either of these criteria is acceptable and center specific.

12. **What is the sequela of brain death on other organs?**
Progressive central nervous system ischemia results in various pathophysiologic changes. Ischemia of the cerebrum results in vagal activation leading to bradycardia and hypotension. Cushing reflex, which is a mixed vagal and sympathetic response, presents as bradycardia and hypertension, and is a direct result of ischemia of the Pons. Finally, ischemia of the medulla results in an autonomic sympathetic surge, which is an attempt to maintain cerebral perfusion pressure. Autonomic sympathetic surge manifests as an intense catecholamine surge directly increasing systemic vascular resistance, which leads to a decrease in left ventricular output and an increase in left atrial pressure. Redistribution of blood volume from profound vasoconstriction leads to an increase in venous return, leading to pulmonary hypertensive crisis.
    Subsequent brainstem herniation, should it occur, results in spinal cord sympathetic deactivation, low cardiac output, and systemic vasodilatation with resulting shock state.
    Plasma levels of adrenocorticotrophic hormone, cortisol, vasopressin, triiodothyronine, and thyroxine are reduced from damage to the hypothalamus and pituitary gland. Nearly 80% of brainstem-dead organ donors develop diabetes insipidus.

13. **What are the effects of brain death on hemodynamics?**
Hemodynamic collapse following the cessation of all brain function is complex. Contributing factors include hypovolemia secondary to the treatment of intracranial hypertension, diabetes insipidus and/or

Table 69-3. University of Wisconsin Donation after Cardiac Death Evaluation Tool

CRITERIA	ASSIGNED POINTS	PATIENT SCORE
Spontaneous Respirations After 10 Min		
Rate >12	1	
Rate <12	3	
TV >200 cc	1	
TV <200 cc	3	
NIF >20	1	
NIF <20	3	
No spontaneous respirations	9	
BMI		
<25	1	
25–29	2	
>30	3	
Vasopressors		
No vasopressors	1	
Single vasopressor	2	
Multiple vasopressors	3	
Patient Age		
0–30	1	
31–50	2	
51+	3	
Intubation		
Endotracheal tube	3	
Tracheostomy	1	
Oxygenation After 10 Min		
O_2 sat >90%	1	
O_2 sat 80%–89%	2	
O_2 sat <79%	3	
	Final Score	
Date of extubation	Time of extubation	
Date of expiration	Time of expiration	
	Total Time	

8 to 12 high risk for continuing to breathe after extubation.
13 to 18 moderate risk for continuing to breathe after extubation.
19 to 24 low risk for continuing to breathe after extubation.
BMI, body mass index; TV, tidal volume; NIF, negative inspiratory force.

hyperglycemia-induced osmotic diuresis, cardiac dysfunction from thyroid hormone imbalance, and vasodilation due to reduction in sympathetic outflow and the onset of neurogenic vasoplegia.

14. What is the approach of donation after brain death management in the intensive care unit?
    1. Cardiovascular
       a. In the setting of circulatory shock, strongly consider cardiovascular monitoring (e.g., pulmonary artery catheter vs. serial echocardiogram).

Table 69-4. United Network for Organ Sharing Consensus Committee Criteria for Prediction of Death Within 60 Min of Withdrawal of Life-Sustaining Treatment

RESPIRATORY SUPPORT CRITERIA

Apnea
Respiratory rate <8 or >30 breaths per minute
Positive end-expiratory pressure ≥ 10 and $SaO_2 \leq 92\%$
$FiO_2 \geq 0.5$ and $SaO_2 \leq 92\%$

CIRCULATORY SUPPORT CRITERIA

Left or right ventricular assist device
Venoarterial or venovenous extracorporeal membrane oxygenation
Dopamine ≥ 15 μg/kg per minute
Norepinephrine or phenylephrine ≥ 0.2 μg/kg per minute
Pacemaker unassisted heart rate <30
IABP 1:1 or Dobutamine or dopamine ≥ 10 μg/kg per minute and CI ≤ 2.2 L/min per m^2
IABP 1:1 and CI ≤ 1.5 L/min per m^2

LIKELIHOOD OF DEATH WITHIN 60 MIN		
0	Criteria	29%
1	Criteria	52%
2	Criteria	65%
3	Criteria	82%
4–5	Criteria	76%

CI, Cardiac index; *IABP*, intra-aortic balloon pump; *SaO₂*, arterial oxygen saturation.

  b. Target mean arterial pressure greater than or equal to 60 mm Hg.
  c. If hypovolemia is suspected, consider crystalloid (e.g., 0.9% normal saline or lactated Ringers) or colloid (e.g., albumin 5%) bolus.
  d. There is insufficient data to recommend a vasopressor or inotrope of choice in nonhypovolemic shock. However, dopamine (which cohort studies suggest improves subsequent kidney and cardiac graft function) and vasopressin (which maybe preferred in the setting of diabetes insipidus) are considered favorable agents.
  e. Avoid high doses norepinephrine and phenylephrine, if possible, because alpha properties may be detrimental to cardiac function.
  f. In resistant hypotension, consider thyroid hormone replacement (see below).
2. Respiratory
  a. Use protective lung ventilation: tidal volume 6 to 8 mL/kg and positive end-expiratory pressure (PEEP) 5 to 8 cm H$_2$0.
  b. Target a pH 7.35 to 7.45, PaO$_2$ greater than or equal to 80 mm Hg, and PaCO 35 to 45 mm Hg.
  c. Institute "ventilator care bundle" (e.g., head of bed elevation, thromboembolism prophylaxis).
  d. Consider ventilator recruitment maneuvers, if atelectasis-related hypoxia is suspected.
3. Fluids and electrolytes
  a. Avoid hypernatremia (goal sodium <155 mEq/L), which has been shown to be detrimental to liver allograft function.
  b. Maintain urine output 0.5 to 2.5 mL/kg per hour with fluid infusion and pressors as needed.
  c. Monitor for diabetes insipidus (suggested by urine output >4 mL/kg per hour, low urine osmolality, and serum hypernatremia).
    i. If hypotensive, consider vasopressin (0.01–0.04 IU/min).
    ii. If normotensive, consider desmopressin (initial dose of 1–4 μg intravenous [IV]; dependent on response, may repeat or continue 1–2 μg IV q6.).
4. Hormone replacement
  a. Consider giving methylprednisolone IV (may consider and center-dependent on preference 250–1000 mg) after brain death is confirmed to aid in reducing inflammation and improving donor graft function.
  b. If donor is hemodynamically unstable despite vasopressors, or in potential cardiac donors with reduced left ventricular ejection fraction ($<45\%$), consider thyroid hormone

replacement: triiodothyronine (T3) 4.0 μg IV bolus followed by 4 μg/h infusion or levothyroxine (T4) 20 μg IV bolus followed by 10 μg/h infusion.

   c. Hyperglycemia management per institutional guidelines as for other critically ill patients

15. What are some of the statistics for organ donation and transplantation?
   • Every 11 minutes, a patient is added to the transplant waiting list (e.g., lung, kidney, heart).
   • Every day, approximately 75 patients receive an organ transplant. Yet every day approximately 20 patients die waiting for a transplant.
   • As of May 4, 2009, the percentage of recipients who were still living 5 years after solid organ transplantation was as follows.
      • Kidney: 69.3%
      • Heart: 74.9%
      • Liver: 73.8%
      • Lung: 54.4%
   • In 2008, 60% of living donors were women. Sixty percent of deceased donors were men.
   • In 2008, 67% of all deceased donors were white, 16% were black, 14% Hispanic, and 2.5% Asian.
   • As of November 2010, patients on the national waiting list were 45% white, 29% black, 18% Hispanic, and 6% Asian.
   • In 2007 (the most recent data), nearly 2.5 million people died in the United States. Yet only 8085 of these people donated their organs.
   • OPTN data show a progressive increase in the rate of organ recovery from DCD donors (844 DCD donors in 2008 compared with 268 in 2003).
   • Currently, more than 86 million people in the United States have indicated a wish to become a donor. Although impressive at first, this still will not be nearly enough to address the growing demand (see Fig. 69.1).

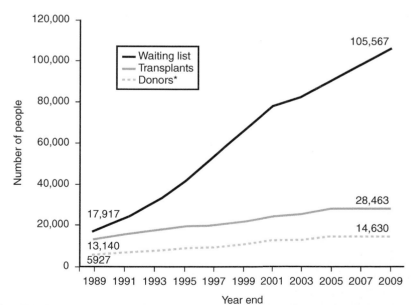

Figure 69-1. Over the past two decades, the gap between the number of patients waiting for a transplant and the number receiving a transplant has continued to widen. The substantial difference between the number of donors and the number of patients waiting for a transplant is one factor that contributes to waiting time from listing to transplantation. *Data include deceased and living donors. (From the University of Wisconsin Organ Procurement Organization: organdonor. gov/aboutStatsFacts.asp.)

KEY POINTS: ORGAN DONATION

1. All patients with impending brain death or withdrawal of care should be screened for the possibility of organ donation.
2. To diagnose brain death, all confounding factors must be excluded.
3. DCD is an ethically acceptable manner in which terminally ill patients can be considered for organ donation.
4. Hemodynamic collapse has resulted in exclusion of approximately 25% of potential organs donated.
5. Strategies in the ICU, optimizing the management of donors after brain death, can increase the number of organs available for transplantation.
6. Implementing protocols for DCD.
7. The gap between those patients awaiting transplants and those donating organs is widening exponentially—the vast majority of those on the transplant list will die waiting.

WEBSITES

Association of Organ Procurement Organizations: aopo.org
Organ Procurement and Transplantation Network: optn.transplant.hrsa.gov
United Network for Organ Sharing: unos.org
U.S. Government Information on Organ and Tissue Donation and Transplantation: organdonor.gov

BIBLIOGRAPHY

1. Bernat JL, D'Alessandro AM, Port FK, et al. Report of a national conference on donation after cardiac death. *Am J Transplant.* 2006;6:281-291.
2. Cypel M, Sato M, Yildirim E, et al. Initial experience with lung donation after cardiocirculatory death in Canada. *J Heart Lung Transplant.* 2009;28:753-758.
3. Truog RD, Miller FG. The dead donor rule and organ transplantation. *N Engl J Med.* 2008;359:674-675.
4. Wijdicks EF, Varelas PN, Gronseth GS, et al. Evidence-based guideline update: determining brain death in adults: report of the Quality Standards Subcommittee of the American Academy of Neurology. *Neurology.* 2010;74:1911-1918.
5. Steinbrook R. Organ Donation after Cardiac Death. *NEJM.* 2007;357:209-213.
6. Shah VR. Aggressive Management of Multiorgan Donor. *Transplant Proc.* 2008;40:1087-1090.
7. Lewis J, Peltier J, Nelson H, et al. Development of the University of Wisconsin donation after cardiac death evaluation tool. *Prog Transplant.* 2003;13:265-273.
8. DeVita MA, Brooks MM, Zawistowski C, et al. Donors after cardiac death: validation of identification criteria (DVIC) study for predictors of rapid death. *Am J Transplant.* 2008;8:432-441.
9. Citerio G, Cypel M, Dobb GJ, et al. Organ donation in adults: a critical care perspective. *Intensive Care Med.* 2016;42:305-315.
10. Kotloff RM, Blosser S, Fulda GJ, et al. Management of the potential organ donor in the ICU: Society of Critical Care Medicine/American College of Chest Physicians/Association of Organ Procurement Organizations Consensus Statement. *Crit Care Med.* 2015;43:1291-1325.
11. Kotsch K, Ulrich F, Reutzel-Selke A, et al. Methylprednisolone therapy in deceased donors reduces inflammation in the donor liver and improves outcome after liver transplantation: a prospective randomized controlled trial. *Ann Surg.* 2008;248:1042-1050.
12. Follette DM, Rudich SM, Babcook WD. Improved oxygenation and increased lung donor recovery with high-dose steroid administration after brain death. *J Heart Lung Transplant.* 1998;17:423-429.
13. Buell JF, Beebe TM, Trofe J, et al. Donor transmitted malignancies. *Ann Transplant.* 2004;9:53-56.
14. Buell JF, Trofe J, Sethuraman G, et al. Donors with central nervous system malignancies: are they truly safe? *Transplantation.* 2003;76:340-343.
15. Zibari GB, Lipka J, Zizzi H, et al. The use of contaminated donor organs in transplantation. *Clin Transplant.* 2000;14:397-400.
16. Freeman RB, Giatras I, Falagas ME, et al. Outcome of transplantation of organs procured from bacteremic donors. *Transplantation.* 1999;68:1107-1111.
17. Theodoropoulos N, Jaramillo A, Ladner DP, et al. Deceased organ donor screening for HIV, hepatitis B and hepatitis C viruses: a survey of organ procurement organization practices. *Am J Transplant.* 2013;13:2186-2190.
18. Seem DL, Lee I, Umscheid CA, et al. PHS guideline for reducing human immunodeficiency virus, hepatitis B virus, and hepatitis C virus transmission through organ transplantation. *Public Health Rep.* 2013;128:247-343.
19. Kucirka LM, Sarathy H, Govindan P, et al. Risk of window period HIV infection in high infectious risk donors: systemic review and meta-analysis. *Am J Transplant.* 2011;11:1176-1187.
20. Dhillon GS, Levitt J, Mallidi H, et al. Impact of hepatitis B core antibody positive donors in lung and heart-lung transplantation: an analysis of the United Network for Organ Sharing Database. *Transplantation.* 2009;88:842-846.

CHAPTER 70

DISASTER MEDICINE, BIOTERRORISM AND EBOLA

Jean Kwo and Daniel W. Johnson

1. **What is disaster medicine?**
   A medical disaster occurs when the destructive effects of natural or man-made forces overwhelm the ability of a given area or community to meet the demand for healthcare. Disaster medicine encompasses the provision of care to survivors of disasters as well as leadership in disaster preparation, disaster planning, disaster response, and disaster recovery.

2. **What are the two general categories of disasters?**
   Natural and man-made are the two categories of disasters.

3. **What are the most commonly encountered disasters?**
   Floods, hurricanes, earthquakes, industrial accidents, acts of terror, and epidemic outbreaks of communicable diseases.

4. **Who assumes leadership and responsibility during a disaster?**
   Local police, fire, or emergency medical service (EMS) agencies along with local authorities initially take charge during a disaster. If the event overwhelms the capabilities of the local government and agencies, the state emergency management agency takes over. The Federal Emergency Management Agency (FEMA) is part of the Department of Homeland Security (DHS) and is the lead federal agency for emergency management. FEMA supports, but does not override, state authorities.

5. **What constitutes disaster response?**
   Disaster response is made up of the decisions and actions taken during a disaster to (1) prevent any further loss of life and/or property, (2) restore order, and (3) begin recovery/rebuilding. The four phases of a disaster response are outlined in Table 70.1.

6. **What is the Incident Command System?**
   The Incident Command System (ICS) is a modular system that provides a command structure to disaster scenes. It assembles the key components of a response (i.e., fire, EMS, law enforcement)

Table 70-1. The Four Phases of a Disaster Response

PHASE	TASKS
Chaos	
Initial response/reorganization (crisis management)	• Establish command post • Needs assessment • Security and safety procedures • Casualty evacuation to CCAs
Site clearing	• Search and rescue/recovery • Clearing debris • Casualty distribution from CCAs to hospital • Initial hospital medical care
Late/recovery	• Rebuilding infrastructure • Definitive hospital medical care/secondary casualty distribution • Provider and casualty mental health follow-up • Postevent critique and analysis of disaster response • Community recovery

CCA, Casualty collection area.

Table 70-2. Triage Categories

RED	Immediate—life-threatening injuries requiring urgent intervention
YELLOW	Delayed—not life-threatening but urgent injuries that can tolerate a delay before further medical care is needed
GREEN	Minimal—not life-threatening and not urgent injuries; also known as the walking wounded
BLACK	Expectant—unsalvageable injuries due to either severity or limits to resources or dead

to an event at a location in close proximity to the scene. Five functional requirements are inherent to the organization: command, operations, planning, logistics, and finance and administration. Although the ICS is commonly a prehospital concept, many medical centers have a hospital emergency ICS (HEICS) set up in the event of a disaster or mass casualty situation.

7. **What is triage?**
   Triage is a concept originating with the French (*trier,* to sort) during the Napoleonic Wars when Baron Dominique-Jean Larrey popularized a system for sorting wounded soldiers in the field and prioritizing which casualties to evacuate first. The principle of triage implies making the most efficient use of available resources. Thus, often the most critically ill patients are evacuated last to ensure that injured casualties who have a greater chance of survival receive expedited medical treatment. See Table 70.2 for triage categories.

8. **Why is triage beneficial in the disaster response?**
   There are three major reasons why triage is beneficial in the disaster response:
   - Triage identifies victims who need rapid medical care to save life or limb.
   - With identification of minor injuries, triage reduces the urgent burden on medical facilities and organizations. On average, only 10% to 15% of disaster casualties are serious enough to require overnight hospitalization.
   - By providing for the equitable and rational distribution of casualties among the available hospitals, triage reduces the burden on each to a manageable level, often even to "nondisaster" levels.

9. **What is the Crisis Standards of Care?**
   A pandemic or other catastrophic disaster may strain medical resources and thereby require a shift in care that was previously focused on the individual patient to one which is focused on doing the most good for the greatest number. Rather than doing everything possible to try to save every life, in a disaster, it will be necessary to allocate scarce resources to save as many lives as possible. This "crisis care" is simply what a prudent person would do with the scarce resources at hand.

INJURIES ASSOCIATED WITH DISASTERS AND MANAGEMENT

10. **What are common categories of injuries encountered among disaster victims?**
    Burns, blast injuries, crush injuries, fractures, and cardiopulmonary/systemic effects of biologic or chemical agents.

11. **What is the mechanism of a blast injury?**
    A bomb explosion generates a blast wave that consists of two parts. There is an initial shock wave of high pressure followed by a blast wind. When explosions occur indoors, there is increased damage due to reverberation and reflection of the blast wave from walls and rigid objects.

12. **What are the four categories of blast injury?**
    See Table 70.3.
    1. Primary: Injuries resulting from the direct effects of pressure.
    2. Secondary: Injuries resulting from flying debris affecting any body part.
    3. Tertiary: Injuries resulting from effects due to blast wind.
    4. Quaternary: Injuries not due to primary, secondary, or tertiary injuries. These include exacerbations or complications of pre-existing medical conditions.

Table 70-3. Injuries Due to Blasts

TYPE	CAUSE OF INJURY	EXAMPLE
Primary	Barotrauma	Tympanic membrane rupture, pulmonary contusion, pneumothorax, pneumomediastinum, bowel rupture/ischemia, solid organ (liver, kidney, spleen) rupture/hemorrhage, traumatic brain injury, globe (eye) rupture
Secondary	Flying debris	Fractures, penetrating wounds to head/thorax/abdomen
Tertiary	Blast wind	Crush and compartment syndromes, traumatic brain injury
Quaternary	Other	Burns, inhalation injury due to toxins or dust

13. **What are the organs most commonly involved in primary blast injuries?**
    Primary blast injuries are caused by barotrauma and involve air-filled organs and air-fluid interfaces. The tympanic membrane is the structure most frequently injured by blasts. The lung is also susceptible to primary blast injury. Disruption of the alveolar-capillary interface can result in pulmonary hemorrhage, contusion, pneumothorax, hemothorax, pneumomediastinum, and subcutaneous emphysema. Systemic acute gas embolism and rupture of the colon can also occur as a result of blast injury.

14. **Describe the management of blast lung.**
    Blast lung is clinically diagnosed by the presence of respiratory distress, hypoxia, and *butterfly* or *batwing* infiltrates (perihilar infiltrates caused by the reflection of the blast wave of mediastinal structures). If patients require mechanical ventilation, the Acute Respiratory Distress Syndrome Network (ARDSNet) protocol is appropriate as high inspiratory pressures increase the risk of air embolism or pneumothorax. Conservative fluid management may decrease the development of pulmonary edema.

15. **What is crush syndrome?**
    Compression of the extremities or other parts of the body can lead to muscle swelling and ischemia. Crush syndrome results from breakdown of muscle cells leading to an influx of myoglobin, potassium, and phosphorus into the systemic circulation. The syndrome is characterized by shock due to hypovolemia, hyperkalemia leading to cardiac arrhythmias, metabolic acidosis due to lactic acid, and acute renal failure due to deposition of myoglobin in the renal tubules. Acute respiratory distress syndrome can occur due to release of inflammatory mediators causing capillary leak. Patients are also at risk for infection and sepsis.

16. **What is the treatment of crush syndrome?**
    Early, aggressive fluid resuscitation with crystalloid at the scene is critical. Fluid should be given to achieve a urine output of greater than 200 mL/h. Continuous electrocardiographic monitoring should be started early because of the risk of arrhythmias associated with hyperkalemia. Additionally, potassium, calcium, and phosphorus levels should be followed serially as well as acid–base status. There is no high-quality evidence to support the use of bicarbonate infusions to alkalinize the urine to a pH of greater than 6.5 to decrease myoglobin deposition. Even with adequate fluid resuscitation, up to a third of patients may develop acute renal failure and require renal replacement therapy.

17. **What are the four properties of hazards within the chemical-biological weapon spectrum?**
    1. Toxicity—toxic effects of agent.
    2. Latency—time between exposure and appearance of toxic effects.
    3. Persistency—ability of toxic agent to remain in the environment.
    4. Transmissibility—ability to be spread from the environment to humans, or from human to human. This may result from direct physical contamination of the victim or due to infectious spread.
       Toxicity and latency determine the management of the victim, whereas persistency and transmissibility determine the management of an incident.

18. **What are some of the chemical agents that may be encountered in a disaster situation?**
    Industrial accidents as well as acts of terror may result in massive release of chemical agents. Nerve agents (e.g., sarin) and organophosphate pesticides inhibit acetylcholinesterase and result in cholinergic crisis: meiosis, increased salivation, muscle cramps and fasciculations, cardiac arrhythmias, and paralysis of the respiratory muscles. Mustards and arsenicals are blistering agents that can produce

Table 70-4. Examples of Toxic Agents

TYPE	EXAMPLE	SYMPTOMS	TREATMENT
Nerve Agents	Sarin Organophosphate	Meiosis, salivation, broncho-constriction, muscular twitches/cramps, tremors, convulsions, respiratory depression, and respiratory muscle paralysis	Atropine Pralidoxime Diazepam
Blistering Agents	Mustards Lewisite	Skin/mucus membrane blisters and bullae, eye damage, tracheobronchitis, broncho-spasm, necrosis/sloughing/blockage of trachea and bronchi	Supportive care: treat skin injuries like burn injuries; severe respiratory tract involvement may require intubation. Specific treatment for Lewisite poisoning: 2,3-dithiocaptopropanol or British Anti Lewisite (BAL)
Blood Agents	Cyanide	Mental status changes, cardiac arrhythmias, convulsions, coma, respiratory failure	Supplemental oxygen, intubation, and mechanical ventilation. Early use of antidotes: Amyl nitrite, sodium nitrite, 4-dimethylaminophenol (DMAP)
Choking Agents	Chlorine Phosgene	Pulmonary edema	Supplemental oxygen, intubation, and mechanical ventilation

burn-like injuries to the skin and upper respiratory tract and lungs. Agents such as cyanide impair cellular respiration. Chlorine and phosgene gas are respiratory irritants and can lead to pneumonitis and pulmonary edema. See Table 70.4.

19. What is bioterrorism?
    Bioterrorism is the deliberate use of viruses, bacteria, or other pathogens to cause illness or death in people, animals, or plants. These agents can be spread through the air, through water, or in food. These pathogens may be manipulated to increase their ability to cause disease, make them resistant to current medicines, or to increase their ability to be spread into the environment. The process of deliberately altering pathogens to make them more harmful or more easily transmittable is known as "weaponization."

20. How does the Centers for Disease Control categorize bioterrorism agents?
    The Centers for Disease Control (CDC) places bioterrorism agents into three categories, depending on how easily they can be spread and the severity of illness or death they cause.
    1. Category A agents are those that pose the highest risk to the public and national security because (1) they can be transmitted easily from person to person, or (2) they are associated with high mortality, or (3) they may cause public panic and social disruption, or (4) they require special action for public health preparedness.
    2. Category B agents are (1) moderately easy to spread, or (2) they result in moderate morbidity and mortality, or (3) require specific enhancements of CDC's laboratory capacity and enhanced disease monitoring.
    3. Category C agents are emerging pathogens that could be engineered for mass spread in the future and have the potential for high morbidity and mortality rates and major health impact.
    See Table 70.5 for examples of these agents.

21. What are some of the challenges in dealing with disasters involving infectious agents?
    There may be an appreciable delay between exposure to an infectious agent (either natural or used as a biologic weapon) and manifestation of signs and symptoms of disease. Thus, clinics, doctors' offices, and hospitals are mostly likely to be the first responders. Large numbers of exposed, ill patients can rapidly overwhelm healthcare systems' infrastructure and supplies. Health officials will also need to deal with fear and panic in the community.

Table 70-5.	Bioterrorism Agents
Category A	Anthrax *Variola* major (smallpox) *Yersinia pestis* (plague) *Clostridium botulinum* toxin (botulism) *Francisella tularensis* (tularemia) Filoviruses—Ebola virus, Marburg virus Arenaviruses—Lassa virus, Junin virus
Category B	*Coxiella burnetti* (Q fever) *Brucella* species (brucellosis) *Burkholderia mallei* (glanders) *Rickettsia prowazekii* (Typhus fever) Viral encephalitis (Eastern equine, Western equine, Venezuelan equine) Epsilon toxin of *Clostridium perfringens* Food/waterborne pathogens (*Salmonella* sp, *Shigella dysenteriae*, *E. coli* O157:H7, *Vibrio cholera*, *Cryptosporidium*)
Category C	Hantavirus Tickborne hemorrhagic fever viruses Tickborne encephalitis viruses Yellow fever Multidrug resistant tuberculosis

22. What is anthrax?
Bacillus anthracis is an encapsulated, gram-positive, spore-forming bacterium that can cause pulmonary, meningeal, cutaneous, and gastrointestinal disease. Anthrax spores may be aerosolized when used as a biological weapon leading to pulmonary and meningeal disease. Once in the body, the anthrax spores are phagocytized by alveolar macrophages and carried to mediastinal lymph nodes. There, the spores germinate and cause disease through the production of toxins leading to systemic disease and shock.

23. What are the symptoms of inhalational anthrax?
Early symptoms are nonspecific with fever, cough, myalgia, malaise, and mimic viral illnesses. However, after a short period of apparent recovery, fever, respiratory failure, acidosis, and shock develop. Routine laboratory tests are usually nonspecific. The earliest clue to diagnosis may be radiographic findings of a widened mediastinum and pleural effusions that rapidly progress to a large size. Anthrax meningitis results from hematogenous seeding and occurs in up to 50% of patients with inhalational anthrax. Patients with anthrax meningitis may need steroids and anticpileptic agents to control edema and seizures. The mortality rate is as high as 67% to 88% even with antimicrobial or antiserum treatment.

24. What is the treatment of anthrax?
If anthrax is suspected, antibiotic treatment should be started immediately while awaiting results of diagnostic testing. In patients with systemic disease, the CDC recommends treatment with two or more antimicrobial drugs. One of these drugs should have bactericidal activity and the other should be a protein synthesis inhibitor to reduce toxin production. First-line drugs with bactericidal activity include fluoroquinolones and carbapenems. Protein synthesis inhibitors include linezolid or clindamycin. Treatment should be continued for 2 or more weeks or until the patient is clinically stable. Because of β-lactam resistance, cephalosporins are contraindicated for the treatment of anthrax.

25. What is the treatment of anthrax meningitis?
Patients who are suspected to have anthrax meningitis should be treated with three or more antimicrobial drugs. At least one of these agents should have bactericidal activity, at least one should be a protein synthesis inhibitor, and all of these agents should have good central nervous system (CNS) penetration. Treatment should be continued for at least 2 weeks or until the patient is clinically stable, whichever is longer. Any suspected infection with anthrax warrants consultation by an Infectious Disease specialist.

26. Where can I find more information about bioterrorism agents?
The CDC maintains a website containing information about specific bioterrorism agents: https://emergency. cdc.gov/agent/agentlist.asp.

27. What infectious disease has the greatest potential to cause a catastrophic pandemic?
According to the CDC, influenza is the most worrisome pathogen with regard to potential for global outbreaks causing mass casualties.

28. Why do pandemics of influenza occur?
Influenza virus A and B cause respiratory illness. These illnesses occur seasonally, typically in the winter months in regions with temperate climates and during rainy seasons in tropical climates. Influenza pandemics are associated with high attack rates and severe illness. They occur in association with influenza A viruses that have hemagglutinin (HA) and neuraminidase (NA) subtypes that have not previously circulated in humans. This results in a lack of immunity and susceptibility to infection and disease. It is believed that these new viruses likely arise within waterfowl, swine, and other animals.

29. What is the burden of disease associated with influenza?
Seasonal flu in the United States results in 114,000 to 624,000 hospitalizations per year based on population-based surveillance data from the 2010 to 2013 flu seasons. Of those, 18,000 to 95,000 require intensive care unit (ICU) admissions. Flu results in 4915 to 27,174 deaths per year. It affects the elderly most; 54% to 70% of hospitalizations and 71% to 85% of deaths occurred among adults over the age of 65.

30. How is influenza activity monitored in the United States?
The CDC collect virologic surveillance data from public health and clinical laboratories, outpatient illness surveillance data from enrolled outpatient healthcare providers, mortality data, hospitalization data, and geographical data from state and territorial epidemiologists for a national picture of influenza activity. This data is reported weekly in FluView (http://www.cdc.gov/flu/weekly/index.htm). Surveillance is necessary to detect influenza strains that may lead to pandemics, to guide national responses to flu activity, to guide treatment by detecting antiviral resistance, and to target interventions to the segments of population most affected by influenza.

31. What are the pulmonary complications of influenza?
Pulmonary complications are the most frequent serious complications of influenza. Influenza can cause a primary viral pneumonia and ARDS. In patients with severe pneumonia, multisystem organ failure can occur with need for vasopressors and renal replacement therapy. During the 2009 H1N1 influenza pandemic, 70% of critically ill patients required mechanical ventilation and 6% required extra-corporeal membrane oxygenation. Almost 40% of these patients required vasopressors and 20% of patients died. Secondary bacterial pneumonia and ventilator-associated pneumonia can also occur. Viral infections can also exacerbate asthma and chronic obstructive pulmonary disease (COPD).

32. What are the extrapulmonary complications associated with influenza?
The incidence of acute myocardial infarction and cardiovascular mortality increases when influenza is circulating. Excess influenza deaths due to cardiovascular disease are reported to be around 35% to 50%. The mechanism is likely related to the acute inflammatory and procoagulant effects of the flu virus. The virus can also cause direct cardiac complications such as myocarditis and pericarditis. Neurologic complications occur mostly in children and can include encephalopathy, encephalomyelitis, aseptic meningitis, focal neurologic deficits, and Guillain–Barré syndrome.

33. Who is at risk for complications of influenza?
Young children (<2 years), adults over the age of 65, pregnant women, and people with chronic medical conditions (see Table 70.6) are at higher risk of serious flu complications.

34. What are the recommendations for treatment of influenza?
The CDC recommends using the NA inhibitors oseltamivir, zanamivir, and peramivir for the treatment of influenza (see Table 70.7 for dosing recommendations). Treatment is recommended for patients with suspected or confirmed influenza requiring hospitalization or who have progressive, severe, or complicated illness and should not be delayed for results of diagnostic testing. Though the evidence for benefit is strongest when treatment is started within 48 hours of illness onset, treatment should be started even if the patient presents greater than 48 hours after illness onset.

35. What is Ebola?
Ebola is a filovirus that causes Ebola virus disease (EVD). EVD is a severe illness most commonly causing fever, diarrhea, vomiting, headache, myalgias, malaise, dehydration, and electrolyte

Table 70-6. Chronic Medical Conditions that Increase the Risk of Complications with Influenza

Chronic pulmonary disease (including asthma)
Cardiovascular disease (except hypertension alone)
Renal disease
Hepatic disease
Hematological disorders (including sickle cell disease)
Diabetes mellitus
Neurologic and neurodevelopment conditions (e.g., cerebral palsy, epilepsy, stroke, moderate to severe developmental delay, muscular dystrophy, or spinal cord injury)
Immunosuppressed patients (caused by medications or HIV infection)
Morbid obesity (BMI ≥40)

BMI, body mass index.

Table 70-7. Neuraminidase Inhibitor Dosing Recommendations

DRUG	DOSAGE
Oseltamivir	75 mg PO twice daily for 5 days
Peramivir	600 mg IV once
Zanamivir	10 mg inhaled twice a day for 5 days

IV, Intravenous; PO, by mouth.

depletion. This constellation of problems can progress to cause multiorgan system failure and death. Since its discovery in 1976, 26 sporadic outbreaks of the disease have occurred in Africa. The 2014 West African outbreak was the largest by far, with over 28,000 people contracting the disease.

36. **What is the treatment for Ebola virus disease?**
Prior to 2014, EVD was thought to be nearly universally fatal. The 2014 outbreak prompted an international coalition of health providers and investigators to attempt various therapies to address EVD. In resource-rich areas, the mainstays of EVD treatment include: strict isolation, aggressive repletion of fluids and electrolytes, administration of nutrition (enteral if tolerated, parenteral if necessary), and antibiotic therapy for secondary bacterial infections. The mortality rate of patients in West African Ebola treatment units ranged from 37% to 74%. In contrast, patients evacuated to Europe or the United States had a mortality rate of 18.5%.

37. **How do healthcare workers protect themselves from Ebola?**
Healthcare workers must utilize extensive personal protective equipment (PPE) with strict adherence to predefined policies and procedures. All skin and mucous membranes must be protected to ensure zero contact between the healthcare provider and bodily fluids containing Ebola virus. Drills and simulations are beneficial in preparing for the care of patients with EVD or other highly infectious diseases. The National Ebola Training and Education Center (NETEC) was established to provide hospitals with necessary didactic and hands-on training. The NETEC web site is: http://netec.org. Additional educational resources for PPE and other pertinent topics can be found at: http://www.nebraskamed.com/biocontainment-unit/ebola.

38. **What is the plan for the next Ebola outbreak?**
A vaccine against Ebola virus has been developed and initial studies demonstrate excellent efficacy and a tolerable side-effect profile. When the next Ebola outbreak occurs, an international coalition of healthcare providers will broadly distribute and administer the vaccine to persons within the affected area. Within the United States, a network of 10 regional Ebola and other special pathogen treatment centers have conducted extensive preparation and training in order to be ready for the next outbreak. Analysis of the 2014 Ebola epidemic has allowed clinicians and researchers to greatly improve preparedness for future outbreaks.

ACKNOWLEDGMENT

The authors wish to acknowledge Drs. Sarah Mooney, MBBCh, MRCP, Christopher Grace, MD, FACP, John R. Benjamin, MD, MSc, and Edward E. George, MD, PhD, for the valuable contributions to the previous edition of this chapter.

KEY POINTS: DISASTER MEDICINE, BIOTERRORISM AND EBOLA

1. During large-scale disasters, FEMA is designed to support, but not override, the authority of state agencies.
2. "Triage" refers to a system for sorting injured and ill persons in the field and prioritizing which casualties to evacuate first to ensure the most efficient use of available resources.
3. The four properties of hazards within the chemical-biological weapon spectrum are: toxicity, latency, persistency, and transmissibility.
4. Public health efforts aimed at containing influenza outbreaks are essential in the prevention of disastrous pandemic spread, as influenza is the single greatest infectious threat to global health.
5. Safe and effective treatment of EVD requires focused preparation and strict adherence to pre-defined protocols for PPE.

BIBLIOGRAPHY

1. Chavez LO, Leon M, Einav S, et al. Beyond muscle destruction: a systematic review of rhabdomyolysis for clinical practice. *Crit Care.* 2016;20:135.
2. Baker DJ. Critical care requirements after mass toxic agent release. *Crit Care Med.* 2005;33:S66.
3. Ganesan S, Raza SK, Vijayaraghavan R. Chemical warfare agents. *J Pharm Bioallied Sci.* 2010;2:166.
4. Karwa M, Currie B, Kvetan V. Bioterrorism: preparing for the impossible or the improbable. *Crit Care Med.* 2005;33:S75.
5. Bower WA, Hendricks K, Pillai S, et al. Clinical framework and medical countermeasure use during an anthrax mass-casualty incident. *MMWR Recomm Rep.* 2015;64:1.
6. Hendricks KA, Wright ME, Shadomy SV, et al. Centers for Disease Control and Prevention expert panel meetings on prevention and treatment of anthrax in adults. *Emerg Infect Dis.* 2014;20. doi:10.3201/eid2002.130687.
7. Reed C, Chaves SS, Daily Kirley P, et al. Estimating influenza disease burden from population-based surveillance data in the United States. *PLoS One.* 2015;10:e0118369.
8. Rothberg MB, Haessler SD. Complications of seasonal and pandemic influenza. *Crit Care Med.* 2010;38:e91.
9. Warren-Gash C, Smeeth L, Hayward AC. Influenza as a trigger for acute myocardial infarction or death from cardiovascular disease: a review. *Lancet Infect Dis.* 2009;9(10):601.
10. Fiore AE, Fry A, Shay D, et al. Antiviral agents for the treatment and chemoprophylaxis of influenza: Recommendations of the Advisory Committee on Immunization Practices (ACIP). *MMWR Recomm Rep.* 2011;60:1.
11. Johnson DW, Sullivan JN, Piquette CA, et al. Lessons learned: critical care management of patients with Ebola in the United States. *Crit Care Med.* 2015;43:1157.
12. Uyeki TM, Mehta AK, Davey RT Jr, et al. Clinical management of Ebola virus disease in the United States and Europe. *N Engl J Med.* 2016;374:636.

CHAPTER 71

ALLERGY AND ANAPHYLAXIS

Susan A. Vassallo

HISTORY

1. When was anaphylaxis first described?

   In 2641 BC, a wasp from the Hymenoptera order (wasps, bees, ants, sawflies) stung Pharaoh Menes. The events were described in hieroglyphics, and this is believed to be the first recorded death by anaphylaxis. Another important event occurred during a cruise on the yacht of Prince Albert of Monaco when the prince asked Professor Charles Richet to apply his immunology skills in the study of the Portuguese man-of-war (*Physalia* or jelly). This invertebrate lives in the Mediterranean Sea and is highly poisonous. In the early 1900s Richet worked at the Musée Océanographique de Monaco. Along with Paul Portier, he extracted the *Physalia* poison with glycerol, injected dogs with this mixture, and was able to reproduce the symptoms of *Physalia* poisoning (1902). He expected a second injection would be harmless, but instead his dogs "showed serious symptoms: vomiting, blood diarrhea, syncope, unconsciousness, asphyxia and death" (Nobel Lecture, 1913). Richet created the word *anaphylaxis* to describe this phenomenon. *Phylaxis* is "protection" in Greek, and the prefix *ana* implies away from protection. Anaphylaxis therefore means "that state of an organism in which it is rendered hypersensitive, instead of being protected." Richet was awarded the Nobel Prize in Physiology and Medicine in 1913 for his discovery of anaphylaxis.

EPIDEMIOLOGY

2. How often does anaphylaxis occur worldwide?

   The incidence of anaphylaxis ranges from one to three people per 10,000. This includes allergic reactions to food, drugs, latex, and Hymenoptera. Lethal anaphylaxis probably occurs in 0.65% to 2.0% of recorded allergic events or in one to three per million people.

3. How often does anaphylaxis occur in the perioperative environment?

   Anaphylaxis during anesthesia is a rare event. The incidence ranges from 0.5 to 16 in 10,000 anesthetics and varies from country to country. These numbers reflect studies done in the United States, United Kingdom, France, Germany, Spain, Australia, New Zealand, and Singapore. The Groupe d' Étude des Réactions Anaphylactoïdes Périopératoires (GERAP) in Nancy, France, has the largest experience in analyzing serious allergic reactions during anesthesia. Since 1990 they have published 10 reports that describe the patterns of 5200 anaphylactic events. When you look at these reviews together, more reactions occurred in women, in patients with a pre-existing history of allergy or atopy, and in patients previously exposed to anesthesia.

MECHANISMS OF ANAPHYLAXIS

4. What are the immune mechanisms that lead to anaphylaxis?

   The final common pathway for anaphylaxis is mast cell activation and subsequent release of vasoactive mediators—both preformed and newly generated substances. Preformed mediators include histamine and tryptase stored in mast cell granules. Newly generated mediators are synthesized at the time of antigen exposure and include leukotrienes (LTC_4, LTD_4, LTE_4), prostaglandins (PGD_2), platelet-aggregating factor (PAF), and cytokines. In the past, the leukotrienes were not well defined and were simply called "slow-reacting substances of anaphylaxis," or SRS-A. It is now known that leukotrienes, prostaglandins, and PAF are much more potent bronchoconstrictors than histamine.

5. How are immunologic reactions in anaphylaxis classified?

   The Gell and Coombs classification (1963) described four types of immunologic reactions (Table 71.1). A fifth type of reaction, termed *idiopathic*, was added to the classification system several years later.

Table 71-1. Gell and Coombs Classification of Immunologic Reactions

TYPE	DESCRIPTION	MEDIATOR
I	Immediate hypersensitivity	IgE usually
II	Cytotoxic or cytolytic	IgG, IgM
III	Immune complex disease	Antigen-antibody
IV	Delayed hypersensitivity	T cells
V	Idiopathic	Unknown

Ig, Immunoglobulin.

Table 71-2. Classification of Clinical Manifestations of Anaphylaxis During Anesthesia

CLASS	CLINICAL MANIFESTATIONS
I	Generalized cutaneous signs: erythema, urticaria with or without angioedema
II	Moderate multiorgan involvement with cutaneous signs, hypotension and tachycardia, bronchial hyperreactivity (cough, ventilatory impairment)
III	Severe life-threatening multiorgan involvement that requires specific treatment: collapse, tachycardia or bradycardia, cardiac arrhythmias, bronchospasm; the cutaneous signs may be absent or occur only after the arterial blood pressure recovers
IV	Circulatory or respiratory arrest
V	Death due to a lack of response to cardio-respiratory resuscitation

From Kroigaard M, Garvey LH, Gillberg, et al. Scandinavian clinical practice guidelines on the diagnosis, management and follow-up of anaphylaxis during anaesthesia. *Acta Anaesthesiol Scand.* 2007;51: 655-670.

6. How are anaphylactic reactions during anesthesia classified?
   See Table 71.2.

7. What substances activate mast cells?
   - Immunoglobulin (Ig) E (IgE) antibodies. IgE antibodies fixed to mast cell surfaces are cross-linked on exposure to an antigen. This initiates cell degranulation and release of mediators.
   - IgG and IgM antibodies. Immunologists have created *knockout mice* that lack the gene for synthesis of IgE antibody. These mice still can develop anaphylaxis via IgG antibodies and complement.
   - Complement-mediated reactions. Complement is the term given to plasma and cell membrane proteins that activate the release of inflammatory mediators. Complement activation occurs as a cascade of reactions. IgG or IgM antibody-antigen binding, heparin-protamine complexes, and radiocontrast dye activate the classic pathway. Endotoxins, certain drugs, and radiocontrast dyes can activate the alternate pathway.
   - Activated T cells can stimulate mast cell degranulation in a delayed hypersensitivity reaction.
   - Direct mast cell activation. Direct mast cell activation can occur in the absence of antibodies or complement. Drugs such as morphine, vancomycin, and d-tubocurarine can cause histamine release, especially if administered quickly.
   - Bradykinin is involved in the systemic inflammatory response system and in angioedema associated with angiotensin-converting enzyme inhibitors.

CAUSES OF ANAPHYLAXIS

8. How frequently do neuromuscular blocking drugs cause anaphylaxis, and what is the mechanism?
   Neuromuscular blocking drugs (NMBDs) long have been considered the most common cause of intraoperative anaphylaxis in adults. This is true in all published studies from Australia, New Zealand, the

United Kingdom, France, Norway, Belgium, and Spain. These drugs have accounted for 54% to 69% of reactions, depending on the study. Within this drug class, succinylcholine and rocuronium are the most common causes. Succinylcholine is a quaternary ammonium ion and is a flexible molecule that can cross-link two IgE molecules more easily than nondepolarizing muscle relaxants with a rigid backbone (e.g., pancuronium or vecuronium).

There are five important points to remember when considering allergy, anaphylaxis, and NMBDs:
- Quaternary and tertiary ammonium ions are present in many drugs, cosmetics, and food products. Sensitization can occur outside of the operating room, and a serious reaction can occur with first exposure to an NMBD.
- Cross-sensitivity between NMBDs can occur in up to 60% of people.
- NMBDs can cause adverse reactions without IgE antibody mediation. This mechanism of action is via direct mast cell degranulation and release of histamine and other inflammatory mediators. Isoquinolinium compounds such as d-tubocurarine, metocurine, atracurium, and mivacurium are more likely to cause mast cell degranulation.
- Anaphylaxis to NMBDs is reported more frequently in Europe, especially in France, and less commonly reported in the United States. An important study has challenged the results of previous French skin test studies. This investigation found that undiluted rocuronium and vecuronium extracts produced a positive wheal and flare response in 50% and 40% of nonatopic anesthesia-naïve volunteers, respectively. However, a dilution of 1:1000 did not yield any skin response at 15 minutes. Although their study was small (30 healthy adults), the authors questioned the reliability of skin prick testing with undiluted solutions of rocuronium and vecuronium when making the diagnosis of allergy. An accompanying editorial supported the recommendations for using dilute test extracts and suggested that the incidence of NMBD allergy may be overestimated.
- No demonstrated evidence exists for improved outcomes with preoperative screening of sensitivity to NMBDs.

9. How common are latex allergies?
Latex is now the fourth most common cause of perioperative anaphylaxis. Latex is harvested from the *Hevea brasiliensis* tree and is used in hundreds of medical products. Latex anaphylaxis still occurs in some countries where sterile and nonsterile latex gloves predominate the healthcare environment. Certain subsets of patients have a higher risk of latex allergy:
- Children with myelodysplasia or bladder exstrophy or children who have had multiple surgeries
- Healthcare workers exposed to latex
- Atopic individuals who have asthma, allergic rhinitis, and certain food allergies (e.g., bananas, kiwi, avocado)
- Workers in the rubber industry
    Latex allergy can present as a type I immediate hypersensitivity reaction mediated by IgE antibodies with the prototypical features of anaphylaxis: hypotension, tachycardia, bronchoconstriction, or cardiovascular collapse. Latex allergy also can present as a type IV T cell–mediated delayed hypersensitivity reaction that is due to chemicals added as accelerators in the manufacture of latex gloves.

10. How often are antibiotics involved in anaphylaxis?
Penicillin is still the most common cause of anaphylaxis within the general population of the United States. It is the leading cause of death from anaphylaxis, and it accounts for a few hundred fatalities each year. Most reactions occur in patients with history of prior exposure to penicillin.
    Penicillin is a low-molecular-weight drug. Penicillin can produce four types of the reactions described in the Gell and Coombs classification. It is immunogenic only after binding to tissues and forming a protein hapten complex. The β-lactam ring of penicillin opens to form a penicilloyl group, which is termed the *major determinant*. Derivatives of penicillin are formed in small amounts and are termed *minor determinants*. IgE antibodies specific for these derivatives also can mediate anaphylaxis to penicillin.

11. How do you treat the patient who reports a reaction to penicillin? Is it safe to administer a cephalosporin?
- Patients with an allergy to penicillin have three times the risk for having anaphylaxis to any other drugs.
- A patient with a history of penicillin allergy should not receive antibiotics with a similar molecular structure.
- A patient with a positive skin test to penicillin should not receive cephalosporins.
- Most patients who report an allergy to penicillin had never been skin tested.

- Some authors suggest that it appears to be safe to administer cephalosporins to patients who claim to be allergic to penicillin. However, no conclusion can be made concerning patients who report severe or anaphylactic reactions to penicillin, because these patients were excluded from studies.
- A formal allergy evaluation can be invaluable in the management of patients who report a history of penicillin allergy. An algorithm has been published for specific care in the hospital environment.

12. How frequent is anaphylaxis to propofol?

The original preparations of propofol contained Cremophor EL and caused hypersensitivity reactions on injection. Today, both the brand and generic formulations contain propofol, soybean oil, glycerol, and sodium hydroxide. The trade brand (Astra Zeneca) contains egg lecithin and the preservative disodium edetate. The generic brands contain egg yolk phospholipid and sodium metabisulfite as a preservative.

Most studies report an incidence of propofol anaphylaxis of 1 in 60,000. One group in France has reported an incidence of 1%. Propofol can cause adverse reactions via IgE antibodies. Occasionally it is associated with nonspecific local histamine release, rash, pruritus, or flushing.

A frequent question regarding propofol is the potential for cross-sensitivity in a patient who is allergic to eggs. The egg lecithin in propofol is purified egg yolk, and most people with egg allergy are sensitive to ovalbumin, the primary protein in egg white. Theoretically, there should be no risk of cross-sensitivity. During phase I trials, propofol was inadvertently given to people with egg allergies without obvious complications. However, the manufacturers of propofol warn that it should not be given to people with egg allergies or soybean allergies. The advantages and disadvantages of propofol administration in patients with egg allergies should be considered.

13. How frequent is anaphylaxis to heparin?

Heparin is a large-molecular-weight acidic mucopolysaccharide, and it is derived from bovine or porcine lung. Type 1 IgE immediate hypersensitivity reactions have occurred in humans, although they are rare. More commonly, heparin can induce thrombocytopenia (HIT), which is mediated by IgG and IgM antibodies directed against platelet factor 4 antigen. This is a delayed adverse reaction usually seen after a few days of heparin therapy. HIT is very rare when low-molecular-weight heparin is used.

14. Are there cases of anaphylaxis to skin and oral disinfectants?

Chlorhexidine is used commonly as a disinfectant before surgery or invasive procedures, including central line placement. Allergy to chlorhexidine is usually mild and limited to cutaneous reactions. In the past few years, reports of intraoperative anaphylaxis to this compound have increased. Typically, hypotension, tachycardia, and cardiovascular collapse occur 24 minutes after application. Because chlorhexidine is also used in toothpastes, mouthwashes, contact lens solutions, and topical antiseptic ointments, significant potential exists for exposure and sensitization to this chemical in the general population.

PRESENTATION OF ANAPHYLAXIS

15. What happens to the patient when anaphylaxis occurs?

Histamine, a preformed mediator, causes vasodilatation, resulting hypotension, and reflex tachycardia. Increased vascular permeability causes edema and urticaria. Cytokines (e.g., tumor necrosis factor), PGD_2, the leukotrienes, and PAF are also potent vasodilators.

Bronchoconstriction, increased mucus secretions, and airway edema can occur in varying stages. A patient might complain of rhinitis, dyspnea, wheezing, or agitation. An anesthetized patient may have decreased airway compliance and increased inspiratory pressure.

Vasodilation causes erythema, and increased vascular permeability can lead to a wheal and flare, which is an area of local edema and redness. In more severe episodes, angioedema can occur. An awake patient might complain of itching, nausea, abdominal pain, or cramping.

MANAGEMENT OF ANAPHYLAXIS

16. How should anaphylaxis be treated?
See Box 71.1.

Box 71-1. Management of Anaphylaxis

1. Remove antigen if detected.
2. Administer 100% oxygen.
3. Administer intravenous fluids.
4. Discontinue antibiotic infusion; discontinue blood, fresh frozen plasma, platelet transfusion, if in progress.
5. Adjust epinephrine dose for the clinical scenario:
   For bronchospasm: Start at low doses 0.1–0.5 mcg/kg IV (or 5–10 mcg), and increase as needed.
   For hypotension: Start at 1–5 mcg/kg IV, and increase as needed.
   For an infusion: Start at 0.05–0.1 mcg/kg per minute IV (or 0.5–5 mcg/min), and increase as needed.
   For cardiac arrest: Pediatric: 10 mcg/kg (0.1 mL/kg of a 1:10,000 solution).
   Adult: 0.5 to 1 mg; titrate to response, as higher doses may be needed.
6. Vasopressin is not included in the 2016 American Cardiac Life Support Guidelines for cardiac arrest. However, it has been used when anaphylaxis is refractory to epinephrine therapy.
   Start with low doses: 5–10 units IV, and increase to 40 units if necessary.
   Infusion dose: 0.4 units per minute.
7. Secondary therapy: antihistamine
   Famotidine: 20 mgs IV
   H_1: diphenhydramine: 0.5–1 mg/kg IV
   Optional: H_2: ranitidine: 1 mg/kg IV
8. Secondary therapy: steroids (dose for anaphylaxis)
   Hydrocortisone: 1–1.5 mg/kg IV

Methylprednisolone: 1 mg/kg IV

DIAGNOSIS OF ANAPHYLAXIS

17. What tests can confirm or negate the diagnosis of anaphylaxis in a patient?
    In vitro tests:
    - **Histamine.** Histamine has a very short half-life, on the order of minutes. Histamine levels are not performed usually because it is easy to miss the peak, especially if the anesthesia care team is resuscitating the patient.
    - **Tryptase.** Serum tryptase is a protease, and it is a marker only for mast cell degranulation. Its half-life is 2 hours, and the level may remain elevated for a few hours after an acute event. However, occasionally tryptase can be released by mast cells without evidence of IgE, IgG, or IgM antibody mediation. Tryptase levels do not always increase during vancomycin administration or with a peanut food allergic reaction.
    - **IgE, IgG, IgM levels.** Total antibody levels are not measured routinely unless there is a concern of immunologic disease (such as multiple myeloma) or absence of certain antibody classes (e.g., congenital IgA deficiency).
    - **Radioallergosorbent test (RAST).** A radioactive marker is used to identify IgE antibodies to a specific antigen. The key point is to isolate and test for the active antigen; otherwise a false-negative result might occur. A substance can have several antigenic components. For example, at least 16 natural rubber latex antigens exist. In the past, in general, RAST was considered less reliable (lower sensitivity and lower specificity) than skin testing, although the reliability has improved significantly since the introduction of the Pharmacia CAP RAST method.
    - **Enzyme-linked immunosorbent assay (ELISA).** This test uses enzyme activity rather than radio-activity to measure IgE levels for a specific antigen. Both RAST and ELISA have false-positive and false-negative rates, specific for each test and antigen. The availability of a test and its clinical utility can be very different things.
      - **Antigens RAST** for measurement of IgE antibodies is available for some NMBDs, propofol, morphine, meperidine, penicillin, barbiturates, aprotinin, protamine, and latex.
      - **ELISA** looking for IgE antibodies and IgG antibodies is available for most of these drugs. Both RAST and ELISA have turnaround times of 4 to 7 days because they must be sent out to regional immunology laboratories.
      In vivo tests:
    - In vivo tests include subcutaneous and intradermal skin tests, provocation tests, and challenge tests, which are performed in an allergist's office. The tests must be done at least 2 to 6 weeks after a suspected allergic reaction because recent mast cell degranulation may have depleted

mediator stores. If skin tests are performed shortly after a reaction, there is the possibility of a false-negative result. Antihistamines must be discontinued 5 days before skin testing. Skin testing can demonstrate whether hypersensitivity is mediated by antibodies; skin tests do not evaluate whether a nonantibody-mediated sensitivity reaction has occurred (e.g., nonspecific mast cell degranulation, which is a side effect of some medications).

- Skin tests are available for NMBDs, propofol, fentanyl, latex, chlorhexidine, and local anesthetics. Skin testing before planned local anesthetic use is helpful, especially if the diagnosis is unclear. Although skin testing is the best available method for identification of sensitivity to NMBDs, it is not infallible. Anaphylaxis to cisatracurium after negative skin testing has occurred. The sensitivity and specificity of skin tests to NMBDs are greater than 95%. No skin tests exist for cefazolin, hydromorphone, or midazolam.
- Penicilloyl polylysine (Pre-Pen) is a commercially available skin test reagent to look for IgE antibodies associated with penicillin. It is positive in up to 85% of patients with β-lactam allergy. The remaining 15% of allergic patients react to minor determinants. These antigens are not commercially available and are prepared in a few specialty centers only for in-house use. Curiously, the anaphylactic reactions are seen more commonly in patients who react to the minor determinants of penicillin.

THE FUTURE

18. Is there any role for anti-IgE therapy in acute anaphylaxis?

Omalizumab (Xolair; Genentech) is a monoclonal IgG antibody that binds to the Cε3 domain of IgE. It is a second-line drug in patients with moderate to severe asthma.

TNX-901 is a humanized IgG1 monoclonal antibody against IgE; it inhibits the binding of IgE to mast cells and basophils. This drug has been studied in people with peanut allergy and was associated with an increase in the threshold of sensitivity to oral peanut challenge.

Sublingual epinephrine for the treatment of anaphylaxis is under investigation.

Old antigens such as sodium metabisulfite may re-surface; new antigens such as sugammadex may emerge. Genomic identification of patients at risk for anaphylaxis may be on the horizon.

KEY POINTS: ALLERGY AND ANAPHYLAXIS

1. Five possible immunologic reactions are involved in anaphylaxis, including immediate hypersensitivity, cytotoxicity, immune complex disease, delayed hypersensitivity, and idiopathic.
2. Several antigens can activate mast cells and cause anaphylaxis including antibodies (IgE, IgG, IgM), drugs directly activating mast cells, complement-mediated reactions, bradykinin, and activated T cells.
3. Penicillin is still the most common cause of anaphylaxis in the general population.
4. Patients who have anaphylaxis have vasodilation and increased endothelial permeability that leads to hypotension, tachycardia, edema, erythema, and urticaria. Bronchoconstriction leads to hypoxia and tachypnea.
5. Epinephrine is still the first-line therapy in the treatment of anaphylaxis. Its alpha-1 agonist effects cause vasoconstriction, which counters hypotension and airway edema.
6. Its beta-1 agonist effects cause chronotropy and inotropy. Its beta-2 agonist effects cause bronchodilation and decrease mediator release.

BIBLIOGRAPHY

1. Baumgart KW, Baldo BA. Cephalosporin allergy. *N Engl J Med.* 2002;346:380-381.
2. Brozovic G, Kvolik S. Anaphylactic reaction after rocuronium. *Eur J Anaesthesiol.* 2005;22:72-73.
3. Cohen SG. The Pharaoh and the wasp. *Allergy Proc.* 1989;10:149-151.
4. de Leon-Casasola OA, Weiss A, Lema MJ. Anaphylaxis due to propofol. *Anesthesiology.* 1992;77:384-386.
5. Dhonneur G, Combes X, Chassard D, Merle JC. Skin sensitivity to rocuronium and vecuronium: a randomized controlled prick-testing study in healthy volunteers. *Anesth Analg.* 2004;98:986-989.
6. Garvey LH, Rode-Petersen J, Humus B. Anaphylactic reactions in anaesthetized patients four cases of chlorhexidine allergy. *Acta Anaesthesiol Scand.* 2001;45:1290-1294.
7. Goodman EJ, Morgan MJ, Johnson PA, Nichols BA, Denk N, Gold BB. Cephalosporins can be given to penicillin-allergic patients who do not exhibit an anaphylactic response. *J Clin Anesth.* 2001;13:561-564.
8. Gouel-Chéron A, Harpan A, Mertes PM, Longrois D. Management of anaphylactic shock in the operating room. *Presse Med.* 2016;45(9):774-783.
9. Guyer AC, Saff RR, Conroy M, et al. Comprehensive allergy evaluation is useful in the subsequent care of patients with drug hypersensitivity reactions during anesthesia. *J Allergy Clin Immunol Pract.* 2015;3(1):94-100.

10. Kay AB. Advances in immunology: allergy and allergic diseases. First of two parts. *N Engl J Med.* 2001;344:30-37.
11. Kay AB. Advances in immunology: allergy and allergic diseases. Second of two parts. *N Engl J Med.* 2001;344:109-113.
12. Laxenaire MC. Epidemiology of anesthetic anaphylactoid reactions. Fourth multicenter survey (July 1994–December 1996). *Ann Fr Anesth Reanim.* 1999;18:796-809.
13. Laxenaire MC. Substances responsible for peranesthetic anaphylactic shock. A third French multicenter study (1992–1994). *Ann Fr Anesth Reanim.* 1996;15:1211-1218.
14. Leung DY, Sampson HA, Yunginger JW, et al. Effect of anti-IgE therapy in patients with peanut allergy. *N Engl J Med.* 2003;348:986-993.
15. Levy JH. Anaphylactic reactions to neuromuscular blocking drugs: are we making the correct diagnosis? *Anesth Analg.* 2004;98:881-882.
16. Meng J, Rotiroti G, Burdett E, Lukawska JJ. Anaphylaxis during general anesthesia: experience from a drug allergy centre in the UK. *Acta Anaesthesiol Scand.* 2017;61(3):281-289.
17. Mertes PM, Laxenaire MC. Adverse reactions to neuromuscular blocking agents. *Curr Allergy Asthma Rep.* 2004;4:7-16.
18. Mertes PM, Volcheck GW, Garvey LH, et al. Epidemiology of perioperative anaphylaxis. *Presse Med.* 2016;45(9):758-767.
19. Moneret-Vautrin DA, Morisset M, Flabbee J, Beaudouin E, Kanny G. Epidemiology of life-threatening and lethal anaphylaxis: a review. *Allergy.* 2005;60:443-451.
20. Oettgen HC, Martin TR, Wynshaw-Boris A, Deng C, Drazen JM, Leder P. Active anaphylaxis in IgE-deficient mice. *Nature.* 1994;370:367-370.
21. O'Sullivan S, McElwain JP, Hogan TS. Kinin-mediated anaphylactoid reaction implicated in acute intra-operative pulseless electrical activity. *Anaesthesia.* 2001;56:771-772 [comment].
22. Richet C. *Nobel Prize Presentation Speech, 1913. Nobel Lectures, Physiology or Medicine, 1901–1921.* Amsterdam: Elsevier; 1967.
23. Tacquard C, Collange O, Gomis P, et al. Anaesthetic hypersensitivity reactions in France between 2011 and 2012: the 10th GERAP epidemiologic survey. *Acta Anaesthesiol Scand.* 2017;61(3):290-299.
24. Vetter RS. Wasp or hippopotamus? *J Allergy Clin Immunol.* 2000;106:196.

CHAPTER 72

HYPOTHERMIA

Matthew J. Meyer and Edward A. Bittner

1. How is hypothermia defined?

Hypothermia is commonly defined as a core temperature less than 35°C (95°F) and is further classified as follows: mild (>34), moderate (34°C–30°C), and severe (<30°C). In suspected hypothermia, the temperature is best measured via the rectum or esophagus. A rectal probe should be inserted 10 to 15 cm and not placed into cold feces. Care should be taken to use a thermometer without a minimum temperature; many thermometers have a minimum temperature of 35°C.

2. What are the five modes of heat loss?

Heat is lost through the following:
- Radiation
- Evaporation
- Conduction
- Convection
- Respiration

Radiation normally accounts for the majority of heat loss and is dependent on the ambient temperature and the amount of body surface exposed. Evaporation from the skin and respiratory tract accounts for approximately a quarter of heat loss. Conduction and convection account for the remaining fraction of heat loss, with a small contribution from inspiration of cold air.

In patients lying uninsulated on the ground or immersed in cold water, conduction may account for the majority of heat loss. Accidental hypothermia usually results from increases in heat loss through one of the mechanisms listed previously. However, it may also be caused by decreased heat production (as can occur in hypothyroidism or adrenal insufficiency) or impaired thermoregulation (as sometimes occurs with central nervous system injury or certain toxic ingestions).

3. What is the significance of shivering?

Shivering is an intrinsic mechanism for augmenting heat production in response to hypothermia. It occurs at core temperatures between 32°C and 37°C. Shivering can result in a fivefold increase in basal metabolic rate but cannot continue when muscles fatigue, their glycogen stores are depleted, or body temperature falls below 32°C. The cessation of shivering in a patient still exposed to the cold should be considered an ominous sign of progressive hypothermia. In a patient with a compromised coronary circulation, shivering may lead to myocardial ischemia and should be monitored, or treated, accordingly.

4. What is the J wave?

Also known as the Osborn wave, or hypothermic hump, the J wave is a hypothermia-related elevation of the J point at the junction of the QRS complex and ST segment (Fig. 72.1). J waves appear at temperatures at or below 33°C. As the temperature decreases further, they increase in size. The J wave is neither specific, nor sensitive, nor prognostic in hypothermia. Automated electrocardiographic interpretation software may misinterpret the J wave as ischemic injury (ST elevation), and it is important to evaluate the electrocardiogram (EKG) carefully.

5. What is core temperature afterdrop?

Core temperature afterdrop is the phenomenon of continued decrease in core temperature when a patient with hypothermia is removed from the cold. It likely results from a combination of thermal equilibration between the relatively warmer core and colder extremities and an increase in convective heat loss due to peripheral vasodilation. It can be avoided by confining active external rewarming to the torso and stabilizing core temperature before thawing frozen extremities. Limiting activity, which stimulates peripheral blood flow, may also be helpful.

6. Which patients with hypothermia should receive cardiopulmonary resuscitation?

Cardiopulmonary resuscitation (CPR) should be instituted immediately in the patient with hypothermia with no signs of life and no verifiable spontaneous circulation. Tissue destruction, dependent lividity,

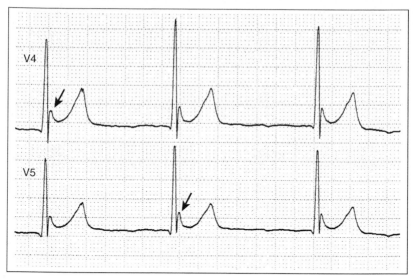

Figure 72-1. J waves in lateral leads during moderate hypothermia.

rigor mortis, and fixed dilated pupils are not reliable indicators of death in hypothermia. A Doppler device to detect blood flow or an ultrasound machine to visualize cardiac activity may be useful to identify otherwise difficult-to-detect perfusion. Even extremely limited perfusion and circulation may be sufficient to meet the reduced metabolic needs in hypothermia. Because mechanical agitation is a possible source of arrhythmias in hypothermia, unnecessary CPR (as can occur if a profound hypothermic bradyarrhythmia is not appreciated) may be especially detrimental to the patient with hypothermia. Once CPR is initiated, it should be continued until the patient has return of spontaneous circulation, cardiopulmonary bypass (CPB) is initiated, or the patient remains without return of spontaneous circulation despite reaching a core temperature greater than 35°C. Many cases of prolonged CPR of patients with hypothermia have been documented. Guidance is provided by the aphorism that "you're not dead until you're warm and dead."

7. You said mechanical agitation can cause arrhythmias. Is it acceptable to endotracheally intubate? What about central venous or pulmonary artery catheterization?
   The hypothermic heart may be particularly irritable and the placement of either an endotracheal tube or central venous catheter may trigger arrhythmias. Regardless, if either an endotracheal tube or central venous catheter is indicated for resuscitation, placement should not be delayed. It will often be necessary to secure the airway with an endotracheal tube because patients with severe hypothermia are obtunded and have depressed airway reflexes, bronchorrhea, and ileus. Insertion of a central venous catheter will often be necessary in patients with severe hypothermia because they may need warming with CPB. When placing a central venous catheter, it may be best to avoid internal jugular or subclavian placement or to be extremely cautious about the depth to which the guidewire and catheter are advanced. It is safest to establish central access via the femoral vein. Pulmonary artery catheters should be avoided because of the potential for induced arrhythmias, as well as a possible increased risk for pulmonary artery rupture.

8. How should arrhythmias be treated in the patient with hypothermia?
   Atrial fibrillation and other supraventricular arrhythmias are common and almost universally benign. They will nearly always resolve with rewarming and should not be treated pharmacologically. Asystole in the patient with severe hypothermia is not as ominous a rhythm as in normothermia and may resolve with rewarming. For ventricular fibrillation (VF), experts have traditionally recommended avoiding pharmacotherapy or repeated attempts at defibrillation until rewarming has been achieved. Pharmacotherapy has traditionally been avoided on the basis of concerns that slowed metabolism of antiarrhythmics and increases in serum levels during rewarming could result in toxic levels. Although

convincing human trials do not exist to support one strategy or another, on the basis of animal data and isolated clinical reports, the American Heart Association endorses the use of standard advanced cardiac life support (ACLS) protocols concurrent with rewarming, including defibrillation and administration of vasopressors during cardiac arrest. The role of antiarrhythmic agents for hypothermic patients is less clear.

9. Aside from the life support measures described, what other initial management should be undertaken?

Volume resuscitation is necessary in most patients with severe hypothermia. Throughout the onset of hypothermia, patients are typically unable to maintain plasma volume both because of impairment of the normal thirst mechanism and because they may not be able to access water. Hypothermia also induces a cold diuresis, with loss of copious dilute urine even in the setting of dehydration. As rewarming reverses peripheral vasoconstriction, hypovolemia may become apparent. In neonates with hypothermia, adequate fluid resuscitation significantly reduces mortality. Such definitive mortality data are lacking in adults, though volume resuscitation does improve hemodynamics. Intravenous administration of 500 to 1000 mL of 5% dextrose in 0.9% sodium chloride is a reasonable starting point for adults, with ongoing resuscitation dictated by clinical response. The hypothermic liver may not be able to metabolize lactate, and therefore lactated Ringers solution is generally avoided. For patients who had a prolonged environmental exposure and may have been deprived of adequate nutrition, electrolytes should be carefully monitored for refeeding syndrome.

10. What are the methods for rewarming patients?

Rewarming can be performed either passively or actively with varying degrees of invasiveness and efficacy. Passive external rewarming is the prevention of further evaporative losses by removing wet or cold clothing—this is the treatment of choice for mild hypothermia (>34°C). Passive external rewarming involves covering the patient with insulating material in a warm environment (ambient temperature >21°C), thereby minimizing heat loss while relying on the patient's own metabolism to generate the heat necessary for rewarming. Active rewarming can be divided into active external rewarming and active core rewarming and involves adding external sources of heat to expedite the rewarming process.

11. How is active rewarming performed?

Active rewarming includes forced air external rewarming, warm water immersion, heating pads, and radiant sources. Active external rewarming is most appropriate for patients with moderate hypothermia (30°C–34°C) and is generally unnecessary for patients with mild hypothermia. There is a concern of core temperature afterdrop with active rewarming attributed to peripheral vasodilation and resulting in a decreased overall rewarming rate. These effects may be mitigated by limiting active external rewarming to patients with brief hypothermic exposures (e.g., witnessed immersion), by restricting rewarming to the trunk, and by combining active external rewarming with active core rewarming. Active core rewarming is most appropriate for patients with severe hypothermia (<30°C) and includes airway rewarming by the administration of heated, humidified inhalant; warmed intravenous fluids; and warm lavage of body cavities (gastrointestinal tract, bladder, peritoneum, pleural cavities, mediastinum). Body cavity irrigation techniques are not tremendously effective, highly invasive, and can have serious technical complications. They should be avoided especially at centers where extracorporeal rewarming techniques are available.

12. Extracorporeal rewarming sounds futuristic and highly technical—what is it?

Extracorporeal rewarming involves removing blood from the patient's circulation, warming it, and reinfusing it. The available techniques include hemodialysis, venovenous rewarming, continuous arteriovenous rewarming, extracorporeal mechanical oxygenation (ECMO), and CPB. Except for ECMO and CPB, these modalities require the patient to have spontaneous circulation. Hemodialysis is widely available, portable, and only requires cannulation of a single blood vessel. It has the added advantages of correcting electrolyte abnormalities and allowing clearance in cases of intoxication with a dialyzable substance. In patients with severe hypothermia and circulatory arrest, CPB or ECMO are the ideal modalities. They provide rapid rewarming and simultaneously offer circulatory support. The principal disadvantages are limited availability, the time required to cannulate major vessels, and the need for anticoagulation. Systems designed for delivering therapeutic hypothermia (see later) can also be adapted to rewarm accidental hypothermia victims. Clinicians should be aware of their own institutional capacities for rewarming a hypothermic patient. While there have been no major studies testing rewarming strategies, a recommended algorithm for rewarming hypothermic patients is presented in Fig. 72.2.

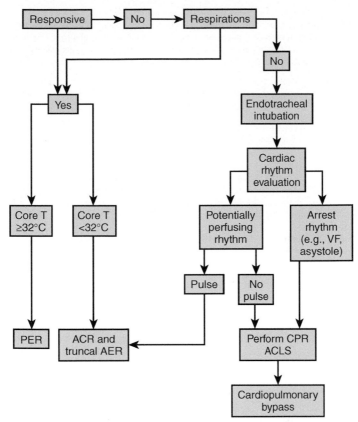

Figure 72-2. Algorithm for initial treatment and method of rewarming in accidental hypothermia. *ACLS*, Advanced cardiac life support; *ACR*, active core rewarming; *AER*, active external rewarming; *CPR*, cardiopulmonary resuscitation; *PER*, passive external rewarming; *T*, temperature; *VF*, ventricular fibrillation.

13. **Which patients with hypothermia should undergo extracorporeal mechanical oxygenation?**
    Any patient with severe hypothermia who is hemodynamically unstable should be considered for ECMO. ECMO is probably the best option for patients with severe hypothermia without spontaneous circulation. Patients must have no contraindication to anticoagulation. Individual centers have established exclusion criteria aimed at identifying those in whom attempted resuscitation is futile; however, none of this data has been rigorously validated. When patients are severely hypothermic their physiology may be profoundly deranged, but these physiologic abnormalities may be survivable: there are case reports of patients surviving after (1) a nadir core temperature of 13.7°C, (2) a peak serum potassium of 11.8 mmol/L, and (3) 6.5 hours of CPR.

14. **What are the therapeutic uses of hypothermia?**
    Therapeutic hypothermia was once accepted as a neuroprotective therapy for adults in cardiac arrest who remained comatose after return of spontaneous circulation. Currently targeted temperature management with avoidance of hyperthermia is the clinical focus, rather than actively instigating hypothermia. Therapeutic hypothermia is still routinely used for cardiovascular surgery requiring circulatory arrest such as aortic arch repairs. It is also under investigation, and used in some centers, for treatment after ischemic cerebral vascular accidents, traumatic brain injury, spinal cord injury, trauma resuscitation, and neonatal asphyxia. The appropriate indications for the use of therapeutic hypothermia in these various disease states are still being defined. Relative contraindications include severe coagulopathy and active bleeding.

15. **What is the usual target temperature in therapeutic hypothermia?**
Few studies directly compare different cooling mechanisms and protocols. Standard cooling regimens (as for return of spontaneous circulation after cardiac arrest) once targeted a core temperature of 30°C to 34°C; however, targeted temperature management now focuses on maintaining patient temperature between 32°C and 36°C for 24 hours or more.

16. **How are patients cooled?**
If cooling must be initiated in an environment (such as the emergency department) where complex, self-regulating cooling equipment is not available, the cooling process can be initiated by placing ice packs around the groin, axillae, head, and neck; administering refrigerated (4°C) intravenous fluids; and covering the patient in a mist of water or alcohol and applying a fan. Intravascular and surface cooling methods have been shown to be equivalent in a retrospective review. Intravascular cooling devices circulate cold water through a specially designed intravascular catheter. Surface cooling similarly circulates cold water through pads applied to the patient's skin. In both systems the cooling device is attached to a patient thermometer that provides feedback control. Unless central blood temperature is measured directly, a lag time will exist between measured temperature (via the esophagus, rectum, tympanic membrane) and true core temperature. This can result in an overshoot below the desired core temperature during induction of hypothermia. The faster the cooling rate, the greater the potential to overshoot.

17. **What should be done if a patient shivers during therapeutic hypothermia?**
Shivering must be suppressed for effective cooling. Some centers use neuromuscular blocking agents to chemically paralyze patients to prevent shivering, though suppression of shivering can be achieved without paralytics in many patients by using medications such as propofol, meperidine, ketamine, dexmedetomidine, and clonidine. Avoiding paralysis has advantages:
- Avoiding mechanical ventilation
- Decreasing the incidence of critical illness polyneuropathy and myopathy
- Allowing clinical monitoring for seizures
- Allowing clinical monitoring of sedation

18. **How long are patients kept in hypothermia?**
Hypothermia is usually discontinued after a specified period of time (usually 24–48 hours) based on the protocol and the indication for cooling. For certain disease processes, such as traumatic brain injury, alternative end points such as the normalization of intracranial pressure have been investigated. The cooling systems (intravascular or surface) described above can be used to regulate rewarming. A typical rate of rewarming is 0.2°C to 0.5°C per hour.

19. **What are the important side effects of therapeutic hypothermia?**
Hypothermia affects nearly every organ system and thus has myriad side effects of variable clinical significance. Electrolyte abnormalities and infectious complications are most likely to concern the clinician. Electrolyte abnormalities commonly require management and must be actively monitored. During cooling, hypomagnesemia and hyperglycemia are common; whereas during rewarming, hypoglycemia and hyperkalemia are dangers. Most centers check electrolyte panels every 30 to 60 minutes during cooling and every 4 to 6 hours during the maintenance of hypothermia. Hypothermia may be immunosuppressive via a number of mechanisms and masks the normal febrile response to infection. Centers may draw routine daily blood cultures during induced hypothermia to monitor for infection. An aggressive stance toward investigation and empiric treatment of other potential infectious sources is appropriate, though routine antibiotic prophylaxis is not justified.

20. **What is the difference between fever and hyperthermia?**
Hyperthermia is an inclusive term of conditions with elevated body temperatures (i.e., heat stroke, malignant hyperthermia, exercise hyperthermia, and fever). Fever is unique because it is the only process that is a regulated rise in body temperature. Fever is coordinated by the immune system through pyrogens that raise the body's temperature set point through action in the hypothalamus. Often fevers are the result of the immune system response to infections, but they can also be stimulated by other disease states that elicit an immunogenic response such as autoimmune diseases and neoplasms. Because fevers are actively managed by the body, they tend to be more difficult to cool than other types of hyperthermia.

21. **When should hyperthermia be treated?**
Hyperthermia, with the exception of fevers, should always be treated to return the patient to near normal body temperature. Hyperthermic conditions like malignant hyperthermia and heat stroke are

the result of the body's inability to effectively reduce increased heat production or accumulation. Fevers, their role in the immune response, and their management are topics of ongoing debate. Fever increases metabolic demand and, consequently, oxygen consumption of different organs, notably the brain and the heart, and may worsen preexisting disease. Fever in patients with traumatic brain injury, ischemic stroke, and postcardiac arrest appears to be associated with poorer neurologic recovery and increased mortality—patients in these subgroups may therefore benefit from treatment. The routine treatment of fevers with antipyretics in patients outside of these subsets may actually be harmful and has been associated with both increased and decreased mortality in some studies.

22. **What happens to patients who are relatively hypothermic after the operating room?**
General anesthesia impairs the body's ability to regulate temperature, and patients can become hypothermic. General anesthesia causes peripheral vasodilation and heat redistributes from the core to the periphery and then from the patient to the environment. Without active external intraoperative rewarming, patients may lose 1°C to 2°C during an average operation. Patients who experience intraoperative hypothermia are at increased risk of coagulopathy and wound infections. Intraoperative hypothermia can also prolong the effect of anesthesia medications and may delay immediate postanesthetic recovery.

ACKNOWLEDGMENT

The authors wish to acknowledge Dr. Peter J. Fagenholz, MD, for the valuable contributions to the previous edition of this chapter.

KEY POINTS: HYPOTHERMIA

1. Rigor mortis, dependent lividity, and fixed pupils do not reliably indicate death in severe hypothermia—no one is dead until warm (>35°C) and dead.
2. Endotracheal intubation and central venous catheter placement should not be delayed when indicated in a hypothermic patient.
3. Cardiac arrest should be treated with standard ACLS in conjunction with rewarming.
4. Therapeutic hypothermia is no longer recommended for patients who remain comatose after return of spontaneous circulation from cardiac arrest. Targeted temperature management (temperature = 32°C–36°C) is the current recommendation.

BIBLIOGRAPHY

1. American Heart Association. *Cardiac arrest in accidental hypothermia.* Available at: http://eccguidelines.heart.org/index.php/circulation/cpr-ecc-guidelines-2/part-10-special-circumstances-of-resuscitation/cardiac-arrest-in-accidental-hypothermia/. Accessed September 15, 2016.
2. American Heart Association. *Part 8: post-cardiac arrest care.* Available at: http://eccguidelines.heart.org/index.php/circulation/cpr-ecc-guidelines-2/part-8-post-cardiac-arrest-care/?strue=1&id=4-1-2. Accessed September 15, 2016.
3. Brown DJ, Brugger H, Boyd J, Paal P. Accidental hypothermia. *N Engl J Med.* 2012;367(20):1930-1938.
4. Cohen JA, Blackshear RH, Gravenstein N, Woeste J. Increased pulmonary artery perforating potential of pulmonary artery catheters during hypothermia. *J Cardiothorac Vasc Anesth.* 1991;5:234-236.
5. Crawshaw LI, Wallace HL, Dasgupta S. Thermoregulation. In: Auerbach PS, ed. *Wilderness Medicine.* 5th ed. Philadelphia: Mosby; 2007:110-124.
6. Danzl DF, Pozos RS, Auerbach PS, et al. Multicenter hypothermia survey. *Ann Emerg Med.* 1987;16:1042-1055.
7. Epstein E, Anna K. Accidental hypothermia. *BMJ.* 2006;332:706-709.
8. Graham CA, McNaughton GW, Wyatt JP. The electrocardiogram in hypothermia. *Wilderness Environ Med.* 2001;12:232-235.
9. Gregory JS, Bergstein JM, Aprahamian C, Wittmann DH, Quebbeman EJ. Comparison of three methods of rewarming from hypothermia: advantages of extracorporeal blood warming. *J Trauma.* 1991;31:1247-1251 [discussion: 1251-1252].
10. Grissom CK, Harmston CH, McAlpine JC, et al. Spontaneous endogenous core temperature rewarming after cooling due to snow burial. *Wilderness Environ Med.* 2010;21:229-235.
11. Holzer M. Targeted temperature management for comatose survivors of cardiac arrest. *N Engl J Med.* 2010;363:1256-1264.
12. Laniewicz M, Lyn-Kew K, Silbergleit R. Rapid endovascular warming for profound hypothermia. *Ann Emerg Med.* 2008;51:160-163.

13. Mattu A, Brady WA, Perron AD. Electrocardiographic manifestations of hypothermia. *Am J Emerg Med*. 2002;20: 314-326.
14. Nakajima Y. Controversies in the temperature management of critically ill patients. *J Anesth*. 2016;30(5):873-883.
15. Nunnally ME, Jaeschke R, Bellingan GJ, et al. Targeted temperature management in critical care: a report and recommendations from five professional societies. *Crit Care Med*. 2011;39:1113-1125.
16. Petrone P, Asensio JA, Marini CP. Management of accidental hypothermia and cold injury. *Curr Probl Surg*. 2014; 51(10):417-431.
17. Pitoni S, Sinclair HL, Andrews PJ. Aspects of thermoregulation physiology. *Curr Opin Crit Care*. 2011;17:115-121.
18. Polderman KH. Mechanisms of action, physiological effects, and complications of hypothermia. *Crit Care Med*. 2009; 37(suppl 7):S186-S202.
19. Polderman KH, Herold I. Therapeutic hypothermia and controlled normothermia in the intensive care unit: practical considerations, side effects, and cooling methods. *Crit Care Med*. 2009;37:1101-1120.
20. Sessler DI. Perioperative thermoregulation and heat balance. *Lancet*. 2016;387(10038):2655-2664.

CHAPTER 73

HEAT STROKE

William J. Benedetto

1. **What is heat stroke?**
   Heat stroke is a life-threatening illness characterized by a core body temperature above 40°C and central nervous system (CNS) dysfunction. The CNS abnormalities may include delirium, lethargy, convulsions, or coma. Anhidrosis (lack of sweating) may or may not be present, depending on the type and presentation of the illness.

2. **What is the pathophysiology of heat stroke?**
   The body gains heat from metabolism and from the environment, and this heat must be dissipated to maintain a normal temperature of 37°C. This process (thermoregulation) relies primarily on cutaneous vasodilatation and evaporation of sweat. When these processes are overwhelmed, core temperature will rise. When the core temperature exceeds 40°C, an acute phase response is elicited from heat-stressed cells including cytokines and heat shock proteins. This acute phase response leads to end-organ damage the degree and extent of which is still being characterized.

3. **What are the two types of heat stroke? How do they present?**
   - Classic heat stroke is associated with high environmental heat and humidity with inadequate cooling. There is generally no history of significant exercise or exertion. Classic heat stroke typically has a slow onset, often developing over days. It generally afflicts the elderly and the chronically ill, who may present with anorexia, nausea, vomiting, headache, dizziness, confusion, and hypotension. Anhidrosis is a common finding. Up to 25% of patients present with hypotension.
   - Exertional heat stroke usually affects young people in good health who are exercising in a hot, humid environment, often with clothing or equipment that restricts cooling. It is rapid in onset; nausea, dizziness, and confusion are common. Fatigue, ataxia, coma, and nuchal rigidity or posturing may also occur. Profuse sweating is a typical finding on examination.

4. **Which populations are at greater risk for heat stroke?**
   - Extremes of age—because of relatively poor temperature regulation in the young and old, especially during heat waves
   - Chronically ill—especially those taking drugs that predispose to heat illness
   - Military recruits—especially Northerners not acclimated to the weather in the Southern region of the United States
   - Athletes—most commonly football players and runners
   - Laborers—especially if water losses have not been replaced
   - Obese individuals—because heat dissipation is compromised

5. **Which medications predispose a person to heat stroke?**
   - Drugs increasing heat production through increased motor activity: cocaine, amphetamines, ephedrine, phencyclidine, lysergic acid diethylamide, alcohol withdrawal
   - Drugs decreasing thirst: for example, haloperidol
   - Drugs decreasing sweating: antihistamines, anticholinergics, phenothiazines, β-blockers

6. **What is the mortality rate of heat stroke?**
   When treatment is prompt and effectively lowers core temperature, mortality in young, healthy patients is minimal. In the setting of delayed effective treatment and significant comorbidities, mortality can be as high as 70%.

7. **What are the common sequelae and complications of heat stroke?**
   Heat stroke can lead to multiorgan dysfunction syndrome, including the following:
   - Encephalopathy
   - Renal failure or rhabdomyolysis (most commonly in exertional heat stroke)

- Acute respiratory distress syndrome
- Myocardial injury and circulatory collapse
- Hepatocellular injury
- Intestinal ischemia and infarction
- Pancreatic injury
- Hemorrhagic complications and disseminated intravascular coagulation, which are common complications and important mechanisms in heat stroke morbidity and mortality

8. Which other diagnoses should be considered in a patient presenting with hyperthermia?
- Other hyperthermic syndromes
  - Malignant hyperthermia
  - Neuroleptic malignant syndrome
  - Drug-induced hyperthermia
- Infections
  - Especially meningitis, encephalitis, and sepsis
- Endocrinopathies
  - Such as thyroid storm and pheochromocytoma
- CNS lesions
  - Hypothalamic bleeding, acute hydrocephalus

9. How can heat stroke be prevented?
Heat stroke is currently more preventable than treatable. Efforts to prevent heat stroke should focus on acclimatization (gradual exposure to higher temperature environments and increasing workloads), rescheduling activities to cooler times of day, increasing consumption of nonalcoholic fluids, and removing vulnerable populations from high-heat areas.

10. What is the most important aspect in the treatment of heat stroke?
Rapid cooling is the main therapeutic goal for treatment of heat stroke. Mortality increases dramatically with even relatively short delays in cooling. Delay in cooling is a better predictor of poor patient outcome than the degree of hyperthermia.

11. What treatment modalities are effective for rapid cooling?
Immersion in ice water is effective, though can be difficult to do and is often poorly tolerated. This modality may not be appropriate in the comatose or combative patient. Aggressive evaporative cooling, consisting of treatment with tepid water spray (40°C [104°F]) and a forced air stream from a fan, has proved successful and is an easy therapy to apply. Ice packs with skin massage to encourage vasodilatation may also be used. Techniques such as iced gastric lavage and peritoneal lavage have also been reported, though the additional cooling may not warrant the increased procedural risks. Though a cooling target has not been clearly established, a core temperature of 39°C or less is considered safe.

12. In addition to cooling, what other treatment is appropriate?
Heat stroke can lead to multiorgan dysfunction, and supportive therapy is indicated, as appropriate:
- Airway protection and mechanical ventilation
- Seizure control with benzodiazepines
- Monitoring of circulatory status and fluid therapy or pressors as needed
- Volume expansion and renal monitoring in the setting of rhabdomyolysis
- Correction of electrolyte abnormalities

13. Which laboratory abnormalities are seen in heat stroke?
- Acid/base disturbance. Classic heat stroke commonly presents with a respiratory alkalosis.
- Exertional heat stroke presents with a respiratory alkalosis and lactic acidosis.
- Hypophosphatemia is common in classic heat stroke, though heat stroke associated with exertion may present with hyperphosphatemia from rhabdomyolysis.
- Hypokalemia is common except in the setting of rhabdomyolysis.
- Serum proteins and hypercalcemia increase because of volume contraction.

14. What prognostic signs predict outcome?
Longer duration of hyperthermia is associated with poorer outcome. Coma, hypotension, hyperkalemia, and an aspartate aminotransferase level greater than 1000 units are associated with a poor prognosis.

15. What steps can be taken to prevent heat stroke?
    • Maintain adequate fluid intake during periods of high temperature, high humidity, or increased activity levels.
    • Decrease levels of activity during time of high heat and humidity.
    • Control ambient temperature and humidity if possible.
    • Dress appropriately for the weather.
    • Use prudence during acclimation to a hotter environment.
    • Adjust dosages of predisposing drugs, if possible, during hot weather.
    • Be aware of symptoms of impending heat stroke.

16. Are medications used to treat heat stroke?
    In general, pharmacologic therapy is NOT indicated for the treatment of classic or exertional heat stroke.
    • Antipyretics are not indicated for the treatment of heat stroke, as the cause of the elevated core temperature is not related to the body's temperature "set-point."
    • Though a preliminary trial suggested some efficacy for dantrolene, further study concluded that dantrolene is *not* indicated for the treatment of heat stroke, except when related to malignant hyperthermia.

KEY POINTS: HEAT STROKE

Diagnostic Criteria for Heat Stroke
1. Exposure to increased heat stress: exercise and/or increased temperature and humidity.
2. Altered mental status.
3. Core (rectal) temperature greater than 40°C.
4. Sweating may or may not be present.

BIBLIOGRAPHY

1. Bouchama A, Dehbi M, Chaves-Carballo E. Cooling and hemodynamic management in heatstroke: practical recommendations. *Crit Care.* 2007;11:R54.
2. Bouchama A, De Vol EB. Acid–base alterations in heat stroke. *Intensive Care Med.* 2002;27:680-685.
3. Bouchama A, Knochel JP. Heat stroke. *N Engl J Med.* 2002;346:1978-1988.
4. Curley FJ, Irwin RS. Disorders of temperature control part II: hyperthermia. In: Irwin RS, Rippe JM, eds. *Intensive Care Medicine.* 5th ed. Philadelphia: Lippincott Williams & Wilkins; 2003:762-777.
5. Leon L, Helwig B. Heat stroke: role of the systemic inflammatory response. *J Appl Physiol (1985).* 2010;109:1980-1988.
6. Marini JJ, Wheeler AP. Thermal disorders. In: *Critical Care Medicine, The Essentials.* Philadelphia: Lippincott Williams & Wilkins; 2006:466-476.
7. O'Connor FG, Casa DJ, Bergeron MF, et al. American College of Sports Medicine Roundtable on exertional heat stroke—return to duty/return to play: conference proceedings. *Curr Sports Med Rep.* 2010;9:314-321.
8. Lin XJ, Li YL, Mei GP, et al. Activated protein C can be used as a prophylactic as well as a therapeutic agent for heat stroke in rodents. *Shock.* 2009;32.524-529.

XIV
TOXICOLOGY

GENERAL APPROACH TO POISONINGS

Jason L. Sanders and Jarone Lee

CHAPTER 74

1. **What are the most common causes of poisoning in adults?**
   - Analgesics (11.9% of poisonings)
   - Sedatives/hypnotics/antipsychotics (10.4%)
   - Antidepressants (6.7%)
   - Cardiovascular drugs (6.1%)
   - Cleaning substances (household; 5.7%)
   - Alcohols (4.6%)
   - Anticonvulsants (3.7%)
   - Pesticides (3.5%)
   - Bites and envenomations (3.3%)
   - Antihistamines (3.1%)

2. **What are the most common causes of poison-associated deaths in adults?**
   - Miscellaneous sedatives/hypnotics/antipsychotics (13.8% of poison-associated deaths)
   - Miscellaneous cardiovascular drugs (13.3%)
   - Opioids (7.9%)
   - Miscellaneous stimulants and street drugs (7.4%)
   - Miscellaneous alcohols (5.6%)
   - Acetaminophen alone (5.1%)
   - Acetaminophen combinations (4.8%)
   - Selective serotonin reuptake inhibitors (SSRI; 3.6%)
   - Miscellaneous fumes/gases/vapors (2.6%)
   - Miscellaneous antidepressants (2.4%)

3. **Should intentional poisonings be assumed *a priori* to have a greater chance of serious harm?**
   - Yes. While only 1.02% and 0.07% of poisonings result in a major effect or death, respectively, intentional poisonings are 32-fold more likely to result in major or fatal effects. This piece of history helps predict clinical course.

4. **What is an initial approach to evaluation and treatment of suspected poisoning, particularly for critically ill patients?**
   History is often unreliable or unavailable. An agent-blind approach is preferable. Focus on airway, breathing, circulation, disability, exposure, and expert consultations (ABCDEs) first:
   - *Airway:* Assess the airway and continuously monitor pulse oximetry. Perform endotracheal intubation if there is doubt about the patient's ability to protect the airway and avoid aspiration. If required, nondepolarizing paralytic (e.g., rocuronium) is preferred to depolarizing paralytic (succinylcholine) if there is risk of existing hyperkalemia (e.g., digoxin overdose, coexisting renal failure). If opioid overdose is suspected, empiric administration of Naloxone should be attempted. Flumazenil is generally avoided even when benzodiazepine overdose is suspected; benzodiazepines are often co-ingested with other compounds for which they are the empiric treatment, and flumazenil can precipitate withdrawal seizures.
   - *Breathing:* Ensure adequate oxygenation and ventilation. In a nonintubated patient with depressed or waxing/waning mental status, if possible, monitor end-tidal CO_2. End-tidal CO_2 illustrates hypopnea and bradypnea, useful for signaling need for additional treatment or stimulation, or when intubation may be necessary. Notably, carbon monoxide poisoning can cause severe hypoxia despite normal pulse oximetry, and methemoglobinemia may display a persistent pulse oximetry of 85% despite severe hypoxia. Beware intubating a patient with severe metabolic acidosis and compensatory respiratory alkalosis (e.g., severe salicylate poisoning), as intubation without ability to maintain adequate minute ventilation may result in cardiovascular collapse.

- *Circulation*: Apply continuous cardiac monitoring and obtain an electrocardiogram.
  - Asystole is treated according to Advanced Cardiac Life Support algorithm.
  - Hypotension can be empirically treated with intravenous (IV) crystalloid. Beware the normally hypertensive older adult who presents normotensive.
  - Bradycardia, along with other electrocardiography (EKG), exam, and lab findings, may suggest underlying cause and treatment approach (Table 74.1).
  - Tachycardia is differentiated by rhythm and interval normality: monomorphic wide complex (often due to sodium channel blockade, treated with IV sodium bicarbonate); polymorphic wide complex (often treated with IV magnesium sulfate); and narrow complex (with hypertension, often due to sympathomimetics or cholinergioo).
- *Disability*: Check finger stick blood glucose. Altered mental status can be caused by hyperglycemia or hypoglycemia. Empiric IV dextrose is required if blood glucose is not rapidly obtainable. Maintain in-line cervical spine immobilization and possibly log-roll precautions if occult trauma is suspected.
- *Exposure*: Ensure adequate safety of patient and staff by following proper decontamination procedures. Undress the patient for full examination and decontamination.
- *Experts*: Early involvement of poison control and toxicology experts is beneficial for assistance with clinical management and public health surveillance. United States poison control centers can be reached 24/7 through a toll-free line (1-800-222-1222). The World Health Organization provides a listing of international poison centers at its website.

5. What are common toxidromes which may help identify the agent underlying poisoning?
   Toxidromes are physiologic syndromes associated with classes of toxins. They may be useful in making the diagnosis of poisoning and initiating treatment (Table 74.2).

6. What laboratory testing is indicated in the poisoned patient?
   Laboratory testing in critically ill poisoned patients should be tailored to the suspected toxin(s) and the findings of the history and physical examination. Laboratory testing should include:
   - Serum electrolytes: Hyperkalemia or hypokalemia increase risk of arrhythmia.
   - Magnesium: If low, inhibits repletion of potassium and increases risk for arrhythmia.
   - Arterial blood gas: Acid-base status predicts intensive care unit (ICU) admission and mortality, guides ventilation, resuscitation, and repletion efforts.

Table 74-1. Trends in Poisonings Causing Bradycardia

AGENT	EKG	CLINICAL FINDINGS	LABORATORY FINDINGS	TREATMENT
Alpha-2 agonists	Sinus bradycardia	Miosis, decreased MS	No patterns	Naloxone
Beta-blocker	First-degree AVB	Decreased MS	Hypoglycemia	Glucagon, IV Calcium
Calcium-channel blocker	Second- and third-degree AVB	Preserved MS	Hyperglycemia	High-dose insulin, IV calcium, Intralipid
Digoxin	Bidirectional ventricular arrhythmia	Change in color vision	Hyperkalemia, elevated digoxin level	Digoxin specific antibody
Organophosphate	Sinus bradycardia	Diarrhea, Urination, Miosis, Bradycardia, Bronchorrhea/Bronchospasm, Emesis Lacrimation Salivation	Decreased RBC cholinesterase activity	Atropine, pralidoxime

AVB, atrial-ventricular block; *EKG*, electrocardiography; *IV*, intravenous; *MS*, mental status; *RBC*, red blood cell. Adapted with permission from Kenneth Bernard, MD, MBA.

Table 74-2. Common Toxidromes

TOXIDROME	CLINICAL FINDINGS	EXAMPLE AGENTS
Cholinergic	Diarrhea, fecal incontinence, enuresis, miosis, tachycardia followed by bradycardia, lacrimation, sialorrhea, sweating, muscle fasciculations followed by weakness and/or paralysis, altered mental status	Organophosphate and carbamate insecticides *Amanita muscaria* Nicotine
Anticholinergic	Agitated delirium, flushing, decreased sweating, tachycardia, mydriasis, urinary retention, decreased peristalsis, hyperthermia	Atropine Benztropine Scopolamine Diphenhydramine
Sympathomimetic	Mydriasis, hyperthermia, seizures, hyperactivity, hypertension, tachycardia, diaphoresis, delusions, piloerection	Cocaine Methamphetamine MDMA
Sympatholytic	Miosis, hypotension, bradycardia or reflex tachycardia, CNS depression	Clonidine Methyldopa Oxymetazoline
Opioid	Miosis, CNS depression, respiratory depression or apnea, may have hypotension	Heroin Morphine Fentanyl Oxycodone
Serotonin syndrome	Mental status changes, autonomic hyperactivity, neuromuscular abnormalities, akathisia, tremor, clonus, muscle hypertonicity, hyperthermia	Sertraline Fluoxetine Citalopram Linezolid Trazodone Meperidine Tramadol
Neuroleptic malignant syndrome	Fever, "lead pipe" muscular rigidity, altered mental status, autonomic dysfunction (in setting of recent treatment with neuroleptics)	Haloperidol Chlorpromazine Promethazine Prochlorperazine Ziprasidone Quetiapine

CNS, Central nervous system; MDMA, methylenedioxymethamphetamine.

- Anion gap: If elevated, suggests metabolic disturbance and possible agent.
- Serum osmolarity: If elevated anion gap, calculating Osmolar gap can suggest toxic alcohol ingestion such as isopropyl alcohol.
- Urinalysis: Casts suggest acute tubular necrosis from intrinsic renal damage. Positive hemoglobin screen without presence of red blood cells suggests rhabdomyolysis. Oxylate crystals suggest ethylene glycol poisoning. Fluorescence under a Wood lamp suggests antifreeze ingestion.
- Liver function tests: May be elevated in acute or chronic alcohol or acetaminophen use.
- Prothrombin time: May be prolonged in acetaminophen overdose-associated liver damage.

7. What is the value of serum and urine toxicology screens in the poisoned patient?
In many hospitals, a *basic* serum toxicology screen includes levels of acetaminophen, salicylate, and volatile alcohols. This is a good starting point when ingestants are unknown, as it includes treatable toxins for which serum levels guide therapy. Quantitative levels of tricyclic antidepressants are of *no* value in determining treatment, and many hospitals use a qualitative screen. Urine drug screens are often used to test for metabolites of drugs of abuse and are often not valuable in making a toxicologic diagnosis. Some hospitals have comprehensive blood or urine toxicology testing that can isolate many obscure compounds. However, the results of these tests often become available long after the window

for appropriate treatment has closed for patients. It is important to know the availability of toxicologic testing at your hospital and to be aware of the limitations of testing. Cross-reactivity with particular assays may also lead to false positives. Treating patients on the basis of their clinical status rather than their test results is often the safest plan.

8. What predicts need for intensive care?
   General criteria for disposition to an ICU includes:
   - $PaCO_2$ >45 mm Hg
   - Need for intubation
   - Postingestion seizures
   - Unresponsiveness to verbal stimuli
   - Nonsinus cardiac rhythm
   - Second- or third-degree atrioventricular block
   - Systolic blood pressure less than 80 mm Hg
   - QRS duration ≥0.12 seconds
   - Age greater than 60 to 65 years
   - Abnormal body temperature
   - Suicidal intent

9. Is there a role for syrup of ipecac in treating poisoning?
   Syrup of ipecac, which induces vomiting, is not recommended in acute poisoning treatment. The American Academy of Clinical Toxicology and the American Academy of Pediatrics recommend against the routine administration of ipecac to poisoned patients in the emergency department and in the home.

10. Is there a role for gastric lavage in the management of the poisoned intensive care unit patient?
    Gastric lavage *(stomach pumping)* involves passage of a large-bore orogastric tube and repeated instillation and aspiration of fluid to remove potentially toxic stomach contents. Usually, there is no role for gastric lavage in the critically poisoned patient. Clinical studies have not confirmed benefit of gastric lavage alone even when performed rapidly (<60 minutes) after ingestion. However, it can be considered in certain, rare cases, such as early (<60 minutes) massive overdoses of drugs without a clear antidote.

11. What is the role of single-dose activated charcoal in the treatment of poisoned patients?
    Activated charcoal reduces the bioavailability of some substances, with the magnitude of reduction declining with increasing time from the ingestion. A single dose of activated charcoal may be useful in the management of some patients, but evidence is insufficient from clinical studies that single-dose activated charcoal improves outcomes in poisoned patients. Consider ICU administration of activated charcoal on a case-by-case basis *only* if the ingested toxin is well adsorbed to activated charcoal (Box 74.1), if the risk of the ingested poison outweighs the aspiration risk of charcoal administration, and if the patient has a patent or protected airway.

12. Does multiple-dose activated charcoal reduce the absorption of poisons from the gastrointestinal tract?
    Multiple-dose activated charcoal (MDAC) is repeated administration of enteral activated charcoal in an effort to increase drug elimination via diffusion along concentration gradients into the gut and preventing the reabsorption of drugs with significant enterohepatic circulation. The process has been referred to as "gastrointestinal dialysis," and drugs amenable to MDAC share some characteristics with dialyzable drugs, including a low (<1 L/kg) volume of distribution and low protein binding. MDAC has demonstrated enhanced elimination of carbamazepine, dapsone, theophylline, quinine,

Box 74-1. Toxins Poorly Adsorbed by Activated Charcoal	
Acids	Inorganic salts
Alcohols including ethanol	Iron
Alkali	Lithium
Ethylene glycol	Pesticides
Heavy metals	Potassium

and phenobarbital. It has been proposed as treatment for a number of other agents, including salicylate and digoxin, and may also be considered for poisoning by sustained-release preparations of drugs.

13. **What is whole-bowel irrigation, and does its use benefit poisoned patients?**
Whole-bowel irrigation (WBI) is the administration of large volumes of polyethylene glycol solution, with the intent of flushing drugs or toxins out of the gastrointestinal tract via liquid stools. Data on the efficacy of WBI for removing drugs from the body are mixed, and clinical evidence is insufficient to recommend its routine use. In addition, the administration of WBI is likely to cause significant discomfort to patients. WBI is possibly an option for expediting the gastrointestinal luminal clearance of sustained-release preparations, toxic heavy metals, or packets of illicit drugs smuggled within the body ("body packers").

14. **What is the role of dialysis in the care of the poisoned patient?**
Drugs amenable to removal via hemodialysis share a number of important characteristics. They must:
- Be small enough and lack charge such that they will cross a dialysis membrane.
- Be highly water soluble and have a small volume of distribution (<1 L/kg is a good rule of thumb) so that they are concentrated in the blood (rather than the tissues) in sufficient quantity for removal.
- Have low protein binding in general, although dialysis can occasionally be used to remove free drug when protein binding is fully saturated in a massive overdose.

15. **Which drugs can be removed from the body via hemodialysis?**
Lithium and salicylate are two drugs commonly removed via hemodialysis in overdose. When considering hemodialysis in a poisoned patient, the risks of the procedure, including venous and/or arterial access, discomfort, transient anticoagulation, and hemodynamic shifts must be weighed carefully against the severity of the poisoning. Acetaminophen can easily be removed by hemodialysis, but this is rarely done, because antidotal treatment with *N*-acetylcysteine usually works well, is noninvasive, and carries less risk to the patient.

16. **What antidotes are commonly useful in the intensive care unit?**
See Table 74.3.

Table 74-3. Antidotes Commonly Used in the Intensive Care Unit

ANTIDOTE	PHARMACOLOGIC EFFECTS	TYPICAL USES
Benzodiazepines	Potentiator of GABA inhibitory neurotransmission in the CNS	Alcohol or sedative/hypnotic withdrawal Antiepileptic Anxiolysis, sedation Relaxation of muscle rigidity Treatment of agitation associated with sympathomimetic or anticholinergic syndromes
Sodium bicarbonate	Can produce alkalemia in the serum and in urine, provides sodium ion load	Treatment of sodium channel blockade due to: tricyclic antidepressants, Class Ia and Ic antiarrhythmics, cocaine, diphenhydramine Serum and urinary alkalinization to prevent tissue distribution and improve renal clearance of: Salicylates
Flumazenil	CNS benzodiazepine receptor antagonist	Reversal of CNS and respiratory depression due to benzodiazepines (in patients *without* history of long-term benzodiazepine use)
Glucose	Cellular energy source	Hypoglycemia Empiric treatment for altered mental status or seizure without clear cause With high-dose insulin infusion for calcium channel blocker poisoning

(Continued on following page)

Table 74-3. Antidotes Commonly Used in the Intensive Care Unit *(Continued)*

ANTIDOTE	PHARMACOLOGIC EFFECTS	TYPICAL USES
Naloxone	Opioid mu, kappa, and delta receptor antagonist	Reversal of respiratory and/or CNS depression suspected to be caused by opiates, opioids
Octreotide	Long-acting somatostatin analog, inhibits pancreatic insulin release	Suppression of drug-induced insulin secretion caused by: Sulfonylureas, quinine
Hydroxocobalamin	Binds cyanide ions to form cyanocobalamin, which is excreted in the urine	Treatment of cyanide toxicity
Physostigmine	CNS and peripheral acetylcholinesterase inhibitor, increasing stimulation of nicotinic and muscarinic ACh receptors	Transient reversal of severe antimuscarinic syndromes *not* caused by cyclic antidepressants
Deferoxamine	Binds free iron in the blood, enhances urinary elimination	Treatment of iron toxicity
Intravenous lipid emulsion	Expands lipid phase in blood, driving lipophilic toxins from tissue into lipid sink	Treatment of local anesthetic toxicity

ACh, Acetylcholine; *CNS,* central nervous system; *GABA,* γ-aminobutyric acid.

17. What additional clinical services should be employed to care for patients with intentional poisonings?

From age 10 to 54, suicide and unintentional injury are two of the top four leading causes of death. As a rule, patients with intentional poisoning should undergo assessment by mental health professionals for assistance with diagnosis and treatment of coexisting mental illness. It is critical to determine eligibility for adjunct care programs and if ingestion is related to physical, mental, or other types of abuse on and/or by the patient.

ACKNOWLEDGMENT

The authors wish to acknowledge Drs. Aaron B. Skolnik, MD, and Susan R. Wilcox, MD, for the valuable contributions to the previous edition of this chapter.

KEY POINTS: GENERAL APPROACH TO POISONINGS

Toxicology
1. A standardized ABCDE approach should be used for all poisoned patients, particularly the critically ill.
2. Stabilization and empiric treatment may precede non-point-of-care diagnostic evaluation.
3. The diagnostic evaluation for the poisoned critically ill patient should be determined by the history and physical examination.
4. Urine and serum toxicology screens vary among hospitals and may not be of significant clinical utility.
5. Syrup of ipecac and gastric lavage no longer have roles in the management of the poisoned patient.
6. Hemodialysis is beneficial in the management of several common poisonings.
7. Poisonings with antidotes must be recognized and treatment initiated promptly.

BIBLIOGRAPHY

1. Alapat PM, Zimmerman JL. Toxicology in the critical care unit. *Chest.* 2008;133:1006-1013.
2. Boyle JS, Bechtel LK, Holstege CP. Management of the critically poisoned patient. *Scand J Trauma Resusc Emerg Med.* 2009;17:29.
3. Brett AS, Rothschild N, Gray R, Perry M. Predicting the clinical course in intentional drug overdose. Implications for use of the intensive care unit. *Arch Intern Med.* 1987;147(1):133.
4. Erickson TB, Thompson TM, Lu JJ. The approach to the patient with an unknown overdose. *Emerg Med Clin North Am.* 2007;25:249-281.
5. Hamdi H, Hassanian-Moghaddam H, Hamdi A, Zahed NS. Acid-base disturbances in acute poisoning and their association with survival. *J Crit Care.* 2016;35:84-89.
6. Hoegberg LC, Bania TC, Lavergne V, et al. Systematic review of the effect of intravenous lipid emulsion therapy for local anesthetic toxicity. *Clin Toxicol (Phila).* 2016;54(3):167-193.
7. Holstege CP, Dobmeier SG, Bechtel LK. Critical care toxicology. *Emerg Med Clin North Am.* 2008;26:715-739, viii-ix.
8. Mowry JB, Spyker DA, Brooks DE, McMillan N, Schauben JL. 2014 Annual Report of the American Association of Poison Control Centers' National Poison Data System (NPDS): 32nd Annual Report. *Clin Toxicol (Phila).* 2015;53(10): 962-1147, doi:10.3109/15563650.2015.1102927.
9. Lee HL, Lin HJ, Yeh ST, Chi CH, Guo HR. Presentations of patients of poisoning and predictors of poisoning-related fatality: findings from a hospital-based prospective study. *BMC Public Health.* 2008;8:7.
10. Mokhlesi B, Leiken JB, Murray P, Corbridge TC. Adult toxicology in critical care: part I: general approach to the intoxicated patient. *Chest.* 2003;123:577-592.
11. World Health Organization. *Poison centres.* Available at: http://www.who.int/gho/phe/chemical_safety/poisons_centres/en/. Accessed October 16, 2016.
12. Wu AH, McKay C, Broussard LA. National Academy of Clinical Biochemistry laboratory medicine practice guidelines: recommendations for the use of laboratory tests to support poisoned patients who present to the emergency department. *Clin Chem.* 2003;49:357-379.

CHAPTER 75

ANALGESICS AND ANTIDEPRESSANTS

Alexis McCabe and Jarone Lee

SALICYLATE TOXICITY

1. **What are the signs and symptoms salicylate poisoning?**
   - **Acute Toxicity:**
     - **Mild:** tinnitus/decreased hearing, nausea, vomiting, diaphoresis, hyperventilation, tachypnea.
     - **Moderate–Severe:** noncardiogenic pulmonary edema, hyperthermia, confusion, delirium, coma, seizures
   - **Chronic Toxicity:** similar to acute poisoning, but more insidious. Often mistaken for sepsis.

   Salicylates stimulate the chemoreceptor trigger zone in the medulla and are highly irritating to the gastrointestinal (GI) tract, resulting in abdominal pain, nausea, vomiting, and occasionally hematemesis; tinnitus and other auditory disturbances from unknown mechanisms that cause toxicity of the cochlea and central nervous system (CNS). Salicylates stimulate the medullary respiratory center causing hyperventilation leading to primary respiratory alkalosis. Uncoupling of oxidative phosphorylation by salicylates causes decreased gluconeogenesis and hyperthermia, thus causing increased oxygen consumption, metabolic rate, and anaerobic glycolysis resulting in organic acid production. Accumulation of organic acids is exacerbated by inhibition of the Krebs cycle, resulting in high anion gap metabolic acidosis. Salicylate-induced increased vascular permeability results in noncardiogenic pulmonary edema and higher brain concentration of the drug.

2. **What constitutes a toxic dose of salicylate and what are some of the sources?**
   The minimal dose required for acute toxicity is 100 mg/kg. Ingestions of greater than 300 mg/kg may be lethal. Other sources of salicylate toxicity besides aspirin include ingestion of aspirin-containing medications such as liquid methyl salicylate (oil of wintergreen), bismuth subsalicylate (Pepto-Bismol)—particularly in children, effervescent antacids, and rarely topical application of ointment containing salicylic acid. Chronic salicylate toxicity may also develop in elderly patients, dehydrated patients, or those taking carbonic anhydrase inhibitors. This can happen even at stable therapeutic doses, depending on the patient's underlying health status and salicylate clearance.

3. **What are the management priorities in treating salicylate poisoning?**
   - Airway, breathing and circulation (ABCs)
   - Volume repletion and correction of metabolic derangements.
   - GI decontamination: after risk/benefit consideration, GI decontamination may be indicated to delay and prevent absorption with administration of activated charcoal, particularly in patients who present early after ingestion or in patients with signs of incomplete absorption (e.g., increasing serum levels).
   - Airway protection and maintenance of respiratory status.
   - Enhanced elimination via prevention of acidemia, alkalinization of urine and extracorporeal methods of clearance with renal replacement therapy.

4. **What signs can portend a poor outcome?**
   The signs of moderate-severe toxicity: hyperthermia, confusion, delirium, coma, seizures, noncardiogenic pulmonary edema in conjunction with severe acidemia can portend a poor prognosis.

5. **What lab values are important to monitor?**
   Management of a salicylate-intoxicated patient requires maintenance of adequate urine output and frequent monitoring of electrolytes, salicylate level, urine pH and blood pH (q1-2h).

6. **What is the effect of salicylate toxicity on electrolytes?**
   Electrolyte balance is imperative. Pay particular attention to glucose management. CNS glucose utilization is increased and CNS glucose concentration may be less than measured serum levels. Hypokalemia

is also a common complication that requires correction. In the setting of hypokalemia, renal reabsorption of potassium via hydrogen ion exchange prevents urinary alkalization, thus decreasing elimination of the drug. Variances in lab analyzers can result in falsely elevated chloride when measured in the presence of salicylates, thus using electrolytes to identify a high anion gap as an indication of possible salicylate toxicity can be unreliable.

7. What is the effect of salicylate toxicity on acid-base status?
   Classically a mixed picture of early primary respiratory alkalosis, elevated anion gap metabolic acidosis and, occasionally, a late respiratory acidosis. Variations can be seen based on amount or timing of ingestion, lab error, or concomitant ingestions. While salicylate toxicity causes acute respiratory alkalosis, it is classically without hypoxia. If a patient is hypoxic, consider noncardiogenic pulmonary edema and co-ingestions. In a patient with respiratory acidosis, consider polysubstance ingestion. Clinical severity can be predicted by serum pH. It is imperative to avoid acidemia, and patients with pH <7.35 are considered to have severe poisoning.

8. What is significant about a salicylate-intoxicated patient's volume status?
   Salicylate-intoxicated patients are typically volume depleted and the degree to which is often underappreciated. Euvolemia should be achieved, as hypovolemia can worsen electrolyte and acid-base disarray via renally mediated sodium and bicarbonate reabsorption and potassium excretion.

9. How does salicylate toxicity cause hematologic abnormalities?
   Platelet function is inhibited and any salicylate-containing product can inhibit vitamin K-dependent clotting factors in toxic concentrations—including decreased production of factor II (prothrombin) and factor VII. The drug also increases capillary endothelial fragility and decreases the amount and function of platelets, although significant bleeding is rare.

10. What is significant about measuring salicylate concentration in a salicylate-intoxicated patient?
    It is important to interpret levels in the context with the patient's overall clinical condition. Many factors can affect salicylate level, including time of exposure, formulation, comorbidities, co-ingestions, reported salicylate concentration units, and patient's pH status. Clinical management should be based on the patient's overall clinical condition and not solely on the salicylate serum level. If the patient's salicylate concentration approaches greater than 90 to 100 mg/dL or greater than 80 to 90 mg/dL with evidence of renal dysfunction, then they need emergent hemodialysis (HD). In chronic toxicity, salicylate concentration may not correlate with patient's clinical acuity.

11. What are important considerations when intubating a salicylate-intoxicated patient?
    Intubation may be indicated in the following: (1) deteriorating mental status; (2) acute lung injury; and (3) in patients with uncontrollable agitation. However, hyperventilation is not in itself an indication for intubation. Sedation and intubation in a salicylate-intoxicated patient can be a precursor to rapid clinical decompensation and increased mortality. Prior to intubation, assess the patient's minute ventilation and pCO_2 to ensure these are maintained via bag valve mask ventilation and then via mechanical ventilation. Concurrent with intubation, administer sodium bicarbonate IV to maintain serum pH of 7.45 to 7.50, as sedation and induction can result in respiratory acidosis and retention of CO_2, causing infiltration of salicylate into the CNS peri-intubation.

12. What is the role of bicarbonate in the treatment of salicylate poisoning?
    Alkalization of serum is important in limiting the distribution of salicylate into tissues, especially the CNS. Furthermore, the ensuing urinary alkalization traps salicylate in its ionized form in the urine and enhances renal clearance. Sodium bicarbonate solutions (typically dextrose 5% with 150 mEq/L 7.5% or 8.4% sodium bicarbonate) should be infused to a goal serum pH of 7.5 to 7.55. This will also help to alkalinize the urine, with a goal urinary pH of 7.5 to 8.0. The rate of infusion should be titrated to maintain a urine output of 2 to 3 cc/kg per hour. To maintain alkaluria, potassium must be replaced aggressively. Often, 30 to 40 mEq/L of potassium chloride is added to sodium bicarbonate infusions to maintain normokalemia.

13. What are the indications for HD in salicylate toxicity?
    Hemodialysis is the preferred method of extracorporeal treatment in salicylate toxicity. Indications are variable in each patient, but should be considered early and often. Indications include, but are not limited to: (salicylate) greater than 100 mg/dL or greater than 90 mg/dL in the presence of impaired renal function; significant CNS alterations such as altered mental status (AMS); seizure; delirium; acute lung injury; new hypoxemia requiring supplemental oxygen or inability to maintain respiratory capacity; significant renal injury not responsive to fluid replenishment; significant hyperthermia; refractory/profound acidemia (serum pH ≤ 7.2) or electrolyte disturbance; contraindication to

volume resuscitation or administration of sodium bicarbonate; and deteriorating clinical condition or rising serum salicylate concentrations (>90 mg/dL or >80 mg/dL w/renal dysfunction) despite adequate resuscitation and sodium bicarbonate administration.

ACETAMINOPHEN TOXICITY

14. What are the signs and symptoms of acetaminophen poisoning?

It is often difficult to recognize, as patients are often asymptomatic after acute ingestion, although some may present with nausea, vomiting, anorexia, or lethargy within hours; very rarely after a massive overdose, patients can present with AMS and metabolic acidosis within 6 hours of ingestion. Twenty-four to 48 hours after overdose, hepatic injury with transaminitis may develop or even acute or hyperacute liver failure with accompanying hyperbilirubinemia, jaundice, coagulopathy, and encephalopathy. Acute renal failure, which is probably multifactorial in origin, may also occur. Acetaminophen toxicity should be considered in any patient with unexplained liver failure.

15. What are predictors of hepatotoxicity?

The most accurate predictor is the serum acetaminophen concentration at 4 to 24 hours after acute ingestion as it relates to the Rumack-Matthew nomogram. Consider hepatotoxicity if ingestion is 7.5 g or 100 mg/kg (whichever is less), co-ingestions especially with diphenhydramine, and presence of medications that increase cytochrome P450 activity.

16. What are the four phases of acetaminophen toxicity?

See Table 75.1.

17. What is the mechanism of acetaminophen-induced hepatotoxicity?

Under therapeutic dosing conditions, most acetaminophen is metabolized in the liver by glucuronidation and sulphation into nontoxic compounds that are excreted in the urine. A very small percentage of acetaminophen is excreted unchanged in the urine. The remainder is metabolized by the cytochrome P-450 system (mostly CYP2E1). During this metabolism, a toxic intermediary, N-acetyl-p-benzoquinone imine (NAPQI), is produced that is rapidly detoxified by hepatic glutathione and ultimately excreted in the urine. The liver has a fixed amount of glutathione, thus in an overdose, it is quickly depleted, leaving the toxic intermediary, NAPQI unmetabolized. This allows NAPQI to accumulate and cause hepatocyte necrosis by binding to hepatic enzymes' sulfhydryl groups.

18. How is the Rumack-Matthew acetaminophen treatment nomogram used?

The Rumack-Matthew treatment nomogram is used to identify patients who have taken a single, acute acetaminophen overdose and who are at risk for hepatotoxicity and require treatment. To use the nomogram, the time of ingestion must be known and a serum acetaminophen level must be drawn at a known time at least 4 hours after ingestion. The time after ingestion is plotted on the x-axis and the acetaminophen level on the y-axis. If the intersection point of these two values falls above the treatment line, the patient is treated with N-acetylcysteine (NAC). In the United States, this treatment line is labeled "possible hepatic toxicity" and corresponds with a 4-hour postingestion

Table 75-1. Time Course and Clinical Stages of Acetaminophen Toxicity

STAGE	TIME COURSE	NAME	SYMPTOMS	SIGNS
1	0–12 (up to 24–36) h	Preinjury	Nausea, vomiting, anorexia, malaise	Elevated serum acetaminophen concentration
2	8–36 h	Liver injury	Nausea, vomiting, RUQ abdominal pain	Transaminitis (AST begins to rise 8–36 h after ingestion)
3	2–4 days	Maximum liver injury	Liver Failure (encephalopathy, coagulopathy, hemorrhage, acidosis)	Hemorrhage, ARDS, sepsis/SIRS, multiorgan failure, cerebral edema
4	>4 days	Recovery	None	Complete hepatic histologic recovery

ARDS, acute respiratory distress syndrome; *AST*, aspartate aminotransferase; *RUQ*, rightupper quadrant; *SIRS*, systemic inflammatory response syndrome. From Adams J. *Emergency Medicine: Clinical Essentials.* Philadelphia, PA: Saunders; 2012.

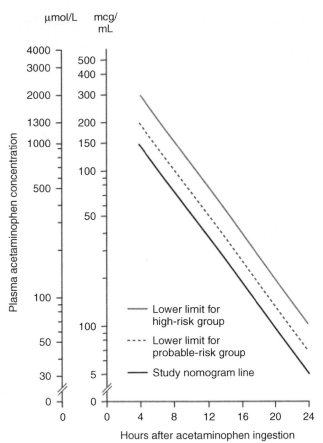

Figure 75-1. The Rumack-Matthew nomogram identifies patients with a single ingestion of acetaminophen at risk for hepatotoxicity. (From Heard KJ. Acetylcysteine for acetaminophen poisoning. *N Engl J Med.* 2008;359:285–292.)

acetaminophen level of 150 mcg/mL (Fig. 75.1). Of note, the U.K. guidelines have been revised to begin NAC with a 4-hour postingestion acetaminophen level of 100 mcg/mL.

19. How does N-acetylcysteine work?
NAC works by replenishing hepatic glutathione stores and acting as a glutathione substitute, allowing the detoxification of NAPQI. This prevents the resulting NAPQI-induced hepatocyte damage and death. It also increases sulphation of acetaminophen, thereby reducing NAPQI formation.

20. What methods are used to administer N-acetylcysteine? Is one better than the other?
Two common regimens exist for treatment and prevention of acetaminophen-induced hepatotoxicity, a 72-hour regimen of oral NAC and a 20-hour regimen of intravenous (IV) NAC. On the basis of the literature at the time of this writing, both regimens seem to have good safety profiles for patients, though more anaphylactoid reactions occur when NAC is administered intravenously and more GI intolerance when administered orally (NAC smells like rotten eggs). Currently, there is no prospective data to suggest that either IV or oral NAC is superior in preventing clinically significant hepatotoxicity (i.e., that resulting in liver failure or need for transplantation). Recent literature suggests a patient-tailored approach.

21. What is the patient-tailored approach?
The NAC treatment protocol was based on an acetaminophen elimination half-life of 21 hours. Often in the setting of acetaminophen overdose, hepatic injury is present, slowing the metabolism and

presumably prolonging its half-life. This is evidenced in documented cases that have showed continued rising of transaminases after completion of 21 hours of treatment. In these cases, current recommendations of the American College of Medical Toxicology state that administering an additional NAC bolus or extending the 6.25 mg/kg per hour infusion may be indicated.

If the patient has evidence of persistent hepatotoxicity after the 21-hour protocol shown by either continued elevations of aminotransferases; presence of predictors of poor prognosis such as decreased pH, increased phosphate, increased lactate, elevated coags, continued elevated serum creatinine; or persistent detection of acetaminophen on laboratory testing, then NAC should be continued. Recommendations go on to further state that given there is no literature establishing a laboratory cut off of acetaminophen, the recommendation is to stop therapy when acetaminophen levels are undetectable and the patient has clinically improved.

22. Is it ever too late to give N-acetylcysteine?

When possible, it is preferred to begin NAC administration within 8 hours of ingestion, but often the timeline can be difficult to establish. Thus, if acetaminophen toxicity is suspected, send a level, but start treatment immediately. Do not delay treatment waiting for the level to result. Beyond 8 hours, NAC may still provide benefit, particularly in the setting of extended-release formulations, multiple ingestions over time, or persistent elevation of liver enzymes after ingestions.

23. Is there a role for HD in acetaminophen toxicity?

Yes. The EXTRIP 2014 workgroup recommends extracorporeal treatments in cases of massive overdose, as standard doses of NAC may not be sufficient. Massive overdose can be presumed in patients who present rapidly after ingestion with signs of mitochondrial dysfunction such as metabolic acidosis and altered mental status before evidence of hepatic injury. Intermittent HD is the preferred method, as it provides rapid correction of acid-base abnormalities and efficient removal of low molecular weight molecules. NAC should be given concurrently during HD, but at higher rates, as NAC is also dialyzable.

24. How does alcohol ingestion affect acetaminophen toxicity?

Acute alcohol toxicity is believed to be protective, as it competes with acetaminophen for CYP2E1, thus decreasing the amount of NAPQI produced. Chronic alcohol ingestion does not appear to increase risk when compared to nonalcoholics after an acute one-time overdose of acetaminophen, although no consensus exists in the literature.

25. What is the recommendation to treat chronic acetaminophen toxicity?

NAC is recommended in patients with detectable acetaminophen levels. It is also recommended in any patient with history concerning for acetaminophen toxicity and elevated transaminases, regardless of the acetaminophen level. Administer NAC for 12 hours, then repeat labs—acetaminophen level and serum transaminases. Treatment may be discontinued if the patient is asymptomatic, the acetaminophen level is undetectable, AND the serum transaminases are normal or have decreased by at least 50% of peak value.

ANTIDEPRESSANT TOXICITY

26. What are the receptor effects and clinical effects of tricyclic antidepressant poisoning?

T   Tremor
C   Cardiovascular
A   Anticholinergic
S   Sedation and Seizures (in predisposed patients)

Tricyclic antidepressants (TCAs) have seven pharmacologic effects. Understanding these effects is helpful in remembering the associated clinical syndrome of TCA toxicity (Table 75.2).

27. How can one quickly identify many tricyclic antidepressants by name?

The name of many TCAs ends in—triptyline or—ipramine. Others include Doxepin, Amoxapine, and Iprindole.

28. What value is the electrocardiogram in patients with tricyclic antidepressant poisoning?

The electrocardiogram is the best early screen for TCA toxicity. Electrocardiographic findings usually manifest within the first few hours of poisoning and allow this potentially fatal diagnosis to be made early. The combination of the following classic electrocardiographic findings in a patient with an unknown ingestion strongly suggests TCA poisoning. These findings include the following:
- Sinus tachycardia
- PR prolongation

Table 75-2. Pharmacologic Effects of Tricyclic Antidepressants

MECHANISM	EFFECT
Presynaptic biogenic amine reuptake inhibition (norepinephrine and serotonin)	Therapeutic antidepressant effect Early sympathomimesis Myoclonus Hyperreflexia
Fast sodium channel influx blockade	QRS duration prolonged PR interval prolonged Right axis deviation Bundle branch blockade Ventricular dysrhythmias Negative inotropy
Potassium channel efflux blockade	QTc prolongation
Muscarinic acetylcholine receptor blockade	Tachycardia Mydriasis Decreased sweating Hyperthermia Flushing Ileus Urinary retention
Histaminic receptor blockade	Sedation
Alpha receptor blockade	Sedation Orthostatic hypotension Miosis Reflex tachycardia
GABA-A receptor blockade	Seizures Status epilepticus

GABA, gamma-aminobutyric acid.

- Widened QRS complex (>100 milliseconds = increased risk of seizures)
- QTc prolongation
- Terminal R complex in aVR >3 mm in height = increased risk of seizures and dysrhythmias
    In addition, electrocardiographic features are predictive of the clinical course and guide treatment in severe toxicity. The risk of seizures increases if the QRS duration is greater than 100 milliseconds, and a terminal R wave greater than 3 mm in aVR predicts an increased risk of both seizures and ventricular dysrhythmias. The presence of either of these findings warrants immediate treatment.

29. How is cardiovascular toxicity of tricyclic antidepressants treated?
    Cardiovascular toxicity of TCAs is treated first with sodium bicarbonate therapy, titrating initial bolus therapy to resolution of QRS prolongation and following this with continuous infusion of bicarbonate solution to alkalinize the serum and provide a loading dose of sodium ions. The goal serum pH is 7.45 to 7.55, and ensure K is monitored q1-2h to prevent hypokalemia. If the patient continues to have QRS prolongation or significant right axis deviation, despite alkalemia, hypertonic saline solution can also be administered with the goal of overwhelming the blocked sodium channels. Synchronous cardioversion should be used in patients with TCA overdose on the basis of current advanced cardiac life support guidelines when indicated. Torsades de pointes can be treated with magnesium sulfate infusion. Despite the QTc prolongation associated with TCA use, the tachycardia due to the antimuscarinic effects of TCAs often limits the likelihood of "R-on-T" phenomena. Finally, in recent years, lipid emulsion rescue has emerged as an antidotal treatment in life-threatening poisoning by lipophilic drugs. All TCAs are highly lipophilic, given their therapeutic targets in the CNS, and animal and human data suggest that TCAs and related compounds respond well to lipid rescue. Patients with known or suspected TCA cardiotoxicity and hemodynamic instability or malignant dysrhythmias are candidates for lipid emulsion therapy.

30. What are some commonly used selective serotonin reuptake inhibitors?
    Fluoxetine, paroxetine, sertraline, citalopram/escitalopram, fluvoxamine

31. What is the classic triad of serotonin syndrome?
    Autonomic instability
    Altered mental status
    Neuromuscular agitation

32. What is the treatment for serotonin syndrome?
    Benzodiazepines. For hyperthermia, the patient may need active cooling methods such as aggressive external cooling, or may need to be intubated, sedated, and paralyzed.

33. What are some common serotonin–norepinephrine reuptake inhibitors?
    Venlafaxine, desvenlafaxine, duloxetine, bupropion

34. What sign of toxicity occurs more often with serotonin–norepinephrine reuptake inhibitors versus selective serotonin reuptake inhibitors?
    Seizures and delayed seizure risk (up to 18 hours). Seizures can happen with therapeutic doses. Treat patients with benzodiazepines. Patients should be monitored for 24 hours, given delayed seizure risk.

ACKNOWLEDGMENT

The authors wish to acknowledge Drs. Aaron B. Skolnik, MD, and Susan R. Wilcox, MD, for the valuable contributions to the previous edition of this chapter.

KEY POINTS: ANALGESICS AND ANTIDEPRESSANTS

1. Patients with salicylate toxicity should start alkalization therapy and have serum salicylate levels checked every 1 to 2 hours.
2. Hemodialysis should be initiated promptly in any patient with salicylate levels over 100 mcg/mL or those with levels greater than 80 mcg/mL with significant clinical deterioration or neurotoxicity.
3. Acetaminophen levels may be plotted on the Rumack-Matthew nomogram only if the patient has had a single, acute ingestion of acetaminophen at a known time with a serum level of at least 4 hours from the ingestion.
4. Any suspected or confirmed acetaminophen-toxic patient should immediately start receiving NAC, by either the oral or IV route.
5. NAC treatment duration should be individualized for each patient.
6. Sodium bicarbonate is the treatment of choice to prevent seizures and arrhythmias in TCA overdose and should be administered as boluses until the QRS is less than 100 milliseconds.

BIBLIOGRAPHY

1. Adams J. *Emergency Medicine: Clinical Essentials*. Philadelphia, PA: Saunders; 2012:1231-1238.e1.
2. Bailey B, Buckley NA, Amre DK. A meta-analysis of prognostic indicators to predict seizures, arrhythmias or death after tricyclic antidepressant overdose. *J Toxicol Clin Toxicol*. 2004;42:877-888.
3. Bradberry SM, Thanacoody HK, Watt BE, Thomas SH, Vale JA. Management of the cardiovascular complications of tricyclic antidepressant poisoning: role of sodium bicarbonate. *Toxicol Rev*. 2005;24:195-204.
4. Body R, Bartram T, Azam F, Mackway-Jones K. Guidelines in Emergency Medicine Network (GEMNet): guideline for the management of tricyclic antidepressant overdose. *Emerg Med J*. 2011;28:347-368.
5. Burns MJ, Friedman SL, Larson AM. Acetaminophen (paracetamol) poisoning in adults: Pathophysiology, presentation, and diagnosis. In: Traub SJ, Grayzel J, eds. *UptoDate*. 2016. Available at: https://www.uptodate.com/contents/ acetaminophen-paracetamol-poisoning-in-adults-pathophysiology-presentation-and-diagnosis?source=search_ result&search=acetaminophen%20overdose&selectedTitle=2~124. Accessed October 1, 2016.
6. Engels PT, Davidow JS. Intravenous fat emulsion to reverse haemodynamic instability from intentional amitriptyline overdose. *Resuscitation*. 2010;81:1037-1039.
7. Ghannoum M, Kazim S, Grunbaum AM, Villeneuve E, Gosselin S. Massive acetaminophen overdose: effect of hemodialysis on acetaminophen and acetylcysteine kinetics. *Clin Toxicol (Phila)*. 2016;54:519-522.
8. Heard KJ. Acetylcysteine for acetaminophen poisoning. *N Engl J Med*. 2008;359:285-292.
9. Heard K, Dart R. Acetaminophen (paracetamol) poisoning in adults: Treatment. In: Traub SJ, Grayzel J, eds. *UptoDate*. 2016. Available at: https://www.uptodate.com/contents/acetaminophen-paracetamol-poisoning-in-adults- treatment?source=related_link. Accessed October 1, 2016.

10. Johnson MT, McCammon CA, Mullins ME, Halcomb SE. Evaluation of a simplified N-acetylcysteine dosing regimen for the treatment of acetaminophen toxicity. *Ann Pharmacother.* 2011;45:713-720.
11. Juurlink DN, Gosselin S, Kielstein JT, et al. Extracorporeal treatment for salicylate poisoning: systematic review and recommendations from the EXTRIP Workgroup. *Ann Emerg Med.* 2015;66:165-181.
12. Khandelwal N, James LP, Sanders C, Larson AM, Lee WM, the Acute Liver Failure Study Group. Unrecognized acetaminophen toxicity as a cause of indeterminate acute liver failure. *Hepatology.* 2011;53:567-576.
13. Levitan R, Lovecchio F. Salicylates. In: *Tintinalli JE, Stapczynski JS, Ma OJ, et al., eds. Tintinalli's Emergency Medicine: A Comprehensive Study Guide.* 8th ed. New York, NY: McGraw-Hill; 2016.
14. Nelson LS, Lewin NA, Howland MA, eds. *Goldfrank's Toxicologic Emergencies.* 9th ed. New York: McGraw-Hill; 2011: 1037-1059.
15. O'Malley GF. Emergency department management of the salicylate-poisoned patient. *Emerg Med Clin North Am.* 2007; 25:333-346.
16. Pierog JE, Kane KE, Kane BG, et al. Tricyclic antidepressant toxicity treated with massive sodium bicarbonate. *Am J Emerg Med.* 2009;27:1168.e3-e7.
17. Sheppard A, Hayes SH, Chen GD, Ralli M, Salvi R. Review of salicylate-induced hearing loss, neurotoxicity, tinnitus and neuropathophysiology. *Acta Otorhinolaryngol Ital.* 2014;34:75-93.
18. Wells K, Williamson M, Holstege CP, Bear AB, Brady WJ. The association of cardiovascular toxins and electrocardiographic abnormality in poisoned patients. *Am J Emerg Med.* 2008;26:957-959.

CHAPTER 76

TOXIC ALCOHOL POISONING

Paul S. Jansson and Jarone Lee

1. **What are the toxic alcohols and how do they differ from ethanol?**
   The toxic alcohols are commonly encountered alcohols that can cause poisoning. They include **methanol, ethylene glycol, isopropyl alcohol,** and **propylene glycol**. Unlike ethanol, which causes immediate toxicity by mechanisms related to central nervous system (CNS) depression (such as respiratory suppression and altered mental status), the pathophysiology of the toxic alcohols is primarily through breakdown to various intermediate metabolites, which can cause specific organ-system damage. Metabolites of methanol cause retinal and optic nerve damage, which can lead to blindness, while metabolites of ethylene glycol damage the kidney, possibly leading to renal failure. Isopropyl alcohol can lead to a hemorrhagic gastritis while propylene glycol can lead to a lactic acidosis.

2. **How are the toxic alcohols metabolized?**
   While each toxic alcohol has its own minor elimination pathway, the majority of the metabolism occurs in the liver, similar to ethanol. The parent compound (e.g., ethanol) is broken down by the enzyme **alcohol dehydrogenase (ADH)** into an intermediate product (e.g., acetaldehyde). The intermediate metabolites are then broken down by a variety of enzymes, depending on the alcohol, to the final elimination products.

3. **How does competitive inhibition play a role in the management of toxic alcohol ingestions?**
   All of the toxic alcohols use ADH as the initial enzyme in metabolism. However, it is clinically useful in coingestions with the toxic alcohols because the administration of fomepizole may be safely delayed until ethanol is metabolized to a concentration of approximately 100 mg/dL. Slowing of ADH is accomplished clinically by competitive inhibition, either by ethanol or fomepizole, a medication that serves as a direct competitive inhibitor of ADH.

4. **Wait, ethanol—like regular alcohol? How does that work?**
   Traditionally, ethanol was used for the management of toxic alcohol ingestions. Ethanol has 10- to 20-fold higher affinity for ADH than the toxic alcohols. At levels higher than 100 mg/dL, ethanol fully saturates ADH receptor sites. Unfortunately, ethanol is difficult to dose (requiring frequent lab checks to ensure that it is kept within a constant range), irritating to veins, and has the unwanted side effect of causing CNS depression. However, it is clinically useful in coingestions with the toxic alcohols because use of fomepizole may be safely delayed until the ethanol level approaches 100 mg/dL.

5. **What is fomepizole?**
   Fomepizole (4-Methyl-1*H*-pyrazole) is a competitive inhibitor of ADH that is safer and more reliable treatment than using ethanol. Similarly to ethanol, it competes with the toxic alcohols for active sites on ADH, slowing the metabolism of alcohols to their toxic intermediates. Fomepizole is given as a loading dose (15 mg/kg IV) followed by periodic injections (10 mg/kg every 12 hours for four doses, followed by 15 mg/kg every 12 hours until the patient is asymptomatic and the toxic alcohol level is undetectable in the blood). Dosing is increased to every four hours if the patient is undergoing dialysis. Side effects are rare, but the medication is expensive.

6. **What other therapies are used in the management of toxic alcohol ingestions?**
   The mainstay of treatment for toxic alcohols involves the prevention of toxic metabolites, either by inhibition of ADH using fomepizole or ethanol, or removal of the parent compound through dialysis. Indications for dialysis include severe metabolic acidosis, large ingestion, any visual change in methanol ingestion, or oliguric/anuric renal failure in ethylene glycol ingestion. Supportive care may also be required for the critically ill, such as the use of vasopressors for hypotension (most alcohols are vasodilators), bicarbonate solutions for acidemia, and intubation for airway protection. As with any poisoning, consultation with a medical toxicologist or poison control center is recommended.

7. **How are toxic alcohol ingestions diagnosed?**
   While a clear clinical history can be the most useful in providing a diagnosis of toxic alcohol ingestion (e.g., the patient brought in by their spouse clutching a jug of antifreeze), diagnosis can be challenging

if the patient presents with altered mental status or is otherwise unable to give a history. Serum alcohol levels can confirm a diagnosis, but are often not readily available in most hospitals. Therefore, a combination of a high index of suspicion, classic laboratory findings, and specific clinical findings can be used to support the diagnosis while waiting for confirmatory testing.

8. What is the osmolal gap and how can it be used to support a diagnosis of toxic alcohol ingestion?
As the alcohol is absorbed from the gastrointestinal tract, it enters the bloodstream as an osmotically active compound, which can be measured by obtaining the serum osmolality. If the measured serum osmolality is significantly different from the calculated serum osmolality, then there is an osmolar gap (osmol gap = measured serum osmolality – calculated serum osmolality). This implies that there is an "unmeasured osmol," most likely the ingested toxic alcohol. The calculated osmolality is derived based on measured concentrations of the most significant osmotically active agents in the blood:

$$Calculated\ Osmolality = 2 \times Na^+ + \frac{BUN}{2.8} + \frac{Glucose}{18} + \frac{Ethanol}{4.6}$$

Although there can be significant person-to-person variability, a normal osmolal gap is less than 10. A gap of greater than 25 increases specificity for a toxic ingestion.

9. How is the anion gap useful in diagnosing a toxic alcohol ingestion?
Similarly to the osmolal gap, the anion gap is a tool to detect unmeasured anions in the blood. The anion gap is calculated using the concentrations of measured anions in the blood as follows:

$$Anion\ Gap = [Na^+] - ([Cl^-] + [HCO_3^-])$$

As the toxic alcohols are metabolized into organic acids (with the exception of isopropyl alcohol), they will increase the anion gap because they are present in the serum as anions. A normal anion gap is usually less than 15 to 18.

10. What is the mountain diagram and how is it useful in toxic alcohol ingestions?
The mountain diagram (Fig. 76.1) refers to the changes in the osmolal gap and the anion gap over time. In early ingestion of the toxic alcohols, the osmolal gap is high as the alcohol is present as an osmotically active agent in the blood. However, as the alcohol is metabolized into an organic acid (except isopropyl alcohol), the osmolal gap decreases and the anion gap anion increases. The mountain diagram is used to visually demonstrate the inverse relationship between the two "gaps."

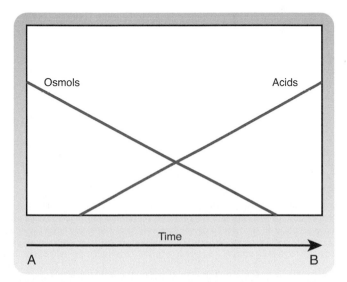

Osmols

Acids

Time

A   B

Figure 76-1. Osmolal gap and anion gap over time. As the parent alcohol is metabolized, the osmolal gap decreases and the anion gap increases. (From Figure 151.4 "Mountain Schematic" in: Mycyk Mark B. Toxic alcohols. In: Adams JG, ed. *Emergency Medicine: Clinical Essentials.* 2nd ed. 2012. Philadelphia: Elsevier.)

11. What is methanol and where is it found?

   Methanol ("wood alcohol") is a colorless, sweet-tasting alcohol that has the highest morbidity and mortality of the toxic alcohols. It was traditionally encountered as the unwanted byproduct of illicit distilling, and is often found in windshield washer fluid, industrial solvents, and canned fuel. It is volatile at room temperatures, so inhalational ingestion and toxicity has been reported.

12. What are the clinical effects of methanol ingestion?

   Methanol itself has little toxicity and causes less CNS depression and inebriation than equivalent doses of ethanol. It is metabolized in the liver by ADH to formaldehyde and then by aldehyde dehydrogenase (ALDH) to formic acid. Formic acid is responsible for most of the direct toxic effects of methanol ingestion. It is directly toxic to the cells of the optic nerve and retina, causing the hallmark visual finding of visual loss (classically described as being "in a snowstorm"). Even small amounts (30 mL/24 g) of methanol can cause permanent vision loss. Formic acid can also affect the brainstem, causing hemorrhages or infarcts in the putamen of the basal ganglia. Damage to the basal ganglia creates neurologic findings similar to those seen in Parkinson disease, including rigidity, tremor, and bradykinesia.

13. Are there any other tricks to the management of methanol ingestion?

   Formate directly halts mitochondrial cytochrome oxidase, slowing cellular respiration and producing a profound metabolic acidosis (often with a pH <7.0 and a serum bicarbonate of <5), in addition to the metabolic acidosis produced by formic acid itself. While the body can attempt to compensate for this profound metabolic acidosis with tachypnea, often bicarbonate infusion will be required to help correct the metabolic derangement. In addition, formic acid is metabolized by a folate-dependent mechanism, so supplementing folic acid can theoretically reduce levels of formic acid.

14. What is ethylene glycol and where is it found?

   Ethylene glycol is a colorless, odorless, and sweet liquid that lowers the boiling point of water, hence its most common use in industrial antifreeze and coolant solutions. Because of its sweet taste, children consume it inadvertently. It is rapidly absorbed from the gastrointestinal tract. Unlike methanol, it is not volatile at room temperature, so inhalation toxicity is extremely rare.

15. What are the clinical effects of ethylene glycol ingestion?

   Similarly to methanol, ethylene glycol itself is relatively nontoxic, but the products of metabolism in the liver are responsible for significant toxicity, particularly oxalic acid. Oxalic acid binds calcium to form calcium oxalate, which precipitates out of the blood into various tissues, including the lungs and heart. This causes pulmonary edema and myocardial depression. Additionally, the crystals accumulate in the renal tubules, causing renal tubular necrosis and renal failure. Crystalluria is therefore the hallmark of ethylene glycol ingestion, although it is not always present. Because calcium oxalate precipitates out of the blood, hypocalcemia may also be seen.

16. Are there any other tricks to the management of ethylene glycol ingestion?

   Oxalic acid is produced from glycolic acid, which has several other breakdown pathways. Supplementation of pyridoxine (vitamin B6; 50 mg IV every 6 hours) and thiamine (vitamin B1; 100 mg IV every 6 hours) can shunt the metabolism of glycolic acid away from the production of oxalic acid. Metabolism of ethylene glycol to oxalic acid and glycolic acid produces an anion gap metabolic acidosis. In these patients, because of the risk of calcium further precipitating calcium oxalate, any hypocalcemia present should be corrected cautiously, and only if causing hemodynamic instability.

17. What is isopropyl alcohol and where is it found?

   Isopropyl alcohol is a clear, colorless liquid commonly sold as "rubbing alcohol" or nail polish remover. After ethanol, it is the most common toxic alcohol ingested. Transdermal toxicity from "sponge bathing" can be seen among children.

18. What are the clinical effects of isopropyl alcohol ingestion?

   The primary clinical manifestation of isopropyl alcohol ingestion is CNS depression. It is two to four times more potent than an equivalent dose of ethanol and lasts two to four times longer. Isopropyl alcohol is a gastrointestinal irritant, so gastritis (occasionally hemorrhagic) and vomiting are common. Because the main metabolic product is acetone, a "fruity" breath odor may be present.

19. Are there any other tricks to the management of isopropyl alcohol ingestion?

   Isopropyl alcohol is converted by ADH to acetone in the liver, which is a ketone. Ketones are not organic acids and do not result in an anion gap. Therefore, ingestion of isopropyl alcohol will increase the osmolal gap, but will not produce the metabolic acidosis present with ingestion of the other toxic alcohols. Because the parent compound is responsible for the majority of the clinical findings, inhibiting its metabolism with fomepizole or ethanol is not indicated.

20. **Are there any other toxic alcohols worth mentioning?**
Propylene glycol is used as a diluent in common medications like phenytoin, lorazepam, and esmolol. It is metabolized to lactic acid and can produce a resultant anion gap metabolic acidosis with hypotension and cardiac dysrhythmias. Toxicity is largely iatrogenic by medication administration and the management is supportive.

ACKNOWLEDGMENT

The authors wish to acknowledge Drs. Aaron B. Skolnik, MD, and Susan R. Wilcox, MD, for the valuable contributions to the previous edition of this chapter.

KEY POINTS: TOXIC ALCOHOL POISONING

- The toxic alcohols are methanol, ethylene glycol, isopropyl alcohol, and propylene glycol. Most toxic alcohol ingestions present with CNS depression. Additionally, methanol can present with blindness, ethylene glycol with renal failure, and isopropyl alcohol with hemorrhagic gastritis.
- Unlike ethanol, the toxic alcohols largely exert their effects through toxic metabolites and not the parent compound.
- Like ethanol, the toxic alcohols are largely metabolized in the liver by ADH.
- The mainstay of treatment for the toxic alcohols is competitive inhibition of ADH by fomepizole or ethanol; in severe cases, dialysis may be required.
- In the early stages of toxic alcohol ingestion, an osmolal gap is present, but in the later stages an anion gap predominates as the osmotically active parent compounds are metabolized (with the exception of isopropyl alcohol) into organic acids.

BIBLIOGRAPHY

1. Mycyk M. Toxic alcohols. In: Adams JG, ed. *Emergency Medicine: Clinical Essentials*. 2nd ed. Philadelphia: Saunders; 2013:1292-1298.
2. White SA. Toxic alcohols. In: Marx JA, ed. *Rosen's Emergency Medicine: Concepts and Clinical Practice*. 8th ed. Philadelphia: Saunders; 2014:2007-2014.
3. Brent J. Fomepizole for ethylene glycol and methanol poisoning. *N Engl J Med*. 2009;360:2216-2223.
4. Kraut JA. Approach to the treatment of methanol intoxication. *Am J Kidney Dis*. 2016;68:161-167.
5. McMartin K, Jacobsen D, Hovda KE. Antidotes for poisoning by alcohols that form toxic metabolites. *Br J Clin Pharmacol*. 2016;81:505-515.

CHAPTER 77

CARDIOVASCULAR MEDICATIONS

Jason L. Sanders and Jarone Lee

1. **What are the common cardiovascular medications used in acutely or critically ill patients?**
   Cardiovascular medications are used to combat common underlying physiologic disturbances, such as hypotension, hypertension, bradycardia, or tachycardia.
   - Hypotension
     - Phenylephrine
     - Norepinephrine
     - Epinephrine
     - Vasopressin
     - Dobutamine
     - Dopamine
     - Methylene blue
     - High-dose insulin
   - Hypertension
     - Nicardipine
     - Esmolol/Labetalol
     - Nitroglycerin
     - Benzodiazepines or phenobarbital
   - Bradycardia
     - Atropine
     - Dopamine
     - Isoproterenol
   - Tachycardia
     - Adenosine
     - Amiodarone
     - Lidocaine

2. **How should an intensivist select which cardiovascular medication to use?**
   Intensivists should be familiar with the characteristics of each cardiovascular medication (Tables 77.1–77.4). They are often powerful and can produce dramatic beneficial and detrimental effects. The medication's effects can be applied to reverse the pathophysiologic disturbances experienced by an individual patient. At times, selection is aided by evidence-based guidelines or consensus on treatment for specific conditions (Table 77.5). Using a first-line agent must always be considered in the clinical context of the specific patient. Allowable dose ranges can vary based on individual clinical experience, clinical context, route of administration, response to medication, and adverse effect.

3. **When using a cardiovascular medication, which patients require continuous monitoring?**
   Cardiovascular medications are typically used only in acutely or critically ill patients. All of these patients require frequent or continuous monitoring due to rapid, often unheralded changes in condition. If possible, monitors should be applied before use of medications, not after, to detect response (or lack thereof) to intervention. Nonetheless, life-saving intervention should not be delayed for insertion of monitoring devices.

4. **What parameters should be monitored and how is monitoring achieved?**
   Minimum monitoring includes cardiac rate and rhythm, blood pressure, and pulse oximetry. Heart rate and rhythm are monitored with continuous telemetry. Be familiar with your institution's guidelines for which patients meet criteria for "low," "moderate," or "high" risk telemetry based on patient pathophysiology. Guidelines dictate when telemetry can be removed and what level of staff must be in attendance when it is removed. Most patients requiring cardiovascular medications are moderate

Table 77-1. Treatments for Hypotension

MEDICATION	RECEPTORS AND OVERALL PHYSIOLOGIC EFFECTS	TYPICAL ADULT DOSE RANGE	ADVERSE EFFECTS
Phenylephrine	Alpha-adrenergic agonist; systemic arterial vasoconstrictor; increases SVR; reduces HR and CO	0.4–9 mcg/kg/min IV	Arrhythmia, reflex bradycardia
Norepinephrine	Alpha >Beta-1 adrenergic agonist; increases vasoconstriction, contractility, HR	0.01–3 mcg/kg/min IV	Arrhythmia, bradycardia, digital ischemia, dyspnea
Epinephrine	Alpha, beta-1, and beta-2 adrenergic agonist; relaxes bronchial smooth muscle; increases HR and SVR	Arrest: 1 mg IV/IO every 3–5 min Anaphylaxis: 0.2–0.5 mg IM every 5–15 min Shock: 0.05–0.2 mcg/kg/min IV	Arrhythmia, hypertension, peripheral ischemia, renal insufficiency, dyspnea
Vasopressin	V1 receptor agonist; increases SVR, MAP; may decrease HR, CO	0.03–0.07 units/min IV	Arrhythmia
Dobutamine	Cardiac beta-1 agonist, vascular beta-2 and alpha-1 adrenergic agonist; increases CO via inotropy and chronotropy	Initial: 0.5–1 mcg/kg/min IV Maintenance: 2–20 mcg/kg/min IV	Ventricular arrhythmia, chest pain, hypotension, hypertension
Dopamine	Low dose: Dopaminergic; renal/mesenteric vasodilation Moderate dose: Dopaminergic, beta-1 agonist; increases HR/CO, renal vasodilation High dose: Dopaminergic, beta-1 and alpha agonist; increases HR, CO, SVR	2–20 mcg/kg/min IV	Arrhythmia, widened QRS complex
Methylene blue	Direct inhibitory effect on endothelial and inducible nitric oxide synthases, blocks cGMP; reduces vasorelaxation and restores vascular tone	1.5–2 mg/kg IV bolus; 0.5–1 mg/kg/h IV infusion	Limb pain, blue-green urine, dysgeusia, nausea, hyperhidrosis, dizziness, discolored skin
High dose insulin	Increases inotropy, maintains euglycemia	1 unit/kg IV bolus followed by 0.5–2 units/kg IV infusion	Hypoglycemia, hypokalemia

cGMP, Cyclic guanosine monophosphate; CO, cardiac output; HR, heart rate; IM, intramuscular; IO, intraosseous; IV, intravenous; kg, kilogram; MAP, mean arterial pressure; mcg, microgram; mg, milligram; min, minute; PO, per os (oral); SVR, systemic vascular resistance.

Table 77-2. Treatments for Hypertension

MEDICATION	RECEPTORS AND OVERALL PHYSIOLOGIC EFFECTS	TYPICAL ADULT DOSE RANGE	ADVERSE EFFECTS
Nicardipine	Calcium channel blocker of smooth muscle and myocardium; smooth muscle relaxation, coronary vasodilation	5–15 mg/h IV	Headache, flushing, angina pectoris, hypotension, nausea, vomiting
Esmolol	Beta-1 adrenergic antagonist; reduces HR and BP	1 mg/kg IV bolus followed by 50–300 mcg/kg/min infusion	Hypotension
Labetalol	Alpha, beta-1, beta-2 antagonist; 1:7 alpha:beta blockade IV; reduces HR and BP	10–20 mg IV bolus, followed by 2–8 mg/min infusion	Hypotension, nausea, dizziness
Nitroglycerin	Relaxes peripheral veins > arteries; reduces cardiac oxygen demand by reducing preload more than afterload; dilates coronary arteries	IV: 5–400 mcg/min SL: 0.3–0.6 mg 2% ointment: ½–2 inches	Headache, hypotension, dizziness
Benzodiazepines or phenobarbital	Potentiate GABA effect	Depends on formulation and route	Sedation, respiratory depression, bradycardia, hypotension, agitation

BP, Blood pressure; GABA, gamma-aminobutyric acid; HR, heart rate; IV, intravenous; kg, kilogram; mcg, microgram; mg, milligram; min, minute; SL, sublingual.

Table 77-3. Treatments for Bradycardia

MEDICATION	RECEPTORS AND OVERALL PHYSIOLOGIC EFFECTS	TYPICAL ADULT DOSE RANGE	ADVERSE EFFECTS
Atropine	Blocks acetylcholine at parasympathetic sites; increases CO	0.5 mg IV push	Not well defined; Arrhythmia
Isoproterenol	Beta-1, beta-2 agonist; increases HR and contractility; dilates peripheral vasculature	2–10 mcg/min IV	Arrhythmia, hypokalemia, dyspnea, pulmonary edema

CO, Cardiac output; HR, heart rate; IV, intravenous; mcg, microgram; mg, milligram; min, minute.

Table 77-4. Treatments for Tachycardia

MEDICATION	RECEPTORS AND OVERALL PHYSIOLOGIC EFFECTS	TYPICAL ADULT DOSE RANGE	ADVERSE EFFECTS
Adenosine	Slows conduction time through AV node; terminates supraventricular tachycardia	6 or 12 mg IV bolus	Arrhythmia, AV block, chest pressure, headache, dizziness, flushing, dyspnea

Table 77-4. Treatments for Tachycardia *(Continued)*

MEDICATION	RECEPTORS AND OVERALL PHYSIOLOGIC EFFECTS	TYPICAL ADULT DOSE RANGE	ADVERSE EFFECTS
Amiodarone	Alpha and beta antagonist; affects Na, K, and Ca channels; prolongs myocardial action potential and refractory period; decreases AV conduction and sinus node function	Pulseless VT/VF: 300 mg IV push followed by 150 mg IV push Arrhythmia: 0.5–1 mg/min	Hypotension, bradycardia, AV block, arrhythmia, nausea, vomiting
Lidocaine	Class Ib antiarrhythmic; suppresses automaticity	1–1.5 mg/kg IV bolus, followed by 1–4 mg/min	Undefined

AV, Atrioventricular; *IV*, intravenous; *kg*, kilogram; *mg*, milligram; *min*, minute; VF, ventricular fibrillation; VT, ventricular tachycardia.

Table 77-5. Cardiovascular Medications by Condition

CONDITION	PREFERRED MEDICATION
Cardiac arrest	Epinephrine IV or IO
Unstable bradycardia	Atropine IV (second line or infusion: dobutamine, isoproterenol)
Unstable VT/VF	Amiodarone IV
Cardiogenic shock from heart failure	Dobutamine IV, epinephrine IV, dopamine IV
Anaphylaxis/Anaphylactic shock	Epinephrine IM or IV
Septic shock	Norepinephrine IV, epinephrine IV, vasopressin IV (used with another vasopressor)
Intracerebral hemorrhage with MAP greater than goal	Nicardipine IV
Aortic dissection with MAP greater than goal	Esmolol IV, labetalol IV
Hypertensive emergency, often with associated flash pulmonary edema, unstable angina, or non-ST elevation myocardial infarction	Nitroglycerin (IV, cutaneous, sublingual), labetalol IV
Alcohol withdrawal with associated tachycardia and hypertension	Benzodiazepine IV or PO, phenobarbital IV or PO
Paroxysmal supraventricular tachycardia	Adenosine IV push
Calcium channel blocker overdose with shock	High dose insulin IV
Ventricular arrhythmia refractory to amiodarone and electrical cardioversion	Lidocaine IV
Refractory shock, vasoplegia associated with cardiac surgery	Methylene blue IV (typically as 4th-line pressor)

IM, Intramuscular; *IO*, intraosseous; *IV*, intravenous; MAP, mean arterial pressure; *PO*, per os (oral); VF, ventricular fibrillation; VT, ventricular tachycardia.

or high risk. Err on the side of caution; life-threatening deterioration is best treated before it occurs and in a controlled setting, not after or in an uncontrolled setting. An electrocardiogram (EKG) should be obtained with any clinical deterioration, which may be signaled by escalating doses of cardiovascular medications. Because of high risk of arrhythmia in any critically ill patient (due to underlying illness and use of arrhythmogenic medications), serial EKGs may be indicated. Blood pressure, especially in critically ill patients, should be monitored invasively with an arterial line. This enables medication titration to meet specific blood pressure goals. Insertion, usually in the radial or femoral artery, should be performed by the most experienced operator or under their guidance due to risk of arterial injury. Continuous pulse oximetry should be applied to all patients. If it is difficult to detect an adequate pulse oximetry waveform, check the equipment, but be wary of cardiovascular and/or pulmonary deterioration impeding noninvasive measurement of pulse oximetry.

5. What types of advanced cardiovascular monitoring are available?
    Advanced cardiovascular monitors provide data beyond heart rate and rhythm, blood pressure, and pulse oximetry. These may include cardiac output, cardiac index, stroke volume, systemic vascular resistance, intracardiac and extracardiac pressures, and more. Devices and methods often rely on measuring flow, pressure, temperature, and time to calculate cardiovascular parameters using first principle equations and patented statistical algorithms. Examples include direct intracardiac catheterization; Doppler ultrasonography (intracardiac, esophageal, transcutaneous); pulse pressure methods (Finapres methodology, arterial manometry, calibrated pulse pressure, statistical analysis of arterial pulse contours); impedance cardiography (measures changes in electrical impedance across the thorax over the cardiac cycle); ultrasound dilution (measures dilution of saline via ultrasound during cardiac cycling); and magnetic resonance imaging. It is important to note: (1) there is no gold standard for measuring these parameters; (2) there is limited data comparing the accuracy and precision of devices and methods; (3) there is limited data on association of measurement with patient outcomes; (4) there are limitations to using each device or method based on patient physiology (e.g., invalid measurements during inspiration or expiration or with mechanical ventilation, with irregular heart rhythm, or valve regurgitation/insufficiency/stenosis); (5) invasive measurement is associated with risk; and (6) devices may be expensive and poorly amenable to use in a crisis. With greater technical development, clinical validation, and outcomes research, these methods may prove beneficial in the future, possibly to sub-populations of the critically ill (e.g., cardiogenic shock), but in general are not widely indicated or employed.

6. How does intracranial pressure monitoring work, and is it useful?
    Acute brain injury, either primary or secondary, can occur when the cerebral perfusion pressure (CPP) is too low or too high. CPP is determined by mean arterial pressure (MAP) minus intracranial pressure (ICP; CPP = MAP − ICP). In general, CPP should be maintained between 60 and 80 mm Hg. When the MAP and ICP are within normal ranges, cerebral arterioles auto-regulate to maintain proper CPP. When the MAP is less than 65 mm Hg or greater than 150 mm Hg, the cerebral arterioles lose their ability to auto-regulate. ICP is typically 7 to 15 mm Hg; above 15 mm Hg is abnormal, and above 20 mm Hg is pathologic. To measure CPP accurately thus requires measurement of the MAP via systemic arterial monitoring and measurement of the ICP.

    Monitoring ICP involves insertion of one of several available devices into the brain or skull by an experienced neuro-proceduralist. An intraventricular catheter is inserted into the lateral ventricle for direct pressure measurement conducted through the cerebrospinal fluid (CSF). It has the added benefit of allowing CSF sampling for analysis and removal of CSF to reduce ICP. A subdural screw is a hollow screw inserted through a hole drilled into the skull and placed through the dura mater. It measures pressure from inside the subdural space. An epidural sensor is drilled through the skull and inserted between the skull and dural tissue; it cannot be used to remove CSF. Theoretically, monitoring and adjusting ICP should aid in the care of patients with acute brain injury. Although many neurointensivists use ICP monitoring to guide treatment, to date there are no class I recommendations that monitoring ICP widely improves patient outcomes, and the utility of the practice is debated.

7. Through what route should cardiovascular medicines be administered?
    Route of administration is based on available access, available forms of medications, indication, acuity, and safety. When no access has been obtained, a few medications can be given sublingually, cutaneously, or intramuscularly. Nitroglycerin can be given sublingually and cutaneously. Epinephrine for early anaphylaxis is famously administered via intramuscular injection, though for treatment of shock requires more invasive administration. If peripheral intravenous (IV) access is obtained, rapid administration of all cardiovascular medications is possible. Relative exceptions include medications which are strong vasoconstrictors—most can be given safely at low doses for shorter periods of time through a peripheral IV, but central venous access is required for longer and higher dose administration. Intraosseous access can be obtained rapidly by trained providers. It also allows administration of all common cardiovascular medications for shorter periods of time. Several medications can be delivered via an endotracheal tube, including epinephrine, atropine, vasopressin, lidocaine, and naloxone, though their pharmacokinetics and dynamics may be unpredictably altered.

8. What are common pitfalls when using cardiovascular medicines in critically ill patients?
Treat the underlying cause before prematurely administering medication, which in theory may improve the dysfunction. For example, in hypovolemic shock due to hemorrhage or profound dehydration, rapid transfusion of blood or crystalloid is indicated before use of vasopressors or inotropes. In septic shock, vasopressors and inotropes are useless without rapid source control and antibiotics. In obstructive shock from pericardial effusion or pulmonary embolism, drain the effusion to reverse tamponade physiology, and administer heparin or thrombolytics for the embolism. In critical aortic stenosis, surgical or percutaneous valve repair is the definitive intervention. In cardiogenic shock due to myocardial infarction from coronary thrombus, cardiac catheterization is critical.

Using medications at doses above the upper limit of physiologic effectiveness increases risk for adverse effects (e.g., arrhythmia, organ ischemia) without improving the underlying physiologic disturbance. If a medication at reasonable doses does not produce significant improvement, the solution is to re-examine the problem and/or change interventions.

ACKNOWLEDGMENT

The authors wish to acknowledge Drs. Aaron B. Skolnik, MD, and Susan R. Wilconx, MD, for the valuable contributions to the previous edition of this chapter.

KEY POINTS: CARDIOVASCULAR MEDICATIONS

1. Cardiovascular medications should be chosen based on their characteristics, evidence of effectiveness in specific conditions, and the pathophysiology of the individual patient.
2. Use of cardiovascular medications necessitates adequate monitoring, including continuous cardiac telemetry, invasive blood pressure monitoring, and continuous pulse oximetry.
3. Advanced monitoring techniques may be helpful in the future for specific patient populations, but in general have not been adequately validated.
4. ICP monitoring may assist in the care of patients with acute brain injury to help maintain adequate CPP.
5. The route of delivery for cardiovascular medications depends on available access, available forms of medications, indication, acuity, and safety.
6. Common pitfalls when using cardiovascular medications include prematurely beginning medications before treating the underlying cause, and using medications at doses above the physiologic upper limit without additional benefit.

BIBLIOGRAPHY

1. Chesnut RM, Temkin N, Carney N, et al. A trial of intracranial-pressure monitoring in traumatic brain injury. *N Engl J Med.* 2012;367:2471-2481.
2. Dellinger RP, Levy MM, Rhodes A, et al. Surviving Sepsis Campaign: International guidelines for management of severe sepsis and septic shock: 2012. *Crit Care Med.* 2013;41:580-637.
3. Hutchinson PJ, Kolias AG, Timofeev IS, et al. Trial of decompressive craniectomy for traumatic intracranial hypertension. *N Engl J Med.* 2016;375:1119-1130.
4. Link MS, Berkow LC, Kudenchuk PJ. Part 7: Adult Advanced Cardiovascular Life Support. 2015 American Heart Association guidelines update for cardiopulmonary resuscitation and emergency cardiovascular care. *Circulation.* 2015;132:S444-S464.
5. Sangkum L, Liu GL, Yu L, et al. Minimally invasive or noninvasive cardiac output measurement: an update. *J Anesth.* 2016;30(3):461-480.
6. Shutter LA, Timmons SD. Intracranial pressure rescued by decompressive surgery after traumatic brain injury. *N Engl J Med.* 2016;375:1183-1184.
7. Su SH, Wang F, Hai J, et al. The effects of intracranial pressure monitoring in patients with traumatic brain injury. *PLoS One.* 2014;9(2):e87432.

CHAPTER 78

NEUROLEPTIC MALIGNANT SYNDROME

Molly L. Rovin and James L. Jacobson

1. **What is neuroleptic malignant syndrome?**
   Neuroleptic malignant syndrome (NMS) is a rare, life-threatening, idiosyncratic reaction associated with antipsychotics (formally known as neuroleptics) and other medications with dopamine antagonism. The usual presentation consists of four primary features:
   - Fever
   - Rigidity
   - Autonomic instability
   - Altered mental status
     Altered mental status is the first presenting symptom in 80% of NMS cases. Mean recovery time after antipsychotic discontinuation is 7 to 10 days, but may be prolonged when long-acting depot antipsychotics are used. For other common features of NMS, see Box 78.1.

2. **How common is neuroleptic malignant syndrome?**
   Recent data suggests the incidence ranges between 0.01% and 0.02%. The incidence of NMS has declined from previous estimates (as high as 3%) due to increased awareness, judicious antipsychotic use, and rapid recognition and treatment.

3. **What is the mortality rate for neuroleptic malignant syndrome?**
   Most cases of NMS will have complete resolution of symptoms when properly treated; however, fatality rates of 10% to 20% have been reported when the disorder is not recognized [*Diagnostic and Statistical Manual of Mental Disorders, fifth edition* (DSM-5)]. Cause of death in NMS is usually a result of cardiac or respiratory arrest (cardiac failure, infarction, arrhythmia, aspiration pneumonia, or pulmonary emboli), myoglobinuric renal failure, or disseminated intravascular coagulation.

Box 78-1. Signs and Symptoms of Neuroleptic Malignant Syndrome

Primary Features

Hyperthermia (association with profuse diaphoresis is a distinguishing feature of NMS)
Altered mental status
Autonomic instability
Extreme generalized rigidity (often called lead-pipe rigidity)

Other Common Features

Creatinine kinase elevation (>4x upper limit of normal)
Tremor
Mutism
Leukocytosis
Labile hypertension (less often hypotension)
Tachycardia
Tachypnea
Dysphagia
Diaphoresis
Sialorrhea
Incontinence

NMS, Neuroleptic malignant syndrome.

4. What is the pathogenesis of neuroleptic malignant syndrome?

   Although the pathophysiology of NMS is poorly understood, dopamine receptor antagonism is thought to play a central role in hypothalamic, nigrostriatal, and mesolimbic/cortical pathways in the brain (Fig. 78.1). It is also hypothesized that other neurotransmitter systems involving γ-aminobutyric acid (GABA), serotonin, and acetylcholine have a contributing role in the initiation and progression of NMS.

5. How is neuroleptic malignant syndrome diagnosed?

   NMS is a diagnosis of exclusion based on an array of clinical features associated with exposure to a dopamine antagonist. Most cases develop within 72 hours, and almost all within 30 days of drug administration. Below is a list of diagnostic criteria proposed from a consensus formed by an international multispecialty panel of NMS experts in 2011. See Box 78.2.

6. What is the differential diagnosis of neuroleptic malignant syndrome?

   The differential diagnosis (which must be excluded in order to conclude that NMS is the likely cause of presenting symptoms) includes central, systemic, and toxic causes of hyperthermia, rigidity, rhabdomyolysis, and altered mental status. See Box 78.3.

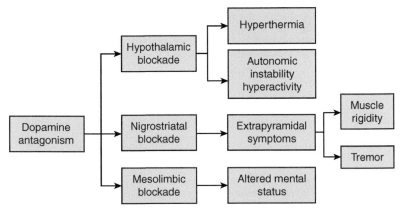

Figure 78-1. Simplified theoretical model for pathogenesis of neuroleptic malignant syndrome.

Box 78-2. Neuroleptic Malignant Syndrome Diagnostic Criteria

This list should be used only as a guide, as no formal diagnostic criteria for NMS currently exists:

1. Exposure to dopamine antagonist, or dopamine agonist withdrawal, within past 72 hours
2. Hyperthermia (>100.4°F or >38.0°C on at least two occasions, measured orally)
3. Rigidity (usually severe and generalized)
4. Mental status alteration (reduced or fluctuating level of consciousness)
5. Creatinine kinase elevation (at least four times upper limit of normal)
6. Sympathetic nervous system lability, defined as at least two of the following:
   Blood pressure instability:
      Elevation: systolic or diastolic ≥25% above baseline, or
      Fluctuation: ≥20 mm Hg diastolic change or ≥25 mm Hg systolic change within 24 hours
   Diaphoresis
   Urinary incontinence
7. Hypermetabolism defined as:
   Tachycardia (rate >25% above baseline)
   AND
   Tachypnea (≥50% above baseline)
8. Negative work up for infectious, toxic, metabolic, or neurologic causes.

NMS, Neuroleptic malignant syndrome.

Box 78-3. Differential Diagnosis of Neuroleptic Malignant Syndrome

Infectious
    Meningitis or encephalitis
    Postinfectious encephalomyelitis syndrome
    Brain abscess
    Sepsis

Psychiatric or Neurologic
    Idiopathic malignant catatonia
    Agitated delirium
    Benign extrapyramidal side effects
    Nonconvulsive status epilepticus
    Structural lesions, particularly involving the midbrain

Toxic or Pharmacologic
    Atropine poisoning from anticholinergics
    Alcohol or sedative withdrawal
    Malignant Hyperthermia (inhalational anesthetics, succinylcholine)
    Parkinsonian hyperthermia syndrome (after abrupt discontinuation of dopamine agonist)
    Salicyl poisoning
    Serotonin syndrome (SSRIs, SNRIs, monoamine oxidase inhibitors, triptans, linezolid)
    Substances of abuse (amphetamines, hallucinogens)

Endocrine
    Thyrotoxicosis
    Pheochromocytoma

Environmental
    Heat stroke

SNRIs, selective serotonin and norepinephrine reuptake inhibitors; *SSRIs,* selective serotonin reuptake inhibitors.

7. **Are there specific laboratory findings for neuroleptic malignant syndrome?**
   No laboratory findings are pathognomonic for NMS, but findings may support or confirm the diagnosis of NMS while excluding other systemic illnesses. Common laboratory abnormalities include the following:
   • Elevated serum creatinine kinase level of 1000 to 100,000 International Units/L
   • Leukocytosis (10,000–40,000/mm^3)
   • Elevated lactate dehydrogenase, alkaline phosphatase, and liver transaminase levels
   • Electrolyte disturbances: hypernatremia, hyponatremia, hyperkalemia, hypocalcemia, hypomagnesemia, and hypophosphatemia
   • Metabolic acidosis
   • Evidence of myoglobinuric acute renal failure: proteinuria, elevated blood urea nitrogen and creatinine levels
   • Low serum iron concentration

8. **Are special diagnostic tests or imaging studies useful?**
   Yes. Brain imaging studies and lumbar puncture are necessary to exclude structural brain disease and infection, though are generally normal in NMS. Electroencephalogram may show diffuse slowing without focal abnormalities, but is not diagnostic for NMS.

9. **Which agents have been implicated in the development of neuroleptic malignant syndrome?**
   First- and second-generation antipsychotic medications have been reported to cause NMS. The most commonly used agents are included below:
   • First-generation antipsychotics: chlorpromazine, fluphenazine, haloperidol, paliperidone, perphenazine, and thioridazine.
   • Second-generation antipsychotics: aripiprazole, clozapine, olanzapine, quetiapine, risperidone, and ziprasidone.
   NMS also has been reported with antiemetic medications such as domperidone, droperidol, metoclopramide, prochlorperazine, promethazine, and trimethobenzamide, as a result of their dopamine antagonism. Abrupt withdrawal of dopaminergic medications (amantadine or L-dopa) and GABA-ergic medications have been reported to precipitate an NMS-like reaction.

10. What are risk factors for development of neuroleptic malignant syndrome?
Several clinical, systemic, and metabolic risk factors have been associated with NMS. Suggested risk factors include:
- History of NMS
- Baseline electrolyte disturbances
- Pre-existing abnormalities in the central nervous system (CNS) dopamine activity or receptor function
- Iron deficiency
- Acute medical or neurologic illness
- Dehydration
- Primary diagnosis of an affective disorder (particularly bipolar disorder and psychotic depression)
- Comorbid substance use disorder
- Acute catatonia
- Psychomotor agitation
- Use of restraints
- Delirium
- Dementia
- Concurrent use of other psychotropic medications, especially lithium
- High doses, rapid dose escalation, and parenteral administration of antipsychotics, or depot formulations of antipsychotics
    Although the variables listed above correlate with the risk of NMS, they are not practical in predicting the development of NMS.

11. Does neuroleptic malignant syndrome have a genetic predisposition?
Recent evidence suggesting genetic vulnerability as a potential risk factor for the development of NMS has been inconsistent. Age and sex alone are not considered independent risk factors; however, younger male patients may be more likely to receive higher doses of antipsychotics to control combative behavioral symptoms, which results in their overrepresentation in NMS case studies.

12. What is the suggested management for neuroleptic malignant syndrome?
Early recognition and diagnosis of NMS is crucial to provide appropriate and prompt treatment. The mainstay of management is to:
- **Stop the offending agent** and other psychotropic agents.
- **Provide the necessary supportive care.** See Box 78.4.
- **Monitor in the intensive care unit (ICU)** as indicated for life-threatening complications. See Box 78.5.

Box 78-4. Supportive Management of Neuroleptic Malignant Syndrome

Aggressive volume resuscitation for dehydration
Most patients are severely dehydrated in the acute phase of the illness.
If creatine kinase (CK) is very elevated, intravenous fluids with urine alkalinization may help prevent or mitigate renal failure from rhabdomyolysis.
Physiologic cooling measures for hyperthermia
Peak and duration of temperature elevation are predictive of morbidity and mortality.
Serial monitoring and correction of electrolyte and metabolic abnormalities
Pharmacologic treatment of markedly elevated blood pressures
Heparin or low-molecular-weight heparin to prevent deep venous thrombosis.

Box 78-5. Life-Threatening Complications of Neuroleptic Malignant Syndrome

Monitor in the Intensive Care Unit for

Cardiac failure	Acute renal failure from rhabdomyolysis
Arrhythmias	Coagulopathies
Myocardial infarction	Disseminated intravascular coagulation
Respiratory failure	Deep venous thrombosis
Aspiration pneumonia	Hepatic failure
Pulmonary embolism	Sepsis

13. What pharmacologic treatments are useful?

In most cases, cessation of antipsychotic medications and supportive medical management are sufficient to reverse the symptoms of NMS. Several empirical off-label treatment approaches can be used in a case-by-case basis:

- Lorazepam 1 to 2 mg parenterally is a reasonable first-line intervention for patients with acute NMS. Recent clinical reports suggest that benzodiazepines (oral or parenteral) may ameliorate symptoms of agitation or catatonia and hasten recovery of NMS.
- Dopamine agonists, such as amantadine and bromocriptine, have been reported to reverse Parkinsonian symptoms, hasten recovery, and decrease mortality rates when used alone or in combination with other pharmacologic agents. Amantadine is generally initiated at 100 mg every 12 hours orally, and can be titrated to a maximum dose of 200 mg every 12 hours. Bromocriptine can be started at 2.5 mg every 6 to 8 hours orally with a maximum daily dose of 40 mg. Be advised that bromocriptine can worsen psychosis and hypotension, as well as precipitate vomiting, and must be used with caution. Abrupt discontinuation of bromocriptine can also precipitate rebound NMS-like symptoms.
- Dantrolene may be useful in cases of extreme hyperthermia, rigidity, and hypermetabolism. Typical dosing is 1 to 2.5 mg/kg intravenously initially and may be increased to 1 mg/kg every 6 hours up to a maximum cumulative dose of 10 mg/kg/day. Side effects may include respiratory impairment and hepatic toxicity.
- Electroconvulsive therapy (ECT) has been shown to be effective when NMS symptoms are refractory to supportive care and pharmacologic treatment. The typical ECT course was six to 10 bilateral treatments with initial response expected in the first few treatments. During ECT, succinylcholine should be avoided in patients with rhabdomyolysis to prevent acute hyperkalemia and cardiovascular complications.

14. Will neuroleptic malignant syndrome recur with subsequent use of neuroleptic medications?

The likelihood of development of NMS after restarting antipsychotic medications once the original episode of NMS has resolved is approximately 30%. To reduce risk of recurrence, allow at least 2 weeks of recovery before restarting any antipsychotic medications. It is best to choose a low-dose and low-potency antipsychotic, and titrate gradually while closely monitoring for subtle signs or symptoms of NMS.

15. Is there any way to decrease the risk of neuroleptic malignant syndrome?

When clinically indicated, reducing antipsychotic dose, avoiding parenteral or depot antipsychotic formulation, avoiding rapid dose escalation, and minimizing other risk factors (e.g., dehydration) may decrease the overall risk for development of NMS. Given that catatonia may be a strong risk factor for the development of NMS, antipsychotics should be avoided in patients with catatonia, if possible, for whom benzodiazepines may be an effective treatment.

16. Are there alternatives to antipsychotic medications for acutely psychotic patients?

A number of alternative treatment options exist for acutely psychotic patients. Benzodiazepines may help reduce agitation in a hyperactive psychotic patient and may potentially lower the absolute dose of antipsychotic needed to manage symptoms. When the primary diagnosis is an affective disorder, aggressive treatment with mood stabilizers or antidepressants is indicated. However, if psychotic symptoms are present in the context of an affective disorder, antipsychotic medications are usually necessary. ECT is also a viable nonpharmacologic alternative for treatment of manic psychosis, depressive psychosis, and catatonia.

17. Are there alternatives to antipsychotic medications for patients with chronic psychotic illnesses?

In chronic psychotic disorders (e.g., schizophrenia, schizoaffective disorder, delusional disorder) there may be no alternative treatment to antipsychotic medications that adequately manages symptoms. Hence, if NMS has occurred, caution is advised on rechallenging with a different class of antipsychotics. Special attention must be paid to second-generation antipsychotics and treatment of reversible risk factors. Efforts must also be made to minimize polypharmacy when clinically indicated.

18. Are malignant hyperthermia and neuroleptic malignant syndrome related?

Malignant hyperthermia (MH) and NMS have similar clinical presentations but different pathophysiologies. MH develops after exposure to inhalation anesthetics, such as halothane, and depolarizing muscle relaxants, such as succinylcholine. MH is characterized by diffuse muscle rigidity, fever, hypermetabolism, elevated creatinine kinase level, hyperkalemia, tachycardia, hypoxemia, metabolic acidosis, and myoglobinuria. MH is caused by a genetic defect in a sarcoplasmic reticulum calcium channel protein, which results in excessive calcium release into skeletal muscle after exposure to triggering medications. Susceptibility to MH is diagnosed by the muscle contracture test. Family studies and muscle contracture testing indicate that **patients with MH do not appear to be at increased risk for NMS, and vice versa.**

19. How is malignant catatonia differentiated from neuroleptic malignant syndrome?
Malignant catatonia (MC) can often be indistinguishable from NMS, with significant symptom overlap. MC tends to have behavioral prodromal symptoms for several weeks consisting of psychosis, agitation, and catatonic excitement, whereas NMS has no known prodromal phase. Motor symptoms of MC frequently include dystonic posturing, waxy flexibility, and stereotyped repetitive movements versus extrapyramidal symptoms characteristic of NMS. Laboratory abnormalities are frequent, but less common in MC than NMS.

20. How is serotonin syndrome differentiated from neuroleptic malignant syndrome?
Serotonin syndrome follows a history of exposure to serotonergic medications, not antipsychotic medications. Clinical features of serotonin syndrome, that are less common in NMS, include: prodromal symptoms (nausea, vomiting, and diarrhea), shivering, mood symptoms (anxiety, euphoria, irritability), hyperreflexia, myoclonus, and ataxia. Tremor and myoclonus are more prominent in serotonin syndrome than NMS. Fever and muscle rigidity, if present, are less pronounced in serotonin syndrome, and elevated creatinine kinase is usually absent.

ACKNOWLEDGMENT

The authors wish to acknowledge Dr. Jennifer M. Hall, DO, for the valuable contributions to the previous edition of this chapter.

KEY POINTS: NEUROLEPTIC MALIGNANT SYNDROME

1. NMS can develop with exposure to any antipsychotic medication—acute or chronic use.
2. When considering the differential diagnosis, the physician should pay particular attention to recent changes in doses and psychotropic polypharmacy.
3. Other dopamine antagonists, such as antiemetic agents, can also cause NMS.
4. Treatment is primarily supportive.
5. In most cases, the most important factors that distinguish NMS from serotonin syndrome are hyperthermia and rigidity.

BIBLIOGRAPHY

1. American Psychiatric Association. *Diagnostic and Statistical Manual of Mental Disorders (DSM-5®).* 5th ed. American Psychiatric Washington, DC: Pub; 2013:709-711.
2. Addonizio G, Susman VL. *Neuroleptic Malignant Syndrome: A Clinical Approach.* St. Louis: Mosby; 1991.
3. Boyer EW, Shannon M. The serotonin syndrome. *N Engl J Med.* 2005;352:1112 1120.
4. Castillo E, Rubin RT, Holsboer-Trachsler E. Clinical differentiation between lethal catatonia and neuroleptic malignant syndrome. *Am J Psychiatry.* 1989;146:324-328.
5. Gurrera RJ, Caroff SN, Cohen A, et al. An international consensus study of neuroleptic malignant syndrome diagnostic criteria using the Delphi method. *J clin Psychiatry.* 2011;72(9):1222-1228.
6. Pope Jr HG, Keck Jr PE, McElroy SL. Frequency and presentation of neuroleptic malignant syndrome in a large psychiatric hospital. *Am J Psychiatry.* 1986;143:1227-1233.
7. Rosebush P, Stewart T. A prospective analysis of 24 episodes of neuroleptic malignant syndrome. *Am J Psychiatry.* 1989; 146:717-725.
8. Shalev A, Hermesh H, Munitz H. Mortality from neuroleptic malignant syndrome. *J Clin Psychiatry.* 1989;50:18-25.
9. Strawn JR, Keck Jr PE, Caroff SN. Neuroleptic malignant syndrome. *Am J Psychiatry.* 2007;164:870-876.
10. Velamoor VR. Neuroleptic malignant syndrome: recognition, prevention and management. *Drug Saf.* 1998;19:73-82.

XV
UNIQUE PATIENT POPULATIONS

CHAPTER 79

CARE OF THE CRITICALLY ILL PREGNANT PATIENT

Stephen E. Lapinsky

1. **What are normal arterial blood gas findings in pregnancy?**
   Pregnancy results in increased ventilation because of elevated carbon dioxide production, as well as an increase in respiratory drive mediated largely by progesterone. These changes cause a low arterial partial pressure of carbon dioxide, at about 30 mm Hg by term. Plasma bicarbonate is decreased to 18 to 21 mEq/L, maintaining the arterial pH in the range of 7.40 to 7.45. Alveolar to arterial oxygen tension difference is usually unchanged, and the mean arterial PO_2 is generally about 100 mm Hg.

2. **How does pregnancy affect hemodynamics?**
   Cardiovascular physiology changes significantly during pregnancy, characterized by an increase in blood volume, an elevation in cardiac output, and a small decrease in blood pressure, resulting in a number of changes in the normal hemodynamic values in the third trimester (Table 79.1). In the supine position, the gravid uterus may produce significant mechanical obstruction of the inferior vena cava, reducing venous return and resulting in a decrease in cardiac output and hypotension. Maternal syncope or fetal distress may result. Supine hypotension syndrome may be avoided by positioning the patient on her left side, or at least with the right hip slightly elevated.

3. **What factors affect oxygen delivery to the fetus?**
   Oxygen delivery to the fetus is determined by the maternal arterial oxygen content, uterine blood flow, and placental function. A number of factors may adversely affect blood flow to the uteroplacental vasculature, which is normally maximally vasodilated. A decrease in maternal cardiac output reduces fetal oxygenation. The maternal response to hypotension does not favor uterine blood flow, and catecholamines (endogenous or exogenous) may aggravate fetal hypoxia by producing uterine vasoconstriction. Uterine blood flow may also be reduced by maternal alkalosis and during uterine contractions.

4. **Are there any special concerns to be considered when inserting an endotracheal tube in a critically ill pregnant patient?**
   The upper airway in pregnancy may be edematous and friable because of the effects of estrogen or placental growth hormone, and aggravated in the presence of preeclampsia producing excessive edema. The nasal route should be avoided, and a smaller endotracheal tube may be necessary. Because of the reduced functional residual capacity and increased oxygen consumption, hypoxemia

Table 79-1. Effect of Late Pregnancy on Pulmonary Artery Catheter Measurements

PARAMETER	CHANGE FROM NONPREGNANT VALUE
Central venous pressure	No change
Pulmonary capillary wedge pressure	No change
Cardiac output	30%–50% increase
Systemic vascular resistance	20%–30% decrease
Pulmonary vascular resistance	20%–30% decrease
Oxygen consumption	20%–40% increase
Oxygen extraction ratio	No change

will develop in a pregnant woman more rapidly than in nonpregnant, critically ill patients during intubation. Intubation should be carried out by the most skilled person available.

Note: The incidence of failed intubation is eight times higher in the obstetric population than in nonobstetric patients.

5. Describe the principles of management of severe pre-eclampsia.

The most important aspect of management is the well-timed delivery of the fetus. Supportive treatment involves fluid management, control of hypertension, and prevention of seizures:

- Patients with pre-eclampsia usually have mild volume depletion and require volume expansion, but excessive fluid administration may result in pulmonary or cerebral edema.
- Hypotension is managed to prevent maternal vascular damage and does not alter the pathologic process of pre-eclampsia. Commonly used regimens include small boluses of hydralazine (5–10 mg intravenous [IV]), boluses or infusion of labetalol, or oral calcium antagonists.
- Seizure prophylaxis should be undertaken with magnesium sulfate, with use of a loading IV bolus of 4 g over a 20-minute period followed by an infusion of 1–2 g/h. Toxic levels (usually >3.5 mmol/L) can cause respiratory muscle weakness and cardiac conduction defects and are usually seen in a patient with associated renal failure. Hypocalcemia during magnesium infusion is common and should not be treated unless symptomatic. The effects of magnesium sulfate (toxic as well as therapeutic) can be reversed with IV calcium.

6. What are the clinical features of the HELLP syndrome?

The HELLP syndrome (i.e., **h**emolysis, **e**levated **l**iver enzyme levels, and **l**ow **p**latelet count) is a complication of pre-eclampsia characterized by multiorgan dysfunction. The diagnostic features are the presence of thrombocytopenia, elevated liver enzymes, and a microangiopathic hemolytic anemia. The patient may present with epigastric or right upper quadrant pain, nausea, and vomiting, with or without other features of preeclampsia. Significant hemorrhage may result from the thrombocytopenia. A rare but catastrophic consequence of HELLP syndrome is hepatic hemorrhage, manifesting with sudden shock or acute abdominal pain.

7. What is acute fatty liver of pregnancy?

This is an uncommon complication of pregnancy manifesting with acute fulminant hepatic failure during the third trimester. Increased awareness of this condition has resulted in earlier diagnosis, with milder liver disease and an improved outcome. The clinical presentation is in the third trimester with malaise, anorexia, and vomiting, followed by abdominal pain and jaundice. The patient deteriorates rapidly with acute liver failure manifested by coagulopathy, hemorrhage, renal failure, and encephalopathy. Management requires urgent delivery of the fetus and supportive therapy for fulminant hepatic failure.

8. How does amniotic fluid embolism present?

Amniotic fluid embolism is a rare but catastrophic obstetric complication usually associated with labor, delivery, or other uterine manipulations. The typical presentation is a sudden onset of severe dyspnea, hypoxemia, and cardiovascular collapse, which may be accompanied by seizures. The maternal presentation is accompanied or preceded by sudden fetal distress. A significant portion of patients die acutely within the first hour. Survivors commonly have a disseminated intravascular coagulopathy and acute respiratory distress syndrome. Several biomarkers have been proposed with poor supporting evidence, but C1 esterase inhibitor deficiency may play a pathogenic role. Management is supportive, and the prognosis for mother and fetus is poor.

9. What are the causes of acute respiratory failure in pregnancy?

The pregnancy-specific diseases (Box 79.1) include amniotic fluid embolism, pulmonary edema resulting from the use of tocolytic therapy or related to preeclampsia, or peripartum cardiomyopathy. Although pregnant patients may have diseases similar to those in nonpregnant patients, pregnancy may increase the risk for venous thromboembolism, acute asthmatic attacks, and gastric aspiration. Changes in immune function in pregnancy predispose to increased severity of influenza pneumonitis, varicella pneumonia, as well as coccidioidomycosis infections. Additionally, pyelonephritis, a common cause of sepsis in pregnancy, can lead to the development of acute respiratory distress syndrome.

10. Does the management of pulmonary embolism differ in pregnant patients?

Investigation of suspected pulmonary embolism is similar to that in nonpregnant patients, beginning with duplex ultrasound. False-positive results may occur because of venous occlusion by the enlarged

Box 79-1. Causes of Respiratory Failure in Pregnancy

Pregnancy-Specific Factors
Amniotic fluid embolism
Tocolytic pulmonary edema
Pre-eclampsia complicated by pulmonary edema
Pulmonary edema due to peripartum cardiomyopathy
Obstetric sepsis with ARDS
Trophoblastic embolism

Risk Increased by Pregnancy
Venous thromboembolism
Asthma
Pulmonary edema due to pre-existing heart disease
Aspiration
ARDS associated with pyelonephritis
Pneumonia (e.g., varicella, influenza)

ARDS, Acute respiratory distress syndrome.

uterus. Ventilation-perfusion scanning and chest computed tomography angiogram can be carried out with a low risk for fetal radiation exposure. Unfractionated heparin and low-molecular-weight heparin are safe and effective in pregnancy. Warfarin is usually avoided because of the risk for embryopathy with first-trimester use, and central nervous system abnormalities and bleeding risk with second- and third-trimester use. Thrombolysis has been used successfully during pregnancy and the postpartum period, but should be limited to life-threatening situations.

11. What are the risks of radiologic procedures in pregnancy?
Estimated fetal radiation exposure varies from less than 0.01 rad (0.1 mGy) for a chest radiograph to about 2 to 5 rad (20–50 mGy) for pelvic computed tomography (Table 79.2). Abdominal shielding with lead and use of a well-collimated x-ray beam can effectively reduce exposure. The potential adverse effects of fetal exposure to radiation are oncogenicity, teratogenicity, and neurologic compromise. A twofold increased risk for childhood leukemia may occur with relatively low-dose fetal radiation exposure (2–5 rad). Teratogenicity is thought to require greater than 10 rad exposure; microcephaly and hydrocephaly have been described after exposure of 10 to 150 rad. Although radiation exposure in pregnancy carries definite risks, the likelihood of any adverse effect is about 0.1% per rad. The perception of risk by patients, family members, and physicians is often vastly higher than the actual risk.

12. How do the manifestations of severe trauma differ in pregnant patients?
Trauma is a common cause of morbidity and mortality in pregnancy. The increased maternal blood volume allows the mother to tolerate moderate blood loss, but this higher volume of hemorrhage necessitates more rapid IV fluid replacement. Fetal or amniotic injury may cause maternal coagulopathy, which can exacerbate hemorrhage. Occult uterine or retroperitoneal hemorrhage always should be considered. Deceleration injuries may precipitate placental abruption after 20 weeks' gestation. In the third trimester, abdominal trauma usually involves the uterus. Other intra-abdominal organs may be compressed in the upper abdomen, and injury in this area may cause significant organ damage. Physical signs of peritonism may be reduced because of stretching of the peritoneum. The bladder is at increased risk for injury as it extends above the pubis, and it should be remembered that some degree of ureteric dilation is normal in pregnancy. The fetus is at risk for morbidity resulting from

Table 79-2. Estimated Fetal Radiation Exposure During Radiographic Studies with Appropriate Shielding

RADIOGRAPHIC STUDY	ESTIMATED FETAL DOSE (RAD)
Chest radiograph	0.001
Ventilation-perfusion scan	0.012–0.050
CT scan of head	0.001
CT scan of chest	0.05–0.1
CT scan of abdomen or pelvis	2–5

CT, Computed tomography.

maternal hypotension, direct injury, fetomaternal hemorrhage (identified by the Kleihauer-Betke test), or placental abruption.

13. **Is management of cardiac arrest different for pregnant patients?**
Management of cardiac arrest in pregnancy follows usual protocols with some modifications. Because cardiopulmonary resuscitation in the supine position may cause impaired venous return, the uterus should be manually displaced to the left. New guidelines recommend manual displacement over left lateral tilt because the latter may reduce the effectiveness of chest compressions. IV access should be established above the diaphragm, and a difficult airway should be anticipated. No change in pharmacologic therapy is necessary, and drugs should not be withheld when clinically indicated. Consider calcium administration if the mother was receiving a magnesium sulfate infusion. Electrical defibrillation may be performed in pregnancy after removal of any fetal monitoring device. When initial attempts at resuscitation have failed, perimortem cesarean section should be considered if the fetus is at a viable gestation (e.g., uterine fundus above the umbilicus) and no return of spontaneous circulation has occurred within 4 minutes. Ideally, delivery should occur within 5 minutes of cardiac arrest for optimal fetal outcome. Cesarean section has been reported to reverse aortocaval compression and allow successful resuscitation of both the mother and infant.

14. **How is massive obstetric hemorrhage managed?**
Supportive measures include adequate venous access, rapid volume replacement, and blood product support. A dilutional coagulopathy should be anticipated. Ultrasound allows assessment of the uterine cavity for retained placental fragments that necessitate uterine curettage. Uterine massage and intramuscular methylergonovine (which should be avoided in the presence of hypertension) are used for uterine atony. Oxytocin infusion is administered in a dose higher than that used for augmentation of labor (e.g., 20–40 units in 1000 mL normal saline solution at a rate up to 250 ml/hr). Prostaglandin analogs are effective; carboprost tromethamine is given by intramuscular or intramyometrial injection in a dose of 0.25 mg, which may be repeated. Intrauterine balloon tamponade is a valuable adjunctive intervention. Prohemostatic drugs such as tranexamic acid are valuable if administered within 3 hours. If bleeding remains uncontrolled, more invasive approaches may be required. These include radiologic arterial embolization and surgical exploration to repair lacerations, to reduce blood flow by arterial ligation, or, if necessary, to remove the uterus.

15. **Which cardiac lesions present problems in pregnancy?**
The changes in cardiovascular physiology in pregnancy may result in decompensation in a patient with pre-existing heart disease because of the rise in cardiac output reaching a peak at about 28 weeks, 40% to 50% above baseline levels. Cardiac lesions limiting cardiac output (e.g., mitral stenosis, aortic stenosis) therefore present a significant risk for precipitating pulmonary edema or hypotension in the third trimester. This risk is particularly high during labor because of the tachycardia and volume shifts associated with delivery. Pulmonary hypertension is associated with significant morbidity and mortality because of the limitation of cardiac output and the inability to respond to postpartum fluid shifts. Congenital heart abnormalities are generally better tolerated in pregnancy unless complicated by pulmonary hypertension. Pregnancy may also predispose the patient to the development of cardiomyopathy.

16. **Does termination of pregnancy improve the outcome of a critically ill mother?**
An understanding of the physiologic effects of late pregnancy may suggest that delivery of the pregnant patient with respiratory failure will improve the mother's condition. However, this has not been found to be true for all patients; some improvement in oxygenation and/or compliance may occur in select patients. If the fetus is at a viable gestation and is at risk because of severe maternal hypoxia, there may be a benefit from removing the fetus from the intrauterine environment. However, delivery is usually not appropriate solely in an attempt to improve maternal oxygenation or ventilation. Consultation by a neonatologist is essential to evaluate fetal risks or benefits, and obstetric indications should determine the mode of delivery. Although cesarean section allows more rapid delivery, the increased physiologic stress may be associated with a higher mortality in critically ill patients.

KEY POINTS: CARE OF THE CRITICALLY ILL PREGNANT PATIENT

Causes of admission to the intensive care unit (ICU) because of pregnancy-specific conditions:

1. Respiratory failure can result from amniotic fluid embolism, pre-eclampsia, heart failure, or respiratory infection.
2. Hepatic dysfunction may occur, including acute fatty liver of pregnancy or HELLP syndrome.
3. Renal failure (e.g., pre-eclampsia or HELLP syndrome, idiopathic postpartum renal failure) may prompt admission to the ICU.
4. Hypertensive complications in the form of pre-eclampsia may occur.
5. Pregnant patients might require intensive care because of hemodynamic compromise, such as obstetric hemorrhage or obstetric sepsis.

BIBLIOGRAPHY

1. ANZIC Influenza Investigators and Australasian Maternity Outcomes Surveillance System. Critical illness due to 2009 A/H1N1 influenza in pregnant and postpartum women: population based cohort study. *BMJ.* 2010;340:c1279.
2. Clark SL, Cotton DB, Lee W, et al. Central hemodynamic assessment of normal term pregnancy. *Am J Obstet Gynecol.* 1989;161(6 Pt 1):1439-1442.
3. Conde-Agudelo A, Romero R. Amniotic fluid embolism: an evidence-based review. *Am J Obstet Gynecol.* 2009;201:445.e1-e13.
4. Lavonas EJ, Drennan IR, Gabrielli A, et al. Part 10: Special Circumstances of Resuscitation: 2015 American Heart Association Guidelines Update for Cardiopulmonary Resuscitation and Emergency Cardiovascular Care. *Circulation.* 2015;132(18 suppl 2):S501-S518.
5. Georgiou C. Balloon tamponade in the management of postpartum haemorrhage: a review. *BJOG.* 2009;116:748-757.
6. Ker K, Shakur H, Roberts I. Does tranexamic acid prevent postpartum haemorrhage? A systematic review of randomised controlled trials. *BJOG.* 2016;123(11):1745-1752.
7. Lapinsky SE. Cardiopulmonary complications of pregnancy. *Crit Care Med.* 2005;33:1616-1622.
8. Lapinsky SE, Kruczynski K, Slutsky AS. State of the art: critical care in the pregnant patient. *Am J Respir Crit Care Med.* 1995;152:427-455.
9. Lapinsky SE, Rojas-Suarez JA, Crozier TM, et al. Mechanical ventilation in critically-ill pregnant women: a case series. *Int J Obstet Anesth.* 2015;24:323.
10. Lowe SA. Diagnostic radiography in pregnancy: risks and reality. *Aust N Z J Obstet Gynaecol.* 2004;44:191-196.
11. Marik PE, Plante LA. Venous thromboembolic disease and pregnancy. *N Engl J Med.* 2008;359:2025-2033.
12. Munnur U, de Boisblanc B, Suresh MS. Airway problems in pregnancy. *Crit Care Med.* 2005;33(suppl 10):S259-S268.
13. Oxford CM, Ludmir J. Trauma in pregnancy. *Clin Obstet Gynecol.* 2009;52:611-629.
14. Ratnapalan S, Bentur Y, Koren G. Doctor, will that x-ray harm my unborn child? *CMAJ.* 2008;179:1293-1296.
15. Siu SC, Colman JM. Heart disease and pregnancy. *Heart.* 2001;85:710-715.
16. te Raa GD, Ribbert LS, Snijder RJ, et al. Treatment options in massive pulmonary embolism during pregnancy: a case-report and review of literature. *Thromb Res.* 2009;124:1-5.
17. Tamura N, Kimura S, Farhana M, et al. C1 esterase inhibitor activity in amniotic fluid embolism. *Crit Care Med.* 2014;42:1392.

CHAPTER 80

CARE OF THE OBESE PATIENT

Hui Zhang and Lorenzo Berra

1. **How is obesity defined?**
   Obesity is defined as an excess of body weight which compared to the predicted body weight of a subject, utilizing height as a determining factor. Body mass index (BMI) is the measurement used to describe the relationship between height and weight. BMI is determined according to the following formula:

   $$BMI = (weight)/(height)^2 = kg/m^2$$

   As shown in Table 80.1, BMI has been stratified into eight different classifications ranging from normal to hyperobese.

   Over the past decades, obesity has become a U.S. healthcare emergency encompassing all age groups. Recent U.S. surveys published in *JAMA* reveal the age-adjusted prevalence of obesity in 2013 to 2014 was 35.0% among men, 40.4% among women,[2] 8.1% among infants and toddlers,[3] and 17.0% among 2 to 19 year olds.[4] The severe obese group (BMI >40 kg/m^2) accounts for approximately 6.4% of the population. Obesity prevalence has been shown to differ among different ethnical populations. For example, the prevalence of grade 3 obesity has the lowest prevalence in Asian groups followed by the non-Hispanic White, Hispanic, and non-Hispanic Black groups. Almost 25% of patients admitted to an intensive care unit (ICU) have a BMI greater than 30 kg/m^2 and 7.5% of patients are admitted with a BMI ≥ 40 kg/m^2 (severe obese).

   According to recent estimates, U.S. healthcare costs attributable to overweight and obesity in 2005 range from UDS$147 billion to nearly USD$210 billion per year.

2. **What prevalent systemic and organ-specific derangements are caused by obesity?**
   The presence of excessive fat causes chronic inflammation, insulin resistance, increased metabolic work, and increased carbon dioxide production and oxygen consumption. Altogether, these changes may lead to hypertension, diabetes, dyslipidemia, and cardiac hypertrophy. The common major organ-specific derangements are listed in Box 80.1.

   Obesity is a major risk factor for cardiovascular disease. The mechanism of obesity-related cardiovascular disease involves an increase in both preload and afterload. The increased preload is explained by the expansion of blood volume due to redundant adipose tissue (perfused 3 mL of blood per each 100 g of tissue on average). An excessive secretion of steroids and catecholamines enhances the renin-angiotensin endocrine axis, resulting in an increased afterload. Together, these alternations lead to myocardial hypertrophy and diastolic dysfunction and, over time, to heart failure, arrhythmias, or cardiac arrest. Additionally, the presence of atherosclerosis, diabetes mellitus, and systemic hypertension increases the risk for myocardial infarction.

Table 80-1. Classification of Obese

CLASS	BMI (kg/m²)
Normal	20–25
Overweight	25–29
Obesity	30–39
Severe obesity	40–44
Morbid obesity	45–49
Super obesity	50–59
Super-super obesity	60–69
Hyperobesity	≥70

BMI, Body mass index.

Box 80-1. Organ-specified Disease Associated with Obesity

Cardiovascular Disease
Congestive heart failure, hypertension, myocardial infarction, dyslipidemia

Respiratory Disease
Hypoventilation syndrome, obstructive sleep apnea, reduced lung volumes, expiratory flow limitation, air-trapping, auto-PEEP, asthma, respiratory failure

Gastrointestinal Disease
Gastroesophageal reflux, nonalcoholic fatty liver disease, steatohepatitis, gastroparesis, gallstones, biliary tract disease, pancreatitis, hernias

Endocrinal Disease
Diabetes mellitus (type II), metabolic syndrome, polycystic ovarian syndrome, hypothyroidism infertility

Neurologic/Psychological Disease
Stroke, depression, idiopathic intracranial hypertension, disordered eating

Hematologic Disease
Venous thrombosis, pulmonary embolism, hypercoagulable state, chronic venous stasis

Musculoskeletal Disease
Degenerative joint disease, chronic back pain

Immune Disease/Infection
Pressure ulcers, skin infection, delayed wound healing, proinflammatory state

Renal Disease
Cancer
Kidney, esophagus, pancreas, colon, breast, ovary, endometrial, prostate

Adipose tissue can induce a proinflammatory/procoagulatory state in obese patients, increasing complications such as venous thrombosis and pulmonary embolism. In addition, diabetes mellitus and hypertension can be responsible for chronic kidney failure.

More than two-thirds of obese patients have obstructive sleep apnea (OSA). The conditions leading to OSA in obese patients include collapsibility of upper airway and disruption of normal physiologic respiratory drive.

Obesity causes a number of physiologic changes in the respiratory system. During spontaneous breathing, obese patients have reduced lung volumes, especially functional residual capacity and expiratory reserve volume. The mass of the abdomen weighs heavily against the diaphragm, which hinders diaphragmatic excursion, resulting in pulmonary atelectasis and small airways collapse. When the small airways collapse, expiratory flow limitation appears, which can cause dynamic hyperinflation. In other words, the force of body mass collapsing lung tissue also collapses airways, resulting in a counterintuitive air trapping auto-PEEP (positive end-expiratory pressure) at low lung volume. The increased expiratory flow limitation augments the breathing efforts of obese patients during spontaneous breathing. In addition, obesity hypoventilation syndrome (OHS) is often observed among obese patients. OHS is defined by a combination of BMI greater than 30 kg/m^2 and awake hypercapnia without other diagnosed causes of hypoventilation. When mechanically ventilated, obese patients may develop atelectasis and hypoxia respiratory failure. The major contributing factors to atelectasis are paralysis, sedation, and supine positioning.

3. What are the intensive care unit admission criteria for obese patients?
   In addition to common causes for ICU admission, obese patients might require ICU admission for close monitoring, treatment, and prevention of secondary adverse events that might be difficult to monitor, treat, or prevent on a regular floor. The ICU admission criteria for obese patients are listed in Box 80.2.

4. How are obese patients assessed upon admission to the intensive care unit?
   On admission to the ICU, BMI, body fat distribution, and history of snoring, sleepiness, and headaches should be collected. The degree of self-mobilization and physical daily activity should also

---

Box 80-2. The Intensive Care Unit Admission Criteria for Obese Patients

Severe obstructive sleep apnea (OSA) or obesity hypoventilation syndrome (OHS) and/or noninvasive mechanical ventilation requirements
Need for respiratory and cardiac monitoring
Difficult glycemic control
Intraoperative surgical or anesthetic complications such as bleeding, cardiovascular or respiratory event, and accidental lesions

---

be assessed as well as the risk for deep venous thrombosis and pulmonary embolism. A plan for noninvasive versus invasive ventilation management should be discussed with the ICU team and the patient. The most common complication in critically obese patients is acute respiratory failure. Particular attention must be paid to gas exchange and breathing efforts, which may prompt mechanical ventilation. The past use and the levels of continuous positive airway pressure (CPAP) and noninvasive ventilation (NIV) should be investigated and continued to be used. In the presence of a history suggestive of OSA/OHS, intermittent/nocturnal noninvasive bilevel positive airway pressure (BiPAP) or CPAP should be used, regardless of the patient's status.

5. What are the concerns associated with the respiratory system of obese patients?
   In obese patients, a difficult airway might be present, which may be due to the increased tongue size, smaller pharyngeal area, redundant pharyngeal tissue, increased neck circumference, and increased chest and abdominal girth. The changes of respiratory mechanics and functions in obese patients are shown in Table 80.2.
   The implementation of methods to minimize possible risk is crucial. Many factors must be taken into consideration as possible predictors for difficult mask ventilation in obese patients, such as the following: (1) BMI greater than 30 kg/m^2 as well as presence of a metabolic syndrome; (2) short neck; (3) higher neck circumference (e.g., >41 cm in women and >43 cm in men); (4) Mallampati score III/IV; and (5) mandibular protrusion.

Table 80-2. Changes of Respiratory Mechanics and Functions in Obese Patients

PHYSIOLOGIC CHANGES	CHALLENGES FOR RESPIRATORY MANAGEMENT
Excessive oropharyngeal adiposity	Upper airway obstruction
Increased risk of pharyngeal collapse during sleep	Frequent sleep apnea/obesity hypoventilation syndrome
Decreased compliance (chest wall >lung)	Decreased compliance during mechanical ventilation
Increased airway resistance	—
Increased work of breathing	—
Increase in resting VO_2	Frequent hypoxemic events
Decrease in FRC and EELV	Atelectasis
FRC <closing capacity	Rapid oxygen desaturation
Small airway closure	—
Alveolar collapse	—
Ventilation-perfusion (V/Q) mismatch	—
Increased PA-aO_2, Decreased PaO_2	—

EELV, End-expiratory lung volume; *FRC*, functional residual capacity; *PaO_2*, arterial partial pressure of oxygen; *PA-aO_2*, alveolar to arterial partial pressure of oxygen; *VO_2*, oxygen consumption; *V/Q*, ventilation/perfusion

An effective standard of measure that can be easily adopted to predict difficult intubation in obese patients and manage the airways accordingly is the so-called El Ganzouri risk index (EGRI).[5] It includes the following: (1) mouth opening, (2) thyromental distance, (3) Mallampati class, (4) neck movement, (5) ability to prognath, and (6) body weight and history of difficult intubation, each of them scored from 0 = low, 1 = medium, to 2 = high risk. The following procedure is recommended: If EGRI is between 0 and 3, intubation difficulties are considered low, and the intubation can proceed with standard devices. If EGRI is between 4 and 7, a video laryngoscope is suggested to improve visibility of the larynx during intubation. If EGRI is higher or equal to 8, an awake intubation with fiberscope is recommended. Another important parameter to be considered before intubation is the noninvasive measurement of oxygen saturation (SpO_2) in ambient air. If SpO_2 is lower than 95%, a preoperative arterial blood gas analysis might be obtained to assess pCO_2, standard bicarbonate for diagnosis assessment of OSA and OHA.

6. What are recommended methods for bag-mask ventilation and oxygenation before intubation in morbidly obese patients?
   The recommended method for bag-mask ventilation and oxygenation before intubation in morbidly obese patients is to place the patient in a 25- to 45-degree head-up position or reverse Trendelenburg position to shift the weight of the chest wall inferiorly and improve diaphragmatic excursion and also facilitate visualization of the vocal cords during direct laryngoscopy. In normal-weight anesthetized subjects, atelectasis is enhanced by the use of 1.0 fraction of inspired oxygen (FiO_2) during induction compared with the use of 0.3 FiO_2 as a result of absorption atelectasis. Lower concentrations of oxygen could reduce the atelectasis, but also reduce the safe apnea period during intubation. As a result, preinduction with 1.0 FiO_2 and application of 10 cm H_2O CPAP is recommended.

7. What is the noninvasive ventilation recommendation for obese patients?
   The NIV should always be attempted when the patient's neurologic status is sufficient, but O_2 therapy alone is ineffective at correcting hypoxemia or when hypercapnia complicates the respiratory failure.
   The following steps should be followed when NIV is applied:
   1. Explain the indications of NIV and the possible outcomes (requirements of intubation or prolonged use of NIV) to the patient. Explain to the patient that he or she is not allowed to drink during NIV.
   2. Perform an arterial-blood gas (ABG) to assess baseline gas exchange.
   3. Fit the mask appropriately. Check the patient with the most comfortable mask.
   4. Suggested initial settings are 10 cm H_2O of pressure support and 10 cm H_2O of PEEP.
   5. Monitor vital signs, gas exchange, respiratory rate, V_T, and comfort of the patient.
   6. Gradually increase PEEP in 2 cm H_2O increments to improve airway patency and oxygenation (SpO_2 >90%). Monitor hemodynamics.
   7. Gradually increase pressure support in 2 cm H_2O increments to improve V_T (until 6–8 mL/kg of ideal body weight [IBW]), reduce the respiratory rate (<25 breaths per minute), reduce ventilatory distress, and improve CO_2 clearance.
   8. Check gas exchange at 60 minutes. If noticeable improvement has been observed and there is no clinical deterioration, NIV can be continued. If NIV did not improve oxygenation or hypercapnia, the patient should be intubated and mechanically ventilated.

8. What are the effects of body positioning during ventilation?
   In the supine obese patient, lung volumes are reduced by the cranial displacement of the diaphragm and the gravitational effect of the abdominal contents upon the diaphragm and the thoracic cavity. The neuromuscular blocking use during the ventilation decreases diaphragmatic muscle tone, which further enhances the atelectasis induced by the abdominal contents. Lemyze et al.[6] observed in critically ill, mechanically ventilated obese patients that placing them in the sitting position constantly and significantly relieved expiratory flow limitation and auto-PEEP, resulting in a dramatic drop in alveolar pressures. Dixon et al.[7] observed that obese patients preoxygenated in a 25 degrees head-up position achieved 23% higher oxygen tensions than patients preoxygenated in the supine position. Pelosi et al.[8] found that prone positioning improved pulmonary function, increased functional residual capacity (FRC), lung compliance, and oxygenation compared with supine position in obese patients during general anesthesia.

9. How is tidal volume calculated in mechanically ventilated obese patients?
   Ventilator settings should be determined based on the patient's predicted body weight (PBW) or IBW and not based on actual or total body weight (TBW) to avoid barotrauma, as an increased BMI does not reflect increased lung size. There are different equations and formulas to calculate the predicted

or IBW. The most widely used formulas are listed below. These are the formulas used by the NIH/ NHLBI ARDS Network in their landwork study and the term PBW = IBW:

$$PBW\ man = 50.0 + 0.905 \times [(Height\ in\ cm) - 152.4]$$
$$PBW\ woman = 45.5 + 0.905 \times [(Height\ in\ cm) - 152.4]$$

10. How are the ventilation mode settings determined?
The optimization of mechanical ventilation is essential to minimize complications for the obese patients in ICU. There is no evidence of superiority of volume- versus pressure-controlled ventilation. Theoretically, pressure-controlled ventilation could lead to a more homogeneous air distribution within different lung compartments. However, volume-controlled ventilation may allow for better control of tidal volumes during surgical procedures where chest wall elastance is affected (e.g., abdominal surgery) and pressure-controlled ventilation in thoracic surgery when one-lung ventilation is indicated. Further, the most important aspect for optimizing gas exchange and minimizing possible ventilator-induced lung injury during mechanical ventilation is the level of pressure reached at end inspiration and end expiration. These are effectively the same in both pressure- or volume-controlled ventilation. The settings of mechanical ventilation of the obese patient are shown in Box 80.3.

11. What are lung recruitment maneuvers followed by a decremental PEEP trial and how are they performed?
In order to reverse atelectasis, a lung recruitment maneuver with a decremental PEEP trial is necessary. A recruitment maneuver is the temporary application of an end-expiratory pressure that is significantly greater than pleural pressure. The applied pressure gradient needs to be high enough to open collapsed alveoli that have opening pressure higher than the normal ventilating peak pressure. The lung recruitment maneuvers (RMs) in obese, mechanically ventilated patients are effective measures in improving respiratory compliance and oxygenation without side effects on hemodynamic. The lung RM can reverse the formation of atelectasis and persist without adequate levels of PEEP during the mechanic ventilation. It is suggested to perform a recruitment maneuver whenever PEEP is increased or after a PEEP discontinuation. A recruitment maneuver followed by a decremental PEEP trial can be performed as follows:
1. Assess hemodynamic stability of the patient.
2. Switch to pressure control ventilation with the following settings:
Pressure control: +15 cm H_2O
PEEP: +10 cm H_2O
Respiratory rate: 10 breaths per minute
I/E ratio: 1:1
3. If the patient is stable, after 30 seconds increase PEEP by 5 cm H_2O (PEEP: +15 cm H_2O).
4. Check oxygenation and hemodynamics.
5. If the patient is stable, after 30 seconds increase PEEP by 5 cm H_2O (PEEP: +20 cm H_2O).
6. Check oxygenation and hemodynamics.
7. If the patient is stable, after 30 seconds increase PEEP by 5 cm H_2O (PEEP: +25 cm H_2O).
8. Check oxygenation and hemodynamics.

Box 80-3. Mechanical Ventilation of the Obese Patient

Mode: Pressure or volume ventilation
Tidal volume: 6 mL/kg PBW averagely, range 4–8 mL/kg PBW
Inspiratory time: 0.6–1.0 second
Plateau pressure: Less than 28 cm H_2O, unless TPP measured, then TPP >20 cm H_2O
Driving pressure ≤15 cm H_2O
Rate only limited by the development of auto-PEEP
Minute volume: 10 L/min or greater
Lung recruitment maneuver with decremental PEEP trial to set PEEP
FiO$_2$ set to main target PaO$_2$
Position: Reverse Trendelenburg position
Noninvasive ventilation for 24–48 h after extubation

PBW, Predicted body weight; *TTP*, transpulmonary pressure.

9. Switch to volume control and perform a decremental PEEP trial. Set ventilator setting similar to that before RM, but keep PEEP at 25 cm H_2O and FiO_2 at 1.0. Measure total respiratory compliance (Crs) after 3 to 5 minutes.
10. Decrease PEEP to 21 cm H_2O after 3 to 5 minutes and measure Crs.
11. Decrease PEEP to 19 cm H_2O after 3 to 5 minutes and measure Crs.
12. Decrease PEEP to 17 cm H_2O after 3 to 5 minutes and measure Crs.
13. Continue this process until the best Crs PEEP can be identified.
14. Recruit the lung again and set PEEP at the best Crs PEEP plus 2 cm H_2O.
15. Decrease the FiO_2 to the lowest level maintaining partial pressure of arterial oxygen (PaO_2) in the target range.

12. **How should obese patients be extubated?**
There is no consensus and scientific data on the best approach for ventilator weaning of obese patients. As the beneficial effects of PEEP and position in this population have become more clear, it is advisable that PEEP should be carefully reduced only after the FiO_2 has stabilized at approximately 0.40. In addition, it is suggested to reduce pressure support level gradually while keeping the PEEP level stable and eventually reduce the PEEP to 8 to 10 cm H_2O. It would be best to extubate these patients while they are on PEEP and start noninvasive CPAP or bilevel positive airway pressure immediately after extubation. NIV then can be weaned in the following 48 to 72 hours.

13. **What are the prophylaxis and course of treatment of venous thromboembolism for obese patients in the intensive care unit?**
The risk of venous thromboembolism (VTE) is increased in obese patients. Some indexes have been proposed to predict the risk of VTE in obesity after surgery, such as the Caprini score—when higher than or equal to 4—represents a threshold for high to moderate risk. Aminian et al. identified 91,963 patients who underwent bariatric operations between 2007 and 2012, and they stratified the postbariatric patients into moderate risk (<0.4%), high risk (between >0.4 and <1% or one of the following: past history of deep vein thrombosis (DVT) or pulmonary embolism (PE), congenital or acquired hypercoagulable conditions [e.g., positive factor V Leiden, prothrombin 20210A], and relevant chronic venous insufficiency), and very high risk (>1%) of DVT[1]. Based on these findings, it was recommended that patients with high or very high attributed risk are suitable to extended prophylaxis (two additional weeks under anti-thrombotic agents; see Table 80.3 for drugs and dosages).

14. **What biases are noted in the treatment of morbidly obese patients?**
Negative attitudes and opinions toward the morbidly obese, which is so-called bias against the patient, can result in actions or lack of actions that may greatly affect a patient's health. Not having standard supplies and equipment, such as hospital gowns, examination tables, or blood pressure cuffs large enough to accommodate morbidly obese patients, can create an uncomfortable environment. Patients' perceptions of being stigmatized by healthcare providers, specifically nurses, can lead to feelings of shame, marginalization, and anxiety. Regardless of healthcare personnel's opinions or the reasons for the patients' obesity, the priority is to provide the best quality of care while ensuring dignity and remaining compassionate and empathetic.

15. **What are the concerns when placing the central venous catheter in obese patients?**
Many morbidly obese patients require a central venous catheter (CVC). However, CVC placement can be challenging because anatomical structures may be difficult to locate and standard-sized catheters may not be long enough for appropriate placement. Practitioners should use ultrasound to accurately locate veins and minimize complications. Although the Trendelenburg position is the preferred position for placement of an internal jugular CVC due to the resulting higher central venous volume and larger vein caliber which can prevent air embolus, this position could also result in an acute deterioration of cardiopulmonary status due to reduced lung volumes, diminished pulmonary reserve, intra-abdominal pressure, and elevated right ventricular pressures. The Trendelenburg position should be used with caution.

16. **What are the risk factors associated with decubitus ulcers and how can they be avoided?**
Several factors predispose obese patients to loss of skin integrity, including decreased blood and oxygen supply due to increased adipose tissue and an increase in perspiration and skin moisture, increasing the risk for bacterial and fungal invasion. Nurses should conduct a thorough wound evaluation, especially in high-risk areas such as the sacrum, buttocks, elbows, and heels, and perform a risk assessment by means of an instrument such as the Braden Scale, which is the standardized approach for assessing risk when an obese patient is admitted to the ICU.

Table 80-3. Recommendation for Anticoagulant Therapy used in Postbariatric Surgery

	VTE PROPHYLAXIS	VTE TREATMENT
Heparin	• Preferred in renal failure • 5000 U 2/3 times a day • Adjusted doses up to 15,000 U Bid without increasing bleeding	• Use based on TBW • Monitoring by APTT —
Enoxaparin	BMI 30–49 kg/m^2: 0.5 mg/kg or 40 mg Q12 h BMI >50 kg/m^2: 0.5 mg/kg or 60 mg Q12 h	BMI 30–49 kg/m^2: 1 mg/kg Q12 h based on ADW Avoid daily dosing regimens
Dalteparin	• 2500 IU SC 1–2 h preoperative, then 2500 units SC qd • High risk of thromboembolic complications 5000 U SC evening before surgery then 5000 units qd (first dose may be evenly split in a preoperative and postoperative dose) — —	200 units IU/kg SC qd for 30 days Months 2–6: 150 units/kg SC qd Avoid to exceed 18,000 units/D Treatment duration: 5–10 days Severe mobility restriction: 5000 units SC Qd Thrombocytopenia: Dose Reduction • Plts 50,000–100,000/mm^3: Reduce daily • Dose by 2500 units until 100,000/mm^3 • Plts <50,000/mm^3, discontinue • Until >50,000/mm^3 Renal impairment, severe: dose reduction • CrCl <30 mL/min: monitor anti-Xa level to determine appropriate dose

APTT, activated partial thromboplastin time; BMI, Body mass index; Plts, platelet; SC, subcutaneous; TBW, total body weight; VTE, venous thromboembolism.
Pompilio CE, Pelosi P, Castro MG. The Bariatric patient in the intensive care unit: pitfalls and management. Curr Atheroscler Rep. 2016;18(9):55.

The key to preventing decubitus ulcers is pressure redistribution, which involves appropriate use of pressure-reducing devices and positioning of patients. The frequency of repositioning should be based on the patient's activity level and risk for skin breakdown. According to recommendations, patients should be turned within a 2-hour interval, because skin erythema and ischemic changes can occur in healthy adults in less than 2 hours on a standard mattress. The quality of skin perfusion is important and mechanisms employed to avoid bad perfusion include prompt treatment of hypotension, limiting vasoconstrictive agents, improving cardiac output, and revascularization of distal tissues. Skin should be kept clean and dry while avoiding excess dryness and scaling. Deep skin folds, such as those under pendulous breasts, groin folds, or under a pannus must be closely monitored, dried thoroughly, and kept as open to air as possible. Correcting malnutrition and promoting early mobility are equally important steps in preventing decubitus ulcers.

17. **What difficulties are presented when administering drugs to obese patients?**
   Differences in proportion of adipose and lean muscle tissue and fluid status can greatly affect pharmacokinetics, absorption, distribution, metabolism, and excretion of drugs. The total blood volume and cardiac output are increased in obese patients, which can cause alterations in plasma protein binding. Hepatic clearance is usually normal or even increased in obese patients and renal clearance can increase because of increases in kidney weight, renal blood flow, and glomerular filtration rate. Volume of distribution in obese patients is dramatically different than that in normal-weight patients, and the extent of change is based on the intrinsic characteristics of a medication, such as molecular size, degree of ionization, extent of lipid solubility, protein binding, and ability to cross biological

membranes. Obesity can alter activity through the cytochrome P-450 pathway, affecting drug clearance. Standard creatinine clearance values may also be inaccurate in morbidly obese patients, and depending on whether IBW or TBW is used in calculations, the values may be overestimated or underestimated. Dosage of renal excreted drugs should be adjusted on the basis of measured creatinine clearance.

18. **What is metabolic response to critical illness in obese patients?**

Regardless of the inducing cause of illness, there is a common hypermetabolic, inflammatory response to physiologic stress which can affect protein, lipid, and carbohydrate utilization throughout the body. Obesity can exaggerate this effect during critical illness because of its proinflammatory state.

Hyperglycemia is a frequent complication of critical illness and the end product of increased counter regulatory hormone such as glucagon, glucocorticoids, and catechcholamines and inflammatory cytokine release, leading to accelerated hepatic gluconeogenesis, lipolysis, and peripheral insulin resistance. It is especially important to control the glucose level in obese patients, given the increased prevalence of diabetes and insulin resistance. The excess glucose can lead to increased lipogenesis, hepatic steatosis, and increased CO_2 production, which will increase work of breathing. Therefore, regular insulin needs to be added to total parenteral nutrition (TPN) solution.

Obese patients have increased levels of hormones and substrate, such as amino acids and free fatty acids (FFAs), when they are fast. Elevations in FFAs signify insulin resistance, which will cause increased lipolysis, impaired skeletal muscle FFA oxidation, and reduced suppression of plasma FFA by insulin. Obese patients are ineffective in using serum FFAs and triglyceride-rich adipose during critical illness. Studies show that obese patients derive energy mainly from catabolism of lean mass. Fat-free mass catabolism typically persists despite the nutrition support in ICU. Hence, hypocaloric, high-protein nutrition is a preferable approach in obese patients for the promotion of endogenous fat oxidation and shift away from utilization of fat-free mass as the predominant fuel source.

19. **What nutritional support is optimal for obese patients admitted to the intensive care unit? What are the contraindications of nutritional support?**

Early enteral nutrition in severely obese patients must be implemented because it helps in alleviating the pre-existing oxidative stress state. Otherwise, the fast will exacerbate the loss of lean body mass and induce the development of sarcopenia.

The 2009 Consensus statement issued jointly by the Society of Critical Care Medicine (SCCM) and the American Society for Parenteral and Enteral Nutrition (ASPEN) endorses hypocaloric feeding of critically ill obese patients with enteral feeds, with the goal to provide no more than 60% to 70% of target energy requirements or 11 to 14 kcal/kg actual body weight per day with BMI between 30 and 50 kg/m² and 22 to 25 kcal/kg ideal weight for patients with BMI above 50 kg/m². Based on nitrogen balance data from studies on hypocaloric feeding, the ASPEN/SCCM guidelines also recommend administration of protein in the range of at least 2.0 g/kg IBW per day for class I and II obese patients (30–39.9 kg/m²) and at least 2.5 g/kg IBW per day for class III obesity (>40 kg/m²). There are relatively few contraindications to hypocaloric feeding, other than conditions precluding the use of high-protein nutrition such as progressive renal failure or hepatic encephalopathy, or conditions in which full caloric loads are preferred, including history of hypoglycemia, diabetic ketoacidosis, or severe immunocompromised state. Otherwise, hypocaloric nutrition should always be considered for the obese ICU patient.

Contraindications include patients with severely unstable hemodynamic status and patients who have not had adequate fluid replacement because such patients may be predisposed to bowel ischemia. Other contraindications include bowel obstruction, severe and protracted ileus, major bleeding in the upper part of the gastrointestinal tract, intractable vomiting or diarrhea, gastrointestinal ischemia, and a high-output fistula.

REFERENCES

1. Aminian A, Andalib A, Khorgami Z, et al. Who Should Get Extended Thromboprophylaxis After Bariatric Surgery?: A Risk Assessment Tool to Guide Indications for Post-discharge Pharmacoprophylaxis. Ann Surg. 2017;265(1):143-150.
2. Flegal KM, Kruszon-Moran D, Carroll MD, et al. Trends in obesity among adults in the United States, 2005 to 2014. JAMA. 2016;315(21):2284-2291.
3. Ogden CL, Carroll MD, Kit BK, et al. Prevalence of childhood and adult obesity in the United States, 2011-2012. JAMA. 2014;311(8):806-814.

4. Ogden CL, Carroll MD, Lawman HG, et al. Trends in obesity prevalence among children and adolescents in the United States, 1988-1994 through 2013-2014. *JAMA*. 2016;315(21):2292-2299.
5. el-Ganzouri AR, McCarthy RJ, Tuman KJ, et al. Preoperative airway assessment: predictive value of a multivariate risk index. *Anesth Analg*. 1996;82(6):1197-1204.
6. Lemyze M, Mallat J, Duhamel A, et al. Effects of sitting position and applied positive end-expiratory pressure on respiratory mechanics of critically ill obese patients receiving mechanical ventilation*. *Crit Care Med*. 2013;41(11): 2592-2599.
7. Dixon BJ, Dixon JB, Carden JR, et al. Preoxygenation is more effective in the 25 degrees head-up position than in the supine position in severely obese patients: a randomized controlled study. *Anesthesiology*. 2005;102(6):1110-1115 [discussion: 1115A].
8. Pelosi P, Croci M, Calappi E, et al. Prone positioning improves pulmonary function in obese patients during general anesthesia. *Anesth Analg*. 1996;83(3):578-583.

CHAPTER 81

ONCOLOGIC EMERGENCIES

Dusan Hanidziar

1. **What is oncologic emergency?**
   Oncologic emergency is a serious, often life-threatening complication of cancer or cancer therapy that requires emergent evaluation and treatment. Oncologic emergency may be the initial clinical manifestation of previously undiagnosed cancer.

2. **Classify oncologic emergencies and provide examples for each class.**
   - Metabolic: tumor lysis syndrome, hypercalcemia, syndrome of inappropriate antidiuretic hormone (SIADH), lactic acidosis
   - Mechanical (structural): acute obstructive hydrocephalus, cerebral edema, spinal cord compression, superior vena cava (SVC) syndrome, malignant pericardial effusion
   - Hematologic: leukostasis, disseminated intravascular coagulation, thrombosis and thromboembolism, hyperviscosity syndrome
   - Infectious: neutropenic fever and sepsis
   - Complications of antineoplastic therapy: cytopenias, cardiac toxicity, neutropenic enterocolitis (typhlitis), hemorrhagic cystitis, pneumonitis, cytokine release syndrome (CRS), anaphylaxis

METABOLIC EMERGENCIES

3. **What are the main features of tumor lysis syndrome?**
   Tumor lysis syndrome results from rapid breakdown of malignant cells and release of their contents into the circulation, typically due to initiation of a cytotoxic therapy. Laboratory abnormalities include hyperkalemia, hyperuricemia, hyperphosphatemia, and hypocalcemia. Cardiac (dysrhythmias), renal (acute renal failure), and neurologic (seizures) complications may result.

4. **Can tumor lysis syndrome be prevented?**
   Yes. Prophylactic measures, including intravenous fluid loading and correction of electrolyte abnormalities, are aimed at preventing cardiac dysrhythmias and acute renal failure. Rasburicase (recombinant urate oxidase) is highly effective in normalizing plasma uric acid levels.

5. **By what mechanisms do tumors cause hypercalcemia?**
   Malignancy-associated hypercalcemia results from (1) parathyroid hormone-related protein (PTHrP)-production by a tumor (80% cases), (2) osteolysis from bone metastasis, (3) calcitriol production by a lymphoma, or (4) ectopic PTH secretion.

6. **What are the classic electrocardiographic findings in patients with hypercalcemia?**
   Electrocardiographic (EKG) findings in clinically significant hypercalcemia include prolonged PR interval, widened QRS complex, shortened QT interval, bundle branch block, and bradydysrhythmias leading to cardiac arrest when serum calcium exceeds 15 mg/dL.

7. **What interventions are effective in the treatment of hypercalcemia?**
   - Intravenous fluid administration: hypercalcemia leads to osmotic diuresis and hypovolemia; therefore, restoring intravascular volume is an important initial step in management. Normal saline is usually administered.
   - Bisphosphonate therapy: pamidronate and zoledronate are first-line agents to treat malignancy-associated hypercalcemia. They inhibit bone hydroxyapatite dissolution and osteoclastic resorption, decreasing plasma calcium levels within 2 to 4 days.

8. **Which tumors are associated with syndrome of inappropriate antidiuretic hormone?**
   Many different tumors can actively produce antidiuretic hormone (ADH) and cause hyponatremia, but it is most commonly found in patients with small-cell lung cancers. Certain chemotherapy drugs, as well as nausea itself, are potent triggers of excessive ADH secretion.

9. Which patients with cancer are at risk of developing lactic acidosis?
   Type B lactic acidosis is a very rare, but life-threatening complication of cancer, most commonly seen in patients with hematologic malignancies characterized by a high proliferative rate, such as lymphomas and leukemias. An increased production of lactic acid by cancer cells and impaired lactate clearance (liver and renal dysfunction) are the underlying mechanism.

10. How does lactic acidosis manifest?
    Patients typically present with otherwise unexplained deterioration in respiratory status (tachypnea). Laboratory investigations reveal anion gap metabolic acidosis and markedly elevated lactate. Aggressive treatment of the underlying malignancy (chemotherapy) and supportive therapy (bicarbonate infusion, renal replacement therapy) are the mainstay of the treatment.

MECHANICAL (STRUCTURAL) EMERGENCIES

11. How do the patients with brain metastases commonly present?
    Patients may present with signs and symptoms of increased intracranial pressure, such as headache, vomiting, and altered mental status. They may also exhibit focal neurologic signs such as hemiparesis, aphasia, and seizures.

12. What is the treatment of brain metastases?
    Depending on the location, size, and number of metastases, treatment options include surgical resection, whole brain radiation, stereotactic radiosurgery, and chemotherapy. Dexamethasone reduces intracranial pressure by decreasing vasogenic cerebral edema.

13. What are the causes of hydrocephalus in oncologic patients?
    Diagnosis of acute hydrocephalus should be considered in any patient who presents with altered mental status, ataxia, headache, or vomiting. In adult oncologic patients, obstructive hydrocephalus can be caused by leptomeningeal carcinomatosis or brain metastases with intraventricular extension.

14. What is the diagnostic workup of new-onset back pain in a patient with cancer?
    Back pain is the initial symptom in 95% patients with malignant spinal cord compression. Magnetic resonance imaging (MRI) of the entire spine is the most sensitive and specific modality to diagnose spinal metastasis.

15. How does malignant spinal cord compression manifest?
    Compressive myelopathy, most often due to epidural metastasis, manifests with pain, motor weakness, paraplegia, sensory dysfunction, and bowel and bladder dysfunction. Rapid progression of neurologic deficit is typical for cord infarcts.

16. What is the most important predictor of outcome in a patient with compressive myelopathy?
    The onset of neurologic deficit in a patient with spinal metastasis is considered a medical emergency. The most important predictor of outcome is the severity of neurologic deficit when the treatment is instituted. Corticosteroids in addition to radiation or surgery are the mainstay of acute treatment.

17. Discuss the signs and symptoms of superior vena cava syndrome.
    Most frequent signs are facial edema and distended neck and chest veins. Most common symptoms are dyspnea at rest and cough.

18. What tumors cause superior vena cava syndrome?
    SVC syndrome is the result of the mechanical obstruction to the venous blood flow due to the external compression or invasion of SVC. Lung cancers (both small and non-small cell) and lymphomas may compress the SVC. Venous thrombosis secondary to cancer and in patients with central venous access can lead to SVC syndrome.

19. How is superior vena cava syndrome treated?
    Patients with cerebral edema and airway edema due to venous congestion require emergent treatment (usually SVC stent). Depending on tumor type, stents, chemotherapy, steroids, or radiation are employed in nonurgent cases. Anticoagulation is initiated in cases of thrombosis.

20. What are the clinical signs suggestive of malignant pericardial effusion?
    Exertional dyspnea is the most common presenting symptom of malignant pericardial effusion. Sinus tachycardia is common.

21. Discuss echocardiographic findings of pericardial tamponade.
Two-dimensional echocardiogram demonstration of right atrial collapse in late diastole and right ventricular collapse in early diastole are most characteristic of tamponade.

22. How is pericardial tamponade managed?
Emergency bedside pericardiocentesis, preferably under ultrasound control, is required in cases of acute tamponade complicated by circulatory shock.

HEMATOLOGIC EMERGENCIES

23. When does leukostasis develop?
Leukostasis (symptomatic hyperleukocytosis) is a medical emergency most commonly seen in patients with acute myeloid leukemia. Myeloid blasts, adherent to endothelium, obstruct capillary blood flow and tissue perfusion is impaired. White blood cell count in affected patients typically exceeds 100,000/μL.

24. How is leukostasis diagnosed?
Clinical suspicion is the key. Organs most frequently affected by leukostasis are lungs, brain, and kidneys. Depending on the organ involved, leukostasis presents as dyspnea, respiratory failure, altered mental status, renal vein thrombosis, or limb ischemia. When leukostasis is suspected, cytoreductive therapies need to be initiated promptly to prevent morbidity and mortality.

25. What combination of laboratory abnormalities is typical for disseminated intravascular coagulation?
Disseminated intravascular coagulation (DIC) is a known complication of cancer, most common in patients with acute leukemia. Typically, moderate to severe thrombocytopenia is present. Elevated D-dimer levels help distinguish DIC from other causes of thrombocytopenia. Global clotting times (activated partial thromboplastin time [aPTT] and prothrombin time [PT]) are typically prolonged.

26. Why does cancer promote venous thromboembolism?
Solid tumor cells express different procoagulant molecules, including tissue factor and cancer procoagulant. Chemotherapy may enhance the risk of thrombosis by damaging the endothelium. Recent surgery, immobilization, and indwelling vascular catheters further increase the risk.

27. What cancers can cause hyperviscosity syndrome?
Waldenström macroglobulinemia and multiple myeloma are the leading causes. Mucosal or skin bleeding (due to paraprotein-induced platelet dysfunction), visual abnormalities, and focal neurologic deficits should raise the clinical suspicion of hyperviscosity syndrome. Fluid resuscitation and plasmapheresis reduce patient morbidity by decreasing serum viscosity.

INFECTIOUS EMERGENCIES

28. Define neutropenic fever.
Neutropenic fever is defined as a single oral temperature over 38.3°C (101°F) or a sustained temperature (over a 1-hour period) of 38°C (100.5°C) in a patient with an absolute neutrophil count (ANC) of less than 500 cells/μL.

29. What is the significance of neutropenic fever?
Patients with neutropenic fever are at high risk of developing serious infections. Rapid workup and empiric antibiotic therapy is warranted. If not treated promptly, sepsis and septic shock may develop. The lower the ANC, the higher the risk of morbidity.

30. What antibiotic regimen is recommended for patients with neutropenic fever?
High-risk patients require an antibiotic with antipseudomonal activity. Cefepime, ceftazidime, meropenem, and piperacillin-tazobactam are all appropriate. Patients with suspected catheter-related infection, skin and soft tissue infection, or hemodynamic instability also need MRSA coverage.

COMPLICATIONS OF ANTINEOPLASTIC THERAPY

31. Can chemotherapy cause acute cardiac complications?
Yes. Certain chemotherapy agents (anthracyclines, cyclophosphamide, 5-fluorouracil) can cause heart failure, arrhythmias (mostly atrial fibrillation), and acute coronary syndrome.

32. What is typhlitis?

Typhlitis (neutropenic enterocolitis) is a life-threatening, necrotizing enterocolitis which affects primarily neutropenic patients with hematologic malignancies. Mucosal damage due to chemotherapy and neutropenia are likely predisposing factors for bowel wall infection. Therapy needs to be individualized, but commonly includes intravenous fluids, bowel rest, and broad-spectrum antibiotics.

33. What are potential complications of cancer immunotherapy?

Immune checkpoint inhibitors, such as antibodies against CTLA-4 and PD1, enhance patient's own antitumor immunity. Colitis, hepatotoxicity, pneumonitis, and adrenal insufficiency are some of the immune-related adverse events that can complicate the treatment. Patients with severe electrolyte abnormalities, adrenal crisis, or respiratory failure require intensive care. Infusion of T cells that are engineered to recognize and attack tumor cells, so-called CAR T cells (chimeric antigen receptor T cells), is commonly associated with cytokine release syndrome (CRS).

34. What is cytokine release syndrome?

CRS is a potentially life-threating complication of cancer immunotherapy. Monoclonal antibodies and more recently, CAR T cells, are known triggers of CRS. CRS clinically manifests when large numbers of lymphocytes become activated and release proinflammatory cytokines. In severe cases, multiorgan failure (encephalopathy, cerebral edema, seizures, cardiac dysfunction, shock, acute respiratory distress syndrome (ARDS), renal and liver failure, DIC) can develop and patients require intensive care.

ACKNOWLEDGMENT

The authors wish to acknowledge Dr. Marie E. Wood, MD, for the valuable contributions to the previous edition of this chapter.

KEY POINTS: ONCOLOGIC EMERGENCIES

Neutropenic Fever

- ANC of less than 500 cells/μL
- A single oral temperature over 38.3°C (101°F) or a sustained temperature (over a 1-hour period) of 38°C (100.5°C)
- Early antibiotic therapy is required to prevent complications such as sepsis and septic shock

BIBLIOGRAPHY

1. Baldwin KJ, Zivković SA, Lieberman FS. Neurologic emergencies in patients who have cancer: diagnosis and management. *Neurol Clin.* 2012;30(1):101-128.
2. Behl D, Hendrickson AW, Moynihan TJ. Oncologic emergencies. *Crit Care Clin.* 2010;26(1):181-205.
3. Lee DW, Gardner R, Porter DL, et al. Current concepts in the diagnosis and management of cytokine release syndrome. *Blood.* 2014;124(2):188-195.
4. Levi M. Cancer-related coagulopathies. *Thromb Res.* 2014;(133 suppl 2):S70-S75.
5. Levi M. Management of cancer-associated disseminated intravascular coagulation. *Thromb Res.* 2016;(140 suppl 1): S66-S70.
6. McCurdy MT, Shanholtz CB. Oncologic emergencies. *Crit Care Med.* 2012;40(7):2212-2222.
7. Röllig C, Ehninger G. How I treat hyperleukocytosis in acute myeloid leukemia. *Blood.* 2015;125(21):3246-3252.
8. White L, Ybarra M. Neutropenic fever. *Emerg Med Clin North Am.* 2014;32(3):549-561.
9. Wood ME. Oncologic emergencies (including hypercalcemia). In: Parsons PE, Wiener-Kronish JP, eds. *Critical Care Secrets.* 5th ed. St Louis: Elsevier; 2013:404-409.
10. Young JS, Simmons JW. Chemotherapeutic medications and their emergent complications. *Emerg Med Clin North Am.* 2014;32(3):563-578.

POST-INTENSIVE CARE SYNDROME AND CHRONIC CRITICAL ILLNESS

Daniela J. Lamas and Anthony Massaro

CHAPTER 82

1. **What is post-intensive care syndrome?**
   Post-intensive care syndrome, or PICS, is defined as new or worsening function in one or more of the following domains after critical illness:
   - Cognitive function
   - Psychiatric function
   - Physical function

   This can occur regardless of the patient's discharge destination—whether it is home, a skilled nursing facility, or long-term acute care hospital. In general, the PICS definition does not apply to patients who were admitted after suffering traumatic brain injury or stroke. There is no specific time frame after critical illness in which PICS can or cannot occur.
   PICS can also be seen in family members of critically ill patients (see Question 9).

2. **What is the incidence and severity of the cognitive impairment in post-intensive care syndrome?**
   Cognitive impairment after critical illness has been reported from 25 to as high as 78% of survivors. In the largest prospective study looking at this question, the BRAIN-ICU study, investigators enrolled 821 patients admitted to medical or surgical intensive care units (ICUs) with shock and/or respiratory failure requiring mechanical ventilation. At 3 months after discharge, 40% of patients had deficits that were similar to moderate traumatic brain injury, and 26% had deficits that were similar to mild dementia. At 12 months post discharge, the deficits persisted for most patients. In another large study of older patients, the prevalence of moderate to severe cognitive impairment increased more than three times among patients who survived severe sepsis. These declines persisted for at least 8 years.
   The cognitive deficits commonly involve difficulty in one or more of the following domains:
   - Attention/concentration
   - Memory
   - Mental processing speed
   - Executive function

   Current care for patients who have survived critical illness does not include routine screening or testing for these issues.

3. **Do oxygenation "targets" during episodes of respiratory failure impact cognitive recovery?**
   While the relationship remains not entirely clear, inadequate oxygenation during acute respiratory distress syndrome has been identified as playing a central role in the development of long-term cognitive impairment, beginning with work in 1999 that showed that the amount of time spent below normal O_2 saturation (i.e., <90%) correlated with decreased cognitive performance. This association was bolstered by findings from the ARDSNet Fluid and Catheter Treatment Trial (FACTT), a study from the National Institutes of Health-initiated clinical network to carry out multi-center clinical trials of acute respiratory distress syndrome (ARDS) treatments. In ARDS survivors with cognitive impairment at 12 months (of note, 55% of those examined), the average daily PaO2 measures were significantly lower than those of survivors without cognitive impairment (71 mm Hg [IQR, 67–80 mm Hg] vs. 86 mm Hg [IQR, 70–98 mmg Hg]).
   These are associations, not causation, but the evidence raises the possibility that oxygenation targets during episodes of respiratory failure do impact cognitive recovery.

4. **Which psychiatric problems are patients most likely to face after intensive care unit discharge?**
   Depression, **anxiety**, and **posttraumatic stress disorder** (PTSD) are the most common disorders in this population. Studies report widely varying absolute risk. A systematic review of 14 studies found

the median point-prevalence of "clinically significant" depressive symptoms in ICU survivors to be 28%. A review of the literature for PTSD in ICU survivors examined 15 studies and found the median point-prevalence of "clinically significant" PTSD symptoms to be 22%. In survivors from the BRAIN-ICU cohort specifically, 37% of patients experienced symptoms of depression, which largely seemed to be associated with somatic symptoms.

5. What is the most common physical impairment in intensive care unit survivors?
   ICU-acquired weakness is the most common physical impairment—impacting at least 25% of ICU survivors. Herridge et al. demonstrated that ICU survivors had a 24% reduction in walk distance compared to age and sex-matched controls. Worse, ARDS survivors had a 6-minute walk distance that was impaired up to 5 years after ICU. Pointing again to the BRAIN-ICU cohort, 32% of these patients were disabled in their activities of daily living at 3 months. This critical illness-related dysfunction was present in those both with and without pre-existing functional disability, and persisted in most patients up to the 12-month follow-up. These physical impairments mean that patients require significant caregiver support. In a multicenter European study of critical illness survivors, one-quarter of patients were in need of care for more than 50 hours weekly at 6 months, most of which was provided by family members.

6. Do patients who survive ARDS have residual pulmonary dysfunction?
   Patients who survive ARDS do have residual pulmonary dysfunction early on, but most parameters return to normal by about 6 months. The degree of residual dysfunction depends on which aspect of lung function is being measured (i.e., spirometry, volumes, or diffusing capacity). At the time of discharge after an ICU admission for ARDS, around 80% of patients will have a reduced diffusing capacity, but less than a quarter will have spirometry or lung volumes that show obstruction or restriction. For most of these patients, lung volumes and spirometry return to normal by about 6 months and diffusing capacity by 5 years. Only a small percentage is left with residual pulmonary dysfunction.

7. What are the major risk factors for post-intensive care syndrome?
   Overall, the risk factors for PICS have not been clearly defined, and depend on the aspect of PICS that is being studied. Additionally, there are both pre-existing factors and ICU-specific factors that have been implicated in the development of PICS.
   - **Cognitive dysfunction**: The BRAIN-ICU study showed the duration of delirium to be an independent risk factor for cognitive impairment at 6 and 12 months following ICU stay. Additionally, severe sepsis survivors are also more likely to develop cognitive dysfunction compared to survivors of non-sepsis hospitalizations, even after adjustment for premorbid cognitive status. Other studies have cited a broader range of risk factors—including hypoxemia, hypotension, glucose dysregulation, respiratory failure, chronic obstructive pulmonary disease (COPD), and the use of renal replacement therapy. In any of these risks factors, the pathogenesis of cognitive impairment after critical illness is not clear, but is postulated to include ischemia, inflammation, and disruption of the blood-brain barrier.
   - **Psychiatric**: The risk factors for the anxiety, depression, and PTSD that characterize the psychiatric components of PICS are similar to the risk factors for cognitive dysfunction. These include severe sepsis, ARDS, trauma, hypoglycemia, and hypoxemia. ICU-related exposures include sedative and analgesia use. Of note, depression, anxiety, and post-traumatic stress prior to critical illness have been observed to increase the risk for these outcomes after discharge. Additionally, women, those older than 50 years of age, lower education level, and pre-existing disability and unemployment have also been described as risk factors for poor psychiatric outcomes. Of note, glucocorticoids are interestingly associated with a lower risk for PTSD; while the mechanism is unclear, this is thought to be due to reversing the deleterious effects of reduced cortisol.
   - **Physical**: The development of ICU-acquired weakness has been associated with prolonged mechanical ventilation, sepsis, multiorgan system failure, and prolonged periods of bed rest. Steroids have also been associated with ICU-acquired weakness.

8. What can we do about post-intensive care syndrome? Are there any possible treatments?
   Perhaps the best way to reduce the burden of PICS is by working in the ICU to minimize sedation and prioritize early mobility in the ICU. There is mixed evidence on the benefit of cognitive therapy. One pilot study looked at the benefit of twice-daily cognitive therapy for patients in medical and surgical intensive care units and found there to be no benefit. A separate pilot randomized trial investigated adding goal-management training (aimed to improve executive function) into a physical therapy program after discharge, and found that the executive function was improved in the group that received the intervention.

One interesting intervention that has had some possible benefit for prevention of PTSD is the ICU diary, which is a daily recording of events during the critical illness written in lay language by family, clinicians, or both. One study compared the incidence of PTSD at 3 months following discharge among patients who had or had not received an ICU diary at 1 month. Those without the diary were more likely to develop PTSD (13% vs. 5%) than those who had received access to this factual, day-to-day recording of their critical illness.

9. **What is post-intensive care syndrome-family?**
Family members have been referred to as the "collateral damage" of critical illness. Post-intensive care syndrome—family (or PICS-F) refers to the long-term effects of an ICU stay on the patient's family. These include: sleep deprivation, anxiety, depression, post-traumatic stress disorder (PTSD), and complicated grief. This may continue for months or even years after an ICU stay. Studies have shown that at least half of family members of the critically ill suffer anxiety at or soon after discharge, which persists for at least 6 months. Symptoms of depression have been described in about a quarter of family members and PTSD in up to one-third of family members, also lasting at least 6 months after discharge. Risk factors for developing PICS-F have been identified, and include poor communication with staff, being in a decision-making role, lower educational level, and having a loved one who died.

10. **Who are the chronically critically ill?**
This term refers to the 5% to 10% of patients who survive a catastrophic acute medical illness or surgery, but are left with prolonged need for mechanical ventilation. One consensus definition for these patients defined the chronically critical ill as those patients who require 21 or more days of mechanical ventilation for 6 hours or more a day. Another suggested approach to identify these patients for clinical trials has been that patients become chronically critically ill when they have received at least 10 days of mechanical ventilation, and their physician neither expects them to die, nor be liberated from mechanical ventilation within the next 72 hours. While prolonged mechanical ventilation is the hallmark, and thus definitions largely revolve around this, these patients also tend to have recurrent infections, organ dysfunction, profound weakness, and delirium. Their condition brings with it high hospitalization cost, frequent readmissions, and often care in the post-acute arena. Overall cost to the healthcare system is estimated at more than $20 billion annually.

11. **What are the outcomes of the chronically critically ill?**
The outcomes of the chronically critically ill are poor, with 1-year survival of between 40% and 50%. Of those who live, readmission rates are high, most remain institutionalized, and less than 12% are home and independent 1 year after their acute illness. Long-term survival has not improved significantly over the past two decades.

12. **What is the ProVent score?**
The ProVent score is a tool to aid in prognostication amongst the heterogeneous population of patients requiring prolonged mechanical ventilation. This tool uses clinical variables measured at day 21 of mechanical ventilation to determine likelihood of death at 1 year: requirement for vasopressors, hemodialysis, platelet count 150 or lower, and 50 years or older in age. Placing these four predictive models in a simple prognostic score identifies low-risk patients (no risk factors, 15% mortality) and high-risk patients (three or four risk factors, 97% mortality). This score was derived and validated at a university-based tertiary care center, among medical, surgical, and trauma patients requiring mechanical ventilation for at least 21 days.

13. **My patient got a tracheostomy tube and a feeding tube placed and is ready to go to rehab! What does that mean? Where is my patient going?**
In this setting, "rehab" likely refers to a long-term acute care hospital (LTACH). These facilities, defined by the Centers for Medicare and Medicaid Services as acute care hospitals with an average length of stay of 25 days or greater, are among the fastest growing segments of the healthcare system. These facilities grew as specialized hospitals for patients who require prolonged mechanical ventilation. Studies have examined survival among the chronically critically ill who are transferred to LTACHs and have found that these patients have similar survival compared with those who continue to receive their care in an ICU. When it comes to cost, total hospital-related costs in the 180 days after admission were lower among patients transferred to LTACHs, but Medicare payments were higher.

14. **What percentage of patients who are sent to LTACH for long-term ventilator wean are successful in coming off the ventilator?**
This is not an area with a robust body of research; however, a review of the largest observational studies on post-ICU weaning from prolonged mechanical ventilation found that more than half of

these patients can successfully come off the ventilator. Of note, if that occurs, that success is more likely to occur within the first 3 months of long-term acute care hospitalization.

BIBLIOGRAPHY

1. Needham DM, Davidson J, Cohen H, et al. Improving long-term outcomes after discharge from intensive care unit: report from a stakeholders' conference. *Crit Care Med.* 2012;40(2):502-509.
2. Pandharipande PP, Girard TD, Jackson JC, et al., BRAIN-ICU Study Investigators. Long-term cognitive impairment after critical illness. *N Engl J Med.* 2013;369(14):1306.
3. Sukantarat KT, Burgess PW, Williamson RC, et al. Prolonged cognitive dysfunction in survivors of critical illness. *Anaesthesia.* 2005;60(9):847-853.
4. Hopkins RO, Weaver LK, Papa D, et al. Neuropsychological sequelae and impaired health status in survivors of severe acute respiratory distress syndrome. *Am J Respir Crit Care Med.* 1999;160:50-56.
5. Mikkelsen ME, Christie JD, Lanken PN, et al. The Adult Respiratory Distress Syndrome Cognitive Outcomes Study: long-term neuropsychological function in survivors of acute lung injury. *Am J Respir Crit Care Med.* 2012;185:1307-1315.
6. Patel MB, Jackson JC, Morandi A, et al. Incidence and risk factors for intensive care unit-related post-traumatic stress disorder in veterans and civilians. *Am J Respir Crit Care Med.* 2016;193(12):1373.
7. Davydow DS, Gifford JM, Desai SV, et al. Depression in general intensive care unit survivors: a systematic review. *Intensive Care Med.* May 2009;35(5):796-809.
8. Davydow DS, Gifford JM, Desai SV, et al. Posttraumatic stress disorder in general intensive care unit survivors: a systematic review. *Gen Hosp Psychiatry.* 2008;30(5):421.
9. Herridge MS, Tansey CM, Matté A, et al. Functional disability 5 years after acute respiratory distress syndrome. *N Engl J Med.* 2011;364(14):1293.
10. Orme Jr J, Romney JS, Hopkins RO, et al. Pulmonary function and health-related quality of life in survivors of acute respiratory distress syndrome. *Am J Respir Crit Care Med.* 2003;167(5):690.
11. Herridge MS, Cheung AM, Tansey CM, et al. One-year outcomes in survivors of the acute respiratory distress syndrome. *N Engl J Med.* 2003;348(8):683.
12. Iwashyna TJ, Ely EW, Smith DM, et al. Long-term cognitive impairment and functional disability among survivors of severe sepsis. *JAMA.* 2010;304(16):1787.
13. Brummel NE, Girard TD, Ely EW, et al. Feasibility and safety of early combined cognitive and physical therapy for critically ill medical and surgical patients: the Activity and Cognitive Therapy in ICU (ACT-ICU) trial. *Intensive Care Med.* 2014; 40(3):370-379.
14. Jones C, Bäckman C, Capuzzo M, et al. Intensive care diaries reduce new onset post traumatic stress disorder following critical illness: a randomised, controlled trial. *Crit Care.* 2010;14(5):R168.
15. Nelson JE, Cox CE, Hope AA, et al. Chronic critical illness. *Am J Respir Crit Care Med.* 2010;182:446-454.
16. Carson SS. Definitions and epidemiology of the chronically critically ill. *Respir Care.* 2012;57(6):848-856. [discussion: 856-858].
17. Carson SS, Garrett J, Hanson LC, et al. A prognostic model for one-year mortality in patients requiring prolonged mechanical ventilation. *Crit Care Med.* 2008;36(7):2061-2069.
18. Kahn JM, Benson NM, Appleby D, et al. Long-term acute care hospital utilization after critical illness. *JAMA.* 2010;303: 2253-2259.
19. Kahn JM, Werner RM, David G, et al. Effectiveness of long-term acute care hospitalization in elderly patients with chronic critical illness. *Med Care.* 2013;51(1):4-10.
20. Scheinhorn DJ, Chao DC, Hassenpflug MS, et al. Post-ICU weaning from mechanical ventilation: the role of long-term facilities. *Chest.* 2001;120(suppl 6):482S-484S.
21. Griffiths H, Hatch RA, Bishop J, et al. An exploration of social and economic outcome and associated health-related quality of life after critical illness in general intensive care unit survivors: a 12-month follow-up study. *Crit Care.* 2013; 17(3):R100.

CHAPTER 83

INTENSIVE CARE UNIT SURVIVORS

Erin K. Kross, Robert Y. Lee and Catherine L. Hough

1. **What are important long-term outcomes for intensive care unit patients?**
For decades, observational and interventional studies of intensive care unit (ICU) patients focused on only who lived and who died. Now, as ICU mortality has decreased, more patients are surviving their ICU stay, encouraging a new focus on outcomes other than mortality. It is known that patients and families care about more than survival—they care about what life will be like after they leave the ICU. More recently, studies have begun to explore patient-centered outcomes such as functional status and quality of life. The most commonly studied patients are those with respiratory failure and the acute respiratory distress syndrome (ARDS), but sepsis, trauma, and heterogeneous groups of ICU patients are increasingly included in post-ICU studies as well.

2. **What is health-related quality of life, and why is this important for intensive care unit survivors?**
Health-related quality of life (HRQoL) is a multidimensional concept that includes domains related to physical, mental, emotional, and social functioning. It assesses an individual's self-reported physical and mental health and focuses on the impact one's health status has on activities and social engagement. HRQoL is an important patient-centered outcome that can be used to assess recovery from critical illness. Compared to the general population, HRQoL is significantly lower in survivors of critical illness and their family members. In general, this has been explained in large part by low scores related to physical dysfunction. These scores improve over time following critical illness, but often do not return to baseline.

3. **What is post-intensive care syndrome?**
Observational studies of survivors of critical illness have found that most patients have impairments in physical and cognitive function and/or mental health. In order to increase awareness of the struggles of ICU survivors, clinicians and researchers from many professions and specialties have coined the term "post-intensive care syndrome," or PICS (see Fig. 83.1). PICS describes the symptoms and signs of impairment in patient-centered domains which are common after critical illness.

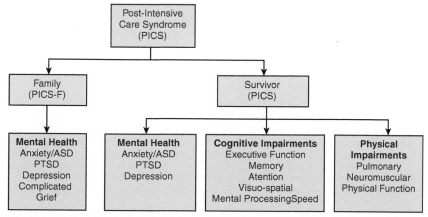

Figure 83-1. Post-intensive care syndrome (PICS) conceptual diagram. *ASD,* Acute stress disorder; *PTSD,* post-intensive care syndrome. (From Needham DM, Davidson J, Cohen H, et al. Improving long-term outcomes after discharge from intensive care unit: report from a stakeholders' conference. *Crit Care Med.* 2012;40:502 [Figure 1, page 505]).

4. Does post-intensive care syndrome affect the families of critically ill patients as well?
   Definitely. Family members of critically ill patients can also be affected by the ICU stay, with the most common problems experienced by family members being psychological distress, such as anxiety, depression, post-traumatic stress disorder (PTSD), and complicated grief. This syndrome has been named PICS-Family, or PICS-F. Both modifiable and nonmodifiable risk factors have been found to be associated with PICS-F. Strategies to improve the frequency and effectiveness of communication, enhance prognostic understanding, and support surrogate decision-making are potential ways to reduce PICS-F.

5. Why should intensive care unit clinicians be concerned about post-intensive care syndrome?
   Thinking about PICS throughout a patient's ICU stay empowers clinicians to provide the best possible patient and family-centered care. Understanding risks for impairment after the ICU allows clinicians to personalize care to promote best outcomes. Additionally, sharing information with family members early in the course of critical illness allows for advanced planning and expectation setting, including preparing for extended institutional stays and difficulty returning to work. In cases where the expected level of function is clearly not acceptable to a patient, knowledge and understanding about PICS may be helpful in determining whether ongoing intensive care is consistent with the patient's goals of care.

6. What types of symptoms are included in post-intensive care syndrome?
   The symptoms of PICS span the domains of physical, cognitive, and mental health. The most common physical symptoms include fatigue, weakness, loss of muscle mass, and pain. Cognitive symptoms include memory loss and forgetfulness, and difficulty with planning and executive function. Symptoms of mental health impairment include nightmares and intrusive thoughts (symptoms of PTSD), anxiety and panic attacks, sadness, and difficulty sleeping.

7. How common are the symptoms of post-intensive care syndrome?
   PICS symptoms are extremely common—in fact, in the first months after critical illness, nearly all patients experience problems with physical and cognitive function. These symptoms initially improve and then plateau after 6 to 24 months, at which point most patients are left with some impairments. For example, among ARDS survivors at 12 months, over 75% will still have physical limitations (such as shorter than expected distance walked on a standardized 6-minute walk test) and cognitive impairment in memory, attention, or concentration. Smaller numbers of survivors will have persisting problems in mental health (25%–50%) and up to 50% of ICU survivors do not return to work in the first year.

8. Are the symptoms of post-intensive care syndrome reflective of pre-existing impairments or new impairments acquired in the intensive care unit?
   There is strong evidence that previously healthy patients may develop new impairments in any of the PICS domains, and that patients with pre-ICU impairments may worsen after critical illness. These findings support the contention that PICS may represent new, or incident, impairment. However, there is also strong evidence that declining health, worsening physical and cognitive function, and worsening mental health are risk factors for critical illness; ICU admission may represent an opportunity to identify pre-existing or worsening impairments. In many ICU populations—especially medical ICUs—the majority of patients may have pre-ICU functional impairments, supporting the idea that much of PICS is new recognition of prevalent impairment.

9. Are the symptoms of post-intensive care syndrome unique to intensive care unit survivors?
   No. It is clear that survivors of acute illnesses and injuries that do not require critical care are also at risk for impairments in physical, cognitive, and mental health. It is not clear if critical illness or its treatments are specific risk factors for PICS.

10. What are the risk factors for long-term physical impairment after intensive care unit?
    Physical impairments after critical illness are sometimes due to the direct effects of the critical illness or injury (e.g., stroke, pelvic fracture, or amputation for necrotizing soft tissue infection). However, physical impairments are also ubiquitous among patients without such a direct link between their critical illness and their resulting physical impairment; in these patients, the impairments are thought to arise from a multitude of physiologic insults in the ICU. ICU-related risk factors for long-term physical impairments include prolonged bed rest, multiorgan failure, and fluid overload. Patient-related risk factors include age and female gender. Pre-existing physical impairment is the most common risk factor for post-ICU physical impairment.

11. What are the risk factors for long-term cognitive impairment after intensive care unit?
    Cognitive impairments after critical illness may be a direct result of primary brain injury (e.g., stroke, trauma), but are also seen commonly in patients without primary brain injury. For patients without

primary brain injury, cognitive impairment after the ICU may be associated with duration of hypoxemia, blood glucose variability, duration of hypotension, duration of delirium, and management with conservative fluid protocols targeting a low central venous pressure during the ICU stay. Surprisingly, in the ARDS population, there is no convincing association between severity of illness/organ failure or age and cognitive impairment.

12. **What are the risk factors for long-term mental health impairment after intensive care unit?**
Several risk factors have been identified for adverse psychological symptoms after critical illness, particularly in ARDS and severe sepsis populations. Some nonmodifiable risk factors include younger age, female gender, lower education level, premorbid alcohol abuse, and pre-existing psychiatric illness including anxiety, depression, and PTSD. Potentially modifiable ICU-based risk factors include hypoglycemia, hypoxemia, and use of ICU sedatives and analgesics.

13. **How can clinicians evaluate for post-intensive care syndrome?**
The evaluation for PICS relies on awareness and the ability to recognize PICS by both critical care clinicians and clinicians outside the ICU. Symptoms are often unrecognized because there is no standardized process of screening or testing for PICS. It is reasonable to consider assessment for cognitive, physical, and mental health signs and symptoms in ICU survivors using a thorough history and physical examination. In appropriate settings, specific testing such as pulmonary function testing, strength or exercise testing, and cognitive testing and/or mental health screening may assist in the diagnosis of PICS. Appropriate referrals may include occupational and physical therapists, neuropsychologists or psychiatrists, and rehabilitation medicine specialists.

14. **What interventions have been proven to prevent or reduce post-intensive care syndrome?**
Two main interventions that may prevent PICS are ICU diaries and a self-help rehabilitation manual. ICU diaries are family- and/or healthcare provider-maintained records of the patient's ICU stay and have been shown to decrease symptoms of PTSD. Education and rehabilitation manuals have been shown to be effective in aiding physical recovery, suggesting that recognizing and normalizing symptoms after critical illness may improve outcomes. There is conflicting evidence regarding the role of early ambulation or physical therapy in the ICU. Several studies have shown that early ambulation or physical therapy in the ICU may improve physical function, while other trials have demonstrated minimal or no benefit.

15. **How can I change delivery of my intensive care unit care in a way that may reduce post-intensive care syndrome?**
Reduction and prevention of PICS for critically ill patients, particularly those receiving mechanical ventilation, may be assisted by use of the ABCDEF bundle approach to care in the ICU (see Box 83.1). This bundled approach promotes strategies that minimize pain, sedation, and delirium; encourages mobility in the ICU and early liberation from mechanical ventilation; and engages and empowers families to be involved in care.

16. **Is there a role for intensive care unit follow-up clinics to treat post-intensive care syndrome?**
There is a lot of interest in the potential role of ICU follow-up clinics in the treatment of PICS. These clinics have been developed at many sites to care for patients and families after critical illness by providing multidisciplinary care for the myriad of post-ICU symptoms and syndromes. However, studies which have investigated the potential benefits of post-ICU clinics have not consistently shown improvement in patient symptoms or outcomes. While these clinics may become an important part of post-ICU care, further investigation is needed to examine which specific clinic-based interventions might improve outcomes for patients with PICS.

Box 83-1. Elements of the ABCDEF Care Bundle

Assess, Prevent, and Manage Pain
Both Spontaneous Awakening Trials (SAT) and Spontaneous Breathing Trials (SBT)
Choice of Analgesia and Sedation
Delirium: Assess, Prevent, and Manage
Early Mobility and Exercise
Family Engagement and Empowerment

17. **What are key knowledge gaps in understanding and reducing post-intensive care syndrome?**
There is still much to learn about post-intensive care syndromes. Critically ill patients include a heterogeneous group of individuals with different premorbid health and functional status, different illness courses and trajectories, and different values and preferences. We are still learning how to optimize our critical care based on patient-specific preferences and focus on outcomes that are truly patient-centered. There also remains much to be learned about the epidemiology and risk factors for PICS while we better understand which patients are at highest risk, which patients have symptoms that may be modifiable, what the best interventions might be for these symptoms, and at which time period these interventions should be targeted.

18. **What potential interventions are coming down the pike?**
There is a great deal of interest in developing and testing interventions to both prevent and treat PICS to improve outcomes for ICU survivors. There is additional observational and descriptive work necessary to fully inform these interventions. Potential intervention targets include both the ICU and the post-ICU periods. Within the ICU, there is hope that intervening on elements posited to be in the causal pathway such as sedation practices, fluid overload, and mobility will improve outcomes. Potential interventions may include optimizing nutrition, advanced exercise programs, and medications fighting anabolic resistance. In the post-ICU period, potential interventions include ICU follow-up clinics, rehabilitation programs, and peer-support models.

KEY POINTS: INTENSIVE CARE UNIT SURVIVORS

- Long-term impairments in physical, cognitive, and mental health are common in intensive care unit survivors, and are referred to as post-intensive care syndrome (PICS).
- Manifestations of PICS include muscle atrophy and weakness, fatigue, pain, memory loss, executive dysfunction, anxiety, depression, difficulty sleeping, and symptoms of PTSD.
- ICU diaries and rehabilitation manuals have been shown to prevent or reduce PICS for both patients and family members.
- Bundled approaches to ICU care that minimize pain, sedation, and delirium; encourage early mobility and early liberation from mechanical ventilation; and promote family engagement in care may also reduce PICS for patients and families.

BIBLIOGRAPHY

1. Davidson JE, Jones C, Bienvenu OJ. Family response to critical illness: postintensive care syndrome-family. *Crit Care Med.* 2012;40:618.
2. Desai SV, Law TJ, Needham DM. Long-term complications of critical care. *Crit Care Med.* 2011;39:371.
3. Herridge MS, Moss M, Hough CL, et al. Recovery and outcomes after the acute respiratory distress syndrome (ARDS) in patients and their family caregivers. *Intensive Care Med.* 2016;42:725.
4. Jolley SE, Bunnell AE, Hough CL. ICU-Acquired Weakness. *Chest.* 2016;150:1129.
5. Long AC, Kross EK, Davydow DS, et al. Posttraumatic stress disorder among survivors of critical illness: creation of a conceptual model addressing identification, prevention and management. *Intensive Care Med.* 2014;40:820.
6. Mehlhorn J, Freytag A, Schmidt K, et al. Rehabilitation interventions for postintensive care syndrome: a systematic review. *Crit Care Med.* 2012;42:1263.
7. Needham DM, Davidson J, Cohen H, et al. Improving long-term outcomes after discharge from intensive care unit: report from a stakeholders' conference. *Crit Care Med.* 2012;40:502.
8. Society of Critical Care Medicine. *ICU Liberation—ABCDEF Bundle.* Available at: http://www.iculiberation.org/Bundles/Pages/default.aspx. Accessed November 28, 2016.
9. Spragg RG, Bernard GR, Checkley W, et al. Beyond mortality: future clinical research in acute lung injury. *Am J Respir Crit Care Med.* 2010;181:1121.

XVI
EMERGING THERAPIES

CHAPTER 84

SEPSIS: EMERGING THERAPIES

Aranya Bagchi

1. **After many decades of research, why is there still no specific antisepsis therapy?**
   Outcomes in the management of patients with sepsis have improved since the turn of the century. However, mortality from sepsis remains at 25% to 30%, and may be as high as 40% to 50% when shock is present. Improvements in the outcomes of patients with sepsis have largely resulted from nonspecific interventions, including fluid resuscitation, early appropriate antibiotic therapy, and source control of the septic focus. Although there are many biologically attractive, potentially therapeutic agents in sepsis, more than 100 phase II and III trials of such agents have failed to date. An important factor in this dismal track record is the difficulty in stratifying patients with sepsis. When patients with pathologies as diverse as necrotizing fasciitis, pneumonia, and toxic megacolon can all be grouped under the umbrella of "sepsis," it seems unsurprising that we have not succeeded in finding a common treatment for these conditions.

2. **What are the current areas of focus in sepsis research that may lead to more effective therapies?**
   This chapter will focus broadly on two areas: innovative approaches that are being applied to better classify patients with sepsis, and emerging technologies and/or biologic agents for the treatment of sepsis. The specific technologies and agents range from cutting-edge advances in next-generation sequencing to the repurposing of drugs that have been used for other conditions. A focus on diagnostic modalities is appropriate, as patient heterogeneity is one of the most important reasons for the failure of the intense research efforts in sepsis to bear fruit.

3. **What is precision medicine? How are the concepts of precision medicine being applied to sepsis?**
   Precision medicine, as defined by the National Institutes of Health, is an approach to disease prevention and treatment that exploits the multiple distinct characteristics of each individual (in genetic makeup, environment, and lifestyle) to maximize effectiveness. The principles of precision medicine have been applied with significant success in oncology, where both diagnosis and treatment are often based on genomic features. Because of the heterogeneity of the patient population in sepsis and the demonstrated failure of multiple "one size fits all" approaches to the treatment of sepsis, precision medicine is an attractive approach toward the diagnosis and management of patients with sepsis. Precision medicine is closely associated with the "-omics" fields (genomics, transcriptomics, metabolomics, etc.). While these areas are likely to be of value in understanding the pathophysiology of sepsis, the data generated by these approaches is typically not "user friendly" for a practicing clinician. Downsizing whole genome profiles to rapidly available biologic "signatures," together with integration of omics data with highly granular physiologic monitor signals and electronic medical record data, may provide powerful tools to stratify patients with sepsis in the near future.

4. **Is there a biomarker that can reliably discriminate between infected and noninfected patients?**
   No. Although biomarkers have been the subject of intense research over decades, and some (such as procalcitonin) have been incorporated in treatment guidelines, no biomarker has been shown to reliably differentiate between infected and noninfected patients. Unfortunately, the lack of a true gold standard for the diagnosis of an infection complicates the interpretation of biomarker studies—for example, only 30% to 40% of patients with sepsis or septic shock have positive blood cultures. Newer technologies such as mass spectrometry to detect microbial proteins or polymerase chain reaction-based methods to detect microbial nucleic acids present the possibility of rapid and accurate diagnosis of infections, although these platforms are not yet ready for routine clinical use.

5. **What is the microbiome? How is it relevant in sepsis?**
   The microbiome refers to the entire microbial population (commensal and pathogenic bacteria, viruses, and fungi), their genes, proteins, and metabolites—in other words, the microbial ecosystem of the body. Changes in the microbiome occur in critical illness, often within hours of a sudden physiologic insult. Recent work indicates that the composition of the microbiome can influence the host response and ultimate outcome. Attempts to re-establish a healthy microbiome are an exciting new treatment

strategy in sepsis and critical illness. The utility of fecal transplantation in the management of recurrent *Clostridium difficile*-associated colitis is an example of the successful manipulation of the microbiome to treat disease.

6. Can analysis of exosomes help in the classification of patients with sepsis?
Exosomes are cell-derived, membrane enclosed vesicles with the potential to transfer proteins, lipids, RNA and DNA between cells. Exosomes have emerged as a novel diagnostic tool in the noninvasive assessment of organ response to injury. Exosomes are highly stable in biologic fluids including blood, plasma, and bronchioalveolar lavage fluid. Studies have shown that, depending on organ/cell of origin and content, exosomes may be protective in sepsis or may contribute to organ injury, and thus may have value in the stratification of prognosis of patients with sepsis. Interestingly, exosomes have also been found to be excellent drug delivery systems, and are currently under investigation as means to deliver therapeutic molecules including proteins and microRNAs. In the not-too-distant future, a patient's own exosomes may be harvested and used as delivery vehicles for drugs used in the management of sepsis.

7. What is the role of mesenchymal stem cells in sepsis and acute respiratory distress syndrome (ARDS)?
Mesenchymal stem cells (MSCs) are one variety of adult stem cells that can be isolated from several sources such as bone marrow, umbilical cord blood, and placenta. Intravenously injected MSCs have the ability to preferentially migrate to injured tissue along chemotactic gradients. MSCs have been shown to have versatile paracrine signaling effects, immunomodulatory activity, and antimicrobial activity. Several preclinical studies have shown that MSCs can reduce the severity of organ injury in both pulmonary and nonpulmonary sepsis. Phase I and IIa clinical trials have been conducted for the use of MSCs in ARDS. While there remain a number of regulatory and quality control issues that have made the conduct of clinical trials with MSCs somewhat challenging, MSCs represent one of the more exciting therapeutic avenues for sepsis on the horizon.

8. Is sepsis a disorder of hyperinflammation or immune suppression?
It depends. Traditional teaching has divided sepsis into two phases—an early systemic inflammatory response (SIRS) phase characterized by an exuberant immune response (think meningococcemia) followed by a prolonged phase of immune suppression or immune paralysis—the compensatory anti-inflammatory response syndrome (CARS). More recent work, however, has shown a more complex picture. Both sepsis and severe trauma are characterized by the activation of about 80% of the leukocyte transcriptome—a "genomic storm," where pro- and anti-inflammatory pathways are activated simultaneously. Therefore, a given patient may exhibit different patterns of hyper- or hypoactive immunity during the course of her illness. The importance of immune suppression in late sepsis, together with the risk for secondary infections, has received a lot of attention. However, a recent Scandinavian trial has shown that although secondary infections are common in critically ill patients, the increase in mortality attributable to secondary infections in patients with sepsis is very modest, only 2.8%.

9. Are immunomodulatory therapies relevant for the management of patients with sepsis?
Based on the discussion above, it is evident that although immune dysregulation is a feature of sepsis, the direction of the dysregulation (hyper or hypo) will differ between patients, and even in the same patient over time. It is therefore important to perform immunophenotyping on a given patient to determine the state of the immune response, which then determines the type of immunomodulatory therapy. Some immunophenotyping methods, such as the quantification of human leukocyte antigen-antigen D related (HLA-DR) antigen expression on monocytes, have been used in clinical studies of patients with sepsis. Based on the immunophenotype, either immune suppressive or stimulating agents may be used in a given patient. Immunosuppressive therapies that are in clinical use include corticosteroids and intravenous immunoglobulin. A number of immunostimulatory therapies are currently being tested in clinical trials, including granulocyte-macrophage colony stimulating factor, interleukin 7 (IL7), antiprogrammed cell death ligand 1 (PD-ligand 1), and thymosin.

10. Are there any new agents for the support of blood pressure or blood flow in septic shock?
A number of agents have been used in recent clinical trials to support blood pressure or improve tissue perfusion in septic shock, with varying degrees of efficacy. A few are briefly mentioned here.
   - **Angiotensin II:** The recent angiotensin II for the treatment of high-output shock (ATHOS-3) trial has shown that angiotensin II significantly improved blood pressure in vasodilatory shock (including septic shock), allowing reductions in catecholamine vasopressor dosage. Angiotensin II may thus be a useful adjunct to vasopressor resistant shock for which currently few options (vasopressin, steroids, methylene blue) exist.

- **Levosimendan:** Levosimendan is a calcium sensitizing inodilator (inotrope and vasodilator) that is approved in many countries, though not in the United States. Unlike catecholamines, levosimendan causes an increase in cardiac output with minimal increases in myocardial oxygen consumption and preserved diastolic function. It also has other, noninotropic effects, including anti-inflammatory and antiapoptotic effects. It thus appears to be an attractive drug for the treatment of septic shock. Unfortunately, a recent large, randomized multicenter trial (LeoPARDS) did not find any benefit to using levosimendan in septic shock. On the contrary, levosimendan was associated with a higher risk of supraventricular tachycardia, and a lower likelihood of successful weaning from mechanical ventilation.

- **Selepressin:** A vasopressin analog that is selective for V_{1A} receptors (V_2 receptors can cause vasodilatation), selepressin has been shown to be associated with better hemodynamics, reduced capillary leakage, and fewer side effects than vasopressin in preclinical studies. A phase II study has been completed, and a large clinical trial is being planned.

- **Thrombomodulin:** Sepsis is associated with dysfunction of the coagulation cascade, and multiple anticoagulants have been tried in sepsis without success, most notably Activated Protein C, which was withdrawn from the market after initial approval. Thrombomodulin, a cofactor of protein C, has shown encouraging results in preclinical studies and in a small phase IIb randomized controlled trial. A subgroup analysis of this trial showed that patients with at least one organ system dysfunction and an international normalized ratio (INR) greater than 1.4 were most likely to benefit—a phase III study is currently underway in this group of patients.

11. Do blood purification strategies help in the treatment of sepsis and septic shock?
    Extracorporeal blood purification methods have been a theoretically attractive treatment modality in the management of septic shock, as data suggest that mortality is related to high concentrations of immunostimulatory or immunosuppressive mediators. Multiple blood purification modalities have been used in patients—here we will briefly discuss two techniques, high volume hemofiltration and Polymyxin B hemoperfusion.

    - **High-volume hemofiltration/Early hemofiltration:** Continuous venovenous hemofiltration (CVVH) is a commonly used technique for renal replacement in critically ill patients who are hemodynamically unstable. Since CVVH has some ability to clear cytokines from plasma, there has been interest in starting CVVH early in the course of septic shock (before traditional renal replacement indications are met). Another approach has been to use higher intensity hemofiltration (effluent rates of 40–50 mL/kg/h instead of the typical 20–25 mL/kg/h). An attractive feature of both approaches is the ability to use equipment that is readily available in ICUs in advanced countries. Unfortunately, large randomized controlled trials for both strategies have not shown any benefit for either strategy. In fact, early initiation of hemofiltration may be associated with worse organ function. Neither modality is recommended for the routine management of septic shock at this time.

    - **Polymyxin B hemoperfusion:** Polymyxin B is an antibiotic that binds strongly to lipopolysaccharide (endotoxin), which is a component of the cell membranes of gram-negative bacteria and a potent inflammatory agent. Polymyxin B hemoperfusion has been used in the management of sepsis in some countries, such as Japan and Italy, for many years. An important trial examining the utility of Polymyxin B hemoperfusion in patients with septic shock and high levels of circulating endotoxin has recently been completed (the Euphrates trial), and the results, when available, will determine whether this technology will be approved in the United States.

KEY POINTS: SEPSIS: EMERGING THERAPIES

1. In spite of decades of research, there is no specific "antisepsis" therapy.
2. A fundamental challenge in sepsis research is to find a biologically relevant way to classify patients—current definitions of sepsis and septic shock include very heterogeneous populations of patients.
3. A strong effort is currently underway using high-throughput technologies (genomics, transcriptomics, etc.) to better define subpopulations of patients with sepsis.
4. Multiple promising drugs for the treatment of sepsis are in late phases of clinical trials and may soon become available for clinical use.
5. Innovative treatment modalities, such as manipulation of the microbiome, use of MSCs, and exosome-mediated drug delivery may significantly change the face of sepsis treatment in the near future.

BIBLIOGRAPHY

1. Alverdy JC, Krezalek MA. Collapse of the microbiome, emergence of the pathobiome, and the immunopathology of sepsis. *Crit Care Med*. 2017;45:337.
2. Cohen J, Vincent JL, Adhikari NK, et al. Sepsis: a roadmap for future research. *Lancet Infect Dis*. 2015;15:581.
3. Gordon AC, Perkins GD, Singer M, et al. Levosimendan for the prevention of acute organ dysfunction in sepsis. *N Engl J Med*. 2016;375:1638.
4. Khanna A, English SW, Wang XS, et al. Angiotensin II for the treatment of vasodilatory shock [e-pub ahead of print]. *N Engl J Med*. 2017;377(5):419-430. doi:10.1056/NEJMoa1704154.
5. Klein DJ, Foster D, Schorr CA, et al. The EUPHRATES trial (Evaluating the use of polymyxin B hemoperfusion in a random-ized controlled trial of adults treated for endotoxemia and septic shock): Study protocol for a randomized controlled trial. *Trials*. 2014;15:218. doi:10.1186/1745-6215-15-218.
6. Matthay MA, Pati S, Lee JW. Concise review: Mesenchymal stem (stromal) cells. Biology and preclinical evidence for therapeutic potential for organ dysfunction following trauma and sepsis. *Stem Cells*. 2017;35:316.
7. Terrasini N, Lionetti V. Exosomes in critical illness. *Crit Care Med*. 2017;45:1054.
8. van Vught LA, Klein Klouwenberg PM, Spitoni C, et al. Incidence, risk factors and attributable mortality of secondary infections in the intensive care unit after admission for sepsis. *JAMA*. 2016;315:1469.
9. Vincent JL. Emerging therapies for the treatment of sepsis. *Curr Opin Anaesthesiol*. 2015;28:411.

INDEX

Page numbers followed by *f* indicate figures; *b*, boxes; *t*, tables.

A

A wave, 84–86, 85f
AAA. *see* Abdominal aortic aneurysm
AAN. *see* American Academy of Neurology
ABCDEF bundle, 22
Abdomen
  abscess, 443
  acute, 440
    causes of, 440
    in immunocompromised patients, 443
    intra-abdominal hypertension and, 442
    intra-abdominal infections and, 443
    mesenteric ischemia and, 443
    Ogilvie's syndrome and, 442
Abdominal aortic aneurysm (AAA), repair of,
    diarrhea following, 444
Abdominal compartment syndrome, 442–443
Abdominal pain
  diabetic ketoacidosis-related, 355
  evaluation of, 441
  imaging studies for, 441
  laboratory tests in, 441
  peritonitis-related, 440
  thoracic conditions and, 441
Abdominal reflexes, brain death and, 404
Abdominal ultrasound, in abdominal pain, 441
ABO systems, 373
Absolute insulin deficiency, 353, 354f
Acalculous cholecystitis, management of, 443
Acetaminophen
  hemodialysis and, 489
  overdose in
    diagnosis of, 346
    management of, 346
    poison-associated death and, 485
    side effects of, 31–32
    for thyroid storm, 367–368t
Acetaminophen toxicity, 494–496
  alcohol ingestion, 496
  chronic, treatment for, 496
  hemodialysis, 496
  hepatotoxicity
    mechanism, 494
    predictors, 494
  patient-tailored approach, 495–496
  phases, 494
  Rumack-Matthew treatment nomogram and,
    494–495, 495f
  signs and symptoms, 494

Acetazolamide, hypokalemia from, 316
Acetylcholinesterase inhibitors, for myasthenia
    gravis, 420
Acid-base disturbances
  differential diagnosis of, 312–313, 313b
  in heat stroke, 480
Acid-base interpretation, 311–313
  anion gap in, 311
  arterial blood gas and serum chemistry values
    in, 312, 312t
  information needed in, 311
Acid burns, 430
Acidosis
  in acute kidney injury, 304t
  definition of, 311
  lactic, cancer and, 534
  metabolic, anion gap, 354
  in renal replacement therapy, 307
Acinetobacter baumannii, 270
Acinetobacter spp.
  in intensive care unit, 265
  sepsis and, 238
ACS. *see* Acute chest syndrome
Actinobacillus actinomycetemcomitans,
    endocarditis and, 244
Activated charcoal, poisoning and, 488b
  multiple-dose, 488–489
  single-dose, 488
Activated partial thromboplastin time (aPTT), 382,
    386
Active core rewarming, 474
Active euthanasia, end-of-life care and, 40
Active external rewarming, 474
Active rewarming, 474
Acute abdomen, 440
  causes of, 440
    in immunocompromised patients, 443
    intra-abdominal hypertension and, 442
    intra-abdominal infections and, 443
    mesenteric ischemia and, 443
    Ogilvie's syndrome and, 442
Acute adrenal insufficiency, 362
Acute asthma, serum potassium concentration in, 316
Acute blood loss, fluid therapy for, 42
Acute chest syndrome (ACS), 190–191
Acute colonic pseudo-obstruction. *see* Ogilvie's
    syndrome
Acute coronary syndrome, management of,
    hypertensive crises with, 299